Flexible and Stretchable Medical Devices

Flexible and Stretchable Medical Devices

Edited by Kuniharu Takei

WILEY-VCH

Editor

Prof. Kuniharu Takei
Osaka Prefecture University
Department of Physics and Electronics
1-1 Gakuen Nakaku
Sakai
599-8531 Osaka
Japan

Cover credit: iStock shawn_hempel

Library of Congress Card No.: applied for

British Library Cataloguing-in-Publication Data
A catalogue record for this book is available from the British Library.

Bibliographic information published by the Deutsche Nationalbibliothek
The Deutsche Nationalbibliothek lists this publication in the Deutsche Nationalbibliografie; detailed bibliographic data are available on the Internet at <http://dnb.d-nb.de>.

Print ISBN: 978-3-527-34183-2
ePDF ISBN: 978-3-527-80484-9
ePub ISBN: 978-3-527-80486-3
Mobi ISBN: 978-3-527-80487-0
oBook ISBN: 978-3-527-80485-6

Typesetting SPi Global, Chennai, India
Printing and Binding C.O.S. Printers Pte Ltd Singapore

Printed on acid-free paper

Contents

Preface

For over 20 years, materials and device applications for flexible and stretchable electronics have been developed by many universities and institutes including industrial companies. This book aims to introduce them, spanning from historical developments to novel device applications including device physics and mechanisms of active device components. To cover all materials and device components for application in medical and healthcare devices, which this book aims to publish, renowned authors have been invited for their contribution to each chapter. We hope that readers can learn not only fundamental device mechanisms, but also novel technologies to realize nonconventional flexible and stretchable electronics. The reason why it was decided to add fundamental mechanism of the flexible devices although this book aims to introduce medical application is because students and new comers to this field can also use this book to study flexible and stretchable electronics. Although a lot of research and developments have been conducted all over the world, innovative breakthrough using the technology is yet to be realized. In moving toward the realization of breakthrough in this field, new ideas from students and new comers are very important to integrate the concepts and technologies introduced in this book. Of course, since this is aimed at medical and healthcare applications, we hope that experts such as doctors, clinical nurse, and medical/healthcare device developers also take a look at this book to understand the currently available technologies. By taking the latest knowledge and understanding as well as the state-of-the-art medical/healthcare devices, it will be our pleasure if any collaboration between them could lead to developing more practical and useful tools. This book may be able to help many engineers and researchers who are involved in materials science, electrical engineering, mechanical engineering, chemistry, medical/neuroscience, and so onto create unconventional ideas from inflexible electronics into flexible electronics. However, since this book covers many fields ranging from materials and device components to device applications, the detailed physics of the materials and devices could not be discussed. If there is something interesting to the readers and if they wish to learn more deeply, please also refer to other textbooks to support the fundamental mechanisms and physics of the devices. This book probably can be a start-up textbook to learn about fundamental flexible and stretchable devices and their applications.We hope this will stimulate many researchers and students to contribute new ideas and to create innovations in the field of flexible and stretchable devices.

Acknowledgments

Finally, I would like to thank all colleagues who agreed with contribution to write the chapters and the Wiley-VCH editorial team to give me a great opportunity to edit this exciting book.

October 2017

Kuniharu Takei
Osaka, Japan

1

History of Flexible and Stretchable Devices

Kuniharu Takei

Osaka Prefecture University, Department of Physics and Electronics, 1-1 Gakuen Nakaku, Sakai, Osaka 599-8531, Japan

Flexible devices such as transistors and transducers have been developed since 1990 by forming organic thin film or transferring inorganic thin film on plastic substrates. From the 1990s to the early 2000s, flexible transistors and light emitting diodes (LEDs) were mainly developed on a flexible substrate using organic materials because organic materials are fundamentally mechanically flexible compared to inorganic films and can be formed by using solution-based or evaporation processes on amorphous plastic substrates [1–4]. However, by utilizing inorganic thin film transfer technique from a bulk wafer to another substrate that was developed by Konagai *et al.* [5] and Yablonovitch *et al.* [6], inorganic-based flexible devices have been also developed since 2000 [7–15]. During the early stages of development of flexible electronics, the fundamental characteristics of devices such as transistors and sensors with relevance to organic and inorganic materials, their electrical characteristics, mechanical reliability, and bendability were deeply studied [7–10]. Although the fundamental properties using similar material systems as well as new material systems are still being investigated [16, 17], the approach for flexible and stretchable electronics is now to develop flexible and/or stretchable device applications [11–15, 17–34]. As device integrations on flexible substrate, Rogers *et al.* developed a paper-like electronic display using organic material-based active matrix backplane in 2001, which was most likely the first demonstration of the material integration for flexible device applications [4]. Following this development, Someya *et al.* demonstrated an artificial electronic skin (e-skin) to detect pressure distributions similar to that in human skin in 2004 [35], and in 2005, his group further developed a pressure and temperature distribution sensing device using organic-based thin film transistors (TFTs) for the active matrix backplane [36]. At the same time, thin film Si TFTs were transferred from silicon-on-insulator (SOI) wafer to a flexible substrate, which allows it to operate TFTs with high mobility and high stability in ambient air [8, 10]. During the 2000s, one of the bottlenecks for flexible electronics using organic materials as the active component was low performance and instability in ambient air. However, subsequent to the demonstration of inorganic-based TFTs, possibilities arose for inorganic material to be flexible electronics. Since

Flexible and Stretchable Medical Devices, First Edition. Edited by Kuniharu Takei.

the Si-based TFTs are a matured technique as the industrial standard for Si-based integrated circuits (ICs), the properties of flexible Si-TFTs show a great performance with a field-effect mobility of 180 cm^2/Vs on a flexible substrate [8]. In 2008, Rogers *et al.* successfully fabricated a highly integrated digital circuit of a four-bit row decoder using carbon nanotube networks as p-type transistors [13]. After several developments of inorganic material formations, device structures, and new organic materials, flexible transistors using both organic and inorganic materials have displayed high potential for flexible electronics due to improvements in their performance and stability. Using the platforms of organic transistors and organic light emitting diodes (OLEDs), active matrix OLED flexible display was demonstrated by Someya *et al.* [37]. In 2010, two e-skin device demonstrations were reported at the same time by Bao *et al.* [19] and Javey *et al.* [20]. Each e-skin has unique structures. The device reported by Javey *et al.* has an inorganic nanowire array active matrix backplane to show high flexibility and performance realized by nanowire printing technique [20], and Bao *et al.* proposed a unique structure to detect tactile pressure with high sensitivity [19]. The flexible and stretchable devices were then applied to medical and neuroscience fields for implantation or *in vivo* experiments by utilizing their flexibility [18, 38–40]. One interesting approach is to use the material such as silk dissolved in water [18, 39]. This eventually allows it to use the sensors and curing devices for the implantation, and it is not necessary to remove it after surgery and curing because it is dissolved in the body, which helps to reduce medical cost and patient load for re-surgery. Subsequent to these developments, many kinds of flexible and stretchable device applications have been developed to date, such as self-healing sensors [23], ultrathin flexible devices [41], photovoltaics devices [30]. In addition, recently, fully printed, multifunctional, low-cost, wearable flexible healthcare devices have been also reported by integrating with multiple sensors for healthcare detections and human activity [42]. However, many demonstrations were often focused on the sensor and transistor integration on flexible and stretchable substrates, and there were still challenges toward moving forward for realizing practical applications. The biggest problem of these devices is how to realize signal processing circuits, wireless systems, and battery because flexible transistors are not capable of building complicated circuits although there has been significant improvements and developments from many groups. To overcome this challenge, in 2016, Javey *et al.* demonstrated a hybrid system integrating flexible chemical sensors and inflexible conventional ICs for signal processing of the sensing results and a wireless system on a flexible printed circuit film [34]. Furthermore, Rogers *et al.* also developed the battery-free hybrid system to monitor health conditions wirelessly by integrating flexible and stretchable antenna and chip-based circuits [43].

In this book, the fundamental physics of electrical components such as flexible and stretchable transistors, memories, and sensors are first introduced to understand the present status of the flexible and stretchable electronics including techniques to fabricate the devices as emerging technologies. After understanding the fundamental characteristics and techniques, medical and healthcare applications using the flexible and stretchable device components are introduced. Especially, skin-mounted healthcare devices, implantable medical devices, and neuroscience

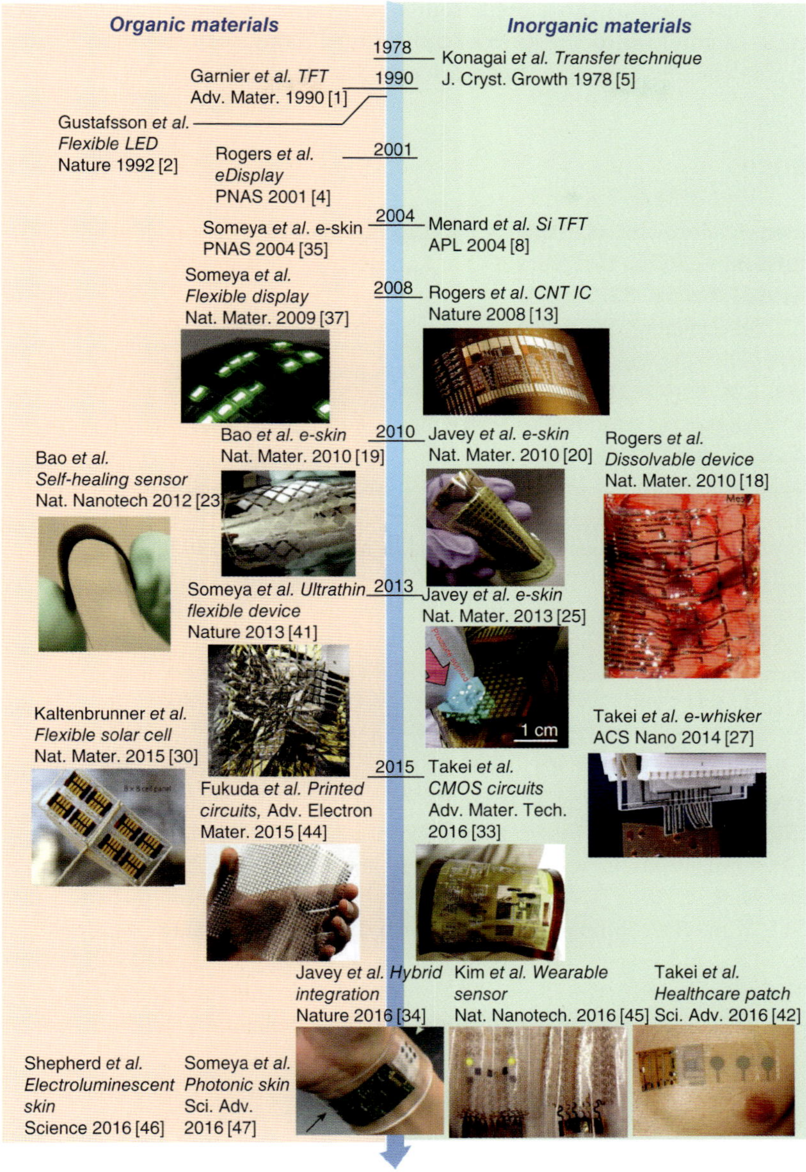

Figure 1.1 History of flexible electronics using organic and inorganic materials. Qing 2008 [13]. Reproduced with permission of Nature Publishing Group; Kim *et al*. 2010 [18]. Reproduced with permission of Nature Publishing Group; Mannsfeld *et al*. 2010 [19]. Reproduced with permission of Nature Publishing Group; Takei *et al*. 2010 [20]. Reproduced with permission of Nature Publishing Group; Tee *et al*. 2012 [23]. Reproduced with permission of Nature Publishing Group; Wang *et al*. 2013 [25]. Reproduced with permission of Nature Publishing Group; Kaltenbrunner *et al*. 2013 [41]. Reproduced with permission of Nature Publishing Group; Harada *et al*. 2014 [27]. Reproduced with permission of American Chemical Society; Kaltenbrunner *et al*. 2015 [30]. Reproduced with permission of Nature Publishing Group; Honda *et al*. 2016 [33]. Reproduced with permission of John Wiley & Sons; Gao *et al*. 2016 [34]. Reproduced with permission of Nature Publishing Group; Lee *et al*. 2016 [45]. Reproduced with permission of Nature Publishing Group; Sekitani *et al*. 2009 [37]. Reproduced with permission of Nature Publishing Group; Fukuda *et al*. 2015 [44]. Reproduced with permission of John Wiley & Sons.

devices are discussed to show the insights into these flexible and stretchable electronics. In addition to the device applications, nanosheet materials for the practical medical and wearable sheets are also discussed (see Figure 1.1).

References

1 Garnier, F., Horowitz, G., Peng, X., and Fichou, D. (1990) *Adv. Mater.*, **2**, 592.
2 Gustafsson, G., Cao, Y., Treacy, G.M., Klavetter, F., Colaneri, N., and Heeger, A.J. (1992) *Nature*, **357**, 477.
3 Garnier, F., Hajlaoui, R., Yassar, A., and Srivastava, P. (1994) *Science*, **265**, 1684.
4 Rogers, J.A., Bao, Z., Baldwin, K., Dodabalapur, A., Crone, B., Raju, V.R., Kuck, V., Katz, H., Amundson, K., Ewing, J., and Drzaic, P. (2001) *Proc. Natl. Acad. Sci. U.S.A.*, **98**, 4835.
5 Konagai, M., Sugimoto, M., and Takahashi, K. (1978) *J. Cryst. Growth*, **45**, 277.
6 Yablonovitch, E., Gmitter, T., Harbison, J.P., and Bhat, R. (1987) *Appl. Phys. Lett.*, **51**, 2222.
7 Hur, S.-H., Khang, D.-Y., Kocabas, C., and Rogers, J.A. (2004) *Appl. Phys. Lett.*, **85**, 5730.
8 Menard, E., Lee, K.J., Khang, D.Y., Nuzzo, R.G., and Rogers, J.A. (2004) *Appl. Phys. Lett.*, **84**, 5398.
9 Sun, Y. and Rogers, J.A. (2004) *Nano Lett.*, **4**, 1953.
10 Ahn, J.H., Kim, H.S., Lee, K.J., Jeon, S., Kang, S.J., Sun, Y., Nuzzo, R.G., and Rogers, J.A. (2006) *Science*, **314**, 1754.
11 Khang, D.-Y., Jiang, H., Huang, Y., and Rogers, J.A. (2006) *Science*, **311**, 208.
12 Sun, Y., Choi, W.M., Jiang, H., Huang, Y.Y., and Rogers, J.A. (2006) *Nat. Nanotechnol.*, **1**, 201.
13 Cao, Q., Kim, H.S., Pimparkar, N., Kulkarni, J.P., Wang, C., Shim, M., Roy, K., Alam, M.A., and Rogers, J.A. (2008) *Nature*, **454**, 495.
14 Ko, H.C., Stoykovich, M.P., Song, J., Malyarchuk, V., Choi, W.M., Yu, C.J., Geddes, J.B. III, Xiao, J., Wang, S., Huang, Y., and Rogers, J.A. (2008) *Nature*, **454**, 748.
15 Yoon, J., Baca, A.J., Park, S.I., Elvikis, P., Geddes, J.B. III, Li, L., Kim, R.H., Xiao, J., Wang, S., Kim, T.H., Motala, M.J., Ahn, B.Y., Duoss, E.B., Lewis, J.A., Nuzzo, R.G., Ferreira, P.M., Huang, Y., Rockett, A., and Rogers, J.A. (2008) *Nat. Mater.*, **7**, 907.
16 Rogers, J.A., Lagally, M.G., and Nuzzo, R.G. (2011) *Nature*, **477**, 45.
17 Wang, C., Takei, K., Takahashi, T., and Javey, A. (2013) *Chem. Soc. Rev.*, **42**, 2592.
18 Kim, D.H., Viventi, J., Amsden, J.J., Xiao, J., Vigeland, L., Kim, Y.S., Blanco, J.A., Panilaitis, B., Frechette, E.S., Contreras, D., Kaplan, D.L., Omenetto, F.G., Huang, Y., Hwang, K.C., Zakin, M.R., Litt, B., and Rogers, J.A. (2010) *Nat. Mater.*, **9**, 511.
19 Mannsfeld, S.C., Tee, B.C., Stoltenberg, R.M., Chen, C.V., Barman, S., Muir, B.V., Sokolov, A.N., Reese, C., and Bao, Z. (2010) *Nat. Mater.*, **9**, 859.

20 Takei, K., Takahashi, T., Ho, J.C., Ko, H., Gillies, A.G., Leu, P.W., Fearing, R.S., and Javey, A. (2010) *Nat. Mater.*, **9**, 821.
21 Kim, D.H., Lu, N., Ma, R., Kim, Y.S., Kim, R.H., Wang, S., Wu, J., Won, S.M., Tao, H., Islam, A., Yu, K.J., Kim, T.I., Chowdhury, R., Ying, M., Xu, L., Li, M., Chung, H.J., Keum, H., McCormick, M., Liu, P., Zhang, Y.W., Omenetto, F.G., Huang, Y., Coleman, T., and Rogers, J.A. (2011) *Science*, **333**, 838.
22 Kim, H.S., Brueckner, E., Song, J., Li, Y., Kim, S., Lu, C., Sulkin, J., Choquette, K., Huang, Y., Nuzzo, R.G., and Rogers, J.A. (2011) *Proc. Natl. Acad. Sci. U.S.A.*, **108**, 10072.
23 Tee, B.C., Wang, C., Allen, R., and Bao, Z. (2012) *Nat. Nanotechnol.*, **7**, 825.
24 Hammock, M.L., Chortos, A., Tee, B.C., Tok, J.B., and Bao, Z. (2013) *Adv. Mater.*, **25**, 5997.
25 Wang, C., Hwang, D., Yu, Z., Takei, K., Park, J., Chen, T., Ma, B., and Javey, A. (2013) *Nat. Mater.*, **12**, 899.
26 Jeong, J.W., Kim, M.K., Cheng, H., Yeo, W.H., Huang, X., Liu, Y., Zhang, Y., Huang, Y., and Rogers, J.A. (2014) *Adv. Healthc. Mater.*, **3**, 642.
27 Harada, S., Honda, W., Arie, T., Akita, S., and Takei, K. (2014) *ACS Nano*, **8**, 3921.
28 Harada, S., Kanao, K., Yamamoto, Y., Arie, T., Akita, S., and Takei, K. (2014) *ACS Nano*, **8**, 12851.
29 Honda, W., Harada, S., Ishida, S., Arie, T., Akita, S., and Takei, K. (2015) *Adv. Mater.*, **27**, 4674.
30 Kaltenbrunner, M., Adam, G., Glowacki, E.D., Drack, M., Schwodiauer, R., Leonat, L., Apaydin, D.H., Groiss, H., Scharber, M.C., White, M.S., Sariciftci, N.S., and Bauer, S. (2015) *Nat. Mater.*, **14**, 1032.
31 Honda, W., Arie, T., Akita, S., and Takei, K. (2015) *Sci. Rep.*, **5**, 15099.
32 Zang, Y., Zhang, F., Huang, D., Gao, X., Di, C.A., and Zhu, D. (2015) *Nat. Commun.*, **6**, 6269.
33 Honda, W., Arie, T., Akita, S., and Takei, K. (2016) *Adv. Mater. Technol.*, **1**, 1600058.
34 Gao, W., Emaminejad, S., Nyein, H.Y., Challa, S., Chen, K., Peck, A., Fahad, H.M., Ota, H., Shiraki, H., Kiriya, D., Lien, D.H., Brooks, G.A., Davis, R.W., and Javey, A. (2016) *Nature*, **529**, 509.
35 Someya, T., Sekitani, T., Iba, S., Kato, Y., Kawaguchi, H., and Sakurai, T. (2004) *Proc. Natl. Acad. Sci. U.S.A.*, **101**, 9966.
36 Someya, T., Kato, Y., Sekitani, T., Iba, S., Noguchi, Y., Murase, Y., Kawaguchi, H., and Sakurai, T. (2005) *Proc. Natl. Acad. Sci. U.S.A.*, **102**, 12321.
37 Sekitani, T., Nakajima, H., Maeda, H., Fukushima, T., Aida, T., Hata, K., and Someya, T. (2009) *Nat. Mater.*, **8**, 494.
38 Kim, D.H., Lu, N., Ghaffari, R., Kim, Y.S., Lee, S.P., Xu, L., Wu, J., Kim, R.H., Song, J., Liu, Z., Viventi, J., de Graff, B., Elolampi, B., Mansour, M., Slepian, M.J., Hwang, S., Moss, J.D., Won, S.M., Huang, Y., Litt, B., and Rogers, J.A. (2011) *Nat. Mater.*, **10**, 316.
39 Hwang, S.-W., Tao, H., Kim, D.-H., Cheng, H., Song, J.-K., Rill, E., Brenckle, M.A., Panilaitis, B., Won, S.M., Kim, Y.-S., Song, Y.M., Yu, K.J., Ameen, A., Li, R., Su, Y., Yang, M., Kaplan, D.L., Zakin, M.R., Slepian, M.J., Huang, Y., Omenetto, F.G., and Rogers, J.A. (2012) *Science*, **28**, 1640.

40 Tao, H., Hwang, S.W., Marelli, B., An, B., Moreau, J.E., Yang, M., Brenckle, M.A., Kim, S., Kaplan, D.L., Rogers, J.A., and Omenetto, F.G. (2014) *Proc. Natl. Acad. Sci. U.S.A.*, **111**, 17385.

41 Kaltenbrunner, M., Sekitani, T., Reeder, J., Yokota, T., Kuribara, K., Tokuhara, T., Drack, M., Schwodiauer, R., Graz, I., Bauer-Gogonea, S., Bauer, S., and Someya, T. (2013) *Nature*, **499**, 458.

42 Yamamoto, Y., Harada, S., Yamamoto, D., Honda, W., Arie, T., Akita, S., and Takei, K. (2016) *Sci. Adv.*, **2**, e1601473.

43 Kim, J., Salvatore, G.A., Araki, H., Chiarelli, A.M., Xie, Z., Banks, A., Sheng, X., Liu, Y., Lee, J.W., Jang, K.-I., Heo, S.Y., Cho, K., Luo, H., Zimmerman, B., Kim, J., Yan, L., Feng, X., Xu, S., Fabiani, M., Gratton, G., Huang, Y., Paik, U., and Rogers, J.A. (2016) *Sci. Adv.*, **2**, e1600418.

44 Fukuda, K., Minamiki, T., Minami, T., Watanabe, M., Fukuda, T., Kumaki, D., and Tokito, S. (2015) *Adv. Electron. Mater.*, **1**, 1400052.

45 Lee, H., Choi, T.K., Lee, Y.B., Cho, H.R., Ghaffari, R., Wang, L., Choi, H.J., Chung, T.D., Lu, N., Hyeon, T., Choi, S.H., and Kim, D.-H. (2016) *Nat. Nanotechnol.*, **11**, 566.

46 Larson, C., Peele, B., Li, S., Robinson, S., Totaro, M., Beccai, L., Mazzolai, B., and Shepherd, R. (2016) *Science*, **351**, 1071.

47 Yokota, T., Zalar, P., Kaltenbrunner, M., Jinno, H., Matsuhisa, N., Kitanosako, H., Tachibana, Y., Yukita, W., Koizumi, M., and Someya, T. (2016) *Sci. Adv.*, **2**, e1501856.

2

Carbon Nanotube Based Flexible and Stretchable Electronics

Le Cai and Chuan Wang

Michigan State University, Department of Electrical & Computing Engineering, East Lansing, MI 48824, USA

2.1 Introduction

Unlike conventional microelectronics/nanoelectronics, whose emphasis is miniaturization for improving processing speed and integration density, marcro-electronics focuses on large-area and low-cost applications and new form factors such as flexible and stretchable devices [1]. Electronic devices that are fabricated on plastic or rubbery substrates such as flexible display, electronic paper, smart packages, skin-like sensors, wearable electronics, implantable medical implements, and many others, could radically change people's perspectives on electronics [2]. The development of those new forms of electronics relies largely on the advancements in materials science. Over decades, amorphous silicon, polysilicon, and organic semiconductors have been extensively studied as the channel materials for thin-film transistors (TFTs), one of the key components in macroelectronics [3]. In recent years, nanomaterials, including quantum dots [4], one-dimensional carbon nanotubes (CNTs), and nanowires [5], as well as two dimensional (2D) materials [6] have attracted numerous research interests in this area because they offer significantly better performance than organic semiconductors and are easier to process than a-Si or polysilicon. In particular, CNTs hold great promise for high performance flexible electronics due to their extremely high carrier mobility, superior mechanical flexibility, and stability [7].

A single-wall carbon nanotube (SWCNT) can be considered as a seamless cylinder formed by rolling up a graphene sheet along a vector $\boldsymbol{C}_h = n\boldsymbol{a}_1 + m\boldsymbol{a}_2$, where $\boldsymbol{a}_1$ and $\boldsymbol{a}_2$ are the basis vectors of the hexagonal crystal lattice of graphene. The indices (n, m) define the two structural parameters, diameter and chirality, of the nanotube. Theoretical calculations indicate that, depending on the indices, the nanotube can have different electrical attributes—metallic for $n–m$ equals multiples of 3, and semiconducting for others. In addition, the bandgap of a semi-conducting nanotube is known to be inversely proportional to its diameter [8].

The unique structure–property relation makes SWCNTs ideal candidates for molecular electronic devices—for example, metallic nanotubes act as inter-connects while semiconducting SWCNTs play the role of channel material for field-effect transistors (FETs) [9]. Additionally, numerous studies have already

Flexible and Stretchable Medical Devices, First Edition. Edited by Kuniharu Takei.

revealed that individual SWCNTs exhibit very exciting electronic properties, which are well beyond their conventional material counterparts. For instance, the current carrying capability of metallic SWCNTs can reach $10^9\,\text{A cm}^{-2}$ (much better than aluminum or copper) while semiconducting SWCNTs can exhibit field-effect mobilities up to $10^4\,\text{cm}^2\,\text{V}^{-1}\,\text{s}^{-1}$ (far exceed silicon) [10]. Nevertheless, devices based on individual SWCNTs suffer from poor uniformity and reproducibility, mainly due to difficulties in reliable synthesis of SWCNTs with homogeneous structural attributes, as well as controllable assembly of SWCNTs over a large area [7, 11]. In addition, novel fabrication methods are needed to render the individual-SWCNT-based devices compatible with current industrial manufacturing processes. On the other hand, macroscale assemblies of SWCNTs, particularly random networks and thin-films, are believed to enable the most realistic applications of SWCNTs in electronics in the short term because they offer not only facile processing but also uniform and reproducible performance due to ensemble averaging [7, 12]. Additionally, SWCNT networks are especially suitable for flexible and stretchable electronics because the lateral deformation of the curvy and entangled SWCNTs can accommodate practically large strains [13]. In fact, there have already been lots of studies demonstrating the great promise of SWCNT networks as the channel materials and/or electrodes in various types of flexible/stretchable electronic devices, such as integrated circuits [14], sensors [13b, 15], organic light-emitting diodes (OLEDs) [16], supercapacitors [17], touch panels [18], and so on.

The widely used strategies for preparing CNT networks and thin films are summarized in Figure 2.1. Generally, they can be classified in two categories: dry processes and solution processes [12]. Dry processes are mainly direct chemical vapor deposition (CVD) growth and dry drawing from vertically aligned CNT arrays [5a]. Direct CVD grown SWCNT films comprise ultralong nanotubes bonded by strong interbundle connections [19], and thereby, possess excellent conductivity, making them suitable for the electrode material of many functional devices like super-fast actuators [24], stretchable supercapacitors [17], and strain sensors [15c]. However, the size of CVD furnaces limit the area of this kind of SWCNT films to typically below $100\,\text{cm}^2$ [19]. Although dry drawing method can, in principle, continuously produce CNT films with unlimited area [20], the direct drawing of SWCNTs from vertical arrays has yet to be realized. Moreover, since there is currently no effective method to grow structurally or electrically homogeneous SWCNTs, the biggest disadvantage of CVD grown SWCNT films is that the as-grown samples typically contain a mixture of CNTs with all types of chirality and metallicity. Therefore, such samples cannot be used as channel materials for transistors until the metallic conduction is eliminated by special process such as electrical breakdown, stripe patterning, or dry filtration [14b, c].

On the other end of the spectrum lies the solution-based process, where several methods have been reported including vacuum filtration [22], rod coating [25], drop coating [14d, 21], and printing [23]. The solution process of CNTs is enabled by successfully dispersing them in suitable organic solvents or in aqueous solution with the assistance of certain types of surfactants [26]. SWCNT thin films obtained by vacuum filtration and rod coating have been used for flexible, stretchable, and transparent electrodes [16b, 27], while printed

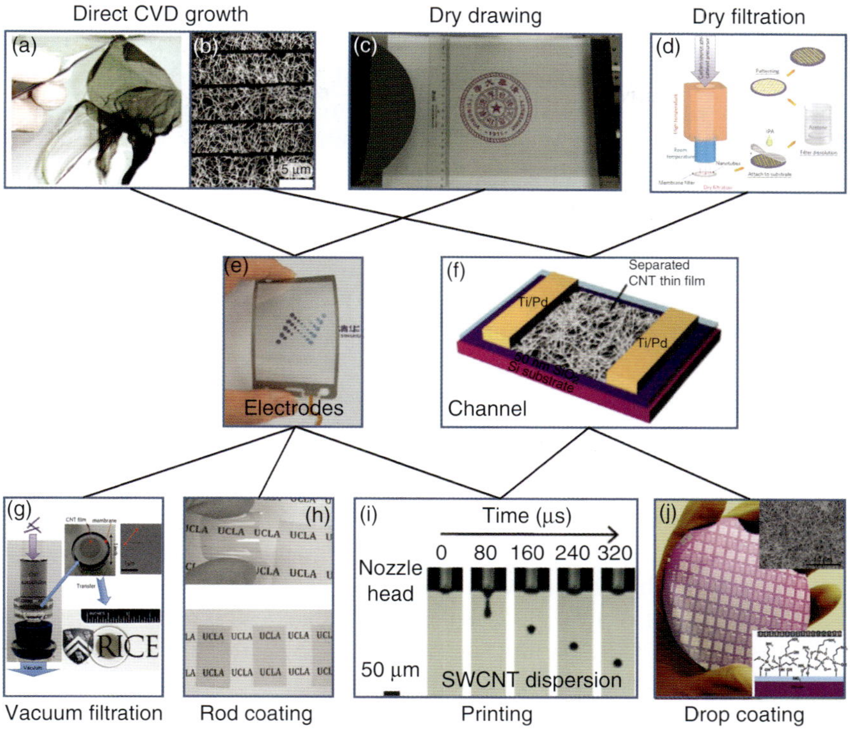

Figure 2.1 Various methods for preparing carbon nanotube networks and representative electronic applications. Dry process (a–d): (a) photograph of directly CVD grown freestanding SWCNT thin film. (Ma *et al.* 2007 [19]. Reproduced with permission of American Chemical Society.) (b) SEM image of CVD grown SWCNT network patterned into strips for channel materials of flexible TFTs. (Cao *et al.* 2008 [14b]. Reproduced with permission of Nature Publishing Group.) (c) Photograph of multi-wall carbon nanotube (MWCNT) thin films obtained using a dry drawing process. (Jiang *et al.* 2011 [20a]. Reproduced with permission of John Wiley & Sons.) (d) Schematics of dry filtration process to collect sparse SWCNT network for flexible TFTs. (Sun *et al.* 2011 [14c]. Reproduced with permission of Nature Publishing Group.) (e, f) Applications of carbon nanotube networks as flexible electrodes (e) (Feng *et al.* 2010 [18]. Reproduced with permission of John Wiley & Sons.) or channel materials for flexible TFTs (f) (Wang *et al.* 2009 [21]. Reproduced with permission of American Chemical Society.). Solution process (g–j): (g) photograph of SWCNT thin film produced by vacuum filtration. (Reproduced from Ref. [22].) (h) Photographs of rod coated SWCNT films with different transmittance. (Yu *et al.* 2011 [16b]. Reproduced with permission of John Wiley & Sons.) (i) Time-dependent snapshot of SWCNT ink droplet during ink-jet printing process. (Okimoto *et al.* 2010 [23a]. Reproduced with permission of John Wiley & Sons.) (j) Photograph of wafer-scale SWCNT TFTs fabricated using drop coated SWCNT network. Insets: SEM image of the SWCNT network and schematic illustration of the surface chemistry used. (Wang *et al.* 2009 [21]. Reproduced with permission of American Chemical Society.)

SWCNT networks have been demonstrated to act as both electrodes and channel materials for TFTs [23a]. One key advantage of solution-based process is low temperature and compatibility with various types of widely used polymeric materials, thus enabling the low cost and large scale deposition onto various flexible and stretchable substrates [7, 12b]. More importantly, through the solution process, it is possible to selectively assemble SWCNTs with the same electronic type or chirality obtained by post-growth purification and separation [28]. With the tremendous progress in SWCNT separation and purification, semiconductor-enriched SWCNTs (sSWCNTs) are now available in large quantities [29], which enables the wafer-scale fabrication of sSWCNT TFTs with high yield and uniform performance [21]. The most significant advantage of using sSWCNT networks for TFT application lies in the unique combination of superior flexibility/stretchability, optical transparency, and low-temperature solution process, which are not possible with conventional polysilicon or amorphous silicon platforms [3a, b]. In addition, compared with organic semiconductors, sSWCNT networks not only offer drastically better air stability but also multiple orders of magnitude improvements in carrier mobility [3c].

The realization of large area flexible/stretchable electronics also relies on the innovations in manufacturing techniques. Conventional microfabrication processes used in semiconductor industry is not desirable due to its high cost, limitation in sample size, and restrictions in substrate material. Alternatively, printing is a promising method with theoretically no restrictions in substrate material and size [30]. In addition, as an additive process, printing produces minimum material waste, and thereby, enables eco-friendly and cost-effective manufacturing. Recently, several groups have reported printed flexible devices and circuits using solution-processed SWCNTs, representing a viable way to large scale and low cost flexible electronics based on SWCNTs [23, 31].

In this chapter, we survey the recent progress on flexible and stretchable electronics with SWCNT networks as either electrodes or channel materials. This chapter is organized as follows. In Section 2.2, we briefly discuss progress made on the high-performance flexible electronics with sSWCNT networks as channel semiconductors. Herein, five examples are presented, namely, flexible TFTs, integrated circuits, flexible displays, electronic skins (E-skins), and X-ray imager. For more detailed and systematic discussion of sSWCNT-based flexible electronics, readers are referred to the recent review papers covering this topic [7, 32]. In Section 2.3, we highlight several applications of SWCNT networks in stretchable electronics, including stretchable conductors and electrodes, sensors, and TFTs. In Section 2.4, we focus on the recently developed fabrication process that is most suitable for large-area flexible/stretchable electronics—printing. The state-of-the-art development of fully-printed SWCNT-based TFTs and integrated circuits are discussed in detail. Lastly in Section 2.5, we conclude with the current challenges and future prospects in this area.

2.2 Carbon Nanotube Networks for Applications in Flexible Electronics

2.2.1 Thin-Film Transistors (TFTs)

TFT plays a critical role in macroelectronics. As discussed previously, sSWCNTs are ideal candidates for the channel material of flexible TFTs because of the unique combination of low temperature processing, mechanical compliance, optical transparency, and superior electrical property. Using high purity sSWCNT solutions, Wang *et al.* obtained wafer-scale nanotube networks with high density and uniformity [21], which subsequently enabled the fabrication of TFTs and logical circuits on both rigid and flexible substrates [14d]. With the assistance of suitable surface chemistry and by controlling the sSWCNT deposition time, the network density can be fine adjusted (as high as 65 tubes/μm^2), which in turn determines the ultimate device performance (Figure 2.2a). Flexible TFTs fabricated on such sSWCNT networks exhibit p-type conduction with on/off current ratio (I_{on}/I_{off}) on the order of 10^4 when the channel length is above 10 µm (Figure 2.2b). In devices with channel lengths of 4 µm, on-current (I_{on}/W) and transconductance (g_m/W) reach 15 $\mu A\ \mu m^{-1}$ and 4 $\mu S\ \mu m^{-1}$, respectively, at a moderate voltage of 5 V. Due to the trade-off between on/off ratio and transconductance, TFTs with large channel lengths (high I_{on}/I_{off}) are ideal for logical circuits while the devices with short channel lengths (large g_m) are suitable for analog and radio-frequency application. In addition, capacitance–voltage (C-V) measurements are performed to precisely determine the gate capacitance which in turn leads to an accurate assessment of the field effect mobility (μ), with a typical value of ~50 $cm^2\ V^{-1}\ s^{-1}$ (Figure 2.2b) [14d], similar to that of low temperature polysilicon (LTPS) and much higher than those of amorphous silicon and organic semiconductors. Furthermore, the use of ultrathin polyimide substrates results in highly flexible TFTs and integrated logical circuits, including inverter, NOR and NAND gates. Such devices and circuits exhibit excellent stability after thousands of bending cycles with curvature radii down to ~1 mm (Figure 2.3).

2.2.2 Integrated Circuits

High-performance TFTs and integrated logical circuits have also been fabricated using random networks of single-walled carbon nanotubes directly grown from CVD methods. Compared with solution-process SWCNTs, CVD-grown SWCNTs often have longer tube length and cleaner surface, which are advantageous for obtaining better carrier mobility owing to fewer inter-tube junctions and less surface scattering. However, since roughly one third of the as-grown SWCNTs are metallic, additional process are needed to suppress the metallic conduction within the SWCNTs network. Cao *et al.* adopt strip patterning to reduce the probability of percolative metallic pathways in the network and obtained transistors with I_{on}/I_{off} as high as 10^5 without significant sacrifice in carrier mobility (~80 $cm^2\ V^{-1}\ s^{-1}$) [14b]. Medium-scale integrated circuits were further demonstrated on plastic substrates. Figure 2.4a,b present the optical image and transient response of a 4-to-16 decoder comprising up to nearly 100 SWCNT TFTs. In another report, Sun *et al.* fabricate TFTs and integrated circuits on transparent and flexible substrates using sparse networks of SWCNTs that are collected from a CVD furnace with a dry filtration method [14c]. The TFTs exhibit field effect mobility and I_{on}/I_{off} of 35 $cm^2\ V^{-1}\ s^{-1}$ and 10^6, respectively. The high electrical performance benefits from the long nanotube lengths (~10 µm) as well as Y-type inter-nanotube junctions which have large contact area and thus low contact resistance. The TFTs were subsequently assembled into a D-flip-flop whose optical images and transient response are shown in Figure 2.4c,d, respectively.

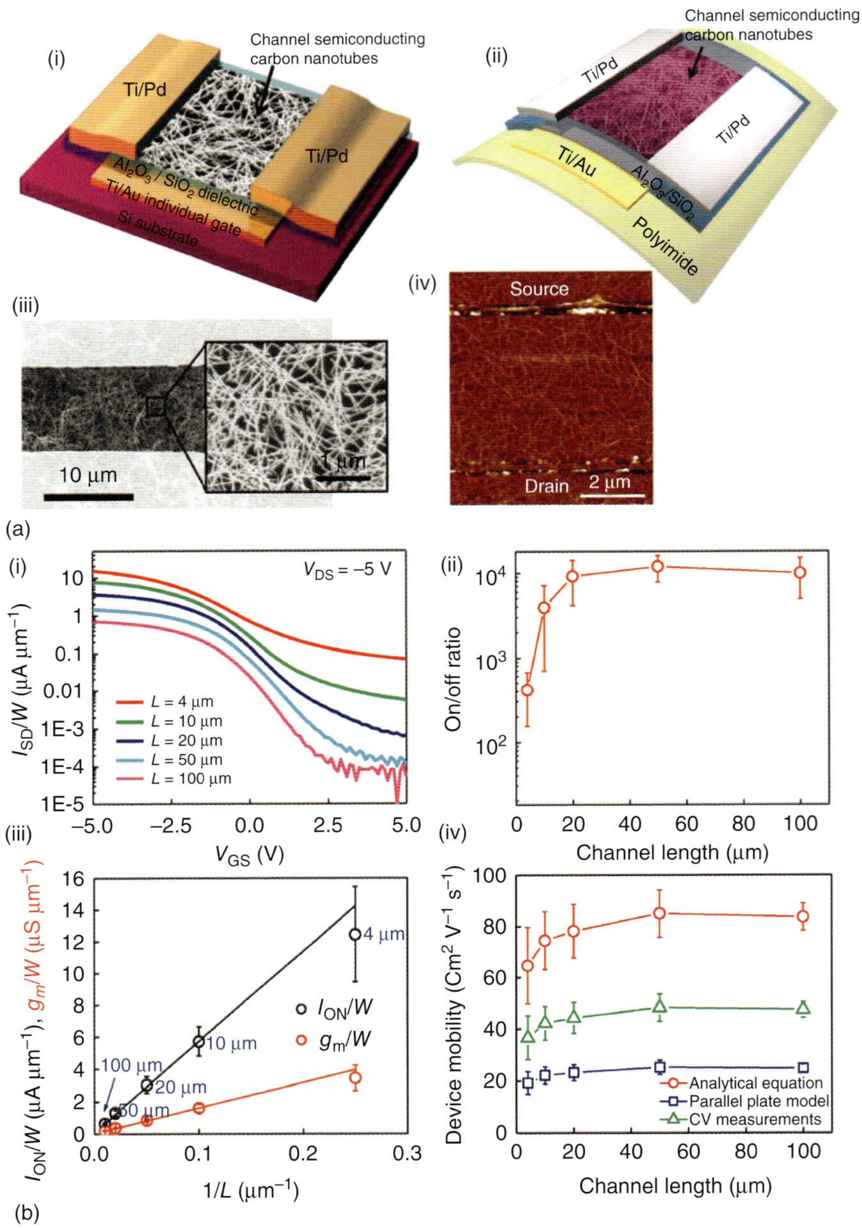

Figure 2.2 High performance TFTs using semiconducting carbon nanotubes (sSWCNTs). (a) Schematics of TFTs on rigid (i) and flexible (ii) substrates. The SEM (iii) and AFM (iv) images of the channel region are also shown. (b) Electrical characteristics of the flexible TFTs. (i) I_d-V_g curves of transistors with different channel lengths; (ii) TFT on/off current ratio as a function of channel length; (iii) normalized on-current and transconductance as functions of reciprocal channel length; (iv) field-effect mobility, calculated based on *C-V* measurement (green), as a function of channel length. Also shown are the mobility obtained using parallel plate model (blue) and cylindrical model (red). (Wang *et al.* 2013 [7]. Reproduced with permission of Royal Society of Chemistry.)

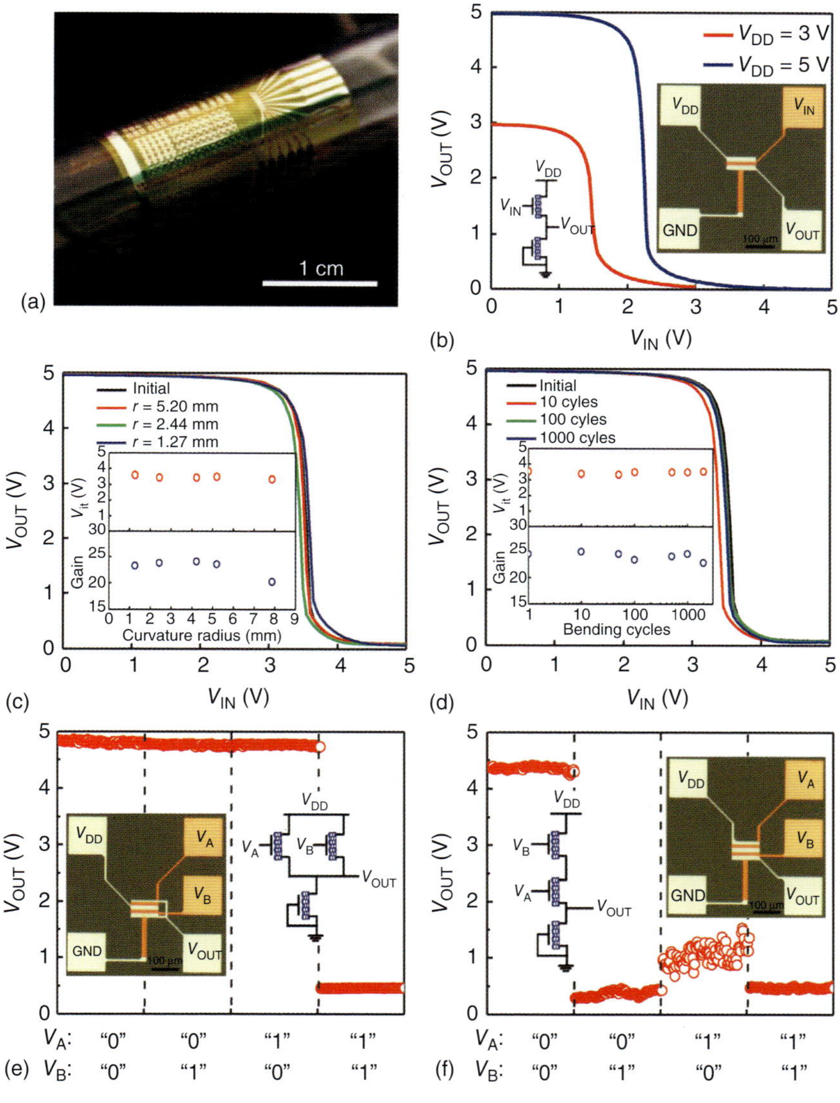

Figure 2.3 Flexible logic gates using CNT-TFTs. (a) Optical image demonstrating the flexibility of the circuits, where the sample is wrapped onto a glass tube with a diameter of 10 mm. (b) Inverter voltage transfer characteristics (VTC) measured with a V_{DD} of 3 or 5 V. Inset shows the schematic and the optical picture of the diode-loaded inverter. (c) Inverter VTC measured while the circuit is bent to various curvature radii. Inset shows the inverter threshold voltage and gain as a function of curvature radius. (d) Inverter durability under cyclic bending test, showing stable performance for up to 2000 cycles. (e, f) Output characteristics of diode-loaded 2-input NOR (e) and NAND (f) gates. V_{DD} is 5 V for both circuits. Insets are the corresponding schematic and optical micrographs. (Wang *et al.* 2012 [14d]. Reproduced with permission of American Chemical Society.)

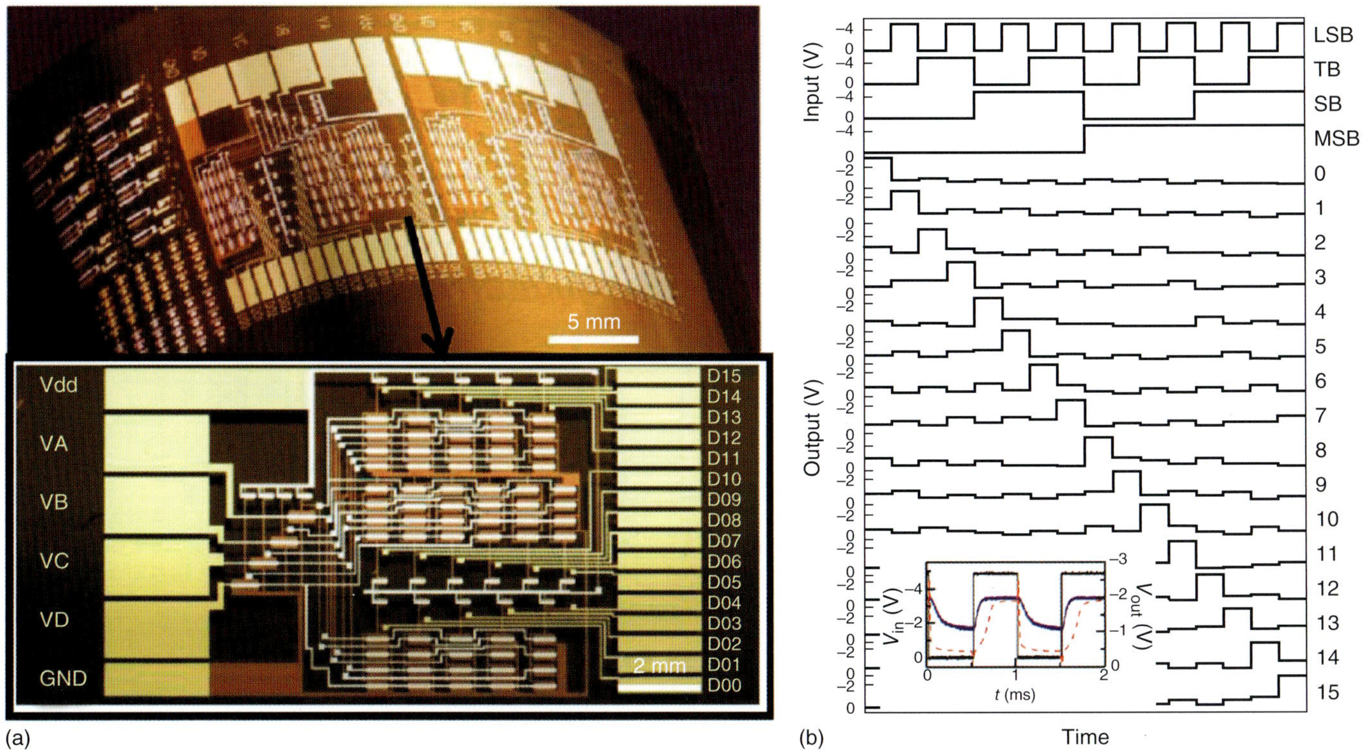

Figure 2.4 More sophisticated flexible integrated circuits using CNT-TFTs. (a) Optical image of a 4-to-16 decoder. (b) Transient response of the decoder. (Cao *et al*. 2008 [14b]. Reproduced with permission of Nature Publishing Group.) (c) Optical images of a D-flip-flop. (d) Transient response of the D-flip-flop. (Sun *et al*. 2011 [14c]. Reproduced with permission of Nature Publishing Group.)

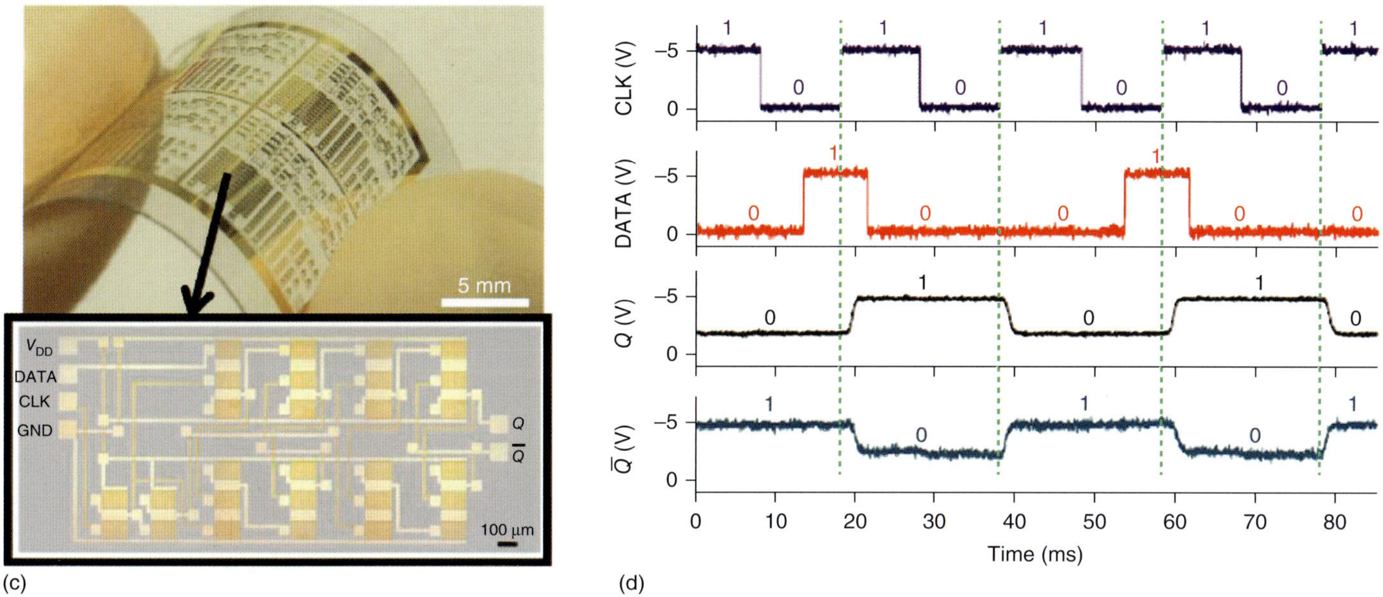

Figure 2.4 (*Continued*)

2.2.3 Active Matrix Backplanes for Flexible Display, E-Skin and Imager

Due to the superior electrical performance and mechanical robustness as well as low-temperature solution process, sSWCNT TFTs are excellent candidates for active matrix (AM) backplane to drive various functional systems like flexible organic light emitting diode (OLED) displays [33], E-skins [34] and X-ray imager [34]. Figure 2.5 presents an example of flexible AMOLED displays where an sSWCNT TFT array is used as the AM backplane [35]. Each pixel is driven by an individual sSWCNT TFT that adopts an interdigitated source/drain configuration to obtain a high output current. The drain electrode of the driving TFT is connected to ITO pad that is sputtered as OLED anode. The emissive layer and Al cathode are subsequently deposited by evaporation. Figure 2.5b–d show the photographs of the single-color (green) and full-color (red, green blue) flexible AMOLED displays under operation. The flexible AMOLED display is further integrated with pressure sensitive rubber (PSR) to realize a user-interactive E-skin [35]. In PSR, carbon black nanoparticles (CB NPs)

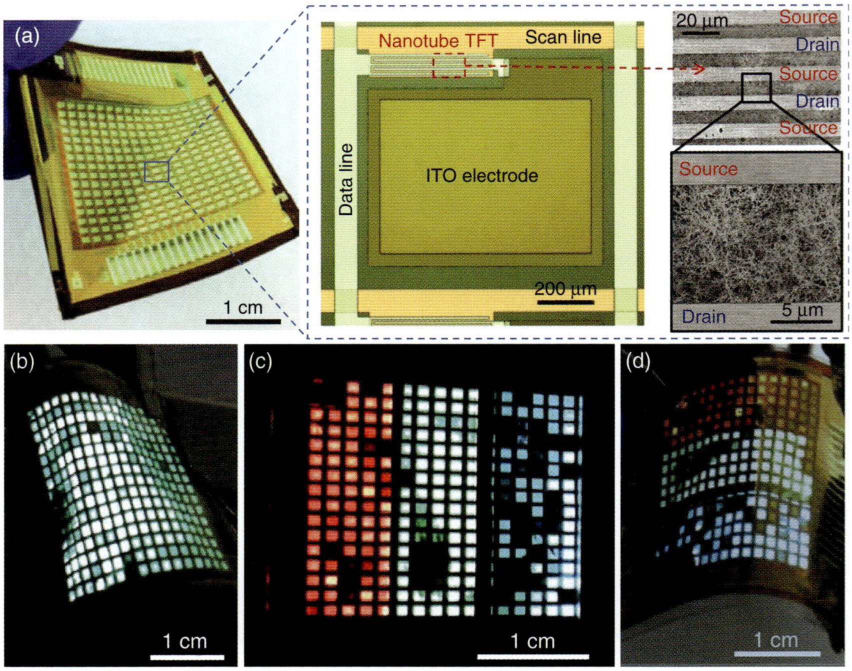

Figure 2.5 Flexible AMOLED display using CNT TFT array as active matrix. (a) Left: photograph of a completed flexible AMOLED display comprising 16 × 16 pixels driven by a CNT TFT active matrix with a size of ~3 × 3.5 cm^2; middle: optical micrograph of one pixel before evaporating the emissive layer; right: SEM image showing the channel region of the CNT TFT. (b) Photograph of a single-color (green) AMOLED display being fully turned on and at bent state, demonstrating a yield, defined as the fraction of lighting pixels, of >97%. The voltages applied to the scan and data lines are −5 and 10 V, respectively. (c, d) Photograph of a full-color (red, green, blue) AMOLED display with all pixels being turned on and at flat (c) and bent (d) states. (Wang *et al.* 2013 [35]. Reproduced with permission of Nature Publishing Group.)

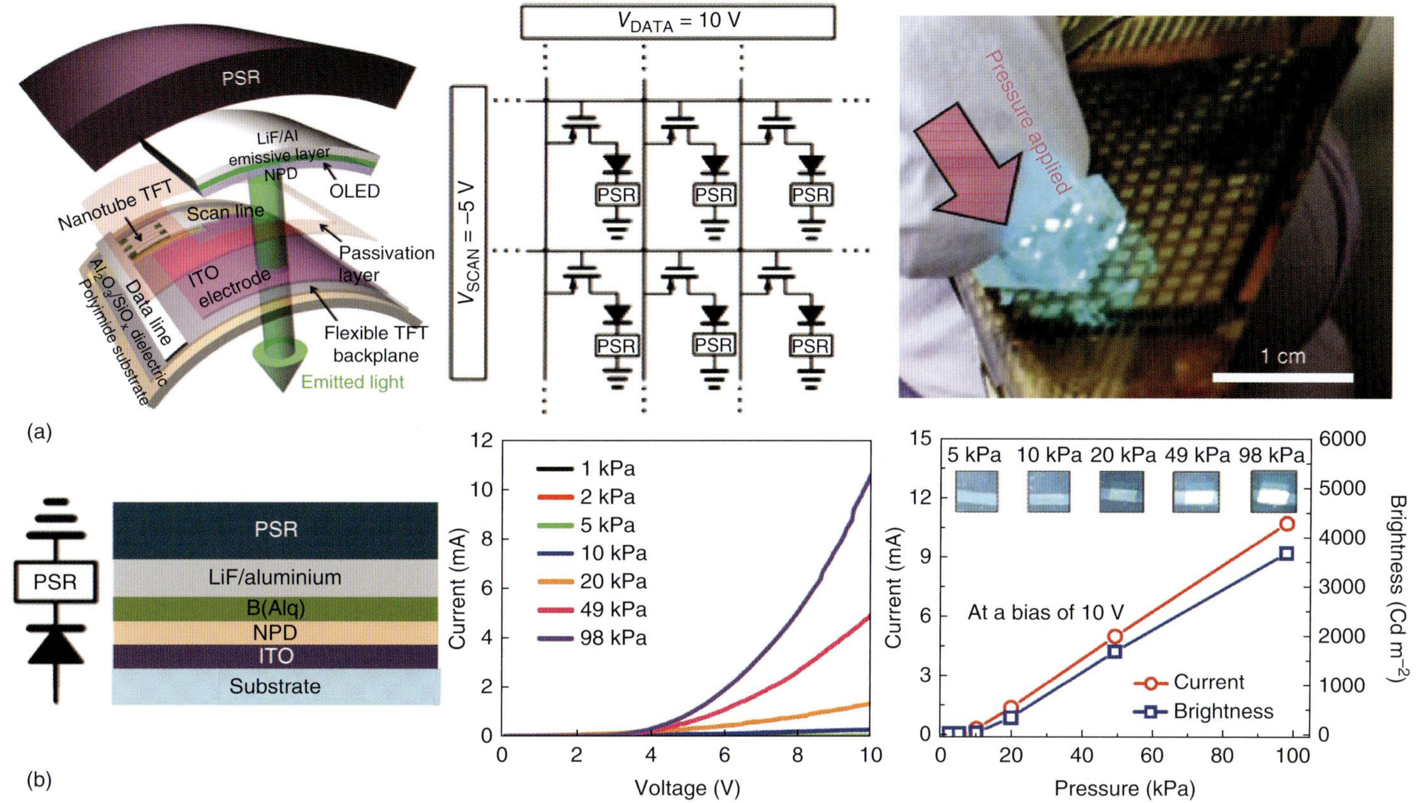

Figure 2.6 User-interactive electronic skin (E-skin) using CNT-TFTs. (a) Left: schematic diagram showing the exploded view of one pixel, consisting of a CNT-TFT, an OLED and a layer of PSR vertically integrated on a polyimide substrate; middle: circuit diagram of the active matrix user-interactive E-skin; right: photograph of a working E-skin. The OLED pixels are turned on locally where the surface is touched and the light intensity reflects the magnitude of the applied pressure. (b) Individual pixel comprising an OLED connected in series to a piece of pressure sensitive rubber (PSR): schematics of the circuit and device structure (left), current–voltage curves under various magnitudes of applied pressure (middle), current and luminance as functions of applied pressure under a bias of 10 V. (d) Optical (middle) and electrical (right) readout from the E-skin system when an L-shaped PDMS slab is used to apply pressure onto the sample. (Wang *et al*. 2013 [35]. Reproduced with permission of Nature Publishing Group.)

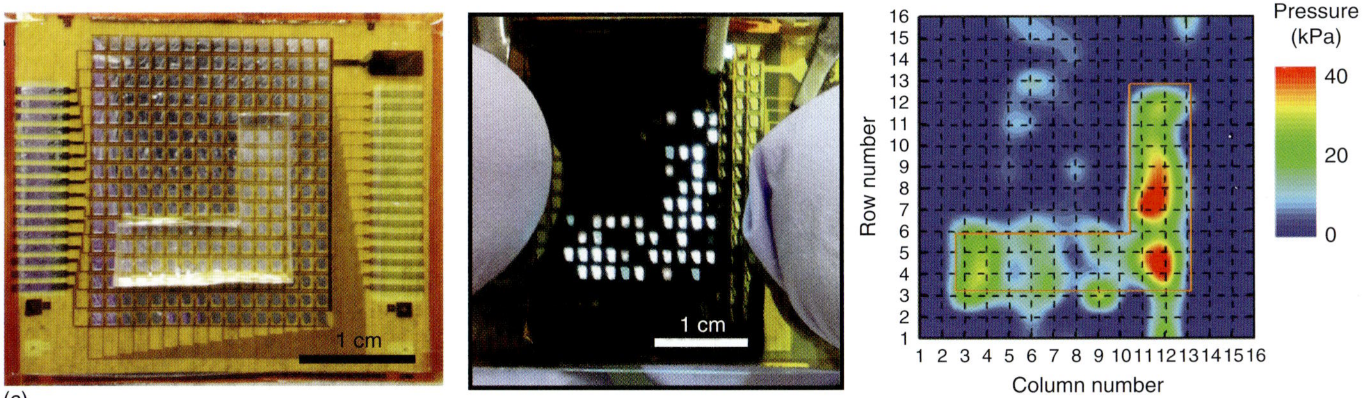

(c)

Figure 2.6 (*Continued*)

are dispersed in rubber matrix as conductive fillers. The CB NPs are brought closer to each other while the PSR is pressed, resulting in a resistance reduction whose magnitude is dependent on the applied pressure. Consequently, the luminance of an OLED can be tuned by the pressure applied on the PSR, as shown in Figure 2.6b. In the integrated interactive E-skin shown in Figure 2.6, the pixels can be turned on locally where the surface is touched (Figure 2.6a, right) and the light intensity of the OLED qualitatively represents the magnitude of the applied pressure, enabling both electrical readout and visual output of the external stimuli with a high spatial resolution (Figure 2.6c). This example represents a system-on-plastic demonstration where three distinct electronic components—carbon nanotube TFT, OLED display, and pressure sensor—are monolithically integrated over large area on a single piece of flexible substrate. Substituting other sensors, such as chemical sensor, light sensor, and temperature sensor, for the pressure sensor used here could allow various functionalities akin or superior to natural skins and find a wide range of applications in smart robotics and security/health-monitoring devices. For instance, a flexible visible light imager can be made by combining the sSWCNT TFT backplane with a flexible photodetector like the P3HT/PCBM bulk heterojunction demonstrated in Figure 2.7 [34]. Similar to the E-skin discussed above, the basic idea is connecting the sensor, the photodetector here, to the drain electrode of the driving sSWCNT TFT. The current is thus determined by the bit line and word line voltages (pixel selection function) as well as the photodetector (sensing element). Laminating a scintillator film (the GOS film in Figure 2.7c) over the flexible AM visible light imager on the irradiation side can further transform the device into a flexible X-ray imager. As shown in Figure 2.7f, the contour of a T-shaped shadow mask can be readily recognized in the two-dimensional intensity profile obtained by measuring the photocurrent of all pixels.

2.3 Carbon Nanotube Networks for Applications in Stretchable Electronics

Mechanical flexibility by itself may not be sufficient for some applications. For instance, a surface with nonzero Gaussian curvature like a sphere or an irregular surface like the elbow could never be comformally covered with a system that is only flexible [36]. Instead, stretchable electronics could fill in. One strategy to realize stretchable devices is based on thin films of conventional bulk semiconductors like Si and GaAs that are configured into wavy or buckling structures and bonded on elastomer substrates [37]. However, this buckling method is rather complicated to fabricate and may not be suitable for large area or mass production. Alternatively, systems that are intrinsically stretchable can be built by using organic materials or nanomaterials with relatively simple processes [38].

Because of the extreme aspect ratio, CNTs are naturally highly curved and entangled in their macro scale assemblies, making them ideal materials for stretchable electronics [38, 39]. *In situ* scanning probe microscopic observations

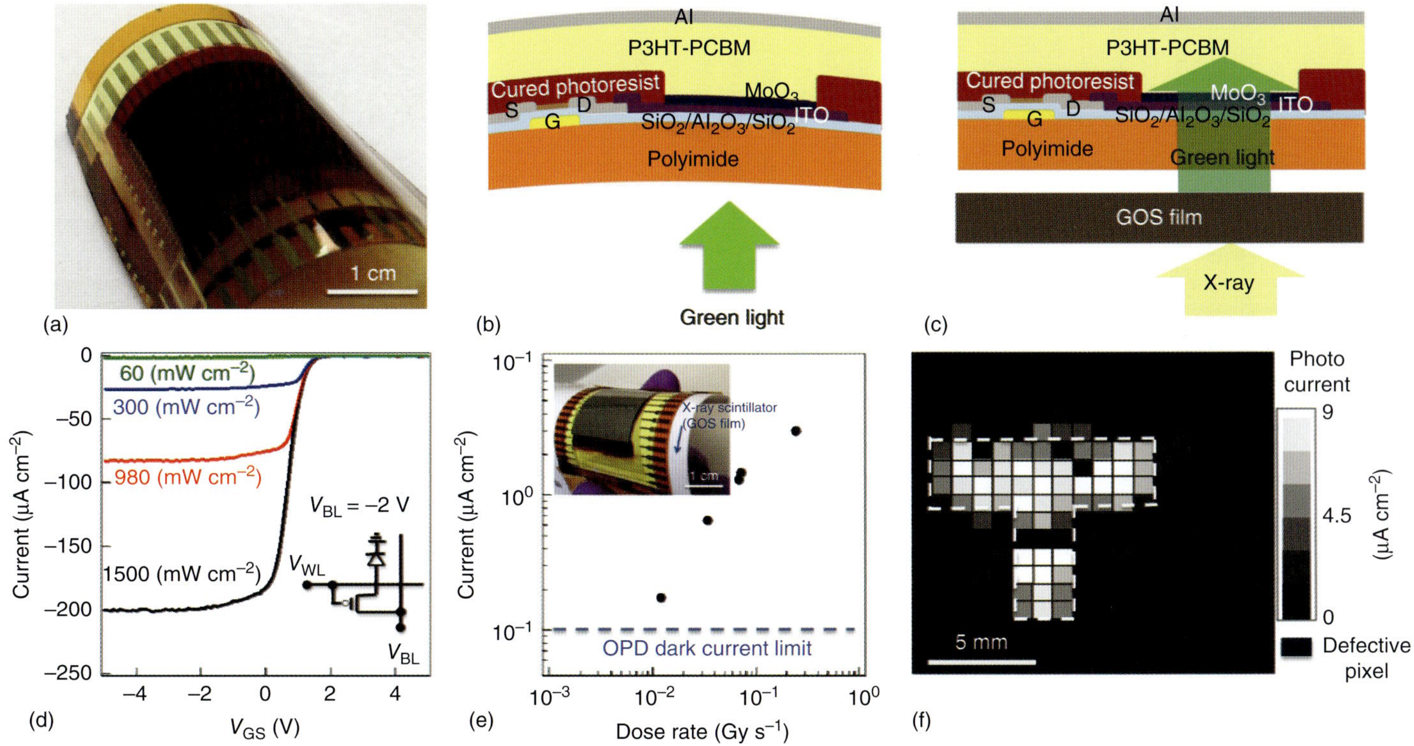

Figure 2.7 Carbon nanotube TFTs enabled flexible active matrix optical and X-ray imagers. (a) Photograph of a flexible imager driven by CNT TFTs being bent. (b, c) Schematics of the device structure and operating mechanism of a green light (b) and X-ray (c) imager. (d) Transfer characteristics of one pixel under different illumination intensities (green light). Inset shows the circuit diagram of a pixel. (e) Measured current of one pixel under a reverse bias of 2 V as a function of X-ray dosage. The dashed line marks the dark current level of the organic photodetector. (f) Two dimensional current profile which successfully reflects the "T"-shaped shadow mask placed between the light source and imager. (Takahashi *et al*. 2013 [34b]. Reproduced with permission of American Chemical Society.)

also reveal that, upon stretching and releasing process, CNTs form wavy structures, either in plane or out of plane [13], that could accommodate further deformations. Generally speaking, metallic nanotubes can be used as stretchable interconnects and electrodes [13b, 16b, 17, 40] while semiconducting nanotubes can take the role of channel materials for stretchable TFTs [14e, f, 34a]. In the following section, we first discuss the CNT stretchable conductors and their applications, and then shift focus to the stretchable transistors with semiconducting carbon nanotubes as channel materials.

2.3.1 Stretchable Conductors

Thin films and networks of carbon nanotubes usually exhibit high optical transparency, which provides additional advantages for the applications as electrodes of stretchable electronic and optoelectronic devices [5a, 12b]. Lipomi *et al.* fabricated highly stretchable and optically transparent electrodes by spin coating SWCNT solutions onto polydimethylsiloxane (PDMS) substrates (Figure 2.8) [13b]. The resistance change of the SWCNT/PDMS stretchable conductors exhibits a unique strain-history-dependent behavior during the initial stretching-releasing tests with progressively increasing strains, implying the strain-dependent evolution of the microscale morphology of the SWCNT network. Systematic electromechanical characterizations reveal that the SWCNT/PDMS stretchable conductors can retain stable conductance after 10 000 cycles of stretching with strains up to 25%. As an application, passive matrix of transparent capacitive sensor arrays with the capability of strain and pressure detection are further demonstrated by using the SWCNT/PDMS stretchable conductors as electrodes.

Although CNT films embedded in elastomers are excellent materials for stretchable electrodes, they are not the best choice for stretchable interconnects that require not only good stretchability and conductivity but also easy processing using direct writing or printing. In this regard, the composites consisting of CNTs and suitable polymeric binders show great promise [39]. Large nanotube lengths and uniform dispersion are desired to obtain composites with good performance. Sekitani *et al.* fabricated printable SWCNT pastes by uniformly dispersing super-growth SWCNTs in a fluorinated rubber with the assistance of an ionic liquid and a high-pressure jet-milling process [40a, b]. Long and fine SWCNT bundles form well-developed conducting networks in the rubber matrix. As shown in Figure 2.9a, fine features of SWCNT stretchable conductors can be patterned by screen printing. The conductivity and stretchability show inverse dependence on SWCNT content—higher SWCNT load leads to better conductivity but lower stretchability. The highest conductivity and stretchability achieved are $102\,\mathrm{S\,cm^{-1}}$ (15.8 wt% SWCNT) and 100% (1.4 wt% SWCNT), respectively. Further improvement of conductivity can be achieved by adding metallic additives in the composite. Chun *et al.* synthesized hybrid composites consisting of micrometer-sized silver flakes and multi-wall carbon nanotubes (MWCNTs) decorated with self-assembled silver nanoparticles [40c]. Silver nanoparticles (~3 nm) with phenyl rings are conjugated with MWCNTs via π–π interaction to produce nAg–MWCNTs that are then mixed with silver flakes

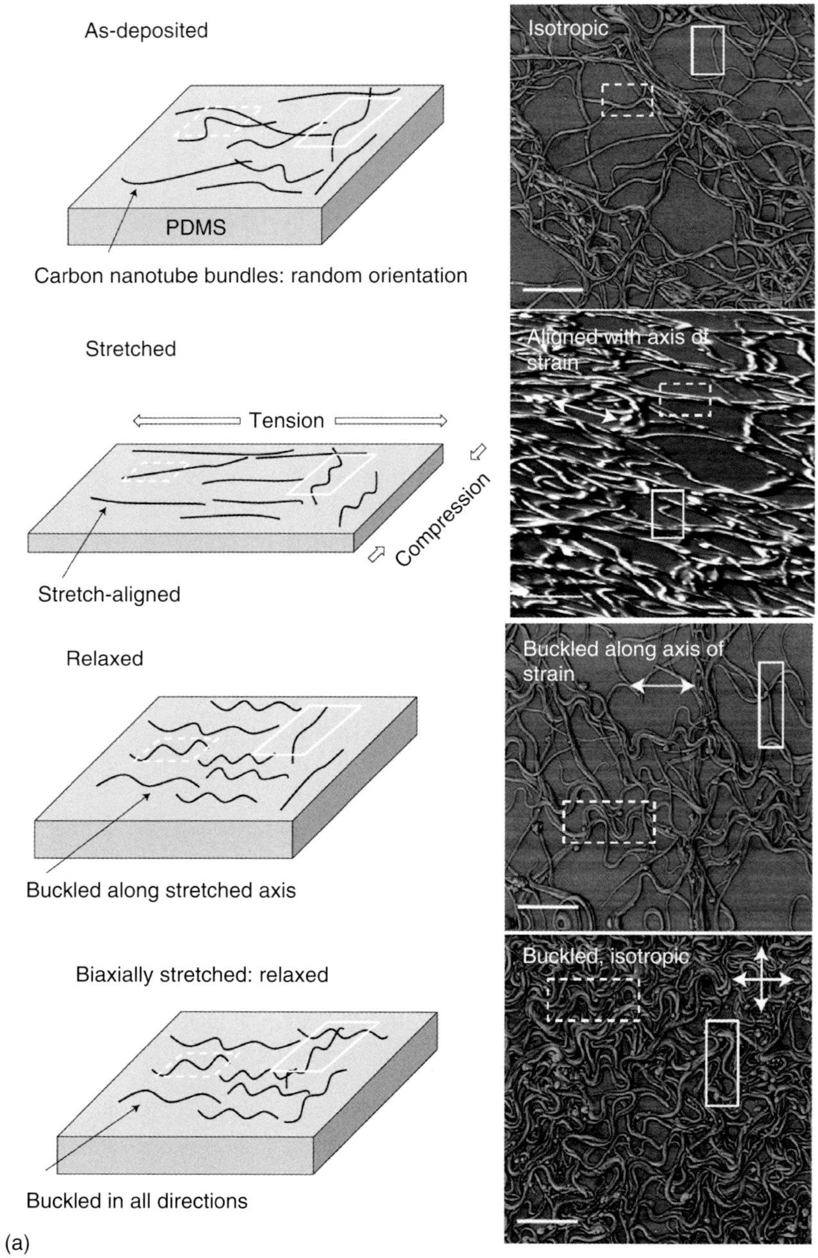

Figure 2.8 Carbon nanotube network as stretchable transparent electrodes for skin-like pressure sensor applications. (a) Schematics (left) and corresponding AFM images (right) showing the microscopic morphology evolution of CNT network on PDMS substrate when subjected to uniaxial and biaxial stretching and releasing tests. (b) Optical images and two-dimensional pressure profile obtained from a transparent pressure sensor array. (Lipomi *et al.* 2011 [13b]. Reproduced with permission of Nature Publishing Group.)

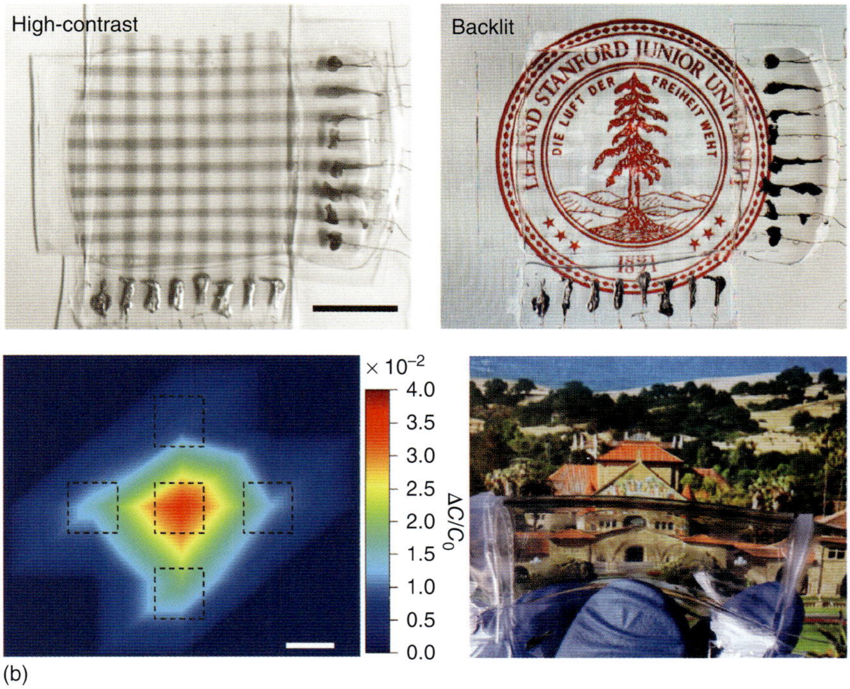

Figure 2.8 (*Continued*)

(Figure 2.9b,d). The nAg–MWCNTs forms an effective electrical network among the silver flakes, which results in a conductivity of as high as 5710 S cm^{-1} at 0% strain and 20 S cm^{-1} at 140% strain.

2.3.2 Stretchable Strain Sensor

Thanks to the above progress in CNT stretchable conductors, several stretchable functional electronic devices have been demonstrated, including strain gauge [15], pressure sensor [13b], OLED [16b, 41], and supercapacitor [17]. In particular, such nanomaterial-based stretchable strain gauges can detect very large strains (typically >30%) that are far beyond the limit of conventional metal foil or semiconductor strain gauges. In addition, the unique mechanical compliance renders them suitable for the applications involving interfacing with biological tissue such as human motion detection, health monitoring and rehabilitation. Figure 2.10 presents two examples of CNT stretchable strain gauges that are used for human motion detection. Yamada *et al.* demonstrated a resistive strain gauge (Figure 2.10a–f) that explores the lateral fracture of as-grown SWCNT arrays, where the controlled opening and closing of cracks lead to reproducible resistive response upon repetitive stretching and releasing [15a]. The device can detect strains as high as 280% with very small amount of overshoot and relaxation.

In another study, Cai *et al.* reported a capacitive strain gauge (Figure 2.10g–k), which is assembled into a parallel-plate capacitor using two layers of CVD-grown

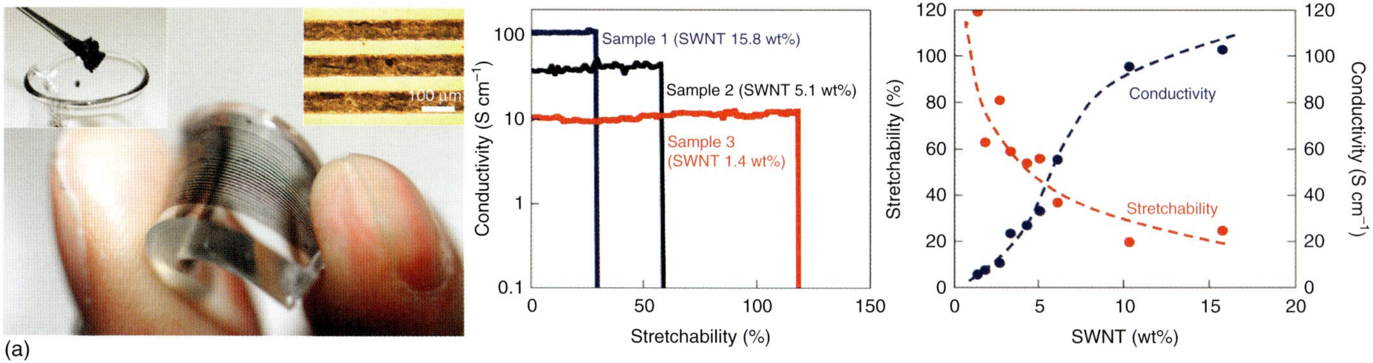

Figure 2.9 Stretchable conductors based on CNT-polymer composites. (a) Elastic conductors comprising super-growth SWCNTs uniformly dispersed in a fluorinated rubber: left, optical images of screen printed patterns with a feature width of 100 μm; middle, conductivity as a function of tensile strain for three samples with different SWCNT content; right, stretchability and conductivity as a function of SWCNT content. (Sekitani *et al*. 2009 [40b]. Reproduced with permission of Nature Publishing Group.) (b–d) Highly conductive and stretchable hybrid composites of silver flake and MWCNTs decorated with self-assembled silver nanoparticles. (b) Diagram of the synthesis process. (c) Conductivity as a function of tensile strain. (d) SEM images of the nanocomposites at a strain of 50%. (Chun *et al*. 2010 [40c]. Reproduced with permission of Nature Publishing Group.)

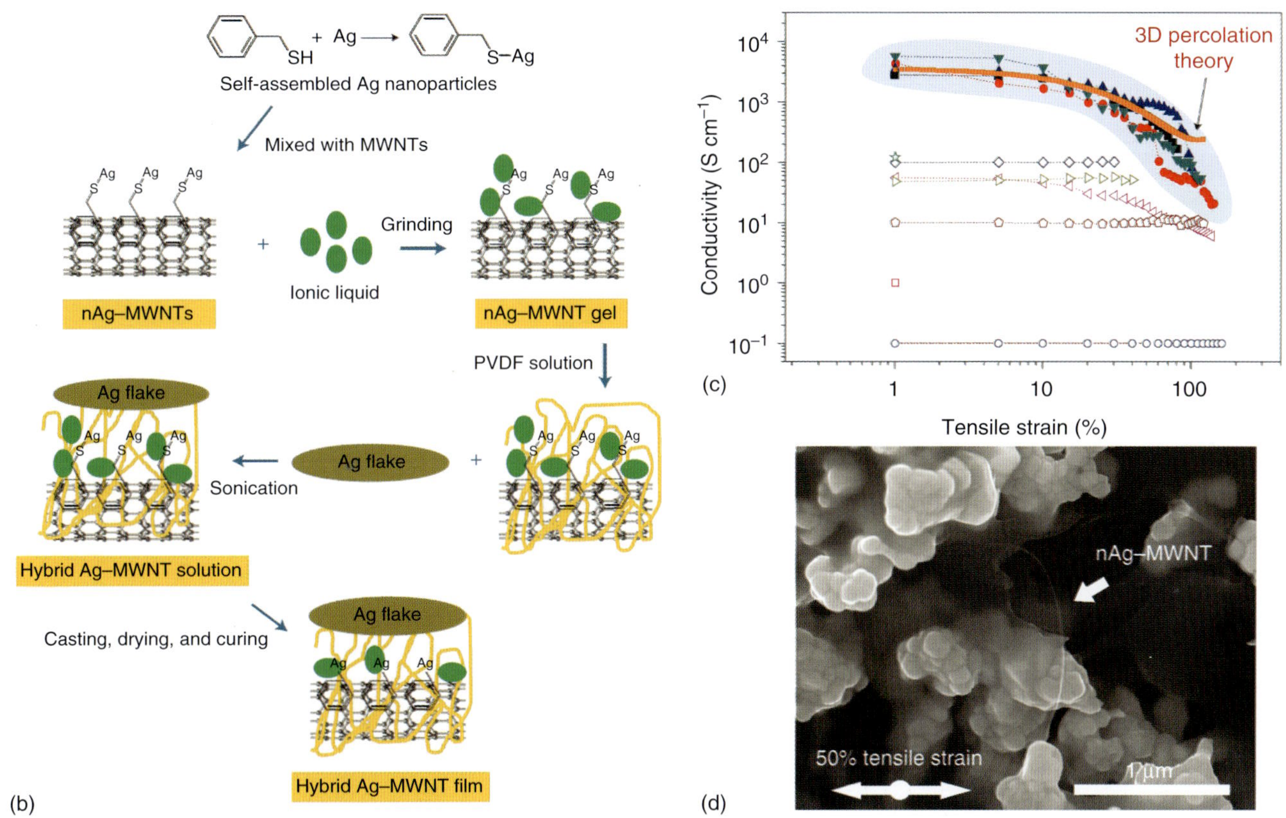

Figure 2.9 (*Continued*)

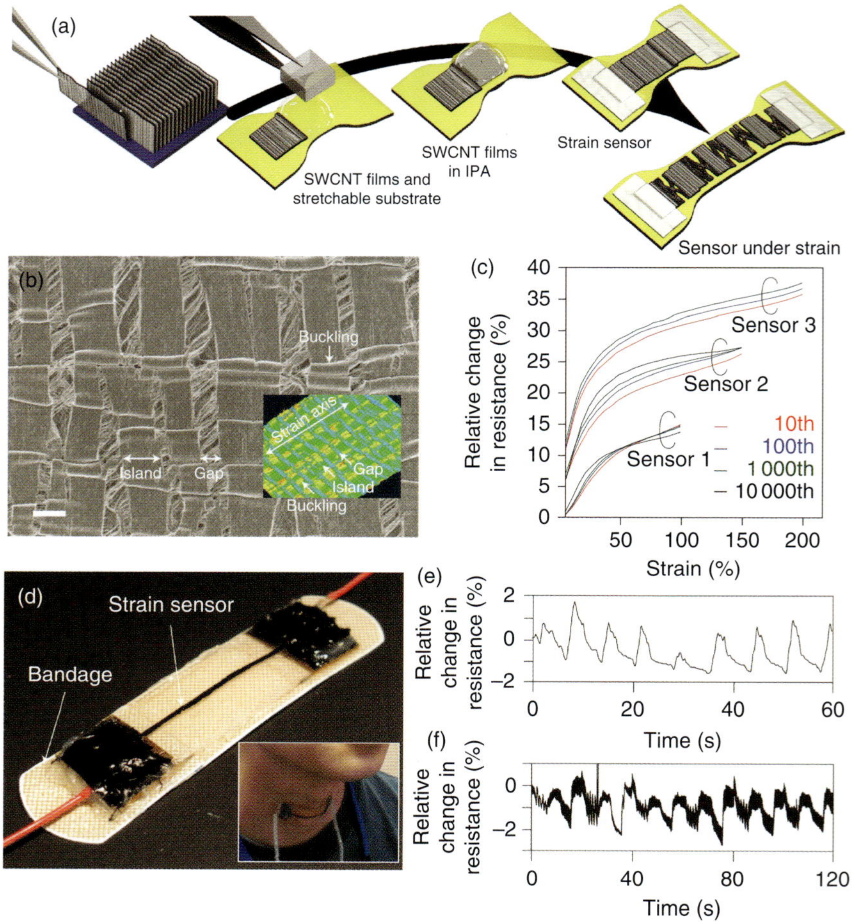

Figure 2.10 Stretchable resistive (a–f) and capacitive (g–k) strain gauges using CNT networks. (a) Schematics of the fabrication process and working mechanism of the resistive strain gauge. (b) *In situ* SEM image of the SWCNT array under a 100% strain, showing the transverse fracture of the film. (c) Relative change in resistance for up to 10 000 stretching cycles with strains of 100%, 150%, and 200%. (d–f) A strain gauge attached to a bandage and adhered to the throat (d) used to detect human breathing (e) and phonation (f). (Yamada *et al.* 2011 [15a]. Reproduced with permission of Nature Publishing Group.) (g) Operating mechanism of capacitive strain gauge using SWCNTs film as stretchable electrodes. (h) Relative changes in resistance of the SWCNT/PDMS composite electrodes under progressively increasing strains. (i) Relative changes in capacitance under stretch-release cycles with progressively increasing strains. (j) Relative changes in capacitance after repeated stretch-release cycles with maximum strain of 100%, 150%, and 200%. (k) Demonstration of using the capacitive strain gauge to monitor the motion of human fingers. Top panel: photographs of a strain gauge attached to the finger with different gestures. Bottom panel: The capacitive response at each corresponding stage. (Cai *et al.* 2012 [40f]. Reproduced with permission of John Wiley & Sons.)

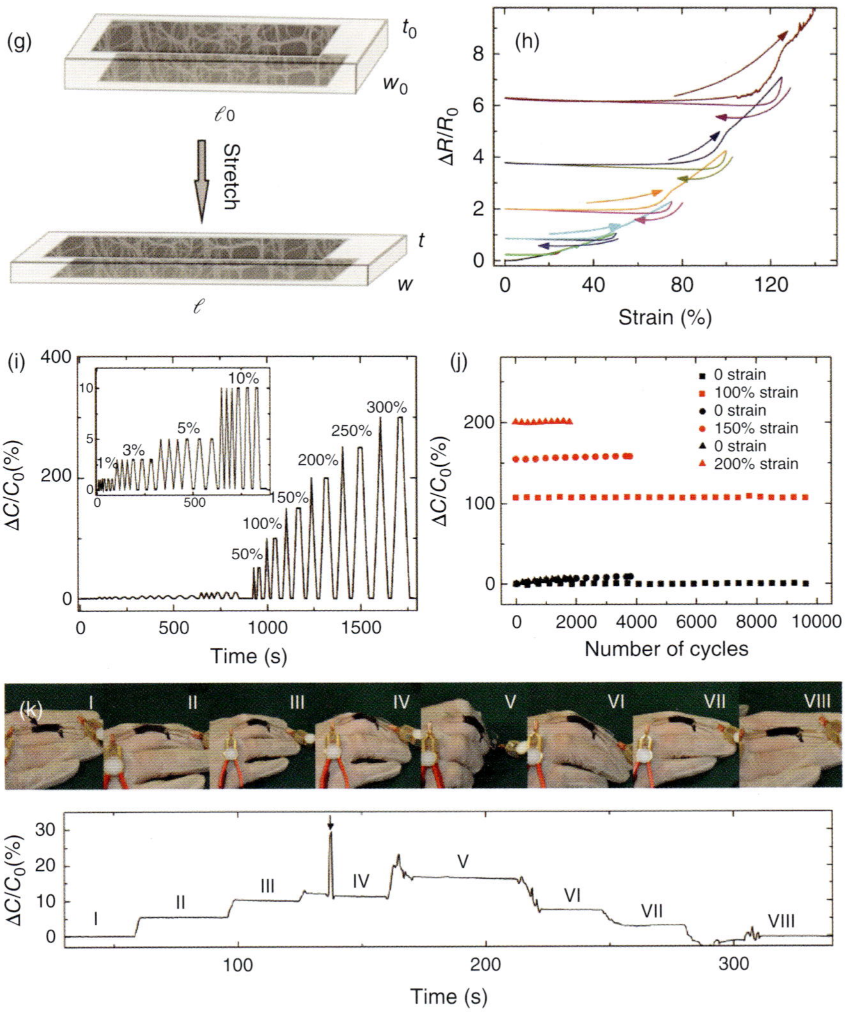

Figure 2.10 (*Continued*)

CNT thin films as stretchable electrodes and a piece of silicone elastomer as the dielectric layer [15c]. When stretched, the Poisson deformation of the elastomer in the device results in an increase of capacitance, which is found to be proportional to the applied strain. Due to the excellent stretchability of the CNT/silicone composite electrodes, the strain gauge exhibits stable and reliable capacitive response throughout the course of repetitive stretching with a maximum strain of up to 300%.

2.3.3 Stretchable Thin-Film Transistors

To date, most of the research effort has been focused on stretchable conductors whereas the potential of using semiconducting SWCNTs as channel materials for stretchable transistors is rarely explored. The hurdles of realizing stretchable

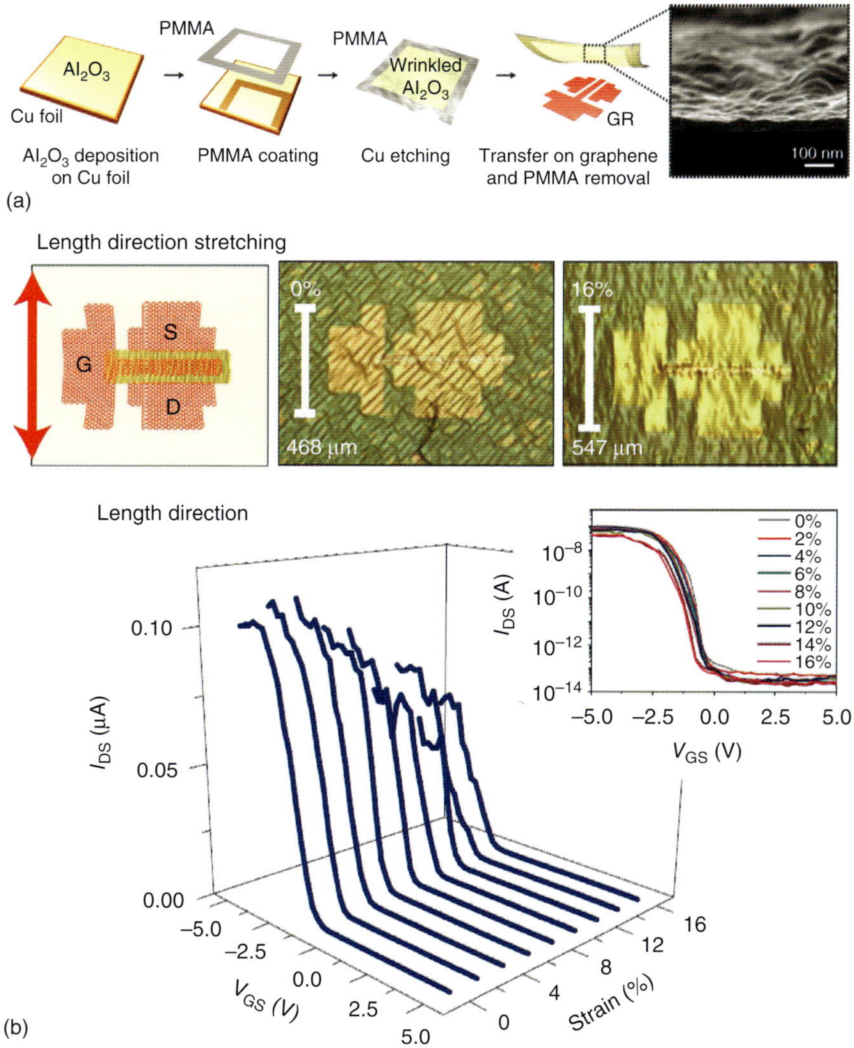

Figure 2.11 Stretchable CNT TFTs enabled by wrinkled Al_2O_3 gate dielectrics. (a) Deposition and transfer of Al_2O_3, which is randomly wrinkled during the transfer process. The SEM image shows the surface morphology of the wrinkled Al_2O_3. (b, c) Schematics, optical micrographs, and transfer characteristics of the fully-fabricated CNT TFTs when stretched along the channel length direction up to a strain of 16% (b) or along the channel width direction up to a strain of 20% (c). (Chae *et al.* 2013 [14e]. Reproduced with permission of Nature Publishing Group.)

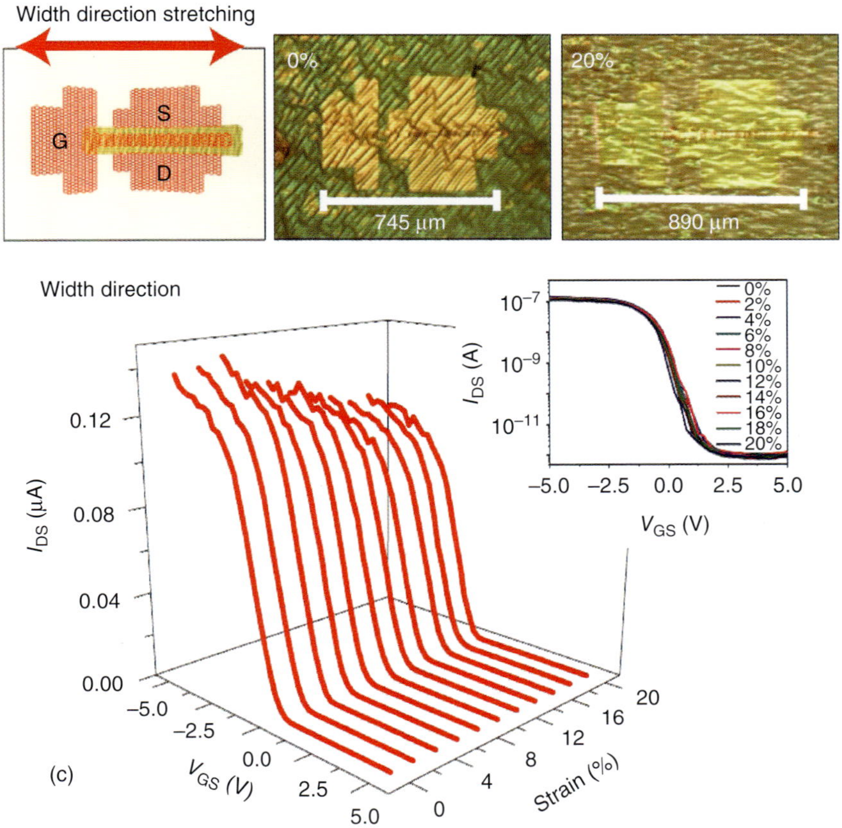

Figure 2.11 (*Continued*)

transistors are manifold. One bottleneck is the gate dielectric material, which is usually brittle. A well-known strategy to make conventional inorganic material stretchable is to induce buckles or wrinkles in the thin films [37a]. Chae *et al.* report that randomly distributed wrinkles can be formed in Al_2O_3 thin film during a transfer process, imparting the film a certain degree of stretchability (Figure 2.11) [14e]. The wrinkled Al_2O_3 is then used as the gate dielectric layer for sSWCNT transistors, which exhibit stable electrical characteristics under a tensile strain up to 20%.

Another approach is to exploit intrinsically stretchable dielectric materials such as polymer electrolyte, ionic liquid, or ion gel [42]. The working mechanism of such type of dielectric materials is that, upon a positive (negative) gate bias voltage, the cations (anions) in the dielectric migrate towards and accumulate at the dielectric/semiconductor interface, which electrostatically induce the accumulation of electrons (holes) in the semiconductor [42]. Xu *et al.* fabricated stretchable SWCNT transistors using ion gel as the dielectric material and achieved a stretchability of over 50% (Figure 2.12) [14f]. Such a high stretchability was achieved by a pre-strain strategy. sSWCNT channel semiconductors and gold electrodes are deposited on a pre-stretched PDMS substrate by transferring and

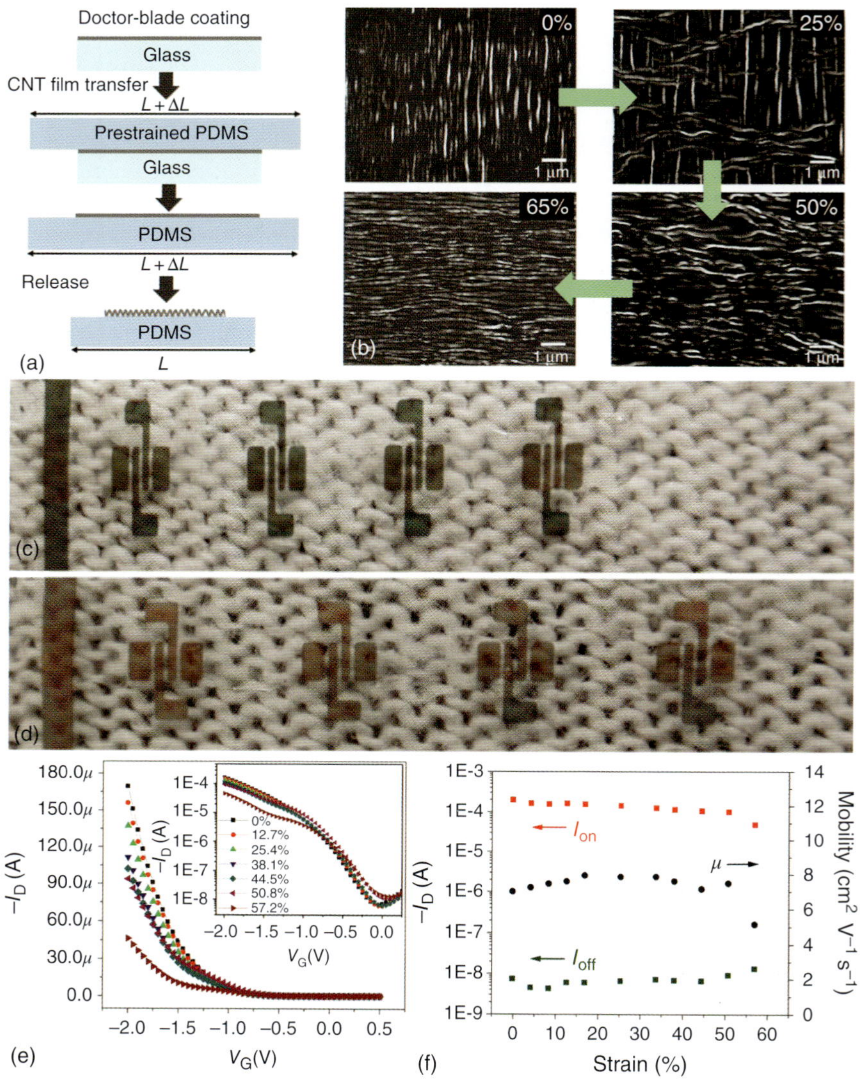

Figure 2.12 Intrinsically stretchable CNT-TFTs. (a) Schematics of the fabrication process where CNT film is transferred to prestrained (50%) PDMS substrate, forming buckled structure after the prestrain in PDMS is released. (b) *In situ* SEM images of the buckled CNT film obtained after prestretched to 25%, 50%, and 65%. (c, d) Photographs of the TFTs before (c) and after (d) stretched to 30%. (e, f) Stretching test showing the transfer characteristics (e), mobility, on-current, and off-current (f) of the CNT-TFTs at various tensile strains up to 57.2%. (Xu *et al.* 2014 [14f]. Reproduced with permission of American Chemical Society.)

thermal evaporation, respectively. Releasing the pre-strain induces wrinkles in both sSWCNT films and gold electrodes, thus enables a high stretchability.

The pre-strain process, however, makes the entire fabrication rather complicated and can be skipped if the evaporated gold is replaced by intrinsically stretchable conducting materials. A straightforward option is to use metallic or unsorted CNTs as the stretchable electrodes while the channel semiconductors are still semiconductor-enriched CNTs. Recently, such all-CNT stretchable TFTs have been fabricated by a process combining microfabrication and inkjet printing [43]. Super-growth CNTs are first dispersed with the assistance of an ionic liquid and then mixed with fluorinated rubber. The dispersion is subsequently spray coated on Si to form an elastomeric conductive film which is patterned by standard microfabrication process. The patterned elastomeric electrode is then embedded and transferred to a PDMS substrate. Next, semiconductor-enriched CNTs are ink-jet printed in the channel regions. To conclude the fabrication process, a piece of ionic gel is laminated over the channel region as gate dielectric. The fabricated TFTs can withstand tensile strains up to 100% while maintaining decent transistor behavior (Figure 2.13).

The use of microfabrication or vacuum facilities does not comply with the concept of green manufacturing. Instead, solution process or printing (discussed in the next section) is needed to realize low-cost and scalable fabrication. Very recently, silver nanowires (AgNWs) and unsorted CNTs, both being readily dispersed in liquid phase, have been used as electrodes to fabricate intrinsically stretchable sSWCNT TFTs exclusively by solution processes [44]. In the first study, AgNWs are spray coated and patterned on an elastomeric substrate, followed by drop casting semiconductor-enriched CNTs, then spin coating a polymeric gate dielectric and finally laminating another AgNWs/elastomer film as gate electrode (Figure 2.14) [44b]; in the second work, unsorted and semiconductor-enriched CNTs are first deposited on Si, and then transferred onto an elastomeric film with spray coated unsorted CNTs as gate electrode and spin coated polymeric gate dielectric (Figure 2.15) [44a]. In both cases, the fabricated devices can be stretched to >50% strains along the channel length or channel width direction. These results represent the state-of-the-art of CNT based intrinsically stretchable TFTs.

In addition to the selection of suitable materials for gate dielectric and electrodes, stable interface between different components also plays a critical role as minute interfacial sliding or delamination may lead to catastrophic failure of the entire device. However, the huge discrepancy in the mechanical and chemical properties of different components poses a great challenge in acquiring a stable interface that can survive long-term operations with large strains (>100%) [36]. For instance, the modulus of SWCNTs can reach 1 TPa [9], more than six orders of magnitude higher than that of common elastomer substrates like PDMS. As a result, the realization of highly stretchable and robust SWCNT transistors still needs extensive cooperation between researchers with expertise in material synthesis, structure design, solid mechanics and fabrication techniques.

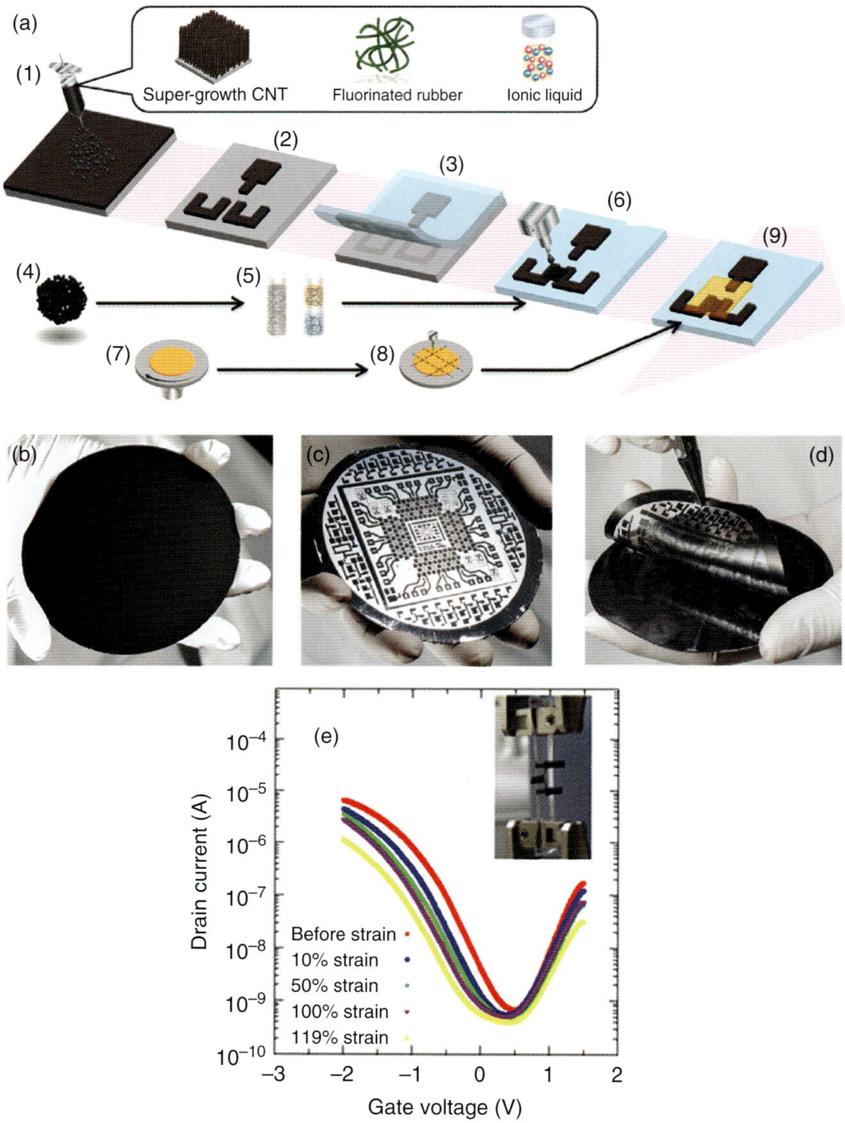

Figure 2.13 Intrinsically stretchable thin-film transistors based on super-growth carbon nanotube electrodes and sSWCNT channel. (a) Schematics of the fabrication process, involving dispersing the super-growth CNTs, spray coating the dispersion, patterning the conductive CNT film and ink-jet printing the semiconducting SWCNTs. (b–d) Photographs of the conductive CNT film just coated on Si (b), after patterning (c) and being peeled off from Si (d). (e) Transfer characteristics of a stretchable TFT while the device is stretched to >110% strain. (Sekiguchi *et al.* 2015 [43]. Reproduced with permission of American Chemical Society.)

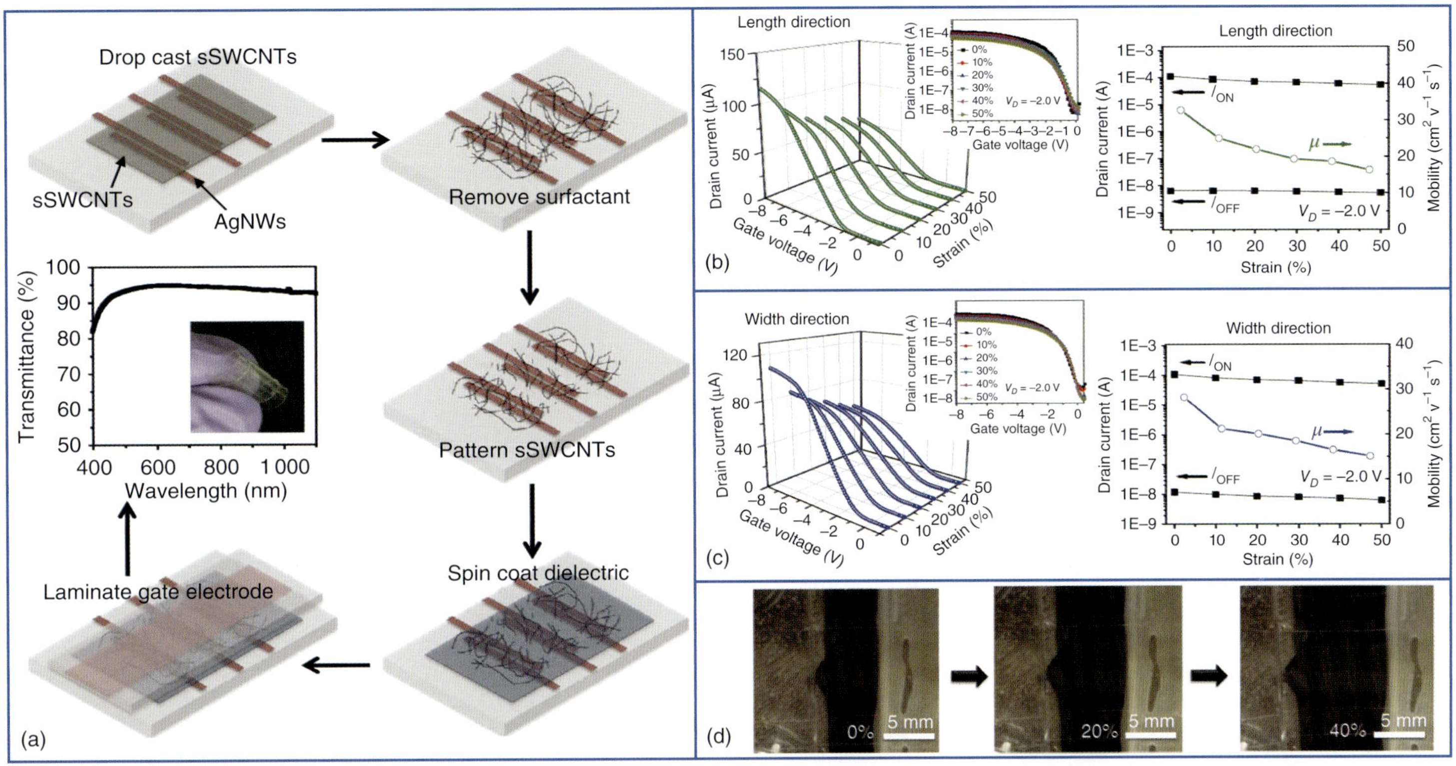

Figure 2.14 Intrinsically stretchable CNT TFTs fabricated by solution process with silver nanowires (AgNWs) as electrodes. (a) Schematics of the fabrication process involving spraying coating AgNWs, drop casting sSWCNTs, spin coating gate dielectric and lamination. (b, c) Electrical characteristics of a device being stretched to 50% strain along the channel length (b) and channel width (c) direction. (d) Optical micrograph of the devices while being stretched to 40% strain along the channel length direction. (Liang *et al*. 2015 [44b], https://www.nature.com/articles/ncomms8647. Used under CC BY 4.0 https://creativecommons.org/licenses/by/4.0/.)

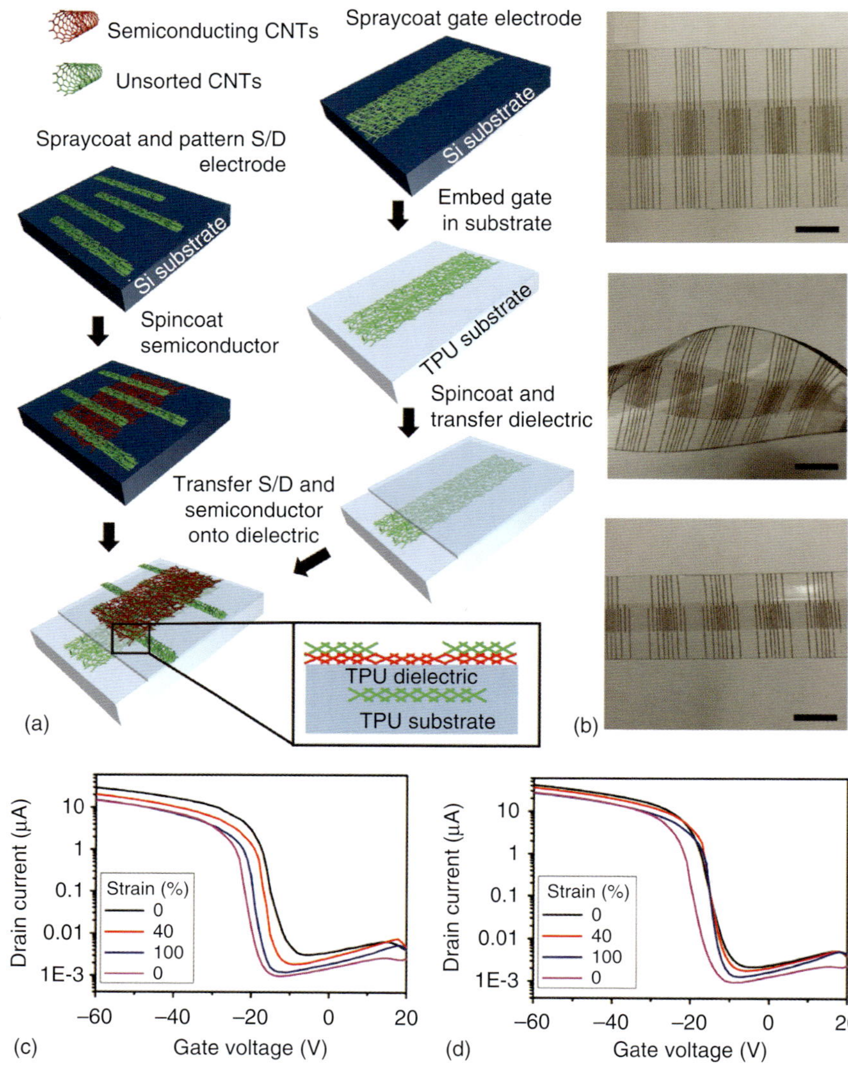

Figure 2.15 Solution processed intrinsically stretchable CNT TFTs with unsorted carbon nanotubes as electrodes. (a) Schematics of the fabrication process involving spray coating unsorted CNTs, spin coating semiconducting CNTs, spin coating gate dielectric and device assembling by transferring. (b) Optical images of the fully fabricated devices. Scale bar, 4 mm. (c, d) Transfer characteristics of a device being stretched to 100% strain along the channel length (c) and channel width (d) direction. (Chortos *et al*. 2015 [44a]. Reproduced with permission of John Wiley & Sons.)

2.4 Scalable Fabrication Process—Printing

Printing as a new manufacturing method for macroelectronics is attracting a great deal of research interests due to the promise of high speed, large scale and low cost production of electronic devices in novel forms [30]. Because no photolithographic patterning or vacuum-based deposition/etching equipment is needed, the cost of electronic devices can be substantially reduced. Additionally, printed electronics can be fabricated on many unconventional substrates, including plastics, papers, textiles, and even rubbers, thus enabling numerous beyond-silicon applications ranging from smart packaging to electronic paper, and from large area smart wallpaper to ubiquitous wearable electronics [2]. Organic semiconductors have been the mainstay in printed electronics for a long time [3c], whereas nanomaterials, among which are quantum dots [4], nanotubes [7], nanowires [45], and two dimensional (2D) nanomaterials [6], are new members of printable functional inks. In fact, many nanomaterials have already significantly outperformed organic semiconductors. For example, the field-effect mobility of printed TFTs using sSWCNTs is generally higher than 1 $cm^2\ V^{-1}\ s^{-1}$ which marks the upper limit for organic semiconductors. In addition to the superior electrical properties, CNTs exhibit excellent mechanical robustness and solution processibility, making them an outstanding material platform for printed flexible and stretchable electronics.

It should be pointed out that, among the three components of a TFT, gate dielectric layer poses a major challenge in printing top-gated TFTs on flexible and stretchable substrates. The widely adopted printable dielectrics are polymers which have rather low dielectric constant, resulting in a large operating voltage. In addition, it is very difficult to get an ultrathin dielectric film with good uniformity and clean interface through printing processes; any pinhole or interfacial trap would lead to poor device characteristics. Besides, the realization of flexibility and stretchability requires the dielectric material to be highly compliant, posing a greater challenge in selecting suitable materials. Two of the promising printable dielectric material platforms that have been studied extensively are ion gels [23b, 31c] and organic–inorganic hybrid dielectrics [31b, d, e, j]. Due to the formation of electrical double layers at the gate/dielectric and dielectric/semiconductor interfaces, ion gel offers very large gate capacitance which is, in principle, independent of the film thickness [42]. Hybrid dielectrics consisting of polymers and inorganic nanoparticles are also excellent platforms for printed and mechanically compliant TFTs because they not only possess high dielectric constant and mechanical flexibility/stretchability but also enable low-cost and scalable solution-based processing [46].

So far, several printing methods have been used to fabricate SWCNT-based devices, such as ink-jet printing [23, 31c, i], screen printing [31b], and gravure printing [31d–g, j]. In the following section, we summarize the state-of-the-art development of printed electronics using CNTs. Although there are several other studies of printed electrical interconnects based on CNTs [40b, c], we focus on the use of CNTs as channel semiconductors though.

2.4.1 Digital Printing—Inkjet and Aerosol Jet

Digital printing is characterized by its mask-free and drop-on-demand (DoD) features, thus provides better adaptability and less material waste. The most widely used digital printing methods are inkjet and aerosol jet printing [30b]. Okimoto *et al.* pioneered the area of inkjet printed SWCNT TFTs by using the same SWCNT material for both contact electrodes and channel semiconductors (Figure 2.16a–e) [23a]. SWCNT networks with low density are used as the channel of the TFT, while more printing runs lead to a higher nanotube density which can be used as the electrodes. They also proposed the utility of ionic liquid as gate dielectric layer to enable the top-gate operation. However, because the ink material is a mixture of metallic and semiconducting nanotubes, very sparse SWCNT network is required for achieving decent on/off current ratio, which unavoidably leads to rather low drive current. Using pre-sorted semiconductor-enriched SWCNTs can lead to devices with both high on/off ratio and large output current. Chen *et al.* demonstrated high-performance back-gated sSWCNT TFTs using an inkjet-like printing method (Figure 2.16f–h) [23c]. The on/off ratio, on-current and mobility reach 10^4, $18\,\mu A\,mm^{-1}$ ($V_{ds} = -0.8\,V$), and $23\,cm^2\,V^{-1}\,s^{-1}$, respectively. They further demonstrated the application of such fully-printed nanotube TFTs in driving a standalone single-pixel OLED (Figure 2.16i).

Ha *et al.* pioneered the field of ionic-gel-gated sSWCNT TFTs by using an aerosol jet printing process (Figure 2.17a,b) [23b]. Gold source/drain and gate electrode arrays are first patterned by conventional photolithography and lift-off processes. Next, semiconducting SWCNTs, ion gel dielectrics, and PEDOT:PSS gate electrodes are printed successively into the channel regions, resulting in flexible TFTs with high hole and electron mobility of 31 and $17\,cm^2\,V^{-1}\,s^{-1}$, respectively. With ion gel dielectrics, the gate operating voltage of the transistors can be very low (<3 V) because of the huge gate capacitance ($>1\,\mu F\,cm^{-2}$). However, due to the small drifting velocity of ions, the switching speed is much lower than conventional dielectrics, which needs further improvement in future. Nonetheless, recently, the same group demonstrated partially printed five-stage ring oscillators with stage delays lower than 5 μs at supply voltages below 3 V, representing an inspiring achievement towards high performance printed circuits using CNTs (Figure 2.17c–e) [31c].

Recently, Cai *et al.* reported highly flexible and foldable CNT TFTs and integrated logic gates fabricated by an all-printing process [47]. As shown in Figure 2.18a, the sSWCNTs, Ag S/D electrodes, PMMA/$BaTiO_3$ gate dielectric layer and Ag gate electrode is printed successively on an ultra-thin polyimide substrate spin-coated on a silicon handling wafer. After finishing printing all components, the substrate is delaminated from the Si wafer, resulting in the ultra-flexible freestanding TFTs and logic gates. The devices can withstand thousands of bending cycles with curvature radii down to 1 mm, as shown in Figure 2.18b,c. Furthermore, the TFTs can survive very aggressive folding tests like squeezing by a tweezer, indicating the excellent flexibility of the hybrid dielectric layer. The electrical performance under folding is actually constrained by the adhesion between Ag electrodes and polyimide substrate since the Ag electrodes

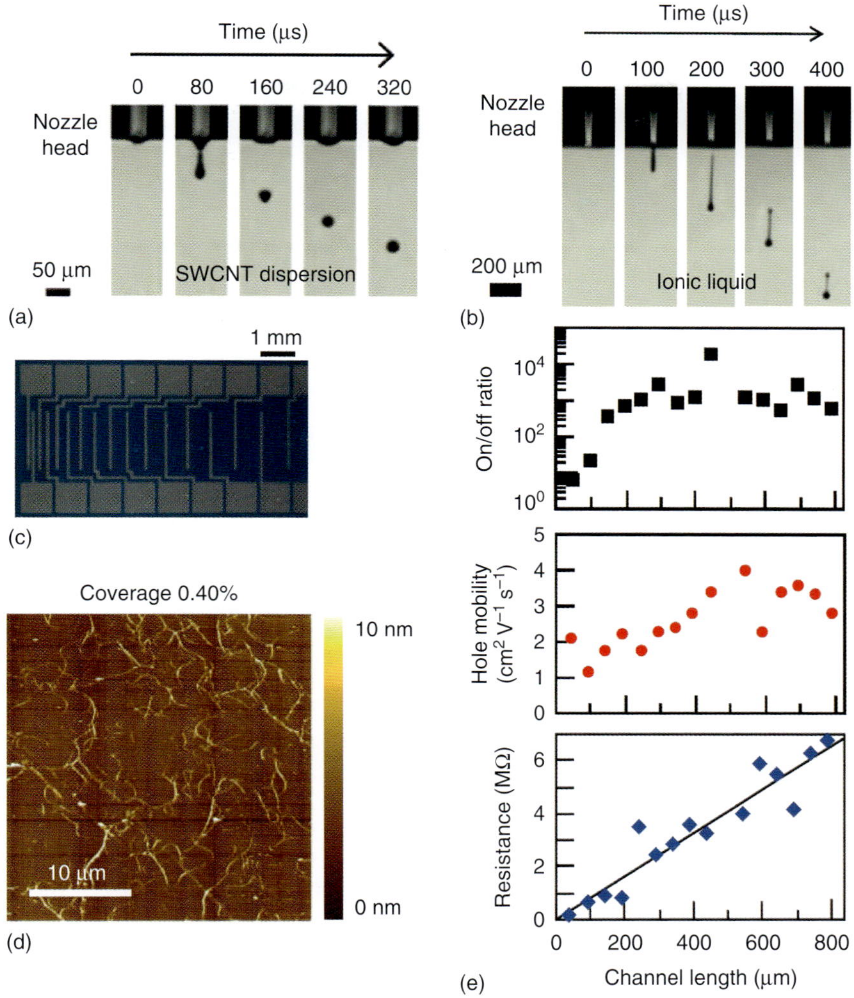

Figure 2.16 Ink-jet printed SWCNT TFTs. (a, b) Snapshots of DMF based SWCNT ink droplet for channel semiconductor (a) and ionic liquid droplet for gate dielectric (b) during the ink-jet printing process. (c) Optical micrograph of ink-jet printed TFT array with gold contact electrodes. (d) AFM image of the printed SWCNT network in the channel of the TFT. (e) Off/off ratio (top), hole mobility (middle), and channel resistance (bottom) as functions of channel length. (Okimoto *et al.* 2010 [23a]. Reproduced with permission of John Wiley & Sons.) (f) Schematics of fabricating polymer electrolyte gated SWCNT TFTs by an ink-jet-like process. (g) Photograph and optical micrograph of fully printed SWCNT TFTs. The SEM image on the right shows the SWCNT network with a high density. (h) Representative transfer (left) and output (right) characteristics of the fully printed SWCNT TFTs. (i) Application of printed CNT-TFT in an OLED control circuit. (Chen *et al.* 2011 [23c]. Reproduced with permission of American Chemical Society.)

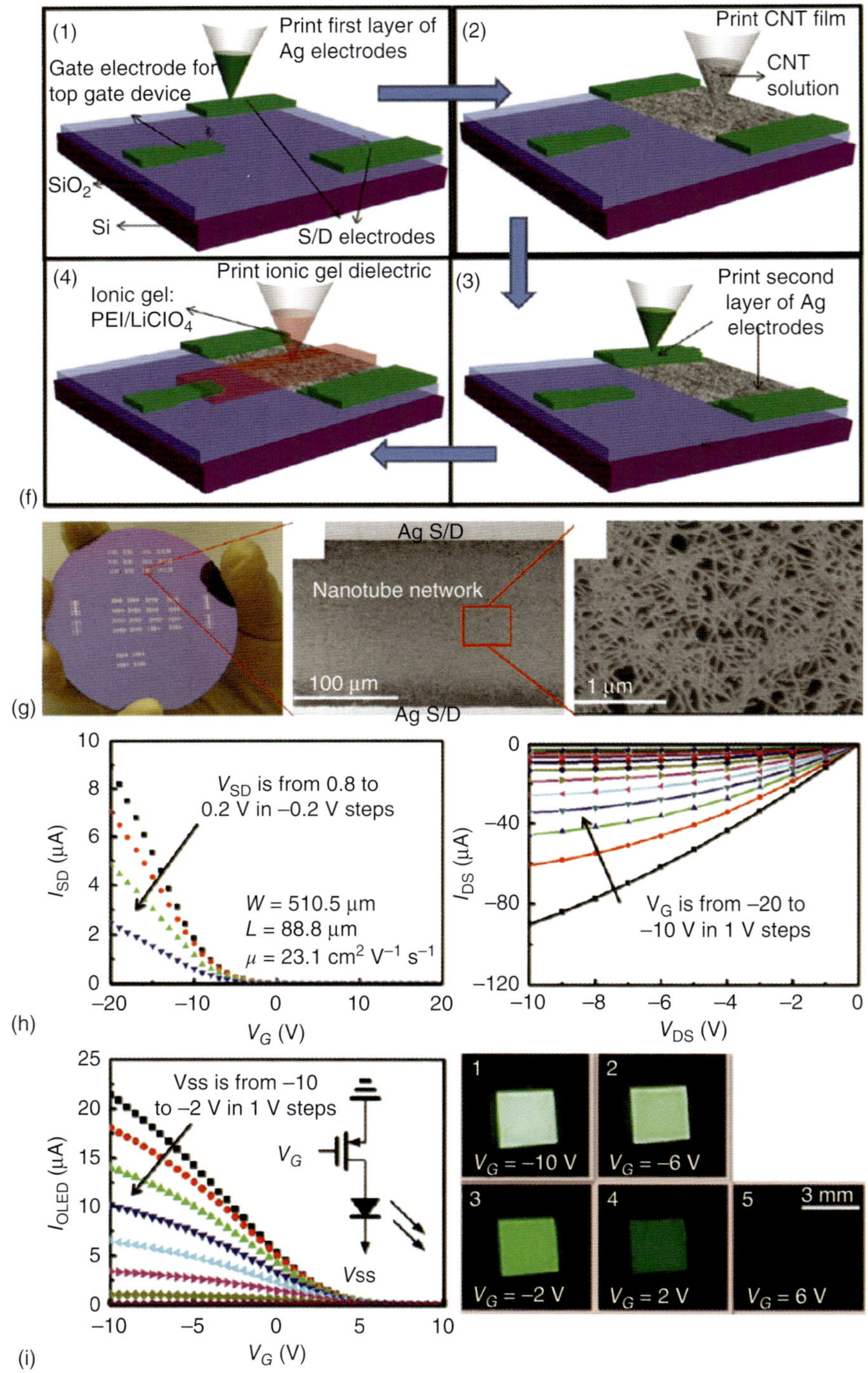

Figure 2.16 *(Continued)*

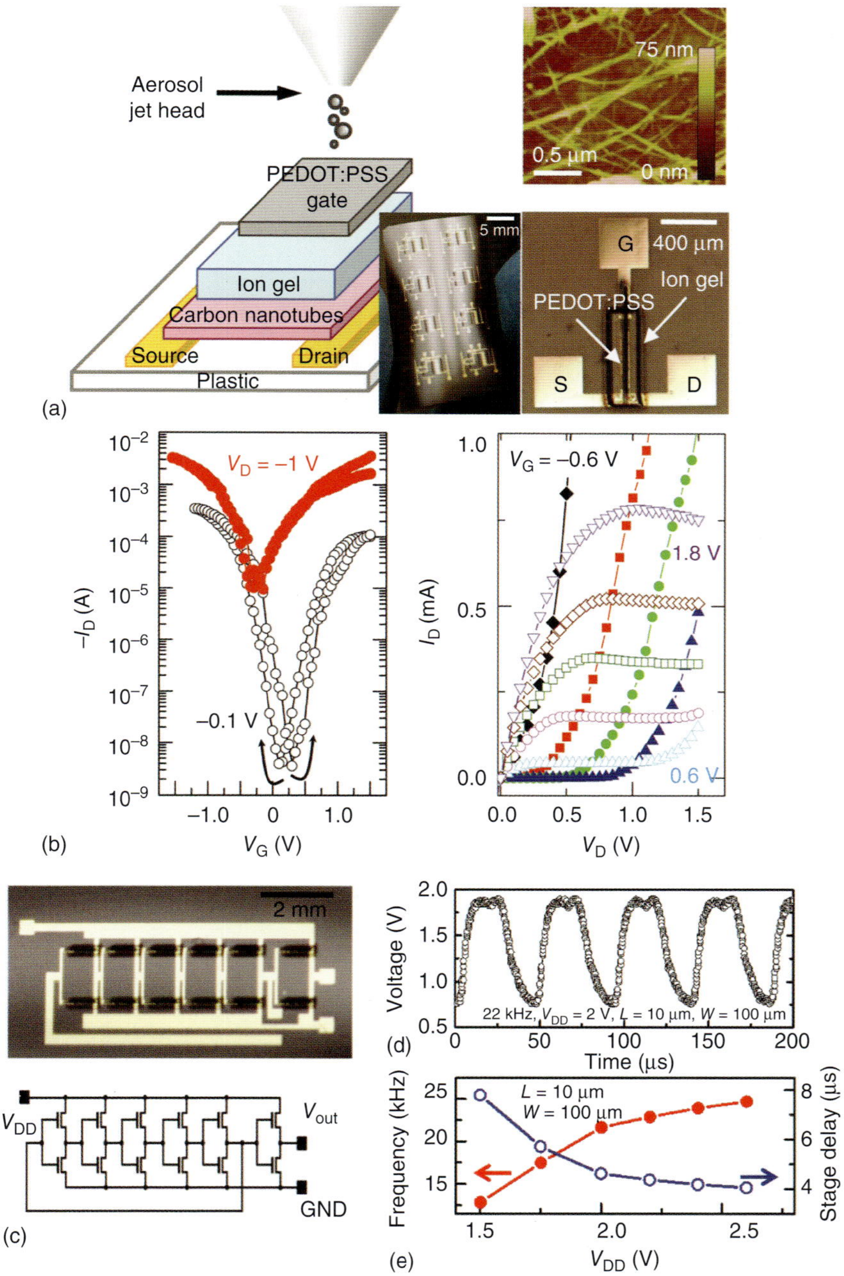

Figure 2.17 Printed CNT-TFT and integrated circuits using ion-gel dielectrics. (a) Schematic diagram and optical micrograph of the printed CNT TFT on flexible substrate with ion-gel dielectric and PEDOT:PSS gate electrode. The top right AFM image shows the printed CNT network. (b) Representative transfer (left) and output (right) characteristics of the printed TFT. (c) Photograph and circuit schematic of a ring oscillator with printed TFTs. (Ha *et al*. 2010 [23b]. Reproduced with permission of American Chemical Society.) (d) Output signal of a ring oscillator driven by a supply voltage of 2 V with a stage delay time of 4.5 μs. (e) Frequency and stage delay times as functions of supply voltage. (Ha *et al*. 2013 [31c]. Reproduced with permission of American Chemical Society.)

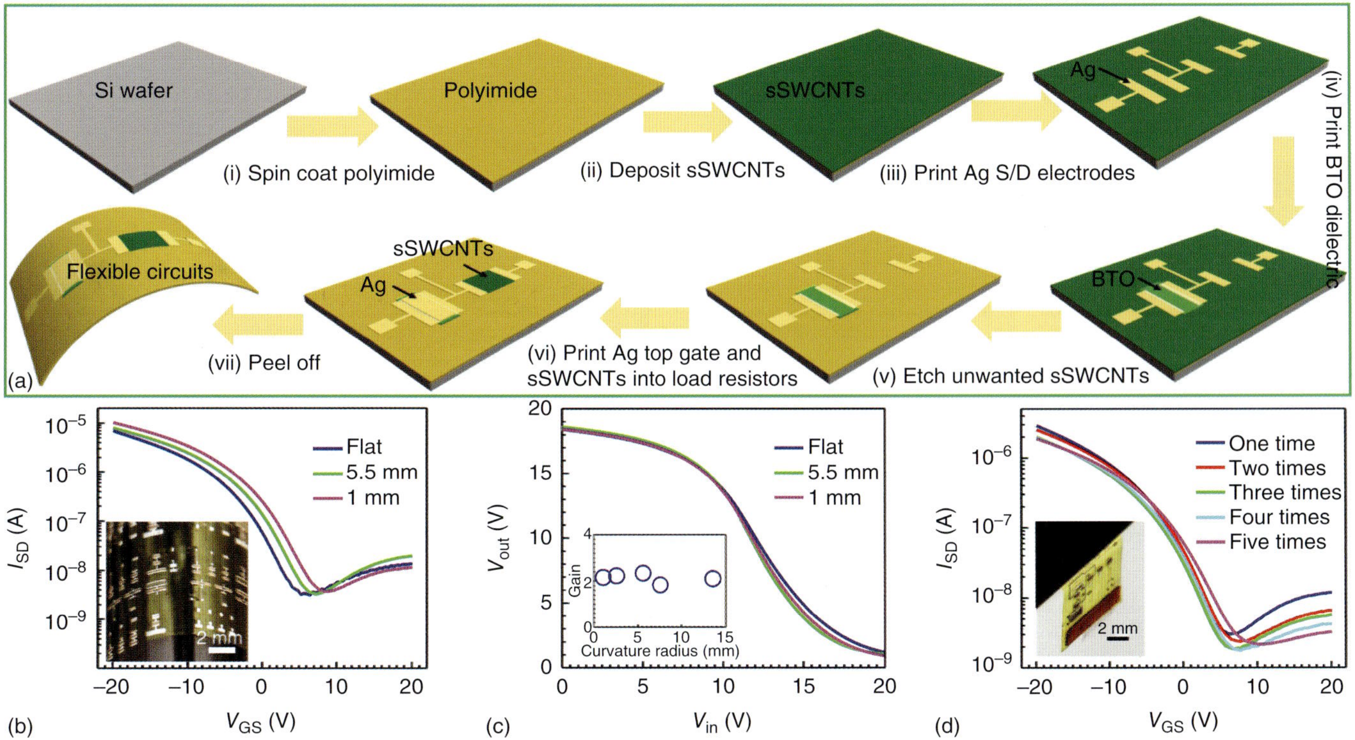

Figure 2.18 Fully-printed highly flexible and foldable CNT TFTs and integrated logic gates. (a) Schematics of the fabrication process. (b) Transfer characteristics of a TFT being bent to different curvature radii. Inset, photograph of the circuits being wrapped around a cylinder with a curvature radius of 13 mm. (c) Voltage transfer characteristics (VTCs) of a resistive loaded p-type only inverter measured at various curvature radii. Inset, inverter gain as a function of curvature radius. (d) Transfer characteristics of a TFT after being folded for multiple times. Inset, optical image of a circuit being folded over the edge of a piece of printing paper. (Cai *et al*. 2015 [47]. Reproduced with permission of John Wiley & Sons.)

delaminate after several folding cycles. Besides, the electrical performance of the logic gates can be fine tuned by printing CNTs in the loading resistor in a layer-by-layer manner, manifesting the unique adaptability of ink-jet printing.

2.4.2 Gravure Printing

Compared with ink-jet printing, gravure printing (roll-to-roll or roll-to-plate) is a more cost-effective way for mass production of electronic devices over large areas. In a series of work by Paru Inc. in South Korea, researchers have demonstrated fully-printed logic gates, half adder, D-flip-flop and one-bit radio-frequency identification (FRID) tags through a gravure printing process [31d, f, g]. In these studies, the silver gate electrodes, $BaTiO_3$/PMMA hybrid dielectrics, semiconducting SWCNTs, and silver source/drain electrodes are sequentially printed onto flexible PET substrates in a roll-to-roll or roll-to-plate manner. For such gravure printing processes, the viscosity and surface tension of the inks and surface chemistry of the substrates are critical and need to be optimized for uniform and reproducible device performance. Beside digital integrated circuit applications, gravure printed SWCNT TFTs have also been incorporated in functional electronic systems such as skin-like sensor arrays. Recently, Yeom *et al.* reported the utility of gravure printed nanotube TFT arrays as active-matrix backplanes for driving large-area compliant tactile sensor arrays (Figure 2.19) [31j]. The active-matrix backplane consists of up to 400 TFTs with high yield (97%) and excellent uniformity. Special attention should be paid to the overlap regions between the column and row selection lines to avoid leakage current between them. The system is capable of detecting pressures ranging from 1 to 20 kPa with a linear sensitivity of 800% kPa^{-1} and spatially mapping the pressure profile (Figure 2.19e). In addition, owing to the mechanical compliance of the hybrid dielectrics, the active-matrix backplane is highly flexible with invariant electrical characteristics when bent to a curvature radius of 1.85 cm.

2.4.3 Printed Complementary Metal–Oxide Semiconductor (CMOS) Devices

Complementary metal-oxide-semiconductor (CMOS) operation is desired for digital logic applications as it provides rail-to-rail swing, large noise margin, and small static power consumption [7]. However, as-grown CNTs typically exhibit p-type behavior in ambient air due to lower Schottky barriers for holes than electrons at the nanotube/metal interfaces for most air-stable metal contacts. Despite of the numerous efforts [48], acquiring air-stable and reproducible n-type CNT transistors in a facile way remains challenging. Alternatively, the heterogeneous integration of p-type CNT and n-type metal oxide transistors is a promising strategy to realize complementary macroelectronic circuits [49]. Many metal oxide semiconductors, including zinc tin oxide (ZTO) and indium zinc oxide (IZO), can be solution processed, thereby opening the possibility of fully-printed hybrid CMOS integrated circuits consisting of p-type SWCNTs and n-type metal oxides [50]. Recently, Kim *et al.* reported high speed, ink-jet printed SWCNT/ZTO hybrid complementary ring oscillators with stage delay of 140 ns, which represents the fastest ring oscillator with printed semiconductors

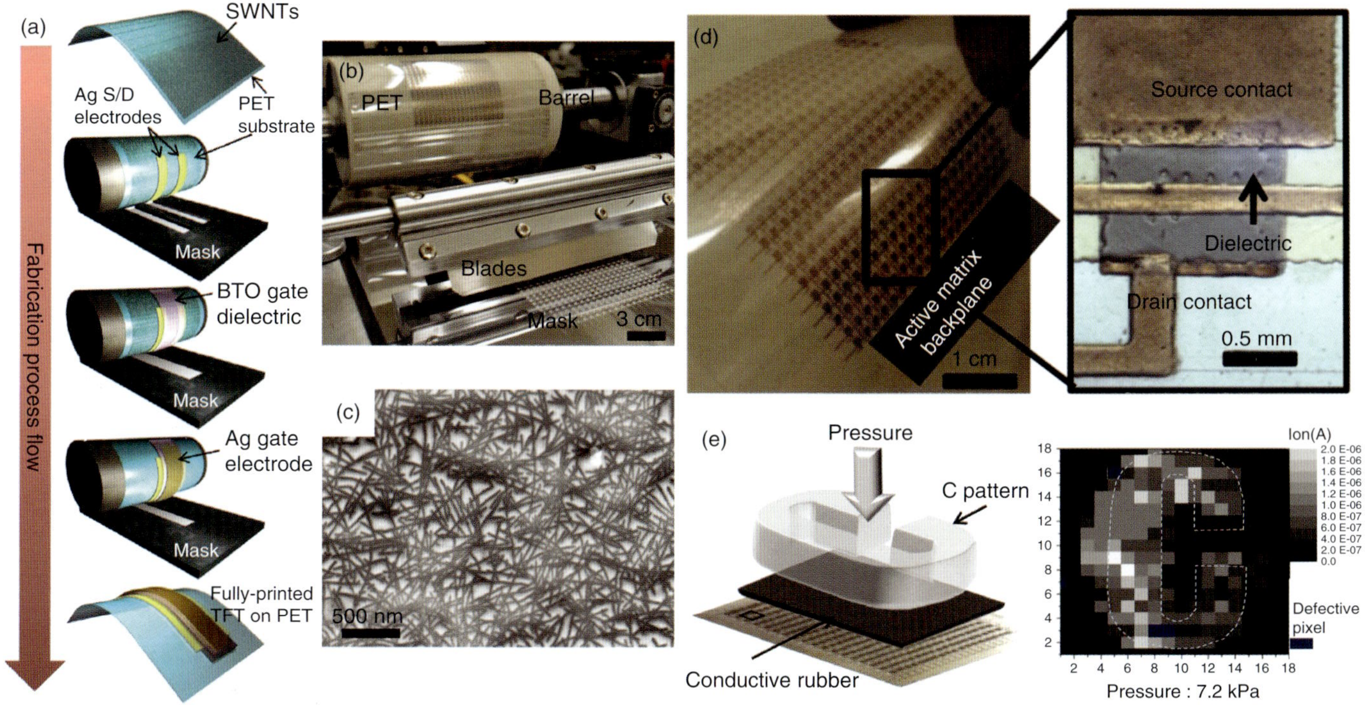

Figure 2.19 CNT-TFTs fabricated using a roll-to-plate printing process for applications in E-skin. (a) Schematics of the simplified gravure printing process (roll-to-plate). (b) Photograph of the roll-to-plate printer. (c) SEM image of the printed CNT network in the channel region of the TFT. (Lau *et al*. 2013 [31e]. Reproduced with permission of American Chemical Society.) (d) Printed flexible active-matrix backplane for E-skin application. Inset: Enlarged view showing a single printed CNT-TFT. (e) Application of the printed active-matrix backplane for E-skin to map the applied pressure profile. (Yeom *et al*. 2015 [31j]. Reproduced with permission of WILEY-VCH Verlag GmbH & Co. KGaA, Weinheim.)

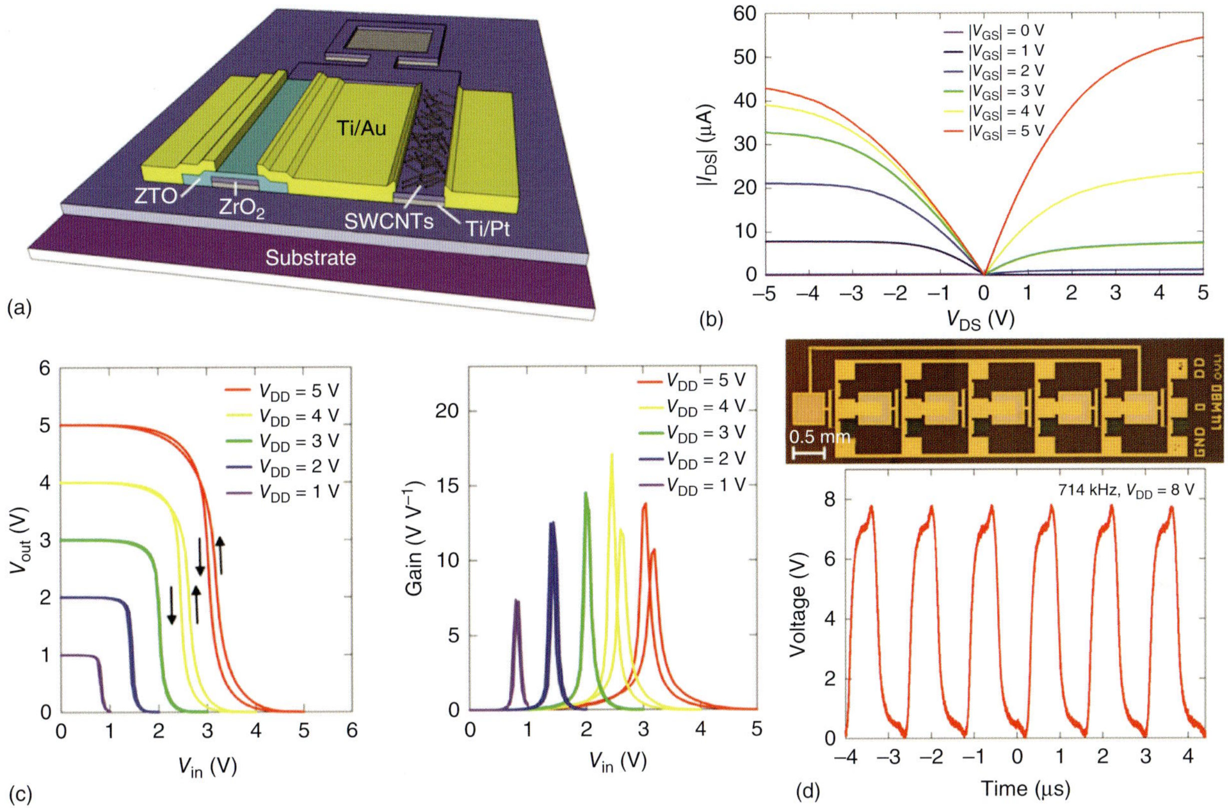

Figure 2.20 Heterogeneous integration of CNT (p-type) and ZTO (n-type) semiconductors for printed complementary integrated circuits. (a) Schematic diagram of the CMOS inverter. (b) Output characteristics of the printed n-type and p-type TFT. (c) VTC (left) and voltage gain (right) of the printed inverter under various supply voltages. (d) Printed 5-stage ring oscillator using the complementary inverters. Top: optical micrograph; bottom: output signal of the oscillator driven by a V_{DD} of 8 V. (Kim *et al*. 2014 [50a]. Reproduced with permission of American Chemical Society.)

to date (Figure 2.20) [50a]. In this study, gate and source/drain electrodes are defined by photolithography and lift-off processes and a double layer of ZrO_2 is deposited by a sol–gel route as the gate dielectric. SWCNTs and ZTO are deposited from solutions using an ink-jet printer. This work indicates that hybrid complementary configuration is a useful approach for achieving fully-printed and sophisticated macroelectronics by circumventing the difficulty in obtaining n-type SWCNT transistors.

2.5 Conclusions and Outlook

Tremendous progress has been made in SWCNT-based flexible and stretchable electronics. Nonetheless, almost no SWCNT-based flexible electronic product is commercially available at this moment [9]. Several challenges remain to be overcome before SWCNT-based electronic devices and systems can be made ready for the applications in consumer markets.

In the materials aspect, although semiconductor-enriched SWCNTs are already commercially available in large quantities, there is still large inhomogeneity in terms of chirality and nanotube length. It is expected that high purity and good homogeneity of the starting material is beneficial for uniform device performance. Additionally, longer nanotubes are desired to reduce the number of tube-to-tube junctions, which could lead to further improvement in device mobility. However, the dissolution and separation of long nanotubes (>10 μm) are not easy. Furthermore, the effects of surfactants on device electrical characteristics require more thorough investigation. The surfactants used to disperse SWCNTs are difficult to remove and can act as barriers for electronic conduction, thus increase the contact and channel resistance. In the future, new surfactant-free methods need to be explored to effectively dissolve SWCNTs without damaging or shortening them. Recent studies of dispersing SWCNTs using superacids or salt-ammonia solutions show promise in this direction [51]. Other problems confronting researchers include methods to obtain air-stable n-type conduction in SWCNTs and improve the uniformity, yield, and stability of SWCNT-based devices.

At the fabrication process end, although printing has been demonstrated to be a promising method for large scale and low cost manufacturing, the printed devices are still far inferior to their counterparts fabricated using conventional microfabrication processes in terms of electrical performance and uniformity. This is mainly caused by the low resolution (typically >50 μm) and poor reproducibility of current printing methods. Future work on printed SWCNT devices should also focus on improving the metal contacts and developing new dielectric materials. Stretchable electronics are relatively new and have attracted significant research interests. Despite the excellent stretchability of both sSWCNT networks and SWCNT thin-film electrodes, the realization of compliant dielectrics and robust interfaces appears to be the bottleneck in this field. Furthermore, fully-printed stretchable systems have yet to be realized. Finally, graphene and other 2D semiconducting materials are also showing increasing potential for flexible/

stretchable electronics [6, 52]. Incorporating SWCNTs with other forms of nanomaterials may lead to some exciting results [14e].

References

1 Reuss, R.H., Chalamala, B.R., Moussessian, A., Kane, M.G., Kumar, A., Zhang, D.C., Rogers, J.A., Hatalis, M., Temple, D., Moddel, G., Eliasson, B.J., Estes, M.J., Kunze, J., Handy, E.S., Harmon, E.S., Salzman, D.B., Woodall, J.M., Alam, M.A., Murthy, J.Y., Jacobsen, S.C., Olivier, M., Markus, D., Campbell, P.M., and Snow, E. (2005) Macroelectronics: perspectives on technology and applications. *Proc. IEEE*, **93** (7), 1239–1256.

2 Forrest, S.R. (2004) The path to ubiquitous and low-cost organic electronic appliances on plastic. *Nature*, **428** (6986), 911–918.

3 (a) Street, R.A. (ed.) (2000) *Technology and Applications of Amorphous Silicon*, Springer-Verlag; (b) Uchikoga, S. (2002) Low-temperature polycrystalline silicon thin-film transistor technologies for system-on-glass displays. *MRS Bull.*, **27** (11), 881–886; (c) Klauk, H. (2010) Organic thin-film transistors. *Chem. Soc. Rev.*, **39** (7), 2643–2666; (d) Street, R.A. (2009) Thin-film transistors. *Adv. Mater.*, **21** (20), 2007–2022.

4 Wang, C.L., Cheng, R., Liao, L., and Duan, X.F. (2013) High performance thin film electronics based on inorganic nanostructures and composites. *Nano Today*, **8** (5), 514–530.

5 (a) Park, S., Vosguerichian, M., and Bao, Z. (2013) A review of fabrication and applications of carbon nanotube film-based flexible electronics. *Nanoscale*, **5** (5), 1727–1752; (b) Liu, X., Long, Y.Z., Liao, L., Duan, X.F., and Fan, Z.Y. (2012) Large-scale integration of semiconductor nanowires for high-performance flexible electronics. *ACS Nano*, **6** (3), 1888–1900.

6 (a) Akinwande, D., Petrone, N., and Hone, J. (2014) Two-dimensional flexible nanoelectronics. *Nat. Commun.*, **5**, 5678; (b) Weiss, N.O., Zhou, H.L., Liao, L., Liu, Y., Jiang, S., Huang, Y., and Duan, X.F. (2012) Graphene: an emerging electronic material. *Adv. Mater.*, **24** (43), 5782–5825.

7 Wang, C., Takei, K., Takahashi, T., and Javey, A. (2013) Carbon nanotube electronics – moving forward. *Chem. Soc. Rev.*, **42** (7), 2592–2609.

8 Saito, R., Dresselhaus, G., and Dresselhaus, M.S. (1998) *Physical Properties of Carbon Nanotubes*, Imperial College Press.

9 De Volder, M.F.L., Tawfick, S.H., Baughman, R.H., and Hart, A.J. (2013) Carbon nanotubes: present and future commercial applications. *Science*, **339** (6119), 535–539.

10 (a) Wei, B.Q., Vajtai, R., and Ajayan, P.M. (2001) Reliability and current carrying capacity of carbon nanotubes. *Appl. Phys. Lett.*, **79** (8), 1172–1174; (b) Durkop, T., Getty, S.A., Cobas, E., and Fuhrer, M.S. (2004) Extraordinary mobility in semiconducting carbon nanotubes. *Nano Lett.*, **4** (1), 35–39; (c) Zhou, X.J., Park, J.Y., Huang, S.M., Liu, J., and McEuen, P.L. (2005) Band structure, phonon scattering, and the performance limit of single-walled carbon nanotube transistors. *Phys. Rev. Lett.*, **95** (14). doi: 10.1103/physrevlett.95.146805

11 Liu, B.L., Wang, C., Liu, J., Che, Y.C., and Zhou, C.W. (2013) Aligned carbon nanotubes: from controlled synthesis to electronic applications. *Nanoscale*, **5** (20), 9483–9502.

12 (a) Cao, Q. and Rogers, J.A. (2009) Ultrathin films of single-walled carbon nanotubes for electronics and sensors: a review of fundamental and applied aspects. *Adv. Mater.*, **21** (1), 29–53; (b) Hu, L.B., Hecht, D.S., and Gruner, G. (2010) Carbon nanotube thin films: fabrication, properties, and applications. *Chem. Rev.*, **110** (10), 5790–5844.

13 (a) Khang, D.Y., Xiao, J.L., Kocabas, C., MacLaren, S., Banks, T., Jiang, H.Q., Huang, Y.Y.G., and Rogers, J.A. (2008) Molecular scale buckling mechanics on individual aligned single-wall carbon nanotubes on elastomeric substrates. *Nano Lett.*, **8** (1), 124–130; (b) Lipomi, D.J., Vosgueritchian, M., Tee, B.C.-K., Hellstrom, S.L., Lee, J.A., Fox, C.H., and Bao, Z. (2011) Skin-like pressure and strain sensors based on transparent elastic films of carbon nanotubes. *Nat. Nanotechnol.*, **6** (12), 788–792.

14 (a) Snow, E., Campbell, P.M., Ancona, M.G., and Novak, J.P. (2005) High-mobility carbon-nanotube thin-film transistors on a polymeric substrate. *Appl. Phys. Lett.*, **86** (3), 033105; (b) Cao, Q., Kim, H.-S., Pimparkar, N., Kulkarni, J.P., Wang, C., Shim, M., Roy, K., Alam, M.A., and Rogers, J.A. (2008) Medium-scale carbon nanotube thin-film integrated circuits on flexible plastic substrates. *Nature*, **454** (7203), 495–500; (c) Sun, D.-M., Timmermans, M.Y., Tian, Y., Nasibulin, A.G., Kauppinen, E.I., Kishimoto, S., Mizutani, T., and Ohno, Y. (2011) Flexible high-performance carbon nanotube integrated circuits. *Nat. Nanotechnol.*, **6** (3), 156–161; (d) Wang, C., Chien, J.-C., Takei, K., Takahashi, T., Nah, J., Niknejad, A.M., and Javey, A. (2012) Extremely bendable, high-performance integrated circuits using semiconducting carbon nanotube networks for digital, analog, and radio-frequency applications. *Nano Lett.*, **12** (3), 1527–1533; (e) Chae, S.H., Yu, W.J., Bae, J.J., Duong, D.L., Perello, D., Jeong, H.Y., Ta, Q.H., Ly, T.H., Vu, Q.A., Yun, M., Duan, X., and Lee, Y.H. (2013) Transferred wrinkled Al_2O_3 for highly stretchable and transparent graphene-carbon nanotube transistors. *Nat. Mater.*, **12** (5), 403–409; (f) Xu, F., Wu, M.Y., Safron, N.S., Roy, S.S., Jacobberger, R.M., Bindl, D.J., Seo, J.H., Chang, T.H., Ma, Z.Q., and Arnold, M.S. (2014) Highly stretchable carbon nanotube transistors with ion gel gate dielectrics. *Nano Lett.*, **14** (2), 682–686.

15 (a) Yamada, T., Hayamizu, Y., Yamamoto, Y., Yomogida, Y., Izadi-Najafabadi, A., Futaba, D.N., and Hata, K. (2011) A stretchable carbon nanotube strain sensor for human-motion detection. *Nat. Nanotechnol.*, **6** (5), 296–301; (b) Cohen, D.J., Mitra, D., Peterson, K., and Maharbiz, M.M. (2012) A highly elastic, capacitive strain gauge based on percolating nanotube networks. *Nano Lett.*, **12** (4), 1821–1825; (c) Cai, L., Song, L., Luan, P., Zhang, Q., Zhang, N., Gao, Q., Zhao, D., Zhang, X., Tu, M., Yang, F., Zhou, W., Fan, Q., Luo, J., Zhou, W., Ajayan, P.M., and Xie, S. (2013) Super-stretchable, transparent carbon nanotube-based capacitive strain sensors for human motion detection. *Sci. Rep.*, **3**. doi: 10.1038/srep03048

16 (a) Liang, J.J., Li, L., Niu, X.F., Yu, Z.B., and Pei, Q.B. (2013) Elastomeric polymer light-emitting devices and displays. *Nat. Photonics*, **7** (10), 817–824;

(b) Yu, Z., Niu, X., Liu, Z., and Pei, Q. (2011) Intrinsically stretchable polymer light-emitting devices using carbon nanotube-polymer composite electrodes. *Adv. Mater.*, **23** (34), 3989–3994.

17 (a) Niu, Z., Dong, H., Zhu, B., Li, J., Hng, H.H., Zhou, W., Chen, X., and Xie, S. (2013) Highly stretchable, integrated supercapacitors based on single-walled carbon nanotube films with continuous reticulate architecture. *Adv. Mater.*, **25** (7), 1058–1064; (b) Yu, C., Masarapu, C., Rong, J., Wei, B., and Jiang, H. (2009) Stretchable supercapacitors based on buckled single-walled carbon nanotube macrofilms. *Adv. Mater.*, **21** (47), 4793–4797; (c) Zhang, N., Luan, P., Zhou, W., Zhang, Q., Cai, L., Zhang, X., Zhou, W., Fan, Q., Yang, F., Zhao, D., Wang, Y., and Xie, S. (2014) Highly stretchable pseudocapacitors based on buckled reticulate hybrid electrodes. *Nano Res.*, **7** (11), 1680–1690.

18 Feng, C., Liu, K., Wu, J.S., Liu, L., Cheng, J.S., Zhang, Y.Y., Sun, Y.H., Li, Q.Q., Fan, S.S., and Jiang, K.L. (2010) Flexible, stretchable, transparent conducting films made from superaligned carbon nanotubes. *Adv. Funct. Mater.*, **20** (6), 885–891.

19 Ma, W., Song, L., Yang, R., Zhang, T., Zhao, Y., Sun, L., Ren, Y., Liu, D., Liu, L., Shen, J., Zhang, Z., Xiang, Y., Zhou, W., and Xie, S. (2007) Directly synthesized strong, highly conducting, transparent single-walled carbon nanotube films. *Nano Lett.*, **7** (8), 2307–2311.

20 (a) Jiang, K.L., Wang, J.P., Li, Q.Q., Liu, L.A., Liu, C.H., and Fan, S.S. (2011) Superaligned carbon nanotube arrays, films, and yarns: a road to applications. *Adv. Mater.*, **23** (9), 1154–1161; (b) Zhang, M., Fang, S.L., Zakhidov, A.A., Lee, S.B., Aliev, A.E., Williams, C.D., Atkinson, K.R., and Baughman, R.H. (2005) Strong, transparent, multifunctional, carbon nanotube sheets. *Science*, **309** (5738), 1215–1219.

21 Wang, C., Zhang, J., Ryu, K., Badmaev, A., De Arco, L.G., and Zhou, C. (2009) Wafer-scale fabrication of separated carbon nanotube thin-film transistors for display applications. *Nano Lett.*, **9** (12), 4285–4291.

22 He, X., Gao, W., Xie, L., Li, B., Zhang, Q., Lei, S., Robinson, J.M., Hároz, E.H., Doorn, S.K., Wang, W., Vajtai, R., Ajayan, P.M., Adams, W.W., Hauge, R.H., and Kono, J. (2016) Wafer-scale monodomain films of spontaneously aligned single-walled carbon nanotubes. *Nat. Nanotechnol.*, **11** (7), 633–638.

23 (a) Okimoto, H., Takenobu, T., Yanagi, K., Miyata, Y., Shimotani, H., Kataura, H., and Iwasa, Y. (2010) Tunable carbon nanotube thin-film transistors produced exclusively via inkjet printing. *Adv. Mater.*, **22** (36), 3981–3986; (b) Ha, M., Xia, Y., Green, A.A., Zhang, W., Renn, M.J., Kim, C.H., Hersam, M.C., and Frisbie, C.D. (2010) Printed, sub-3V digital circuits on plastic from aqueous carbon nanotube inks. *ACS Nano*, **4** (8), 4388–4395; (c) Chen, P., Fu, Y., Aminirad, R., Wang, C., Zhang, J., Wang, K., Galatsis, K., and Zhou, C. (2011) Fully printed separated carbon nanotube thin film transistor circuits and its application in organic light emitting diode control. *Nano Lett.*, **11** (12), 5301–5308.

24 Li, J., Ma, W., Song, L., Niu, Z., Cai, L., Zeng, Q., Zhang, X., Dong, H., Zhao, D., Zhou, W., and Xie, S. (2011) Superfast-response and ultrahigh-power-density electromechanical actuators based on hierarchal carbon nanotube electrodes and chitosan. *Nano Lett.*, **11** (11), 4636–4641.

25 Dan, B., Irvin, G.C., and Pasquali, M. (2009) Continuous and scalable fabrication of transparent conducting carbon nanotube films. *ACS Nano*, **3** (4), 835–843.

26 (a) Bergin, S.D., Nicolosi, V., Streich, P.V., Giordani, S., Sun, Z.Y., Windle, A.H., Ryan, P., Niraj, N.P.P., Wang, Z.T.T., Carpenter, L., Blau, W.J., Boland, J.J., Hamilton, J.P., and Coleman, J.N. (2008) Towards solutions of single-walled carbon nanotubes in common solvents. *Adv. Mater.*, **20** (10), 1876–1881; (b) Islam, M.F., Rojas, E., Bergey, D.M., Johnson, A.T., and Yodh, A.G. (2003) High weight fraction surfactant solubilization of single-wall carbon nanotubes in water. *Nano Lett.*, **3** (2), 269–273.

27 McCarthy, M.A., Liu, B., Donoghue, E.P., Kravchenko, I., Kim, D.Y., So, F., and Rinzler, A.G. (2011) Low-voltage, low-power, organic light-emitting transistors for active matrix displays. *Science*, **332** (6029), 570–573.

28 (a) Hersam, M.C. (2008) Progress towards monodisperse single-walled carbon nanotubes. *Nat. Nanotechnol.*, **3** (7), 387–394; (b) Liu, H.P., Nishide, D., Tanaka, T., and Kataura, H. (2011) Large-scale single-chirality separation of single-wall carbon nanotubes by simple gel chromatography. *Nat. Commun.*, **2**, 309; (c) Tu, X.M., Manohar, S., Jagota, A., and Zheng, M. (2009) DNA sequence motifs for structure-specific recognition and separation of carbon nanotubes. *Nature*, **460** (7252), 250–253.

29 Arnold, M.S., Green, A.A., Hulvat, J.F., Stupp, S.I., and Hersam, M.C. (2006) Sorting carbon nanotubes by electronic structure using density differentiation. *Nat. Nanotechnol.*, **1** (1), 60–65.

30 (a) Arias, A.C., MacKenzie, J.D., McCulloch, I., Rivnay, J., and Salleo, A. (2010) Materials and applications for large area electronics: solution-based approaches. *Chem. Rev.*, **110** (1), 3–24; (b) Singh, M., Haverinen, H.M., Dhagat, P., and Jabbour, G.E. (2010) Inkjet printing-process and its applications. *Adv. Mater.*, **22** (6), 673–685.

31 (a) Beecher, P., Servati, P., Rozhin, A., Colli, A., Scardaci, V., Pisana, S., Hasan, T., Flewitt, A.J., Robertson, J., Hsieh, G.W., Li, F.M., Nathan, A., Ferrari, A.C., and Milne, W.I. (2007) Ink-jet printing of carbon nanotube thin film transistors. *J. Appl. Phys.*, **102** (4), 043710; (b) Cao, X., Chen, H.T., Gu, X.F., Liu, B.L., Wang, W.L., Cao, Y., Wu, F.Q., and Zhu, C.W. (2014) Screen printing as a scalable and low-cost approach for rigid and flexible thin-film transistors using separated carbon nanotubes. *ACS Nano*, **8** (12), 12769–12776; (c) Ha, M., Seo, J.-W.T., Prabhumirashi, P.L., Zhang, W., Geier, M.L., Renn, M.J., Kim, C.H., Hersam, M.C., and Frisbie, C.D. (2013) Aerosol jet printed, low voltage, electrolyte gated carbon nanotube ring oscillators with sub-5 μs stage delays. *Nano Lett.*, **13** (3), 954–960; (d) Jung, M., Kim, J., Noh, J., Lim, N., Lim, C., Lee, G., Kim, J., Kang, H., Jung, K., Leonard, A.D., Tour, J.M., and Cho, G. (2010) All-printed and roll-to-roll-printable 13.56-MHz-operated 1-bit RF tag on plastic foils. *IEEE Trans. Electron Devices*, **57** (3), 571–580; (e) Lau, P.H., Takei, K., Wang, C., Ju, Y., Kim, J., Yu, Z., Takahashi, T., Cho, G., and Javey, A. (2013) Fully printed, high performance carbon nanotube thin-film transistors on flexible substrates. *Nano Lett.*, **13** (8), 3864–3869; (f) Noh, J., Jung, M., Jung, K., Lee, G., Kim, J., Lim, S., Kim, D., Choi, Y., Kim, Y., Subramanian, V., and Cho, G. (2011) Fully gravure-printed D flip-flop on

plastic foils using single-walled carbon-nanotube-based TFTs. *IEEE Electron Device Lett.*, **32** (5), 638–640; (g) Noh, J., Kim, S., Jung, K., Kim, J., Cho, S., and Cho, G. (2011) Fully gravure printed half adder on plastic foils. *IEEE Electron Device Lett.*, **32** (11), 1555–1557; (h) Vaillancourt, J., Zhang, H., Vasinajindakaw, P., Xia, H., Lu, X., Han, X., Janzen, D.C., Shih, W.-S., Jones, C.S., Stroder, M., Chen, M.Y., Subbaraman, H., Chen, R.T., Berger, U., and Renn, M. (2008) All ink-jet-printed carbon nanotube thin-film transistor on a polyimide substrate with an ultrahigh operating frequency of over 5 GHz. *Appl. Phys. Lett.*, **93** (24), 243301; (i) Xu, W., Liu, Z., Zhao, J., Xu, W., Gu, W., Zhang, X., Qian, L., and Cui, Z. (2014) Flexible logic circuits based on top-gate thin film transistors with printed semiconductor carbon nanotubes and top electrodes. *Nanoscale*, **6** (24), 14891–14897; (j) Yeom, C., Chen, K., Kiriya, D., Yu, Z.B., Cho, G., and Javey, A. (2015) Large-area compliant tactile sensors using printed carbon nanotube active-matrix backplanes. *Adv. Mater.*, **27** (9), 1561–1566.

32 Sun, D.M., Liu, C., Ren, W.C., and Cheng, H.M. (2013) A review of carbon nanotube- and graphene-based flexible thin-film transistors. *Small*, **9** (8), 1188–1205.

33 (a) Zhang, J., Fu, Y., Wang, C., Chen, P.-C., Liu, Z., Wei, W., Wu, C., Thompson, M.E., and Zhou, C. (2011) Separated carbon nanotube macro-electronics for active matrix organic light-emitting diode displays. *Nano Lett.*, **11** (11), 4852–4858; (b) Zhang, J., Wang, C., and Zhou, C. (2012) Rigid/flexible transparent electronics based on separated carbon nanotube thin-film transistors and their application in display electronics. *ACS Nano*, **6** (8), 7412–7419.

34 (a) Takahashi, T., Takei, K., Gillies, A.G., Fearing, R.S., and Javey, A. (2011) Carbon nanotube active-matrix backplanes for conformal electronics and sensors. *Nano Lett.*, **11** (12), 5408–5413; (b) Takahashi, T., Yu, Z., Chen, K., Kiriya, D., Wang, C., Takei, K., Shiraki, H., Chen, T., Ma, B., and Javey, A. (2013) Carbon nanotube active-matrix backplanes for mechanically flexible visible light and X-ray imagers. *Nano Lett.*, **13** (11), 5425–5430.

35 Wang, C., Hwang, D., Yu, Z., Takei, K., Park, J., Chen, T., Ma, B., and Javey, A. (2013) User-interactive electronic skin for instantaneous pressure visualization. *Nat. Mater.*, **12** (10), 899–904.

36 Rogers, J.A., Someya, T., and Huang, Y. (2010) Materials and mechanics for stretchable electronics. *Science*, **327** (5973), 1603–1607.

37 (a) Kim, D.-H., Ahn, J.-H., Choi, W.M., Kim, H.-S., Kim, T.-H., Song, J., Huang, Y.Y., Liu, Z., Lu, C., and Rogers, J.A. (2008) Stretchable and foldable silicon integrated circuits. *Science*, **320** (5875), 507–511; (b) Park, S.-I., Xiong, Y., Kim, R.-H., Elvikis, P., Meitl, M., Kim, D.-H., Wu, J., Yoon, J., Yu, C.-J., Liu, Z., Huang, Y., Hwang, K.-C., Ferreira, P., Li, X., Choquette, K., and Rogers, J.A. (2009) Printed assemblies of inorganic light-emitting diodes for deformable and semitransparent displays. *Science*, **325** (5943), 977–981; (c) Kim, D.-H., Xiao, J., Song, J., Huang, Y., and Rogers, J.A. (2010) Stretchable, curvilinear electronics based on inorganic materials. *Adv. Mater.*, **22** (19), 2108–2124.

38 Sekitani, T. and Someya, T. (2010) Stretchable, large-area organic electronics. *Adv. Mater.*, **22** (20), 2228–2246.

39 Yao, S.S. and Zhu, Y. (2015) Nanomaterial-enabled stretchable conductors: strategies, materials and devices. *Adv. Mater.*, **27** (9), 1480–1511.

40 (a) Sekitani, T., Noguchi, Y., Hata, K., Fukushima, T., Aida, T., and Someya, T. (2008) A rubberlike stretchable active matrix using elastic conductors. *Science*, **321** (5895), 1468–1472; (b) Sekitani, T., Nakajima, H., Maeda, H., Fukushima, T., Aida, T., Hata, K., and Someya, T. (2009) Stretchable active-matrix organic light-emitting diode display using printable elastic conductors. *Nat. Mater.*, **8** (6), 494–499; (c) Chun, K.-Y., Oh, Y., Rho, J., Ahn, J.-H., Kim, Y.-J., Choi, H.R., and Baik, S. (2010) Highly conductive, printable and stretchable composite films of carbon nanotubes and silver. *Nat. Nanotechnol.*, **5** (12), 853–857; (d) Shin, M.K., Oh, J., Lima, M., Kozlov, M.E., Kim, S.J., and Baughman, R.H. (2010) Elastomeric conductive composites based on carbon nanotube forests. *Adv. Mater.*, **22** (24), 2663–2667; (e) Zhang, Y., Sheehan, C.J., Zhai, J., Zou, G., Luo, H., Xiong, J., Zhu, Y.T., and Jia, Q.X. (2010) Polymer-embedded carbon nanotube ribbons for stretchable conductors. *Adv. Mater.*, **22** (28), 3027–3031; (f) Cai, L., Li, J., Luan, P., Dong, H., Zhao, D., Zhang, Q., Zhang, X., Tu, M., Zeng, Q., Zhou, W., and Xie, S. (2012) Highly transparent and conductive stretchable conductors based on hierarchical reticulate single-walled carbon nanotube architecture. *Adv. Funct. Mater.*, **22** (24), 5238–5244; (g) Xu, F., Wang, X., Zhu, Y.T., and Zhu, Y. (2012) Wavy ribbons of carbon nanotubes for stretchable conductors. *Adv. Funct. Mater.*, **22**, 1279–1283.

41 Liang, J.J., Li, L., Niu, X.F., Yu, Z.B., and Pei, Q.B. (2013) Fully solution-based fabrication of flexible light-emitting device at ambient conditions. *J. Phys. Chem. C*, **117** (32), 16632–16639.

42 Kim, S.H., Hong, K., Xie, W., Lee, K.H., Zhang, S.P., Lodge, T.P., and Frisbie, C.D. (2013) Electrolyte-gated transistors for organic and printed electronics. *Adv. Mater.*, **25** (13), 1822–1846.

43 Sekiguchi, A., Tanaka, F., Saito, T., Kuwahara, Y., Sakurai, S., Futaba, D.N., Yamada, T., and Hata, K. (2015) Robust and soft elastomeric electronics tolerant to our daily lives. *Nano Lett.*, **15** (9), 5716–5723.

44 (a) Chortos, A., Koleilat, G.I., Pfattner, R., Kong, D., Lin, P., Nur, R., Lei, T., Wang, H., Liu, N., Lai, Y.-C., Kim, M.-G., Chung, J.W., Lee, S., and Bao, Z. (2015) Mechanically durable and highly stretchable transistors employing carbon nanotube semiconductor and electrodes. *Adv. Mater.*, **28** (22), 4441–4448; (b) Liang, J., Li, L., Chen, D., Hajagos, T., Ren, Z., Chou, S.-Y., Hu, W., and Pei, Q. (2015) Intrinsically stretchable and transparent thin-film transistors based on printable silver nanowires, carbon nanotubes and an elastomeric dielectric. *Nat. Commun.*, **6**, 7647.

45 Fan, Z.Y., Ho, J.C., Takahashi, T., Yerushalmi, R., Takei, K., Ford, A.C., Chueh, Y.L., and Javey, A. (2009) Toward the development of printable nanowire electronics and sensors. *Adv. Mater.*, **21** (37), 3730–3743.

46 Ortiz, R.P., Facchetti, A., and Marks, T.J. (2010) High-k organic, inorganic, and hybrid dielectrics for low-voltage organic field-effect transistors. *Chem. Rev.*, **110** (1), 205–239.

47 Cai, L., Zhang, S., Miao, J., Yu, Z., and Wang, C. (2015) Fully printed foldable integrated logic gates with tunable performance using semiconducting carbon nanotubes. *Adv. Funct. Mater.*, **25** (35), 5698–5705.
48 (a) Ha, T.J., Chen, K., Chuang, S., Yu, K.M., Kiriya, D., and Javey, A. (2015) Highly uniform and stable n-type carbon nanotube transistors by using positively charged silicon nitride thin films. *Nano Lett.*, **15** (1), 392–397; (b) Zhang, J., Wang, C., Fu, Y., He, Y., and Zhou, C. (2011) Air-stable conversion of separated carbon nanotube thin-film transistors from p-type to n-type using atomic layer deposition of high-kappa oxide and its application in CMOS logic circuits. *ACS Nano*, **5** (4), 3284–3292; (c) Lee, S.Y., Lee, S.W., Kim, S.M., Yu, W.J., Jo, Y.W., and Lee, Y.H. (2011) Scalable complementary logic gates with chemically doped semiconducting carbon nanotube transistors. *ACS Nano*, **5** (3), 2369–2375.
49 Chen, H., Cao, Y., Zhang, J., and Zhou, C. (2014) Large-scale complementary macroelectronics using hybrid integration of carbon nanotubes and IGZO thin-film transistors. *Nat. Commun.*, **5**. doi: 10.1038/ncomms5097
50 (a) Kim, B., Jang, S., Geier, M.L., Prabhumirashi, P.L., Hersam, M.C., and Dodabalapur, A. (2014) High-speed, inkjet-printed carbon nanotube/zinc tin oxide hybrid complementary ring oscillators. *Nano Lett.*, **14** (6), 3683–3687; (b) Vuttipittayamongkol, P., Wu, F.Q., Chen, H.T., Cao, X., Liu, B.L., and Zhou, C.W. (2015) Threshold voltage tuning and printed complementary transistors and inverters based on thin films of carbon nanotubes and indium zinc oxide. *Nano Res.*, **8** (4), 1159–1168.
51 (a) Davis, V.A., Parra-Vasquez, A.N.G., Green, M.J., Rai, P.K., Behabtu, N., Prieto, V., Booker, R.D., Schmidt, J., Kesselman, E., Zhou, W., Fan, H., Adams, W.W., Hauge, R.H., Fischer, J.E., Cohen, Y., Talmon, Y., Smalley, R.E., and Pasquali, M. (2009) True solutions of single-walled carbon nanotubes for assembly into macroscopic materials. *Nat. Nanotechnol.*, **4** (12), 830–834; (b) Fogden, S., Howard, C.A., Heenan, R.K., Skipper, N.T., and Shaffer, M.S.P. (2012) Scalable method for the reductive dissolution, purification, and separation of single-walled carbon nanotubes. *ACS Nano*, **6** (1), 54–62.
52 (a) Pu, J., Zhang, Y.J., Wada, Y., Wang, J.T.W., Li, L.J., Iwasa, Y., and Takenobu, T. (2013) Fabrication of stretchable MoS_2 thin-film transistors using elastic ion-gel gate dielectrics. *Appl. Phys. Lett.*, **103** (2), 023505; (b) Yan, C., Cho, J.H., and Ahn, J.H. (2012) Graphene-based flexible and stretchable thin film transistors. *Nanoscale*, **4** (16), 4870–4882.

3

Organic-Based Transistors and Sensors

Aristide Gumyusenge[1], Tianbai Xu[2], Xiaozhi Wang[2], and Jianguo Mei[1,3]

[1] Purdue University, Department of Chemistry, 560 Oval Drive, West Lafayette, IN 47907, USA
[2] Zhejiang University, Department of Information Science and Electronics Engineering, Hangzhou 310027, P. R. China
[3] Purdue University, Birck Nanotechnology Center, 1205 W State Street, West Lafayette, IN 47906, USA

3.1 Introduction

With the emerging popularity of wearable electronics, with the high expectations from robotics engineering, with the desire and need for implantable electronics, and the quest to mimic nature in medicine engineering and artificial intelligence, we are seeking to achieve flexible—bendable and stretchable—electronics. Even though silicon remains the highest performing material in electronics, and is still being studied to be rendered thinner and flexible, silicon-based technology seems to lack the desired easy processability for low-cost manufacturing. The research community is thus dedicating tremendous efforts toward coming up with materials that can potentially complement the traditional inorganic systems used in electronics industry, not to rival silicon technology, but fulfilling the needs mentioned above. Among studied materials are organic semiconductors owing to their tunable optical, electronic, and redox properties, in combination with their ability to be processed at ambient conditions, and their biocompatibility [1–5]. The starting point for achieving large-area processing is making flexible transistors and sensors, and eventually, high-performance large-scale flexible electronics can be achieved [6–9]. Organic semiconductors have already shown promising results for commercial devices, and are being investigated for further uses in flexible circuitry [3, 10]. In this chapter, we give an overview of current approaches on achieving flexible all-organic transistors and transistor-based sensors. In the first section, we will introduce how all-organic devices can be achieved in terms of choosing substrates, electrodes, dielectric layer, and operating channel, as well as the device geometry. The second section will focus on the current state-of-the-art design of transistors; the fundamental working principles that ought to be preserved in flexible hybrids will be introduced. The third section will be dedicated to currently studied fabrication techniques suitable for organic-based transistors. In the last section, applications of flexible transistors will be discussed as we review ongoing efforts in transistor-based sensors design.

Flexible and Stretchable Medical Devices, First Edition. Edited by Kuniharu Takei.

3.2 Materials Consideration for Flexible Organic-Based Transistors

To achieve organic flexible transistors and sensors, we first ought to discuss what makes any material suitable for flexible transistors fabrication and then review how performances can be improved. This section will thus attempt to define flexibility at the level of a transistor, discuss the choice of substrates and electrodes, and introduce the choice of the dielectric layers, as well as the organic functional channel layers. Representative literature will be provided for those readers interested in further learning about current efforts in organic-based flexible electronics.

3.2.1 How Flexibility is Achieved

How we define flexibility becomes an important talking point in organic-based electronics as a first step toward deviating from the traditional robust silicon-based technologies. Some material chemists argue that for a material to be considered flexible, this should be an intrinsic property [11–13], while the counterargument suggests that any material could be rendered flexible if made thin enough [14, 15]. The word "flexible" will be used in this chapter to refer to both bendable and stretchable, and the distinction between these two terms will become crucial as we discuss the applications of organic transistors. Flexibility will here be viewed in terms of the physical strain that a device (material) can sustain when bent and/or stretched. Organic materials oftentimes tend to be associated with flexibility—ergo the common appellation of "plastics"—despite many cases that display high crystallinity and brittleness [16]. The organic systems we consider here are those that are able to provide excellent flexibility at the level of all major components of a transistor—substrate, electrodes, and active layer. We herein review materials under investigation for each component toward achieving large-area organic flexible systems.

3.2.1.1 Flexible Substrates

The approach to thin-out the silicon-based technology, of transferring it onto thinner and bendable substrates to fabricate lighter electronics has recently been a key feature in many tech companies. It could thus be envisioned that the same approach could be used to apply existing technology on flexible substrates; flexible TV displays, for instance, could be fabricated. Among substrate candidates, metals such as steel and aluminum have been investigated to be made thinner, therefore flexible [17]. Thin glass is another candidate mostly for groups interested in applying flexibility to displays (e.g., curved and bendable TVs, wearable displays, etc.) Glass provides excellent optical properties desired for displays (transmittance and birefringence), but it showed great difficulty when trying to achieve desired thinness without damaging the rather fragile and brittle glass sheets [18]. The preferred alternatives have been plastic polymer substrates. Plastic substrates have gained more popularity than the last two counterparts, not only because they tend to tolerate strain better, but also because they display several other properties that metals, for instance, cannot provide: easy processability, low melting points (whenever desired), biodegradability, not to forget their low-cost. Plastic substrates have then been used in roll-to-roll processing owing to their ability to be printed in long foldable and pliable sheets at low temperatures [19, 20]. Most of the plastic substrates are based on thermoplastics, as well as other high glass-transition points (Tg) polymers. The most widely used polymers include polyethylene terephthalate (PET), polyethylene naphthalate (PEN), polycarbonates (PCs), and polyimides (PIs) [21–23], to name a few. Depending on their crystallinity, these polymers have thus been advanced as candidates to replace glass in fabrication of devices that require excellent optical properties combined with bendability and/or stretchability. Most newly developed fabrication techniques aim to lower the cost and unsustainability associated with the high temperatures required for metal-based substrates.

3.2.1.2 Flexible Electrodes

The use of metal electrodes remains prominent in electronics due to their excellent electronic properties. It is however worth mentioning that the most popular electrode being gold in competition with other precious metals such as platinum and silver, the cost aspect in device fabrication cannot be undermined. Most research groups take advantage of vapor deposition and sputtering to pattern thin layers of the desired metal onto substrates of choice [24–26]. Using special processing methods, transparent and pliable metal electrodes can be achieved [27–29]. Note that most of these generally used methods require high vacuum and/or high temperatures. The meticulous nature of these methods used to achieve flexibility of metal electrodes thus calls for easier and cheaper alternatives to fabricate flexible electrodes.

A special appraisal is presented on the discovery of charge conductivity in conjugated polymers by Heeger and coworkers [30]. Thanks to their work, conducting polymers have shown to be excellent candidates that can replace metal electrodes in device fabrication [31, 32]. Not only have conducting polymers shown great electronic conductivity, but they have also opened doors to easier and low-cost electrode patterning routes as they can be solution-processed at low temperatures. Free-standing flexible polymer electrodes have been achieved and incorporated in several device designs proving their ability to obviate the use of metals [33–36]. In addition to their plastic properties, conductive polymers show great conductivities, excellent charge, and discharge cycles, as well as low band gaps owing to the conjugated π-system along their backbone [36–38]. These metallic properties have also shown to be greatly enhanced in carbon nanotubes owing to their ability to be fabricated in highly oriented nanowires [39, 40]. Carbon nanotubes have thus been used to be incorporated in flexible arrays for sensing applications [41–43]. Free-standing polymer electrodes are thus being investigated as they are more suitable for low-cost fabrication of flexible electronics—they can easily be patterned as thin films.

In case of special properties that tend to be solely characteristic for metals—magnetism for instance—metal-polymer hybrids have been studied. These hybrids are usually achieved by immersing metal nanoparticles in a polymer medium; this combination affords the desired properties of the

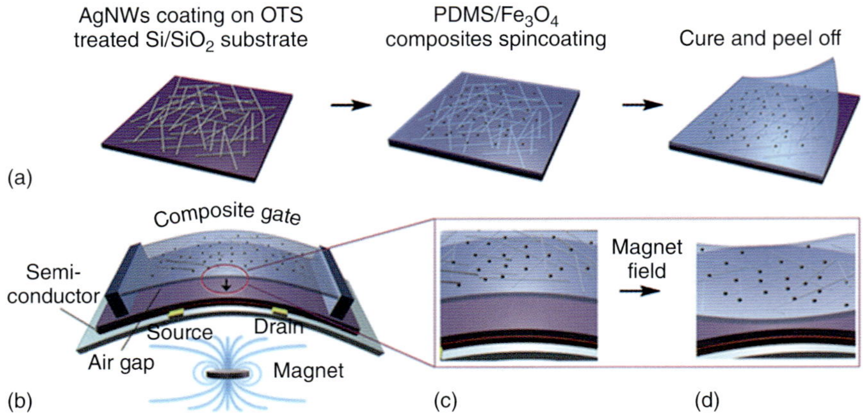

Figure 3.1 Gate electrode engineering achieving highly flexible magnetic sensors using the gate suspension technique. Silver nanoparticles are immersed in a solution of PMDS yielding a magnetically active composite. (Adapted from Ref. [47].)

metal with the flexibility of the polymer. Several composite systems have been explored and polymers such as polyamides, polyacrylamide, and other hydrogels have been used to achieve highly flexible conductive arrays [33, 44–46]. For instance, Zang *et al.* demonstrated a flexible magnetic sensor achieved by taking advantage of gate-electrode engineering. The group incorporated magnetically active nanoparticles (silver nanowires and iron oxide nanoparticles) into polydimethylsiloxane (PDMS), a flexible medium, and flexible composites could be fabricated. Using a gate suspension technique (as depicted in Figure 3.1) a flexible magnetic sensor was achieved [47]. Such sensors would find great applications in soft robotics.

3.2.2 Organic Dielectric Layer

Another crucial component in transistor fabrication is the layering of a dielectric layer on the top of the patterned electrodes. This step remains relevant for charge injection in organic systems [48, 49]. Given how thin the dielectric layer is made, it does not play a crucial role in limiting device flexibility. It has however been shown that by using polymer gate dielectrics in place of the inorganic dielectrics, the overall performance can be significantly improved in thin-film transistors (TFTs) [50]. An effective dielectric layer requires to be a very thin and pinholes-free film of an insulator that can allow electric field injection at low voltages. This task, however, becomes challenging as most polymer insulators tend to yield thicker films (100 nm) and require high voltages [51]. In order to circumvent this leakage issue while retaining thinness, polymers such as poly-4-vinyl-phenol (PVP) [50, 52–55], poly(methyl methacrylate) (PMMA) [51], polystyrene (PS) [56], and polyvinyl alcohol (PVA) [57] have been used. These polymers have showed the ability to be cross-linked achieving desired thinness, uniformity, and of excellent charge injection. Note that instead of relying on traditionally used methods such as vapor deposition, sputtering, and thermal growing as it is the case for inorganic dielectrics—usually silicon (or aluminum) oxides and nitrides [48]—the polymers listed above could be deposited by solution processing. Using all-organic dielectric materials thus becomes more suitable for the fabrication of flexible devices; no harsh conditions are required and desired results can be achieved.

3.2.3 Organic Functional Layer

The use of organic materials in transistor fabrication emerged in the late 1980s with the discovery of (semi)conducting polymers [30, 58, 59]. Ever since, organic semiconductor-based transistor fabrication has seen tremendous attention to the point of achieving performances approaching that of polycrystalline silicon [5, 60]. Polymer backbone engineering, as well as side chain engineering are two crucial tools to improve charge carrier mobility in semiconductor polymer systems. With the manipulation of conjugated backbones, as well as functionality tuning of side chains, charge carrier transport in polymer systems has thus seen tremendous improvements in the past two decades. Mobilities exceeding $40\,cm^2\,V^{-1}\,s^{-1}$ have been achieved [61].

One of the specialties for which organic semiconductors are popular is their ability to be processed as thin films at ambient temperatures. This low temperature processing has made organic thin-film transistors (OTFTs) potential candidates for devices processed on flexible polymeric substrates such as smart paper, radio frequency tags, smart cards, flexible displays, and sensors as will be discussed later in this chapter [62, 63]. In addition, this ease of achieving OTFTs provides an appealing alternative to industry as a way to obviate the meticulous and harsh protocol required for achieving thin layers of silicon [64, 65]. Organic semiconductors from small molecules, to oligomers, and conjugated polymers have shown the ability to be processed into thin films, and several device designs have been studied [2, 4–6]. We will not discuss the material design and engineering for organic semiconductors in detail. We will however revisit what has been accomplished in terms of improving charge carrier transport when we get to transistor designs; materials design and device performance tend to be inseparable in this field.

3.3 State-of-the-Art Designs and Fabrication of Organic-Based Transistors

OTFTs for different applications adopt various designs namely organic field-effect transistors (OFETs) [3, 6, 8], electrolyte-gated organic field-effect transistors (EGOFETs) [66–68], organic electrochemical transistors (OECTs) [66–72], and the list goes on. These designs aim to substitute inorganic materials with organic alternatives as the active layers in transistor fabrication. Using organic materials has promised to decrease, if not completely eliminate, the cost of high temperature ramping that is usually required for inorganic systems. Thin-film processing has also opened doors to several fabrication techniques including screen printing, inkjet printing, and different photolithographic techniques—we will revisit fabrication techniques in later sections. For all the designs discussed further, we will need to keep in mind that charge transport in the channel layer tends to be associated to the first few layers of molecules. This concentration of charge in the bottom layers becomes crucial when choosing the optimal film thickness, as well as strategic electrodes placement for particular transistor designs [62, 64, 65]. In this section, we introduce representative transistor designs, explain their working mechanisms, and discuss their potential applications in organic electronics.

3.3.1 Organic Field-Effect Transistors

3.3.1.1 Structure

OFETs are by far the most widely studied transistor configuration in organic transistors. This design provides amplifying and/or switching of electronic signals, while maintaining a rather simple layout. The first demonstration of a solid-state OFET was reported by Tsumura *et al.* [73], which was around the same time when Kodak research laboratory had just demonstrated an organic light-emitting diode [58, 59]. Since then, the field of OFETs has been widely studied to the extent of improving the primitive charge carrier mobilities from 10^{-5} to higher than tens of $cm^2\ V^{-1}\ s^{-1}$ [4, 6, 61]. An OFET consists of an organic semiconducting layer deposited between two ohmic contacts (source and drain), separated by a thin dielectric layer from a third contact (gate). The gate can be positioned either on the top (top gate) or at the bottom (bottom gate). In some cases, the gate can also serve as the substrate, otherwise, the assembly can be patterned on a substrate (traditionally glass or heavily doped silicon).

Choosing the right device geometry is another crucial step to achieving high performance of a transistor. One of the main challenges in OFET fabrication is to ensure that neither the functional layer nor the electrodes are damaged in the process. Generally, in order to minimize atmospheric and/or harsh environment exposure, electrodes are deposited on a substrate, followed by the channel layer, and then the assembly is protected with a dielectric layer (plus the gate contact). The geometry varies depending on the intended functions of the OFET and the materials of choice. For instance, n-type materials, that is, electron-transporting semiconductors tend to be associated with low air stability. It is thus common to adopt device geometries that encapsulate the semiconductor materials between the more stable layers—insulating layer and/or passivation layer—achieving bottom-contact or top-contact geometries as shown in Figure 3.2.

It is also to be noted that many researchers are investigating the use of the vertical geometries as opposed to lateral planar geometries to increase OFETs performance and device stability [74–78]. In the vertical geometry, the semiconductor layer is sandwiched between the source and drain pads, thus reducing the channel length to the film thickness of the deposited functional layer. This geometry still faces challenges mainly due to the difficulty of charge injection through the source contact, which, in this configuration, becomes significantly close to the gate electrode yielding a capacitive unit. One of the proposed ways around this issue is the use of perforated source contacts. The electric field accumulated at the dielectric–source interface can be allowed to tunnel through the

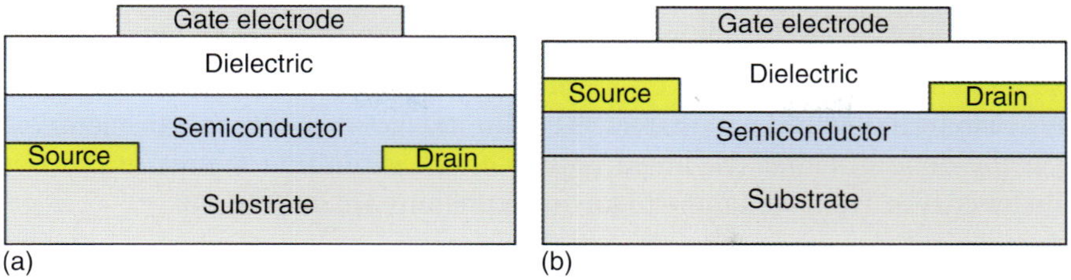

Figure 3.2 Transistor structures preferred for sensitive materials (a) bottom-contact top gate, (b) top-contact top gate. Contact is in reference to the position of source and drain with the semiconductor.

intentionally placed holes within the source electrode. High OFET performances have been achieved and reported affording potential applications for these structures in achieving flexible arrays [79, 80].

3.3.1.2 Performance and Characterization

As previously stated, an OFET is a three-terminal device that operates by switching and/or amplifying a current passing through an organic semiconducting layer deposited between two ohmic contacts (source and drain). This current flow is usually a response to a certain voltage (V_G) applied on a third plate (gate) lying underneath or on the top of the semiconductor layer. The amount of current that is able to flow between the source and drain—through the active layer—subsequently marks the device's performance in terms of its ability to transport charge carriers. The question of whether organic materials could perform to the same level as the inorganic counterparts has been the driving force to finding organic materials with high conductivities, as well as facile processability. With such materials in hand, flexible all-organic transistors can be achieved to fabricate large-area devices for daily uses. OFETs have shown promising results and we hope to be able to say the same for flexible hybrids by the end of this chapter.

Ordinarily, transistor performance is tested by analyzing the channel layer's transductance (or capacitance) as a response to an applied V_G. By applying another voltage (V_{DS}) between source and drain contacts, the performance of the channel layer can be monitored from the decrease in voltage as the current travels through the organic material. Extrapolating transfer and output curves, a few key parameters are usually reported to characterize OFET performance. First, charge carrier mobility (μ), ON/OFF ratio, as well as the threshold voltage (V_{TH}) are to be evaluated. Charge carrier mobility tells how fast the charge carriers can move from one contact to the other, while the ON/OFF ratio shows the difference between currents before the device could be turned on and when the device is switched on. The threshold voltage is an indication of the minimum voltage V_{DS} that has to be applied before the device can be "tuned on". V_{TH} is oftentimes reported with its subthreshold slope (SS) which is the voltage difference required to increase the current between source and drain by a factor of ten. This slope is usually an indication of how fast the device can switch from the OFF state to the ON state. Notice the dependence of the threshold voltage on any fabrication defects, since any holes or leakages—contact resistance—would have to be filled before the device can turn on. Also note that the organic-based systems borrow these parameters from the inorganic systems that are used by physicists to derive the parameters [81]. The extraction of these parameters is normally done in either the linear regime or the saturation regime of the I/V transfer curves, from which the following equations are derived [4]:

$$I_{\mathrm{ds}} = \mu \frac{W}{L} Ci(V_{\mathrm{g}} - V_{\mathrm{t}})V_{\mathrm{ds}},\ V_{\mathrm{g}} - V_{\mathrm{t}} \gg V_{\mathrm{ds}}\ \text{(linear regime)} \tag{3.1}$$

$$I_{\mathrm{ds}}(\text{sat.}) = \mu \frac{W}{L} (V_{\mathrm{g}} - V_{\mathrm{t}})^2,\ V_{\mathrm{g}} - V_{\mathrm{t}} < V_{\mathrm{ds}}\ \text{(saturation regime)} \tag{3.2}$$

Equation (3.1) and (3.2) are compiled for OFET performance characterization. I_{DS} is the current between the source and drain electrodes, μ the charge carrier mobility, mostly referred to as mobility, W and L are the width and the length of the operating channel, respectively, and V_{G} and V_{TH} are the applied gate voltage and the threshold voltage, respectively.

Note the occasional overestimation of charge carrier mobility from the nonlinear slopes of the transfer curve, as shown in Figure 3.3, which tends to be characteristic for many semiconducting polymers including cyclopenta-dithiophene-benzothiadiazole copolymer (CDT-BTZ) (Figure 3.3a), diketo-pyrrolopyrrolethieno[3,2-*b*]thiophene copolymer (DPP-T-TT) (Figure 3.3b), and indacenodithiophene-co-benzothiadiazole (IDTBT) (Figure 3.3c) [82]. The presence of kinks within the transfer curve can lead to inaccurate performance results. The research community in this field is thus debating the linearity of transfer curves is required for accurate charge mobility reporting [83]. Nonetheless, OFETs have shown excellent performances and have shown potential to be applied to large-area processing. The ongoing quest for improving their functionalities has thus enriched the library of (semi)conducting oligo/polymers, and remarkably high charge carrier mobilities have been achieved [61]. For the readers interested in further learning about the evolution of OFETs material engineering, representative examples of highly functionalized materials were reviewed and respective mobility milestones were presented [5].

3.3.2 Modifications of OFETs for Sensing Applications

Several OFETs modifications have been designed in accordance with the desired applications especially in sensing as shown in Figure 3.4. In the next section, we show a few of the proposed designs, explain their working mechanisms, while providing their potential applications in organic electronics. The operating mechanism of OECT will be used to discuss the device performance; the other configurations tend to operate in a similar manner and will not be discussed in detail. Readers may consider the work of Piet Bergveld for more insights on ion-sensitive field-effect transitors [85].

3.3.2.1 Electrolyte-Gated and Ion-Sensitive Organic Field-Effect Transistors

An EGOFET is a proposed device design that slightly differs from an OFET mainly for biological interfacing purposes. In addition to the major components of an OFET, EGOFETs are topped with an electrolyte layer that is

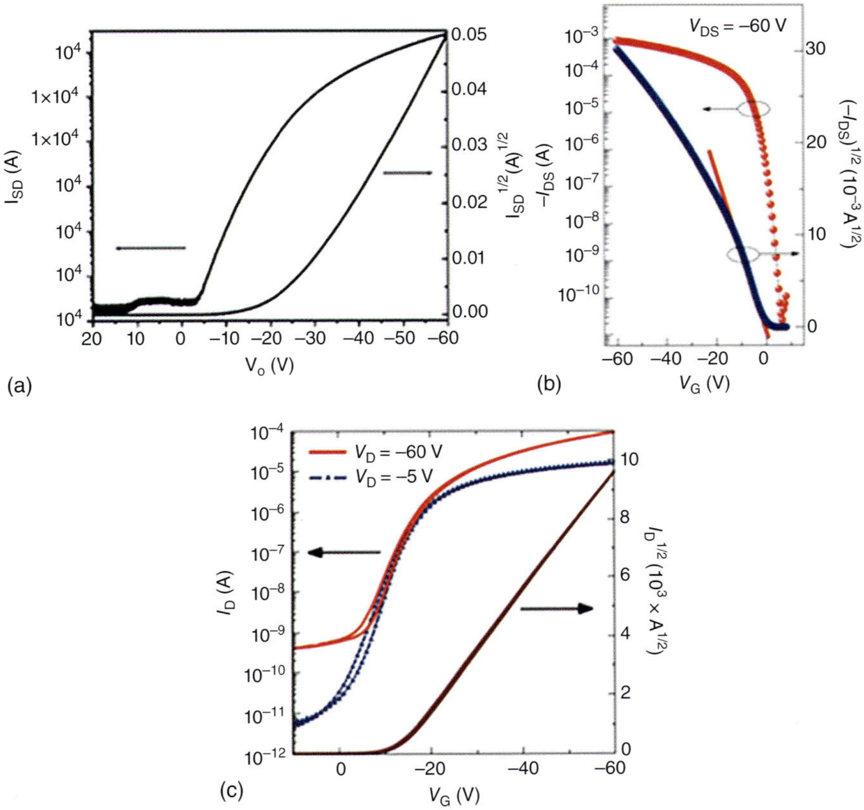

Figure 3.3 Transfer characteristics curves for mobility extraction from high-performance conjugated polymer OFETs showing occasional non-ideal transfer characteristics: (a) CDT-BTZ bottom-gate, top-contact FET. (b) DPP-T-TT bottom-gate, top-contact FET. (c) IDTBT top-gate, bottom-contact FET. (Adapted from Ref. [4].)

meant to interface with charged analytes [84]. This design has mainly been used in designing biosensors as the latter require a soft and benign interface between the device and the physiological environment. This interfacing ability has allowed for the coating of traditional metal electrodes in order to access and monitor neurons activity [86], intra- and extracellular stimulation [68], physiological pH sensing [67], as well as bio-transduction sensing [66, 87]. The working principal of electrolyte-gated transistors relies on the ability of their electrolyte/semiconductor interface to selectively detect any potentiostatic change due to ionic injection in the electrolyte layer. The amplified capacitance of the transistor is usually explained by the formation of a double Helmholtz layer between the electrode/electrolyte interface, and then the electrolyte/semiconductor interface. This double layer formation was extensively studied by Salleo research group at Stanford University [88]. With the combination of the flexibility that was discussed for OFETs—which still applies here—and the "softness" offered by electrolyte coating, EGOFETs have thus been potential candidates for interfacing with physiological tissues.

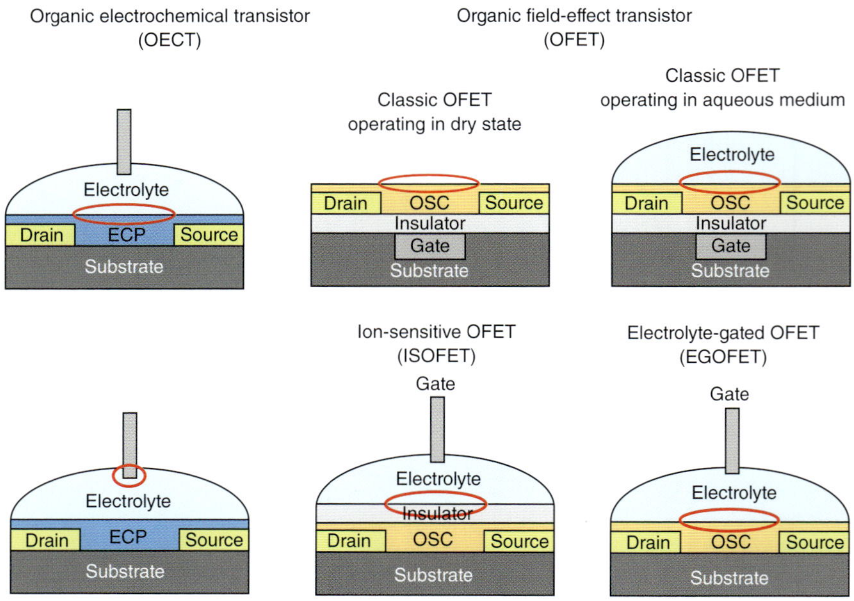

Figure 3.4 Representative modifications of OFET design for sensing applications. The red circle indicates the interface of the functional layer (OSC: organic semiconductor, ECP: electrically conductive polymer) and the electrolyte-sample solution. (Adapted from Ref. [84].)

Ion-sensitive electrolytes have been employed to achieve ion-sensitive organic field-effect transistors (ISOFETs). This OFET modification has been proposed and used for pH sensors [89, 90], various water-soluble metabolites sensing [91, 92], as well as anionic and cationic sensing [93, 94]. The injection of ions at the electrolyte interface can be translated into an electrical signal and the device's response can be monitored. Note that most of the studied electrolytes are in their aqueous phases as depicted in Figure 3.4, and oftentimes need to be contained in a well of inert polymers such as PDMS. Ideally, a solid state electrolyte or a hydrogel would be more applicable for easy manipulation of the device and for flexible arrays. To further improve the device design and sensitivity, a structure that exploits similar working mechanism as an ISOFET (as well as EGOFET) but on a wider spectrum of analytes has been studied, namely OECT.

3.3.2.2 Organic Electrochemical Transistors

This rather newly developed organic transistor design gained its popularity in the past two decades due to its promising ability to interface with the biological systems. OECTs were a timely development after the argument that the field of biomedicine has not fully benefited from the currently available technologies—compared to other fields such as entertainment and telecommunication. The validity of this argument is simply rooted in the fact that the currently available technologies are rather rigid and cannot be in direct contact with the soft and fragile bio-physiological tissues. In efforts to establish the missing link between the soft biological tissues and the robust silicon-based technologies, OECTs have shown promising performances to be suitable candidates [35, 70,

95, 96]. Owing to their ability to translate change in ionic concentration—one of the most common mechanism in signal recognition in physiology—OECTs have been identified as device designs that can render the possible fabrication of implantable technologies. Long-term implantation of high-tech devices would be a crucial addition to fields of bio-medicine and drug delivery.

The ion-detecting ability of OECTs has thus been widely explored to design biomedical devices from glucose sensors to brain activity monitors [35, 96]. Being a newly studied design, OECTs have seen tremendous advancement as researchers started to design ionic-conducting materials that could be matched with the physiological functions. When poly(3,4-ethylenedioxythiophene)-polystyrene sulfonate (PEDOT-PSS) was first synthesized, its unprecedented performance in electro-ionic conductivity allowed the fabrication of improved devices significantly exceeding what had been reported by Wrighton's research in the 1980s [96, 97]. PEDOT-PSS remains the most widely studied electro-ionic conducting polymer for OECTs mostly due to its commercial availability, and also its excellent electrochemical performance [71, 95, 96, 98]. One of the remaining challenges for OECT design, however, is a full understanding of the device's working mechanism. The device's physics becomes complicated due to the combined electronic and ionic conductivity.

3.3.2.3 Operating Mechanisms

All three modifications of OFETs rely on one major working principal: when the electrolyte comes in contact with a charged analyte (or when a voltage is applied), the change in chemical potential within the electrolyte is detected by the underlying (semi)conducting layer. This principal becomes more complicated for an OECT since the later requires a combination of electric conductivity and ionic conductivity of the organic layer (shown as ECP in Figure 3.4 above). The current consensus of an OECT operating mechanism is that upon injection of ions in the electrolyte layer, the latter becomes doped. With the presence of negatively charged sites in the subsequent conducting layer, the anions migrate to de-dope the now positively charged electrolyte layer, leaving behind an electron-conducting layer. This doping and de-doping cycle results in the movement of holes (positive charge carries) correlating to a generated current and detectable potential change. This injection of holes at the source electrode is oftentimes studied in the depletion mode of the device [95]. OECT performance is then evaluated as the ability of the active material to detect change in electrochemical potential at the electrolyte interface, and its ability to translate it into a current flow.

3.4 Fabrication Techniques for Organic-Based Transistors and Sensors

The fabrication technology for flexible organic-based transistors and sensors has been greatly dictated by the materials of choice and the desired structures of the devices. Generally, the gate, source, drain electrodes, and inorganic dielectric layer can be patterned using traditional methods, for example, photolithography or shadow mask [24, 25]. The organic layer, however, requires less harsh fabrication methods employing newly developed "softer" technologies such as transfer printing, inkjet printing, or even direct writing. In addition, many organic materials are incompatible with most solvents used in traditional microfabrication processes, which means appropriate methods have to be predetermined depending on the sensitivity of the material in use. The ultimate goal of being to able to achieve low-cost printing of circuits, techniques such as spin coating, drop casting, inkjet printing, screen printing, gravure printing, to name a few, have been studied [52, 99]. Not only are these methods low-cost, they are also more compatible with achieving flexible, pliable, and even stretchable devices as most of them can be conducted at room temperature. Low temperature processing provides low-cost fabrication and also obviates thermal expansion of flexible substrates; this thermal expansion is oftentimes linked to the misalignment of the different device layers and can affect patterning resolution. These methods have been used to achieve long pliable sheets of integrated circuits [19, 20, 100].

For flexible devices, spin coating and drop casting remain the two most widely used methods in transistor fabrication. The two methods allow for achieving very thin films of the semiconductor layer, especially spin coating, and have shown great results in large-area flexible arrays. However, these methods still rely heavily on the use of organic solvents and remain less appealing to industrial-scale manufacturing. Industrial production prefers a more robust and fast fabrication route: roll-to-roll printing. For roll-to-roll manufacturing, preferred alternatives would be inkjet printing, screen printing, as well as other routes that allow for a continuous process. The organic semiconductor materials can be prepared as inks with proper viscosity and the channel layers can be readily printed. In this case, the channel length and the amount of material needed in transistor fabrication can be determined by the printer's resolution. Much efforts are currently being put into achieving high resolutions as the roll-to-roll printing route promises low-cost manufacturing of desired circuits [19, 53]. Figure 3.5 summarizes the current

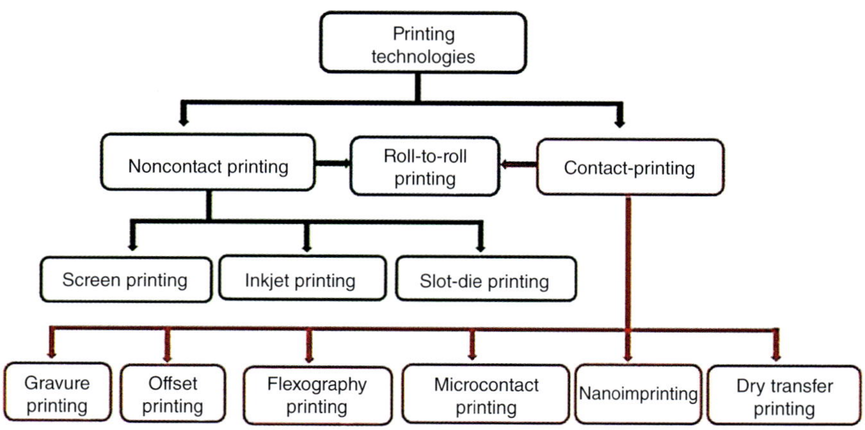

Figure 3.5 Printing technologies for roll-to-roll printing of flexible electronics under investigation. (Khan *et al.* 2015 [101]. With permission from IEEE.)

approaches toward achieving easy and reliable roll-to-roll printing; for the readers interested in further details, a review by Khan *et al.* [101] is recommended.

3.5 Flexible Organic Transistor-Based Sensors

Compared with inorganic systems, organic materials present many advantages in sensing owing to their mechanical properties, electrical properties and their biocompatibility. Throughout the previous sections, we showed different designs of organic-based transistors and we repeatedly hinted on their applications. In this section, we focus on organic-based transistors that have been studied to design sensors. We thus present a few examples of sensors namely for strain, temperature, pressure, as well as bio-analytes using organic materials as active layers. Note that for most sensors under investigation, the use of metal electrodes and/or glass substrates still remains popular, therefore many figures shown in this section are only partially organic.

3.5.1 Flexible Organic Strain Sensors

Flexible strain sensors, different from the traditional strain sensors, put forward a higher demand on material design as well as device geometry. Intrinsically stretchable materials would be ideal choices for strain sensing, but many material candidates lack the ability to combine stretchability with other desired properties—electrical and stability. For organic-based designs, this stretchability remains an issue as most of OTFT-based systems manifest low moduli [16, 102]. If the strain applied on the devices exceeds the crack-on-set strain of the material, cracks will form within the film, and the device will lose its function. Flexible organic-based strain sensors are thus oftentimes fabricated on thin and unstretchable plastic substrates to acquire the required bendability. Generally, strain-sensitive materials, piezoelectric, for example, are used to be incorporated in a device in order to detect applied strain. For instance, Hsu *et al.* designed a flexible strain sensor using an OFET structure patterned on polyvinylidene fluoride (PVDF) [103]. To fabricate the OFET devices on PVDF, a layer of parylene-C was used as the dielectric layer, and an aluminum layer at the bottom acted as a reference electrode. When strain was applied on the device, the PVDF layer could generate an accumulation of charge because of its piezoelectricity. The accumulated charge then acted as the gate voltage and turned-on the channel layer. Different strain conditions induced different drain currents (Figure 3.6b). Using an array of devices, the strain applied on a large area could be detected.

Besides piezoelectric devices, other device structures and different fabrication processes have been introduced for strain sensing. For instance, Nam *et al.* demonstrated a kind of strain sensor based on heptazole TFTs [104] as shown in Figure 3.7. An inverter-type TFT circuit was introduced to measure the large elastic strain (up to ca. 2.5%), owing to excellent mechanical properties of heptazole. Despite the anisotropic electrical properties of heptazole under strain—which caused little current variation under horizontal strain—the

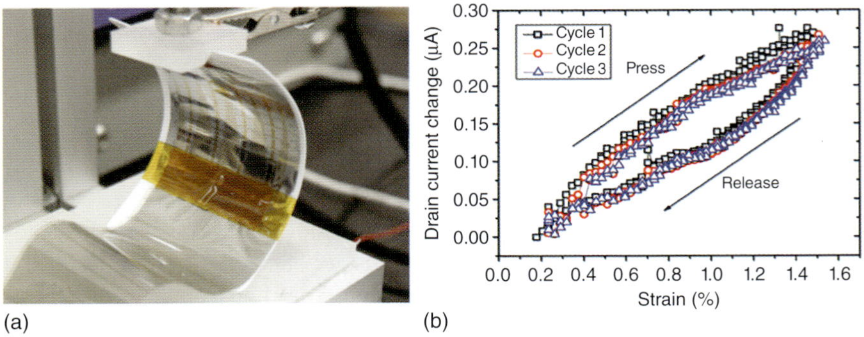

Figure 3.6 Illustration of a piezoelectric-based strain sensor (a) strain is applied from both ends of the sensor, and (b) is the performance of the devices under different strain. (Hsu *et al.* 2011 [103]. With permission from IEEE.)

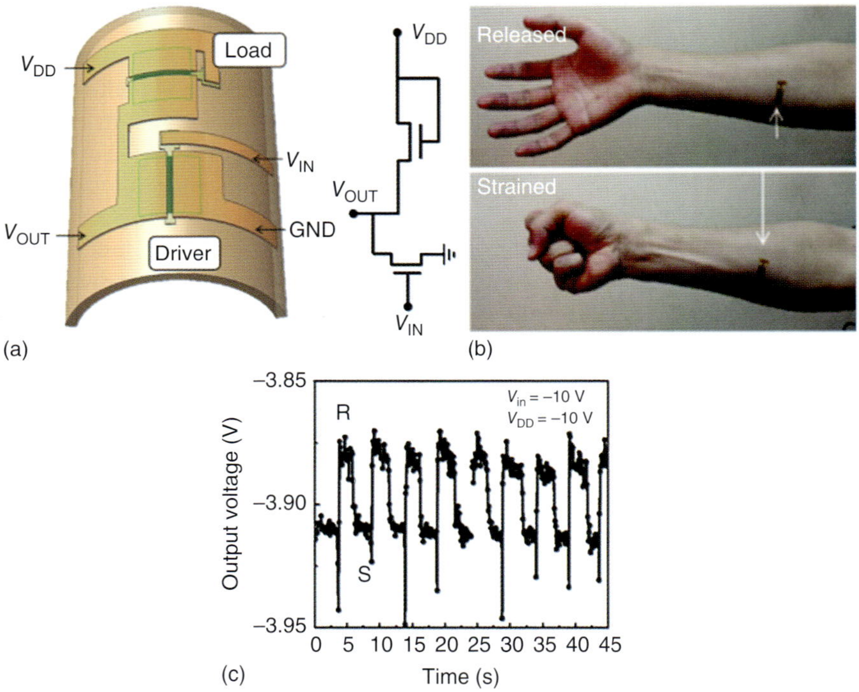

Figure 3.7 Demonstration of an elastic strain sensor based on heptazole: (a) device structure and junctions layout, (b) strain gauge mounted on a fore arm, (c) muscle movement detected by the sensor. (Adapted from Ref. [104].)

current could change dramatically under vertical strain. The performance of the device could be tuned by controlling the orientation of the heptazole. The strain gauge was used to detect the movement of a muscle, as shown in Figure 3.7b.

3.5.2 Flexible Organic Pressure Sensors

As mentioned above, organic materials tend to be delicate and sensitive to harsh conditions. This delicate nature thus makes many organic materials unsuitable for direct use in pressure sensing. In order to achieve organic-based pressure sensors without direct use of the organic functional layer, two methods are generally used. One method is to branch a pressure-sensitive resistor in series with an organic-based amplifier (OFET for instance) [105, 106]. A few thin-film organic pressure sensors have then been demonstrated using the field-effect transistor configuration [107, 108]. In these sensors, the output current will change due to the change in the resistance under applied pressure. These devices tend to be very thin, which allows them to withstand bending. For example, Kaltenbrunner *et al.* presented an ultralightweight pressure sensor that could be bent even to radii as low as 5 μm [23]. In this work, the device was fabricated on a 1 μm-thick plastic foil making it lighter than a similar size feather (as shown in Figure 3.8a). The transistor was patterned in series with a tactile sensor through a "via hole," and all the fabrication processes were compatible with CMOS (complementary metal oxide semiconductor) technology, which showed the potential for large-scale fabrication. The source and drain current could be tuned by the pressure applied on the tactile sensor, and the mapping of the pressure was achieved by scanning the current changes of the array. A second method to achieve a pressure sensor is to incorporate a pressure-sensitive unit as one of the TFT components. For instance, a pressure-sensitive dielectric layer, which can also tune the output current under different pressures (Figure 3.9a) [109, 112].

Most of the flexible organic pressure sensors mentioned above still face a few challenges as the response times are usually poor and the sensitivities tend to be low. In addition, detection methods also remain a challenge as it becomes difficult to directly and accurately monitor the pressure changes within the

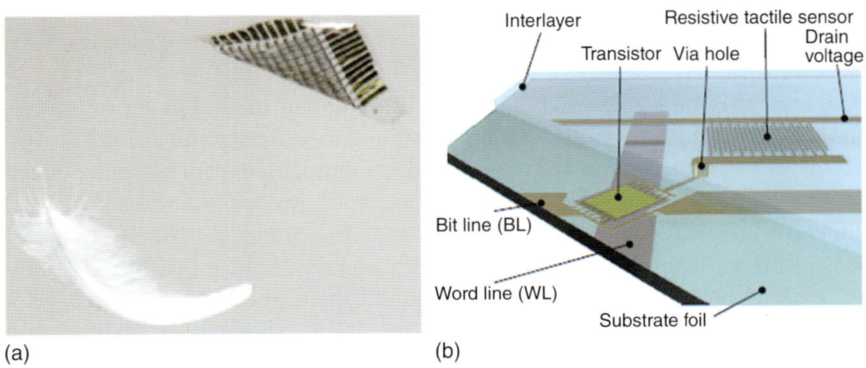

Figure 3.8 An ultralightweight device for pressure sensing (a) device weight compared to a feather in air, (b) structure of a single pressure sensor in the array on a flexible foil. (Adapted from Ref. [23].)

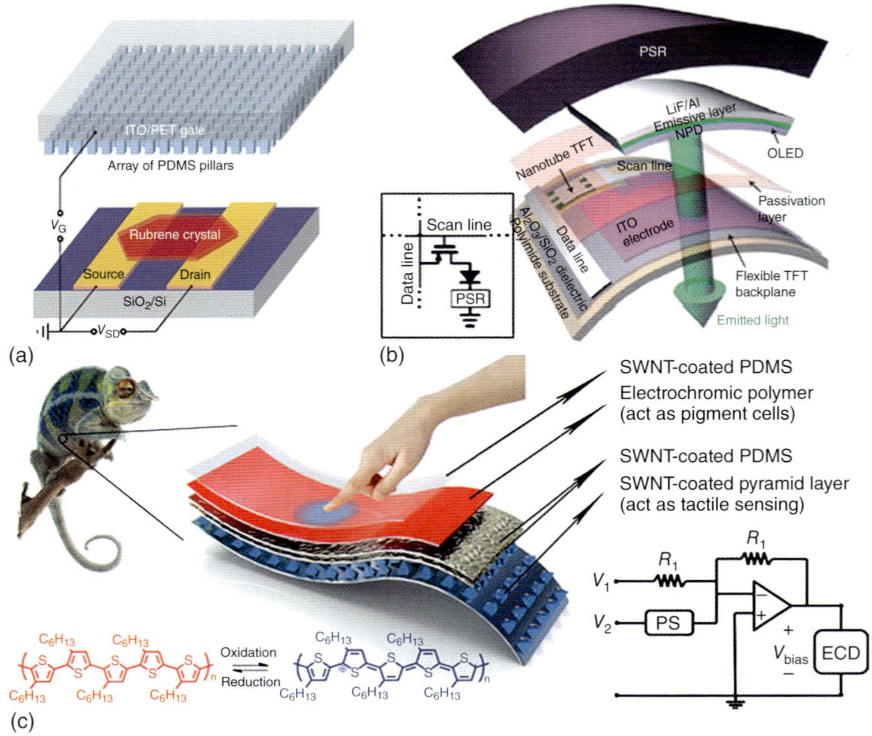

Figure 3.9 (a) A pressure sensor equipped with a flexible and microstructured dielectric layer. (b) Structure of an OLED-based pressure sensor. (c) A kind of pressure sensor mimicking the chameleon's skin. The organic layer is oxidized upon applied pressure resulting into a color change. (Adapted from Refs [109–111].)

device. In their efforts to directly visualize the device's response, Wang *et al.* demonstrated a new kind of flexible pressure sensor [110] by integrating an organic light-emitting diode (OLED) in the sensor. The pressure distribution could directly be displayed according to the pixels (Figure 3.9b). In the area of applied pressure, the OLEDs would turn on and the device's response was evaluated from the intensity of the emitted light.

However, this incorporation of OLEDs within the sensors has its shortcomings as it leads to complex device structures, as well as the robust nature of the device. To address the device complexity issue, a rather simpler concept was introduced by Chou *et al.* as shown in Figure 3.9c. The group proposed an idea of e-skin mimicking chameleon's skin, where an applied pressure would stimulate a color change in the channel layer due to the redox reaction induced within the polymer system [111]. The device's response could then be easily monitored via a color change. Note that the original material, P3HT, showed low stability and this appealing concept is yet to be commercialized. We can however project that this concept could be put to use by addressing device stability using more stable p-type materials, or making use of device passivation.

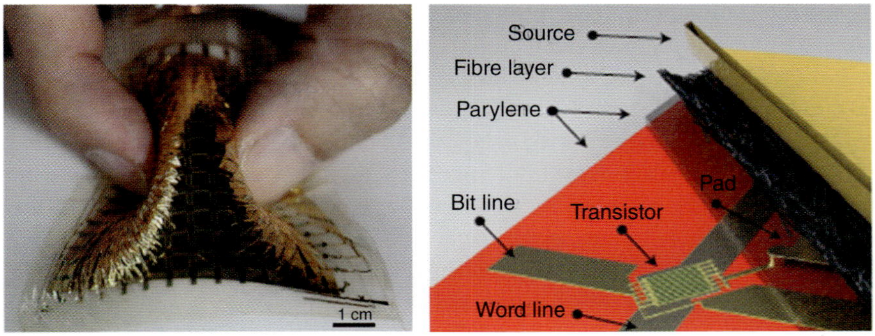

(a) (b)

Figure 3.10 Bending insensitive pressure sensor. (a) Array of nanofibers insensitive to bending strain. (b) Structure of the sensor showing different layers encapsulating a transistor. The fiber layer underlies the source electrode making the device insensitive to bending strain. (Adapted from Ref. [113].)

Another puzzling issue for flexible pressure sensors is that it is oftentimes difficult to distinguish pressure from other mechanical deformations, for instance, bending of the device. Most flexible pressure/strain sensors will respond to both kinds of deformations, in other words the pressure change during the strain test will interfere with the anticipated result and vice versa. In their efforts to obviate the signal interference and stable performance, Lee *et al.* presented a new kind of pressure sensor [113], which is insensitive to bending—the device only responds to normal pressure. The pressure sensor is composed of bending-insensitive nanofibers and TFT arrays as shown in Figure 3.10. The insensitivity of the sensor to strain was mainly attributed to the nanofibrous structures, that is, the alignment of the fibers would change during the bending to help release the strain in each fiber. The device as a whole thus showed insignificant sensitivity to strain while applied pressure could be detected.

3.5.3 Flexible Organic Temperature Sensors

The availability of traditional thermometers might overshadow the need for temperature sensors until one starts considering the need for flexible thermometers—temperature sensors. Ideally, a surgeon should not need an assistant to hold a thermometer during the procedure if a flexible temperature sensor can be directly inserted. Another futuristic example would be having a patch-like sensor that can monitor the thermal activity of, for instance, babies and patients in critical condition. If connected to a monitor system, patients and/or doctors can respond according to continuous monitoring. Here, we turn our focus onto ongoing investigation on designing temperature sensors based on organic materials. Most currently studied flexible organic temperature sensors take advantage of the OTFT structure and the temperature-sensitive resistance [114–116]. Several similarities between these designs and the TFT-based pressure sensors discussed earlier may become easily noticeable to many readers.

Recently, Yokota *et al.* have demonstrated one kind of OTFT-based ultrathin flexible temperature sensor [116]. The sensor shows high sensitivity above 20 mK and a high-speed response time of less than 100 ms, in combination with a working range that can be tuned from 20 to 50 °C. The device design was laid out so that each pixel of the active-matrix-based temperature sensor consisted of an OTFT and a block of acrylate copolymer with graphite particles fillers. The thermal sensitivity of the mixture could be tuned by changing the ratio of the fillers. In principle, any change in temperature within the device leads to a volume change of the copolymer owing to changes in the distances between carbon fillers. This variation in volume can thus be detected as the source-drain current varies and could be monitored as the device's response to temperature change. Since all the materials used in the devices are biocompatible, this sensor design finds potential applications for *in vivo* monitoring.

Highly flexible and stretchable temperature sensors can also be achieved by altering the device structure or by enhancing the elasticity of the thin-film material. For instance, Hong *et al.* presented a stretchable temperature sensor that could work well under 30% biaxial applied strain, showing potential application of the temperature sensor in stretchable electronics [114]. The device design combines carbonanotubes-based active matrices (AM) [110] with a temperature-sensitive resistor to achieve direct temperature monitoring. In order to achieve high flexibility, the interconnecting material for the devices was chosen to be liquid metal—which has been used for stretchable electronic devices. The channel layer consisted of SWCNTs (single wall carbon nanotubes) which are also suitable for stretchable devices (Figure 3.11a). All the devices were first fabricated on PET substrates and then encapsulated by silicon rubber (Ecoflex 00-30) film. The use of such stretchable substrates (devices on high modulus materials, then embedded in low modulus materials) [117] have shown to dramatically release the strain on the devices. Finite element modeling (FEM) analysis was further used to show strain distribution across the devices during the stretch process, thus indicating the effectiveness of the array layout (as depicted in Figure 3.11b).

3.5.4 Flexible Organic Biosensors

As previously mentioned, organic materials have shown abilities to function inside physiological tissues and have so far demonstrated great sensitivities toward various metabolites. OECTs, as well as other modified designs of OFETs, have been used to detect different metabolites including glucose, urea, and ionic concentration, as well as in brain activity [31, 92, 118–124]. With the need for more advanced medical procedures, organic-based sensors provide a rich platform for sensing several metabolites, thus opening doors to newly desired techniques in biomedicine. Organic-based biosensors also offer the ability to be linked with enzymatic activity thus offering most of the required qualities of a sensor—selectivity, sensitivity, viability, quick response time, as well as reproducibility. These properties have thus been exploited in organic-based sensors producing promising results [125, 126]. For instance, Malliaras' group has pioneered the design of OECT-based bio-sensors, and has demonstrated

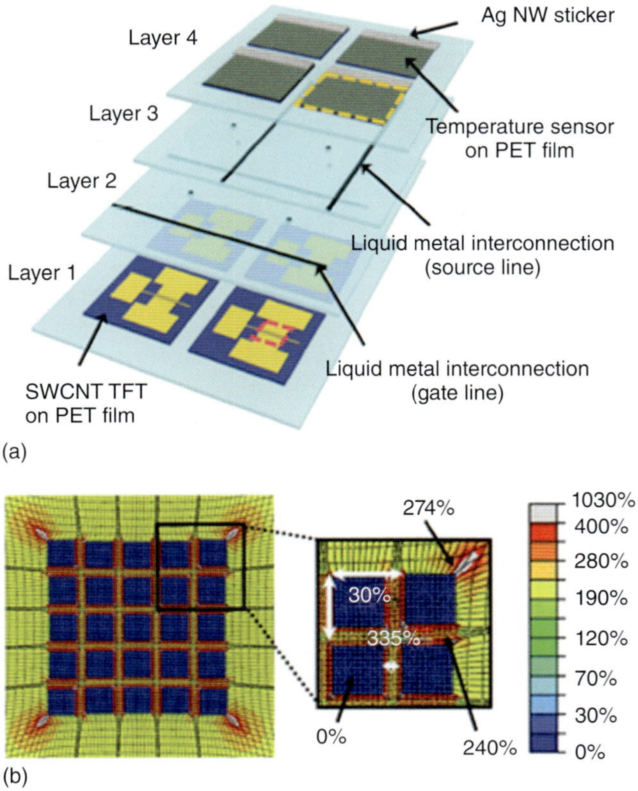

Figure 3.11 (a) Strucrture of a stretchable temperature sensor. (b) Strain distribution of the sensor during the stretching process. (Adapted from Ref. [114].)

applications for soft tissue interfacing. Figure 3.12a shows the layout of an OECT-based glucose sensor utilizing enzymatic sensitivity and selectivity on glucose [96]. The device detects the protons injected in the electrolyte layer as a product of the enzymatic glucose degradation. The device design was later coupled with fluorescent chromophores for direct optical monitoring of glucose levels (as shown in Figure 3.12b) [127]. Furthermore, the group later demonstrated the use of soft organic semiconductors, namely PEDOT:PSS, and achieved flexible and implantable electrodes for electroencephalography (Figure 3.12c) [33, 35]. These flexible arrays showed excellent stability at the brain–tissue interface, in combination with improved neurosignals compared to their inorganic counterparts. These organic-based systems are thus promising in terms of flexible implantable medical device design.

The combination of the properties discussed above allows for organic-based devices to answer questions that could not be answered before particularly in biomedicine. For instance, long-term implantation of the inorganic sensors has been limited by the performance degradation of the sensors due to their rejection by the immune system [35]. Another critical parameter for implantation of the device being their flexibility; rigid devices have the risk of damaging the targeted

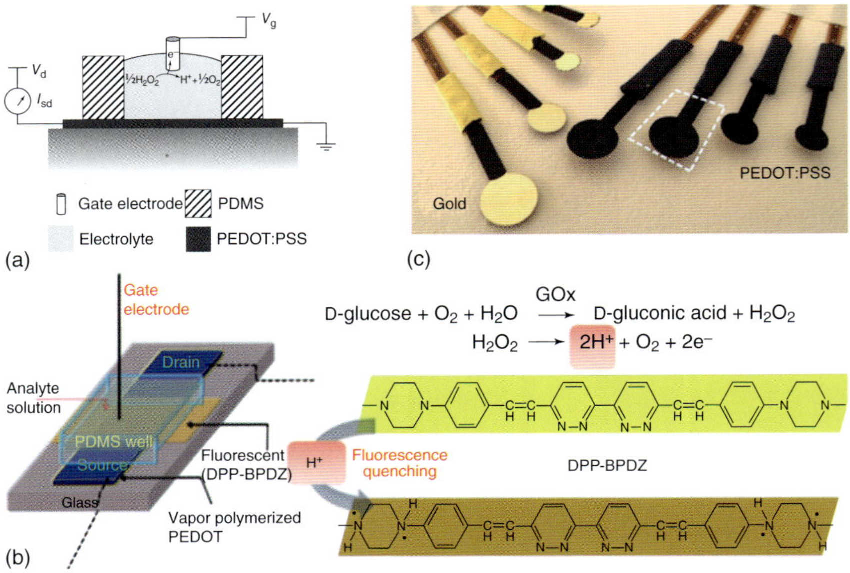

Figure 3.12 (a) Device layout of an organic electrochemical transistor-based biosensor for enzymatic sensing. The presence of analytes can be detected from the change in H^+ at the gate–electrolyte interface. The doping and dedoping of the ionic transporting channel layer is used to detect enzymatic-specific analyte. (b) Glucose monitoring using the detection of proton via fluorescence quenching. (c) Fabricated biocompatible electrodes for brain activity detection. PEDOT:PSS is used to coat the contacts for ionic detection and soft interfacing. (Adapted from Refs [35, 96, 127].)

organs in our bodies. Oftentimes, for brain–machine interface (BMI) applications, traditional devices made by silicon or metal needles arrays have shown to be unsuitable as the devices have to penetrate inside the brain tissue to acquire accurate and updated signals. With this lack of soft interfacing between the physiological world and currently available silicon-based technologies, flexible organic devices find potential applications in biomedicine and long-term implantation. In their efforts to circumvent these challenges for inorganic systems, Rogers' group recently demonstrated a series of work aimed at wireless optogenetics [128, 129]. These systems mainly include flexible needles, μ-ILEDs, microchannel for *in vivo* pharmacology, and wireless control module as shown in Figure 3.13. Notice that these systems are partially organic. The devices could be implanted either in the brain or in the spinal cord of rats and could be controlled by wireless signals from the outside. In principal, the medicine is primarily stored in the reservoirs and will flow through u-fluidic channels to the brain or spinal tissues. At the same time, the u-ILEDs at the tip of the needle will emit light to activate the ion channels of the cell for the injection of the medicine. The joule heaters will be wirelessly activated and will lead to the expansion of the reservoirs until the rupture of a Cu-membranes.

Despite the efforts of the Rogers group, a fully implantable long-term, flexible device is yet to be approved. Plenty of attention still needs to be paid to details

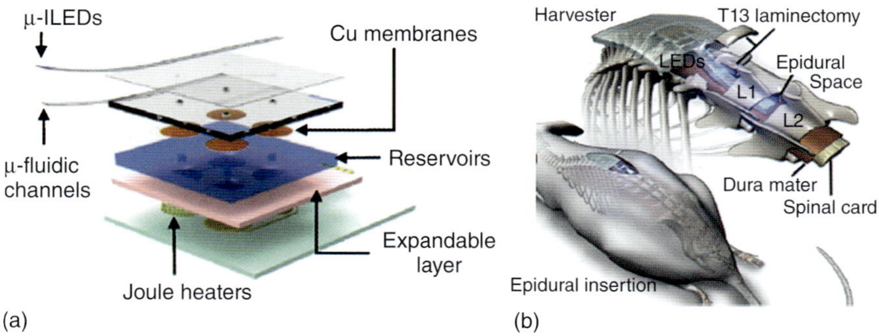

Figure 3.13 (a) Device layer of an μ-ILEDs-based wireless optogenetics system. The joules heaters are separated from medicine reservoirs by an expandable layer. The reservoirs and the encapsulating Cu-membrane can be wirelessly triggered to rupture by the heating and expansion of the expandable membranes. (b) Demonstration of the implatation of the optogenetic device in the spinal cord of a mouse. (Adapted from Ref. [129].)

such as the power source for such a device (implantable batteries [130]), the device's life, and transiency [128, 131, 132], as well as device conformity with physiological tissues; organic-based devices can potentially fulfill these requirements.

3.5.5 Flexible Organic Optical Sensors

There are several ways to design organic-based flexible optical sensors. Depending on the components of the desired devices, organic-based optical sensors can be divided into two main groups: OLED-based devices and devices based on organic wave guide. OLEDs-based sensors are by far the most widely studied structure in optically active electronics while wave-guide-based sensors tend to be coupled to pressure sensors [133]. OLEDs have offered various advantages owing to their rather simple geometry and ease with which they can be achieved on flexible substrates. Flexible displays have been under investigation, and one could safely argue that they might be the next novelistic marketable e-products. All organic-based light-emitting diodes have shown promising results in terms of achieving flexibility, finding applications in e-paper, bendable TVs, wearables, and low-cost monitors [134, 135].

In addition, OLEDs have been studied in combination with organic photodetectors (PDs). This combination of two designs expands the application of these optical sensors to fields requiring continuous monitoring such as healthcare. For instance Bansal *et al.* have demonstrated a wearable optical sensor to medical uses [136]. This sensor could be used in measuring signals from intact muscles to control the movement of active prosthetic devices and tissue oxygenation. In Figure 3.14, the device was fixed in a probe bandage around the upper limb. The wavelength and the location of the PD were carefully chosen to optimize the device performance. With the movement of the muscle, the scattering of the photons was observed to change, which could subsequently be detected by the PDs. In this way, the devices could be used to control a robotic arm.

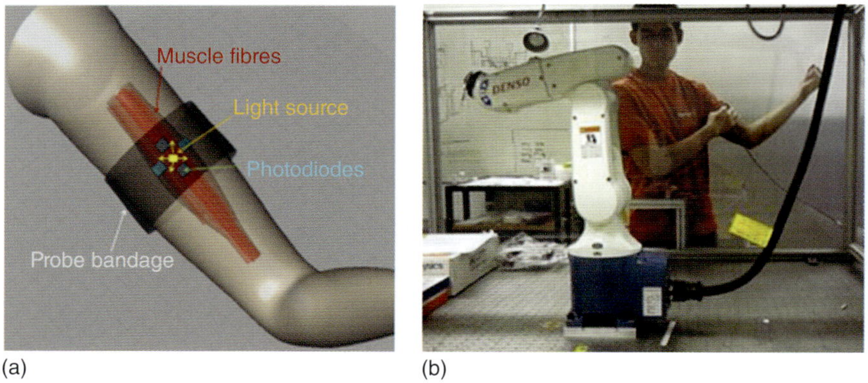

Figure 3.14 Demonstration of an optical sensor based on OLED coupled with a PD; (a) the bandage consists of one light source and four photodiodes to detect the movement of muscle fibres. (b) A robotic arm mimicking the arm movement of a volunteer. (Adapted from Ref. [136].)

3.6 Summary and Outlook

In this chapter, we present an overview of the recent advances in organic-based flexible electronic devices, including transistors and sensors. We have shown that organic transistors are excellent candidates for achieving easily patterned circuits for low-cost flexible electronics. We have also shown that by changing the structure and/or materials used, transistors can be designed for specific sensing platforms such as chemical sensors and biosensors. Different kinds of organic flexible sensors, including pressure, thermal, and optical sensors were demonstrated, and most of the sensors mentioned earlier have shown great potential for healthcare and wearable applications. Unlike inorganic materials, organic materials were demonstrated to be suitable for fabrication techniques including inkjet printing and screen printing to achieve roll-to-roll printing. Some organic materials are even compatible with the standard CMOS process, which shows their potential for large-scale and low-cost fabrication. Another important advantage of the organic-based flexible devices is their biocompatibility; how this feature has attracted special research interest for achieving "soft" devices, especially for implantable devices has been discussed as well.

Up to this point, we have described what has been accomplished in order to achieve flexibility and what materials have been studied for organic-based systems. We have even showed the applicability of some of the ubiquitous assays. We have yet to answer the question of what is next for organic-based devices. And the answer will ultimately be rooted in the fact that many researchers in this field would agree that achieving flexible electronics would revolutionize technology to the same level as silicon has. Not only have organic materials showed the ability to perform to the level of silicon, but also have presented properties that the future of technology is demanding. Performance milestones have already been achieved in flexible organic-based devices meeting the requirement for daily-use devices manufacturing. The research community in this field still ought to focus on the material design, as the intrinsic flexibility of organic materials seems to be taken for granted. Accessing intrinsically flexible (bendable and stretchable) organic semiconductors, organic dielectrics, as well as all transistor components would allow easy fabrication of highly flexible circuitries. A little more attention also ought to be paid to the device engineering in order to overcome resilient challenges such as devices' air stability and device mechanical durability, but nonetheless these platforms are ready to be turned into marketable products. Achieving easy roll-to-roll processing would extremely impact the fields of healthcare, energy, environmental sustainability, and robotics, to name a few. We hope to have guided the readers through current efforts toward achieving all-organic-based transistors and organic transistor-based sensors. We envision the great impact that these devices can potentially have as this seems to be an opportune time to question whether silicon-based technology has reached its apogee.

References

1 Miller, L.S. and Mullin, J.B. (1991) *Electronic Materials: From Silicon to Organics*, Plenum Press, New York.
2 Facchetti, A. (2011) *Chem. Mater.*, **23**, 733.
3 Forrest, S.R. (2004) *Nature*, **428**, 911.
4 Sirringhaus, H. (2014) *Adv. Mater.*, **26**, 1319.
5 Mei, J., Diao, Y., Appleton, A.L., Fang, L., and Bao, Z. (2013) *J. Am. Chem. Soc.*, **135**, 6724.
6 Dimitrakopoulos, C.D. and Malenfant, P.R.L. (2002) *Adv. Mater.*, **14**, 99.
7 Newman, C.R., Frisbie, C.D., da Silva Filho, D.A., Brédas, J.-L., Ewbank, P.C., and Mann, K.R. (2004) *Chem. Mater.*, **16**, 4436.
8 Reese, C., Roberts, M., Ling, M.-M., and Bao, Z. (2004) *Mater. Today*, **7**, 20.
9 Nomura, K., Ohta, H., Takagi, A., Kamiya, T., Hirano, M., and Hosono, H. (2004) *Nature*, **432**, 488.
10 Gelinck, G.H., Huitema, H.E.A., van Veenendaal, E., Cantatore, E., Schrijnemakers, L., van der Putten, J.B.P.H., Geuns, T.C.T., Beenhakkers, M., Giesbers, J.B., Huisman, B.-H., Meijer, E.J., Benito, E.M., Touwslager, F.J., Marsman, A.W., van Rens, B.J.E., and de Leeuw, D.M. (2004) *Nat. Mater.*, **3**, 106.
11 Yu, Z., Niu, X., Liu, Z., and Pei, Q. (2011) *Adv. Mater.*, **23**, 3989.
12 Mei, J. and Bao, Z. (2014) *Chem. Mater.*, **26**, 604.
13 O'Connor, B., Chan, E.P., Chan, C., Conrad, B.R., Richter, L.J., Kline, R.J., Heeney, M., McCulloch, I., Soles, C.L., and DeLongchamp, D.M. (2010) *ACS Nano*, **4**, 7538.
14 Kim, D.-H., Lu, N., Ma, R., Kim, Y.-S., Kim, R.-H., Wang, S., Wu, J., Won, S.M., Tao, H., Islam, A., Yu, K.J., Kim, T.-I., Chowdhury, R., Ying, M., Xu, L., Li, M., Chung, H.-J., Keum, H., McCormick, M., Liu, P., Zhang, Y.-W., Omenetto, F.G., Huang, Y., Coleman, T., and Rogers, J.A. (2011) *Science*, **333**, 838.
15 Li, T., Suo, Z., Lacour, S.P., and Wagner, S. (2005) *J. Mater. Res.*, **20**, 3274.

16 Printz, A.D., Zaretski, A.V., Savagatrup, S., Chiang, A.S.C., and Lipomi, D.J. (2015) *ACS Appl. Mater. Interfaces*, **7**, 23257.
17 Hu, L., Kim, H.S., Lee, J.-Y., Peumans, P., and Cui, Y. (2010) *ACS Nano*, **4**, 2955.
18 Plichta, A., Habeck, A., Knoche, S., Kruse, A., Weber, A., and Hildebrand, N. (2005) *Flexible Flat Panel Displays*, John Wiley & Sons, Ltd, p. 35.
19 Seung, H.K., Heng, P., Costas, P.G., Christine, K.L., Jean, M.J.F., and Dimos, P. (2007) *Nanotechnology*, **18**, 345202.
20 Andersson, P., Forchheimer, R., Tehrani, P., and Berggren, M. (2007) *Adv. Funct. Mater.*, **17**, 3074.
21 Simon, D., Ware, T., Marcotte, R., Lund, B.R., Smith, D.W., Prima, M., Rennaker, R.L., and Voit, W. (2013) *Biomed. Microdevices*, **15**, 925.
22 Vora, R.H., Krishnan, P.G., Goh, S.H., and Chung, T.-S. (2001) *Adv. Funct. Mater.*, **11**, 361.
23 Kaltenbrunner, M., Sekitani, T., Reeder, J., Yokota, T., Kuribara, K., Tokuhara, T., Drack, M., Schwodiauer, R., Graz, I., Bauer-Gogonea, S., Bauer, S., and Someya, T. (2013) *Nature*, **499**, 458.
24 Mattox, D.M. (2010) *Handbook of Physical Vapor Deposition (PVD) Processing*, 2nd edn, William Andrew Publishing, Boston, MA, p. 195.
25 Mattox, D.M. (2010) *Handbook of Physical Vapor Deposition (PVD) Processing*, 2nd edn, William Andrew Publishing, Boston, MA, p. 237.
26 Greer, J.R., Oliver, W.C., and Nix, W.D. (2005) *Acta Mater.*, **53**, 1821.
27 Klauk, H., Huang, J.-R., Nichols, J.A., and Jackson, T.N. (2000) *Thin Solid Films*, **366**, 272.
28 Li, Y.Q., Tang, J.X., Xie, Z.Y., Hung, L.S., and Lau, S.S. (2004) *Chem. Phys. Lett.*, **386**, 128.
29 Salinas, J.-F., Yip, H.-L., Chueh, C.-C., Li, C.-Z., Maldonado, J.-L., and Jen, A.K.Y. (2012) *Adv. Mater.*, **24**, 6362.
30 Shirakawa, H., Louis, E.J., MacDiarmid, A.G., Chiang, C.K., and Heeger, A.J. (1977) *J. Chem. Soc., Chem. Commun.*, 578.
31 Mabeck, J.T. and Malliaras, G.G. (2006) *Anal. Bioanal. Chem.*, **384**, 343.
32 Takamatsu, S., Lonjaret, T., Ismailova, E., Masuda, A., Itoh, T., and Malliaras, G.G. (2015) *Adv. Mater.*, **28**, 4485.
33 Khodagholy, D., Doublet, T., Gurfinkel, M., Quilichini, P., Ismailova, E., Leleux, P., Herve, T., Sanaur, S., Bernard, C., and Malliaras, G.G. (2011) *Adv. Mater.*, **23**, H268.
34 Kim, Y.H., Sachse, C., Machala, M.L., May, C., Müller-Meskamp, L., and Leo, K. (2011) *Adv. Funct. Mater.*, **21**, 1076.
35 Leleux, P., Badier, J.-M., Rivnay, J., Bénar, C., Hervé, T., Chauvel, P., and Malliaras, G.G. (2014) *Adv. Healthc. Mater.*, **3**, 490.
36 Snook, G.A., Kao, P., and Best, A.S. (2011) *J. Power Sources*, **196**, 1.
37 Sekine, S., Ido, Y., Miyake, T., Nagamine, K., and Nishizawa, M. (2010) *J. Am. Chem. Soc.*, **132**, 13174.
38 Ryu, K.S., Lee, Y.G., Hong, Y.S., Park, Y.J., Wu, X., Kim, K.M., Kang, M.G., Park, N.G., and Chang, S.H. (2004) *Electrochim. Acta*, **50**, 843.

39 Baughman, R.H., Zakhidov, A.A., and de Heer, W.A. (2002) *Science*, **297**, 787.
40 Niu, C., Sichel, E.K., Hoch, R., Moy, D., and Tennent, H. (1997) *Appl. Phys. Lett.*, **70**, 1480.
41 Rubianes, M.A.D. and Rivas, G.A. (2003) *Electrochem. Commun.*, **5**, 689.
42 Musameh, M., Wang, J., Merkoci, A., and Lin, Y. (2002) *Electrochem. Commun.*, **4**, 743.
43 Vitale, F., Summerson, S.R., Aazhang, B., Kemere, C., and Pasquali, M. (2015) *ACS Nano*, **9**, 4465.
44 Kim, D.-H., Viventi, J., Amsden, J.J., Xiao, J., Vigeland, L., Kim, Y.-S., Blanco, J.A., Panilaitis, B., Frechette, E.S., Contreras, D., Kaplan, D.L., Omenetto, F.G., Huang, Y., Hwang, K.-C., Zakin, M.R., Litt, B., and Rogers, J.A. (2010) *Nat. Mater.*, **9**, 511.
45 Birthe, R., Conrado, B., Robert, O., Pascal, F., and Thomas, S. (2009) *J. Neural Eng.*, **6**, 036003.
46 Kang, H., Jung, S., Jeong, S., Kim, G., and Lee, K. (2015) *Nat. Commun.*, **6**, 6503.
47 Zang, Y., Zhang, F., Huang, D., Di, C.-A., and Zhu, D. (2015) *Adv. Mater.*, **27**, 7979.
48 Hoerni, J.A. (1962) Google Patents, Method of manufacturing semiconductor devices. US Patent 3025589 A.
49 Facchetti, A., Yoon, M.H., and Marks, T.J. (2005) *Adv. Mater.*, **17**, 1705.
50 Klauk, H., Halik, M., Zschieschang, U., Schmid, G., Radlik, W., and Weber, W. (2002) *J. Appl. Phys.*, **92**, 5259.
51 Noh, Y.-Y. and Sirringhaus, H. (2009) *Org. Electron.*, **10**, 174.
52 Sirringhaus, H., Kawase, T., Friend, R.H., Shimoda, T., Inbasekaran, M., Wu, W., and Woo, E.P. (2000) *Science*, **290**, 2123.
53 Kawase, T., Sirringhaus, H., Friend, R.H., and Shimoda, T. (2001) *Adv. Mater.*, **13**, 1601.
54 Halik, M., Klauk, H., Zschieschang, U., Schmid, G., Radlik, W., and Weber, W. (2002) *Adv. Mater.*, **14**, 1717.
55 Roberts, M.E., Queraltó, N., Mannsfeld, S.C.B., Reinecke, B.N., Knoll, W., and Bao, Z. (2009) *Chem. Mater.*, **21**, 2292.
56 Yoon, M.-H., Yan, H., Facchetti, A., and Marks, T.J. (2005) *J. Am. Chem. Soc.*, **127**, 10388.
57 Jang, Y.; Kim, D. H.; Park, Y. D.; Cho, J. H.; Hwang, M.; Cho, K. *Appl. Phys. Lett.* 2006, **88**, 072101.
58 Tang, C.W. (1986) *Appl. Phys. Lett.*, **48**, 183.
59 Tang, C.W. and VanSlyke, S.A. (1987) *Appl. Phys. Lett.*, **51**, 913.
60 Tseng, H.-R., Phan, H., Luo, C., Wang, M., Perez, L.A., Patel, S.N., Ying, L., Kramer, E.J., Nguyen, T.-Q., Bazan, G.C., and Heeger, A.J. (2014) *Adv. Mater.*, **26**, 2993.
61 Yuan, Y., Giri, G., Ayzner, A.L., Zoombelt, A.P., Mannsfeld, S.C.B., Chen, J., Nordlund, D., Toney, M.F., Huang, J., and Bao, Z. (2014) *Nat. Commun.*, 5.
62 Zang, Y., Huang, D., Di, C.-A., and Zhu, D. (2016) *Adv. Mater.*, **28**, 4549.

63 Sheraw, C.D., Zhou, L., Huang, J.R., Gundlach, D.J., Jackson, T.N., Kane, M.G., Hill, I.G., Hammond, M.S., Campi, J., Greening, B.K., Francl, J., and West, J. (2002) *Appl. Phys. Lett.*, **80**, 1088.
64 Huang, J., Sun, J., and Katz, H.E. (2008) *Adv. Mater.*, **20**, 2567.
65 Defaux, M., Gholamrezaie, F., Wang, J., Kreyes, A., Ziener, U., Anokhin, D.V., Ivanov, D.A., Moser, A., Neuhold, A., Salzmann, I., Resel, R., de Leeuw, D.M., Meskers, S.C.J., Moeller, M., and Mourran, A. (2012) *Adv. Mater.*, **24**, 973.
66 Casalini, S., Leonardi, F., Cramer, T., and Biscarini, F. (2013) *Org. Electron.*, **14**, 156.
67 Buth, F., Kumar, D., Stutzmann, M., and Garrido, J.A. (2011) *Appl. Phys. Lett.*, **98**, 153302.
68 Cramer, T., Chelli, B., Murgia, M., Barbalinardo, M., Bystrenova, E., de Leeuw, D.M., and Biscarini, F. (2013) *Phys. Chem. Chem. Phys.*, **15**, 3897.
69 Nilsson, D., Kugler, T., Svensson, P.-O., and Berggren, M. (2002) *Sens. Actuators, B*, **86**, 193.
70 Rivnay, J., Leleux, P., Sessolo, M., Khodagholy, D., Hervé, T., Fiocchi, M., and Malliaras, G.G. (2013) *Adv. Mater.*, **25**, 7010.
71 Lin, P., Yan, F., and Chan, H.L.W. (2010) *ACS Appl. Mater. Interfaces*, **2**, 1637.
72 Yun, M., Sharma, A., Fuentes-Hernandez, C., Hwang, D.K., Dindar, A., Singh, S., Choi, S., and Kippelen, B. (2014) *ACS Appl. Mater. Interfaces*, **6**, 1616.
73 Tsumura, A., Koezuka, H., and Ando, T. (1986) *Appl. Phys. Lett.*, **49**, 1210.
74 Ma, L. and Yang, Y. (2004) *Appl. Phys. Lett.*, **85**, 5084.
75 Ben-Sasson, A.J., Greenman, M., Roichman, Y., and Tessler, N. (2014) *Isr. J. Chem.*, **54**, 568.
76 Liu, B., McCarthy, M.A., Yoon, Y., Kim, D.Y., Wu, Z., So, F., Holloway, P.H., Reynolds, J.R., Guo, J., and Rinzler, A.G. (2008) *Adv. Mater.*, **20**, 3605.
77 Günther, A.A., Sawatzki, M., Formánek, P., Kasemann, D., and Leo, K. (2016) *Adv. Funct. Mater.*, **26**, 768.
78 McCarthy, M.A., Liu, B., Jayaraman, R., Gilbert, S.M., Kim, D.Y., So, F., and Rinzler, A.G. (2011) *ACS Nano*, **5**, 291.
79 Ben-Sasson, A.J., Avnon, E., Ploshnik, E., Globerman, O., Shenhar, R., Frey, G.L., and Tessler, N. (2009) *Appl. Phys. Lett.*, **95**, 213301.
80 Kim, K., Lee, T.H., Santos, E.J.G., Jo, P.S., Salleo, A., Nishi, Y., and Bao, Z. (2015) *ACS Nano*, **9**, 5922.
81 Pierret, R.F. (1996) *Semiconductor Device Fundamentals*, Addison-Wesley, Reading, MA.
82 McCulloch, I., Salleo, A., and Chabinyc, M. (2016) *Science*, **352**, 1521.
83 Bittle, E.G., Basham, J.I., Jackson, T.N., Jurchescu, O.D., and Gundlach, D.J. (2016) *Nat. Commun.*, **7**, 10908.
84 Kergoat, L., Piro, B., Berggren, M., Horowitz, G., and Pham, M.-C. (2011) *Anal. Bioanal. Chem.*, **402**, 1813.
85 Bergveld, P. (1972) *IEEE Trans. Biomed. Eng.*, **BME-19**, 342.
86 Schmidt, E.M., McIntosh, J.S., and Bak, M.J. (1988) *Med. Biol. Eng. Comput.*, **26**, 96.

87 Huang, W., Diallo, A.K., Dailey, J.L., Besar, K., and Katz, H.E. (2015) *J. Mater. Chem. C*, **3**, 6445.
88 Park, Y.M. and Salleo, A. (2009) *Appl. Phys. Lett.*, **95**, 133307.
89 Loi, A., Manunza, I., and Bonfiglio, A. (2005) *Appl. Phys. Lett.*, **86**, 103512.
90 Bartic, C., Palan, B., Campitelli, A., and Borghs, G. (2002) *Sens. Actuators, B*, **83**, 115.
91 Someya, T., Dodabalapur, A., Gelperin, A., Katz, H.E., and Bao, Z. (2002) *Langmuir*, **18**, 5299.
92 Roberts, M.E., Mannsfeld, S.C.B., Queraltó, N., Reese, C., Locklin, J., Knoll, W., and Bao, Z. (2008) *Proc. Natl. Acad. Sci. U.S.A.*, **105**, 12134.
93 Scarpa, G., Idzko, A.L., Yadav, A., and Thalhammer, S. (2010) *Sensors*, **10**, 2262.
94 Knopfmacher, O., Hammock, M.L., Appleton, A.L., Schwartz, G., Mei, J., Lei, T., Pei, J., and Bao, Z. (2014) *Nat. Commun.*, 5.
95 Bernards, D.A. and Malliaras, G.G. (2007) *Adv. Funct. Mater.*, **17**, 3538.
96 Bernards, D.A., Macaya, D.J., Nikolou, M., DeFranco, J.A., Takamatsu, S., and Malliaras, G.G. (2008) *J. Mater. Chem.*, **18**, 116.
97 White, H.S., Kittlesen, G.P., and Wrighton, M.S. (1984) *J. Am. Chem. Soc.*, **106**, 5375.
98 Kirchmeyer, S. and Reuter, K. (2005) *J. Mater. Chem.*, **15**, 2077.
99 Søndergaard, R.R., Hösel, M., and Krebs, F.C. (2013) *J. Polym. Sci., Part B: Polym. Phys.*, **51**, 16.
100 Shim, G.H., Han, M.G., Sharp-Norton, J.C., Creager, S.E., and Foulger, S.H. (2008) *J. Mater. Chem.*, **18**, 594.
101 Khan, S., Lorenzelli, L., and Dahiya, R.S. (2015) *IEEE Sens. J.*, **15**, 3164.
102 Roth, B., Savagatrup, S., de los Santos, N.V., Hagemann, O., Carlé, J.E., Helgesen, M., Livi, F., Bundgaard, E., Søndergaard, R.R., Krebs, F.C., and Lipomi, D.J. (2016) *Chem. Mater.*, **28**, 2363.
103 Hsu, Y.J., Jia, Z., and Kymissis, I. (2011) *IEEE Trans. Electron Devices*, **58**, 910.
104 Nam, S.H., Jeon, P.J., Min, S.W., Lee, Y.T., Park, E.Y., and Im, S. (2014) *Adv. Funct. Mater.*, **24**, 4413.
105 Someya, T., Sekitani, T., Iba, S., Kato, Y., Kawaguchi, H., and Sakurai, T. (2004) *Proc. Natl. Acad. Sci. U.S.A.*, **101**, 5.
106 Someya, T., Kato, Y., Sekitani, T., Iba, S., Noguchi, Y., Murase, Y., Kawaguchi, H., and Sakurai, T. (2005) *Proc. Natl. Acad. Sci. U.S.A.*, **102**, 12321.
107 Ge, J., Sun, L., Zhang, F.R., Zhang, Y., Shi, L.A., Zhao, H.Y., Zhu, H.W., Jiang, H.L., and Yu, S.H. (2016) *Adv. Mater.*, **28**, 722.
108 Boutry, C.M., Nguyen, A., Lawal, Q.O., Chortos, A., Rondeau-Gagne, S., and Bao, Z. (2015) *Adv. Mater.*, **27**, 6953.
109 Mannsfeld, S.C.B., Tee, B.C.K., Stoltenberg, R.M., Chen, C.V.H.H., Barman, S., Muir, B.V.O., Sokolov, A.N., Reese, C., and Bao, Z. (2010) *Nat. Mater.*, **9**, 859.
110 Wang, C., Hwang, D., Yu, Z., Takei, K., Park, J., Chen, T., Ma, B., and Javey, A. (2013) *Nat. Mater.*, **12**, 899.
111 Chou, H.-H., Nguyen, A., Chortos, A., To, J.W.F., Lu, C., Mei, J., Kurosawa, T., Bae, W.-G., Tok, J.B.H., and Bao, Z. (2015) *Nat. Commun.*, **6**, 8011.

112 Schwartz, G., Tee, B.C., Mei, J., Appleton, A.L., Do Kim, H., Wang, H., and Bao, Z. (2013) *Nat. Commun.*, **4**, 1859.

113 Lee, S., Reuveny, A., Reeder, J., Lee, S., Jin, H., Liu, Q., Yokota, T., Sekitani, T., Isoyama, T., Abe, Y., Suo, Z., and Someya, T. (2016) *Nat. Nano*, **11**, 472.

114 Hong, S.Y., Lee, Y.H., Park, H., Jin, S.W., Jeong, Y.R., Yun, J., You, I., Zi, G., and Ha, J.S. (2016) *Adv. Mater.*, **28**, 930.

115 Trung, T.Q., Ramasundaram, S., Hwang, B.U., and Lee, N.E. (2015) *Adv. Mater.*, **28**, 502.

116 Yokota, T., Inoue, Y., Terakawa, Y., Reeder, J., Kaltenbrunner, M., Ware, T., Yang, K., Mabuchi, K., Murakawa, T., Sekino, M., Voit, W., Sekitani, T., and Someya, T. (2015) *Proc. Natl. Acad. Sci. U.S.A.*, **112**, 14533.

117 Lee, C.H., Ma, Y., Jang, K.-I., Banks, A., Pan, T., Feng, X., Kim, J.S., Kang, D., Raj, M.S., McGrane, B.L., Morey, B., Wang, X., Ghaffari, R., Huang, Y., and Rogers, J.A. (2015) *Adv. Funct. Mater.*, **25**, 3697.

118 Tanese, M.C., Fine, D., Dodabalapur, A., and Torsi, L. (2005) *Biosens. Bioelectron.*, **21**, 782.

119 Bartic, C., Campitelli, A., and Borghs, S. (2003) *Appl. Phys. Lett.*, **82**, 475.

120 Voiculescu, I., Mcgill, R.A., Zaghloul, M.E., Mott, D., Stepnowski, J., Stepnowski, S., Summers, H., Nguyen, V., Ross, S., Walsh, K., and Martin, M. (2006) *IEEE Sens. J.*, **6**, 1094.

121 Choi, S., Lee, H., Ghaffari, R., Hyeon, T., and Kim, D.H. (2016) *Adv. Mater.*, **28**, 4203.

122 Liao, C., Zhang, M., Yao, M.Y., Hua, T., Li, L., and Yan, F. (2014) *Adv. Mater.*, **27**, 7493.

123 Liao, C., Mak, C., Zhang, M., Chan, H.L.W., and Yan, F. (2014) *Adv. Mater.*, **27**, 676.

124 Berggren, M. and Richter-Dahlfors, A. (2007) *Adv. Mater.*, **19**, 3201.

125 Nishizawa, M., Matsue, T., and Uchida, I. (1992) *Anal. Chem.*, **64**, 2642.

126 Macaya, D.J., Nikolou, M., Takamatsu, S., Mabeck, J.T., Owens, R.M., and Malliaras, G.G. (2007) *Sens. Actuators, B*, **123**, 374.

127 Yuna, K., Jaekwon, D., Jeonghun, K., Sang Yoon, Y., George, G.M., Christopher, K.O., and Eunkyoung, K. (2010) *Jpn. J. Appl. Phys.*, **49**, 01AE10.

128 Park, C.W., Kang, S.-K., Hernandez, H.L., Kaitz, J.A., Wie, D.S., Shin, J., Lee, O.P., Sottos, N.R., Moore, J.S., Rogers, J.A., and White, S.R. (2015) *Adv. Mater.*, **27**, 3783.

129 Jeong, J.-W., McCall, J.G., Shin, G., Zhang, Y., Al-Hasani, R., Kim, M., Li, S., Sim, J.Y., Jang, K.-I., Shi, Y., Hong, D.Y., Liu, Y., Schmitz, G.P., Xia, L., He, Z., Gamble, P., Ray, W.Z., Huang, Y., Bruchas, M.R., and Rogers, J.A. (2015) *Cell*, **162**, 662.

130 Bock, D.C., Marschilok, A.C., Takeuchi, K.J., and Takeuchi, E.S. (2012) *Electrochim. Acta*, **84**. doi: 10.1016/j.electacta.2012.03.057

131 Hwang, S.-W., Tao, H., Kim, D.-H., Cheng, H., Song, J.-K., Rill, E., Brenckle, M.A., Panilaitis, B., Won, S.M., Kim, Y.-S., Song, Y.M., Yu, K.J., Ameen, A., Li, R., Su, Y., Yang, M., Kaplan, D.L., Zakin, M.R., Slepian, M.J., Huang, Y., Omenetto, F.G., and Rogers, J.A. (2012) *Science*, **337**, 1640.

132 Hwang, S.-W., Song, J.-K., Huang, X., Cheng, H., Kang, S.-K., Kim, B.H., Kim, J.-H., Yu, S., Huang, Y., and Rogers, J.A. (2014) *Adv. Mater.*, **26**, 3905.

133 Yun, S., Park, S., Park, B., Kim, Y., Park, S.K., Nam, S., and Kyung, K.-U. (2014) *Adv. Mater.*, **26**, 4474.

134 Sekitani, T., Nakajima, H., Maeda, H., Fukushima, T., Aida, T., Hata, K., and Someya, T. (2009) *Nat. Mater.*, **8**, 494.

135 Jain, K., Klosner, M., Zemel, M., and Raghunandan, S. (2005) *Proc. IEEE*, **93**, 1500.

136 Bansal, A.K., Hou, S., Kulyk, O., Bowman, E.M., and Samuel, I.D.W. (2015) *Adv. Mater.*, **27**, 7638.

4

Printed Transistors and Sensors

Kenjiro Fukuda [1,2]

[1] *RIKEN Thin-film Device Laboratory, RIKEN Center for Emergent Matter Science, 2-1, Hirosawa, 2-1 Wako, Saitama 351-0198, Japan*
[2] *Japan Science and Technology Agency, PRESTO, 4-1-8, Honcho, Kawaguchi, Saitama 332-0012, Japan*

4.1 Introduction

Printed electronics has been attracting significant attention from fundamental research groups to industries because the marriage of conductive, insulating, and semiconducting materials with printing technologies enables one to make thin, lightweight, and large-area electronic devices and systems. Organic materials possess intrinsic mechanical flexibility because of their loose Van der Waals bonding between organic molecules, and they make durable flexible organic devices feasible [1]. A recent study reported that high-performance organic thin-film transistors (TFTs) with printed semiconducting layers exhibited high carrier mobilities greater than $10\,cm^2\,V^{-1}\,s^{-1}$ [2]. Such a high mobility will lead to novel applications of printed TFTs, such as flexible displays [3], radio-frequency identification (RFID) tags [4–6], sensors [7], and medical applications [8, 9].

Printing processes require different technologies from conventional vacuum deposition to photolithographic processes used for fabricating electronic devices because the inks and printed patterns are affected by rheological effects. In order to achieve high-performance printed TFTs and integrated circuits, both ink parameters and printing technologies should be carefully selected. Well-known printing methods such as inkjet, screen, and gravure printing, and other novel printing technologies are now being applied to fabricate electronics. Each printing technology requires different ink parameters and offers different resolutions and thicknesses of the formed patterns. Hence, to obtain the desired film, it is vital to consider the most suitable choice of ink and printing method to be employed. The important printing parameters are as follows [10]:

Resolution: Resolution concerns how close together the lines and spaces of printed patterns can be positioned. The resolution of the printing apparatus generally determines the final resolution of the patterns. The resolution of the cliché, or dot sizes in the case of digital fabrication without cliché such as inkjet printing, is an important factor in the resolution of any printing method.

Flexible and Stretchable Medical Devices, First Edition. Edited by Kuniharu Takei.

Accuracy: Accuracy concerns the extent to which repeated printed patterns have the same alignment. Low accuracy makes it quite difficult to form multistack structures with high resolution. In determining the accuracy of printing, both the repeat accuracy of the printing apparatus and the thermal deformation of the target substrate films should be taken into account.

Uniformity over a large area: This parameter focuses on the thickness of the patterns and lines/spaces. Printing methods require the ability to produce uniform patterns over large areas (ranging from several tens of centimeters to several meters). The drying process plays an important role in this uniformity, because most printing processes use solutions or semidried patterns.

Compatibility of inks with printing components: This parameter is concerned with whether a functional ink can be utilized for a certain printing technique. The viscosity of inks constrains the number of suitable printing methods. There are many other ink parameters that determine their compatibility with printing methods, such as the size of particles dissolved in the inks, adsorption of the solvent into the silicone blanket, adaptability of inks to doctor blading, and adhesion strength of the printed patterns to substrates/stamps.

Wettability of target substrate: The wettability concerns the extent to which the target surface is wetted by a functional ink. The wettability is mainly determined by the surface energy of the target substrates. Poor wettability can result in an aggregation of the applied inks, whereas excessive wettability may cause the lines to spread before drying. The surface wettability or surface energy of the substrates can affect the transfer of printed patterns from the blanket.

Throughput: The throughput concerns how quickly a printing technique can form patterns. One of the great benefits of printed electronics technology is mass production at a reasonable cost. The high speed and high quality of printed patterns should be maintained for hundreds of print operations.

In this chapter, the recent progress on fully printed organic circuits and biosensors using such circuits is introduced. Section 4.2 details several printing technologies that have been used for the fabrication of organic TFTs and circuits. In Section 4.3, fabrication processes of fully printed TFTs and specific technologies for printed electronic devices are shown. Finally, the biosensor application that uses printed organic circuits is introduced in Section 4.4.

4.2 Printing Technologies for Electronics

Printing technologies can be classified roughly into two types: printing without form plates (or cliché), and printing with form plates. Noncontact printing technologies that do not use form plates have an advantage over contact printing of allowing on-demand patterning. However, printing technologies with form plates have typically higher printing speeds (or throughput) than printing technologies without form plates, and so are more suitable for mass production. In this section, three kinds of printing technologies that are used for fabrication of printed organic TFTs are introduced.

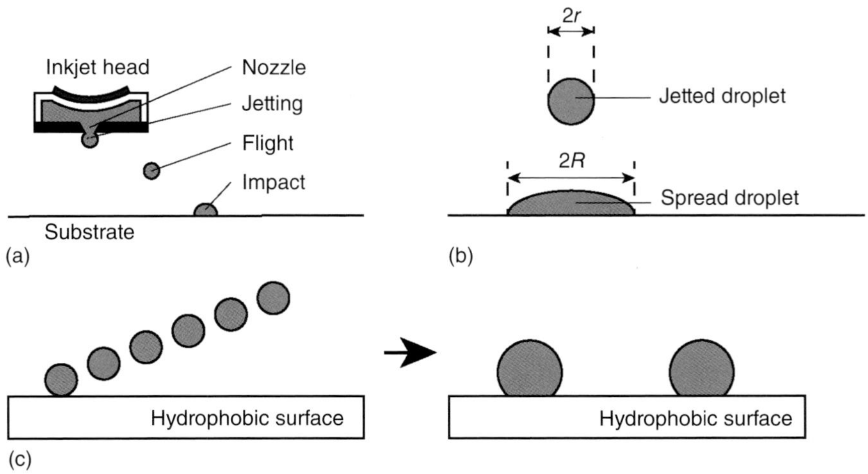

Figure 4.1 (a) Schematic illustration of inkjet process. (b) Ink spreading after application to the hydrophilic substrate. (c) Clumping together of the applied inks onto the hydrophobic surface.

4.2.1 Inkjet Printing

Inkjet printing, which is a representative form of noncontact printing, is widely used for the fabrication of printed electronic devices. Inkjet printing requires low-viscosity inks (approximately $10\,\mathrm{mN\,s^{-1}}$), and therefore typically uses metal nanoparticle inks for electrodes. For organic semiconductors, small-molecule materials are better than polymer materials because solution inks of small molecules tend to have lower viscosity than polymer solution inks. Inkjet printing consists of five processes: ejection from the nozzles, flight, impact on the substrates, ink spreading, and drying of the solvent [11, 12] (Figure 4.1a). The ejection and flight processes are partially controlled by nozzle conditions such as the voltage applied to the piezoelectric actuator, voltage waveform, and cartridge temperature. The typical volume of ink drops jetted from the inkjet head ranges from 1 to 100 pL [13, 14], which corresponds to a diameter greater than 10 μm. The normal flight speed of the droplet ranges from 1 to $10\,\mathrm{m\,s^{-1}}$.

The inkjet cannot control the droplet after ejection from the nozzles. The low viscosity of the ink causes the drop to expand after being deposited on the substrate (Figure 4.1b), which limits the resolution of inkjet-printed patterns. The spreading of the ink is affected by the surface energy of the substrate, substrate temperature, and ink properties. To reduce the spread of the ink, hydrophobic surfaces are preferable. However, excessive hydrophobicity prevents the formation of continuous lines that are absolutely necessary for electronic components because some droplets clump together to a location and can prevent stable patterns (Figure 4.1c) [15]. Figure 4.2 shows the patterns obtained from inkjet-printed silver nanoparticle inks by changing the drop spacing and substrate temperature. At low substrate temperature and small spacing, the line width becomes too large and straight lines cannot be obtained. At high substrate temperature, the spread of droplets can be suppressed and

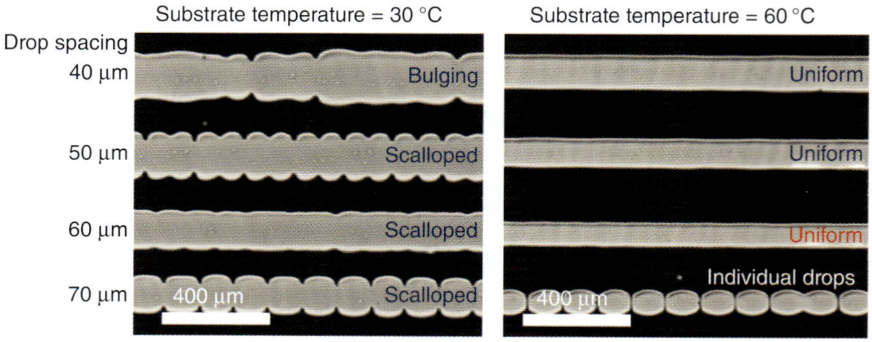

Figure 4.2 Examples of patterns obtained from inkjet-printed silver nanoparticle inks by changing drop spacing and substrate temperature. The surface of the substrate was coated by PVP. A relatively high substrate temperature (60 °C) and appropriate drop spacing (60 μm) enables narrow and uniform lines.

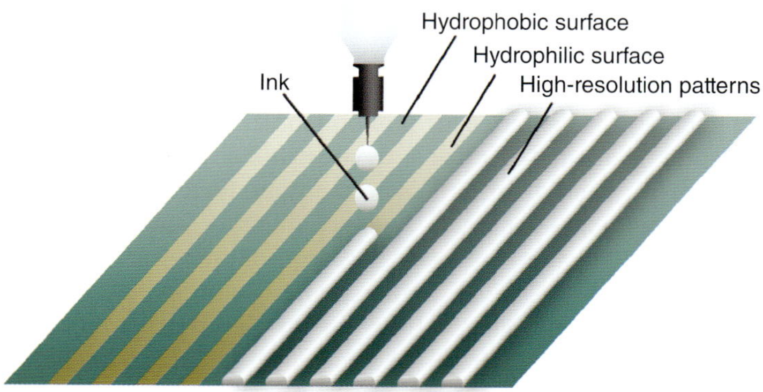

Figure 4.3 Schematic illustration of wettability contrast inkjet printing technique. The inks only remain on the hydrophilic surfaces, and so fine patterning can be obtained when wettability contrast surfaces are used.

straight lines can be formed onto the substrate; however, overly large spacing causes individual drops.

To downscale inkjet-printed patterns, wettability contrast surfaces are often used [16]. Hydrophilic silver nanoparticle ink does not remain on hydrophobic surfaces, whereas the inks that land on hydrophilic areas spread over the edge of the area (Figure 4.3). Thus, inkjet printing with wettablility contrast surfaces can achieve both high-resolution patterning and a high alignment margin. This wettability contrast technique can be applied to not only inkjet printing, but also other printing processes such as gravure printing [17] and spin-coating [18, 19].

4.2.2 Gravure Printing

Gravure printing is a kind of intaglio printing using an engraved plate. This is a very promising printing technique, and has been widely used for the fabrication

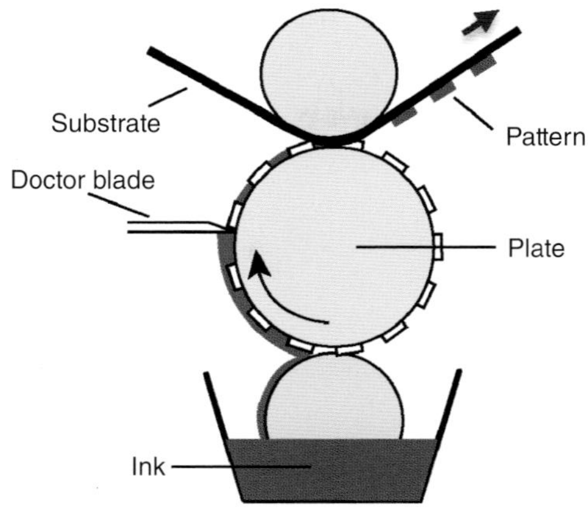

Figure 4.4 Schematic illustration of gravure offset printing.

of electronic devices because it can achieve high printing speeds of the order of 100–1000 m min^{-1} [20–22]. The process of gravure printing can be separated into three parts: ink filling to the form plate, wiping with doctor blade to remove excess ink, and transfer to the target substrate (Figure 4.4). The ink–transfer ratio in gravure printing processes is mainly determined by the capillary number C_a, which is given by [23, 24]:

$$C_a = \frac{\eta U}{\gamma},$$

where η is the apparent viscosity, U is the printing speed, and γ is the surface tension. The feature size of gravure printing is 20 μm [25]. Recently, Subramanian and coworkers reported high-resolution lines/spaces down to 2 μm at a printing speed of 1 m s^{-1} by optimizing the ink viscosity and print speed [24, 26, 27].

4.2.3 Reverse-Offset Printing for High-Resolution Patterning

Reverse-offset printing enables high-resolution patterning, high throughput, and scalability with a feature line width and space of 5 μm [28–30]. This technique can be divided into three parts: first, ink is coated on a silicone blanket (coating step); second, the ink-coated blanket is pressed softly onto an engraved glass surface to remove unnecessary areas of ink (patterning step); finally, the partially dried ink pattern remaining on the blanket is transferred to the substrate (transfer step) (Figure 4.5a). However, patterned inks are transferred onto the blanket in conventional offset printing, whereas reverse-offset printing conducts the patterning process after inking the blanket. Reverse-offset printing uses engraved rigid glass as the form plate and a flat blanket as the donor. Because the blanket absorbs the solvent from the ink coated onto it, semidried patterns on the blanket prevent the pattern from spreading after its transfer onto the substrate. Furthermore, reverse-offset printing enables fine electrodes to be patterned over large areas (Figure 4.5b). We fabricated reverse-offset printed silver electrodes with straight edges and line/space dimensions of 15/0.6 μm [28] (Figure 4.5c). The semidried patterns also enable thin structures with virtually no taper. The thickness of the reverse-offset printed silver electrodes was 100 nm, which is within the favorable range for TFTs and other multilayer stack electronic devices (Figure 4.5d).

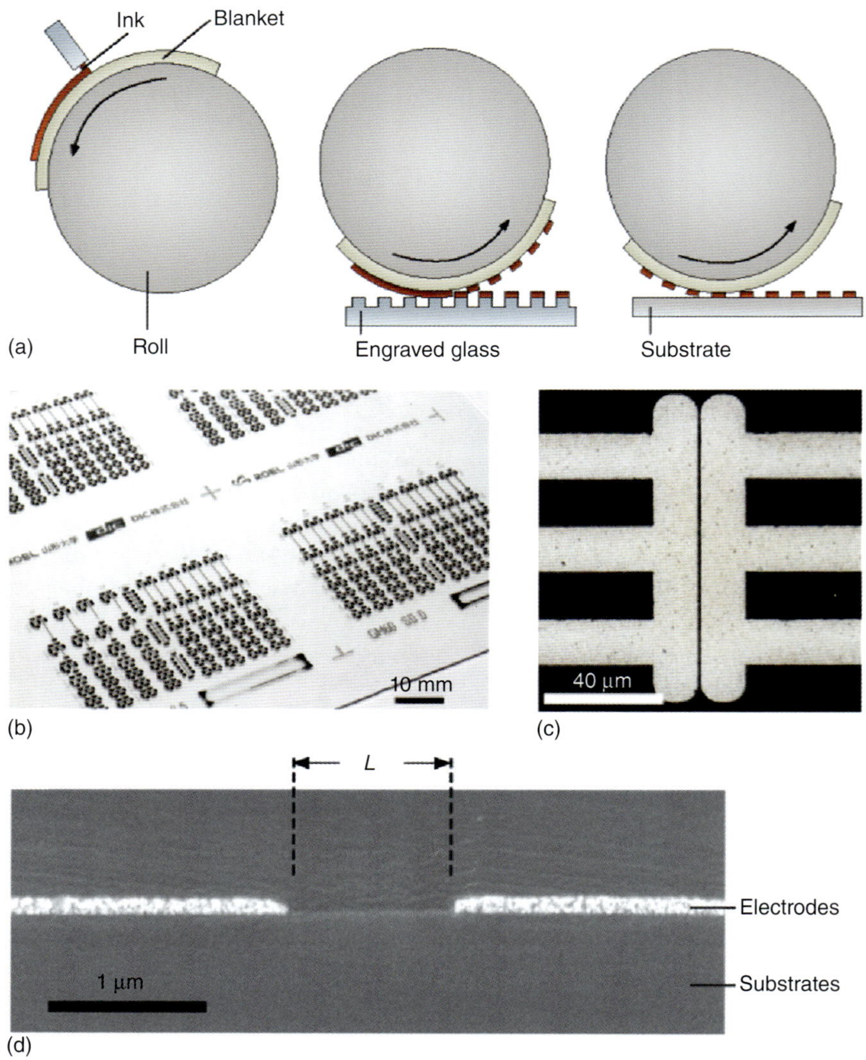

Figure 4.5 (a) Schematic illustration of reverse-offset printing: ink coating (left), patterning (middle), and transfer (right). (b) Top-view photograph of reverse-offset printed electrodes formed on 120 mm × 120 mm glass substrates. (c) Photograph of printed electrodes with a width/spacing of 15/0.6 μm. (d) Cross-sectional SEM image of the printed electrodes. (Fukuda *et al.* 2015 [28]. Reproduced with permission of John Wiley & Sons.)

4.3 Printed Transistors

4.3.1 Fabrication of Fully Printed Transistors

The typical structure and fabrication process of fully printed TFTs are shown in Figure 4.6. To minimize damage to the semiconducting layer, it is preferable that the patterning of the semiconducting layer is the final step of the fabrication

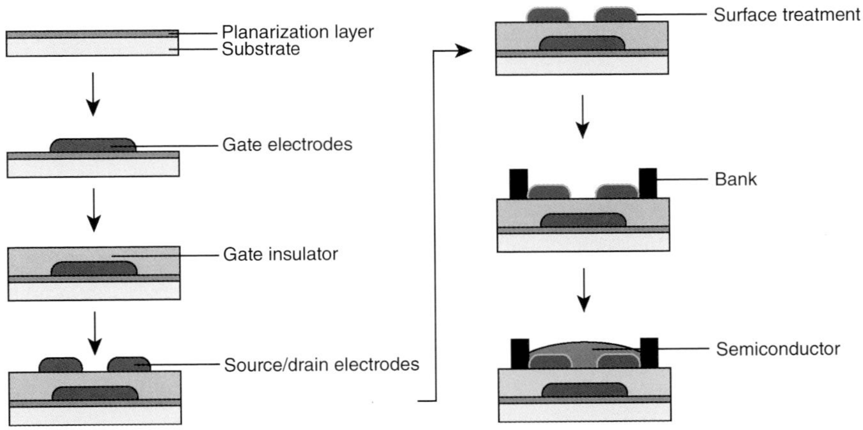

Figure 4.6 Fabrication process of fully printed organic TFTs.

process. To fulfill this demand, we used a bottom-gate and bottom-contact configuration for the TFT architecture. The surface flatness of the substrate directly affects device performance. Typical films such as polyethylene naphthalate (PEN) and polyethylene terephthalate (PET), which are used as base substrates of electronic devices, have a surface roughness comparable to that of Si substrates. However, thinner films have rough surfaces, with a root mean square roughness of more than 10 nm and a maximum height of more than 100 nm for randomly distributed peaks [31]. Therefore, a planarization layer is required for thinner substrate films. The surface wettability of both the substrate and the gate dielectric layer is also an important parameter for printed electronics. Hydrophobic fluoropolymer is often used in organic TFTs with top-gate configurations because the solution of such polymer does not damage the organic semiconducting layers; but such hydrophobic properties or low surface energies make it quite difficult to print appropriate patterns onto the surfaces. Because TFTs have vertically stacked structures, bottom gate electrodes should have thin thickness and uniform flatness to achieve better insulating properties between the bottom electrodes and top source/drain electrodes.

4.3.2 Profile Control of Inkjet-Printed Electrodes

As mentioned in Section 2.1, noncontact printing such as inkjet printing uses low-viscosity inks and thereby suffers from nonuniformity of the obtained patterns because of the so-called coffee-ring effect [32]. When printed ink dries on the surface of a substrate, the solute is generally transported from the center to the edge, and the resulting solute film forms a nonuniform ring-like profile. To suppress the coffee-ring effect and to obtain a flat pattern is one of the most important issues for printed electronics. According to a model that predicts the final shape of a dried thin film [33], solvent evaporation rate (J_s) and diffusion coefficient (D) affect the final shape of the film. The smaller value J_s or the larger value D more readily induces a convex shape. This is because diffusion tends to homogenize the concentration field contrary to the outward flow (Figure 4.7a).

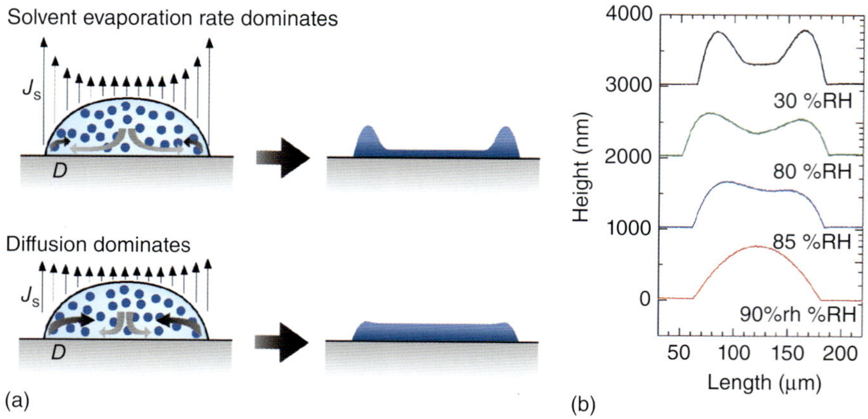

Figure 4.7 (a) Schematic illustration explaining the relation between solvent evaporation speed and final shape of drying films. (b) Profiles of inkjet-printed silver electrodes dried at relative humidity levels 30%, 80%, 85%, and 90 %RH. The drying temperature and drying time were 30 °C and 30 min, respectively. (Fukuda *et al.* 2013 [34]. Reproduced with permission of American Chemical Society.)

In order to control the final shape of inkjet-printed silver electrodes, we focused on how to suppress the J_s of the silver nanoparticle ink [34]. We used silver nanoparticles dispersed in a water-based solvent. Both environmental temperature and humidity decide the J_s of water, therefore we controlled the drying conditions and assessed the dependencies the ambient humidity and drying time on the profiles. The silver nanoparticle ink was patterned with an inkjet printer onto the cross-linked poly-4-vinylphenol (PVP) layers. After printing, the substrates were stored in a drying chamber in which both temperature and humidity were set to constant values. Temperature in the chamber was held at 30 °C, and relative humidity was changed from 30 to 90 %RH, while the storage time was fixed to 30 min. After the drying process, the substrates were heated to 140 °C for 1 h to sinter the silver nanoparticles.

Figure 4.7b shows line profiles (cross-sectional view) of printed silver electrodes dried at various humidity levels. The final shape of the electrodes was changed dramatically by changing only the relative humidity of drying chamber. The cross-sectional profile for a line with ambient humidity of 30 %RH was concave. These nonuniformities in silver electrode thickness are a result of the coffee-ring effect. This concave shape was suppressed by increasing the ambient humidity from 30 to 80 %RH, such that a nearly trapezoidal shape was observed at an ambient humidity level of 85 %RH. Furthermore, for ambient humidity levels of 90 % RH the silver electrodes formed a convex shape. These results clearly show that the water-based silver nanoparticle ink with low viscosity was very sensitive to the ambient humidity levels during the drying process. The uniform profiles can be obtained with appropriate humidity level (in this case, 85 %RH), and so the electrodes can be used for electronic devices with stacked structures.

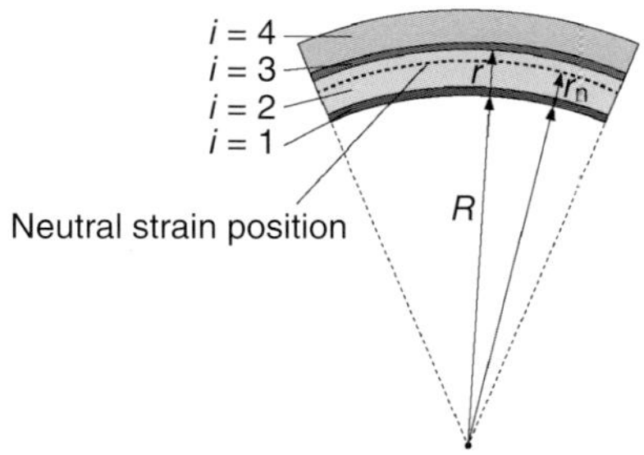

Figure 4.8 Location of the neutral strain position of multilayer stack film.

4.3.3 Mechanical Stability

4.3.3.1 Calculation of Strain in the Devices

The neutral strain position b of a device with multistack layers (Figure 4.8) should be calculated to consider the strain in the device. The neutral strain position b of a multilayer stack with the nth layer on top of the first layer on the bottom is given by [35]:

$$b = \frac{\sum_{i=1}^{n} E_i t_i \left[\sum_{j=1}^{i} t_j - \frac{t_i}{2}\right]}{\sum_{i=1}^{n} E_i t_i} \tag{4.1}$$

where E_i and t_i denote the Young's moduli and thicknesses of the individual layers, respectively. Assuming that the total thickness of the device, $t = \sum_{i=1}^{n} t_i$ is much smaller than the bending radius R, the bending strain at an arbitrary position r from the bottom surface of the device yields:

$$\varepsilon(r) = \frac{r - b}{R + b} \tag{4.2}$$

This equation indicates that locating the device in the neutral strain position can almost cancel the strain on the device, giving it robust mechanical properties [36]. If the substrate is sufficiently larger than the other layers, the strain equation can be simplified as [37, 38]:

$$\varepsilon = \frac{d}{2R} \tag{4.3}$$

Although this equation is often used for the devices with relatively thick (10 μm or more) polymer substrates, Eq. (2) is more appropriate for devices with thin-film bases down to less than 10 μm.

4.3.3.2 Improvement of Adhesion

Adhesion is an important issue for printed silver electrodes, as for other printed conductive materials. Although the adhesion of silver pastes can be improved by introducing a binder polymer [39], silver nanoparticle inks generally contain little or no binder polymers to reduce the resistivity. Weak adhesive strength complicates flexible electronics. However, adding binder polymers to the ink is not advantageous for device electronic performance because such binders often inhibit carrier injection from the electrodes to semiconducting layers [40].

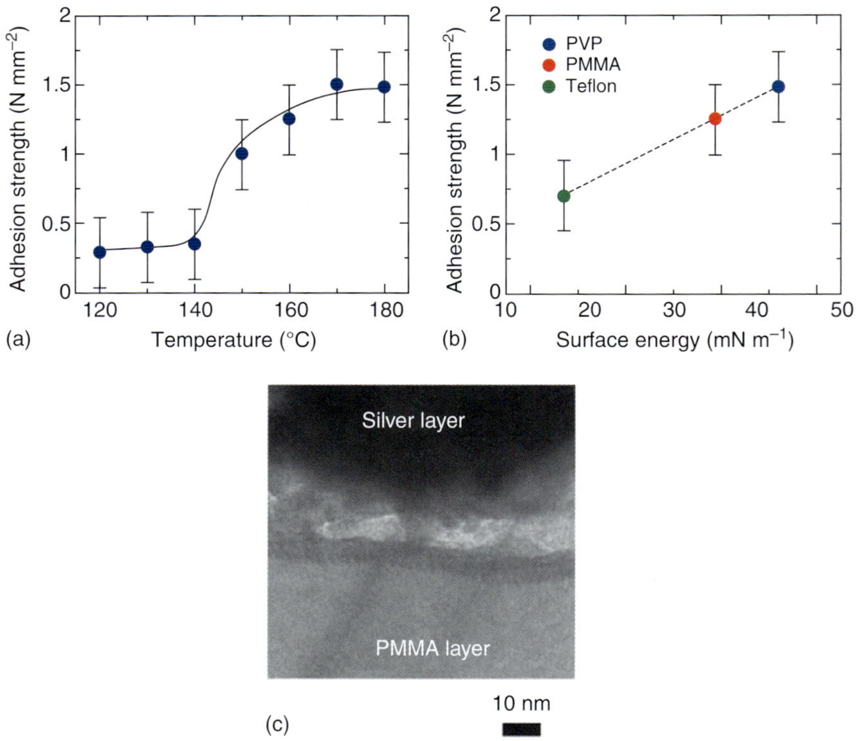

Figure 4.9 (a) Adhesion strength of printed silver electrodes on PVP interlayer as a function of sintering temperature. (b) Relative adhesion strength versus surface energy of the underlayers. (c) Cross-sectional TEM images of the interface between the silver electrode layers and PVP. (Reproduced with permission. Copyright 2015 [41], IOP publishing.)

A polymer interlayer with a low glass transition temperature (T_g) can improve the adhesion of printed silver nanoparticle inks, as the sintering process above the T_g of the polymer interlayer leads to a strong fusion between the printed silvers and polymers [41, 42]. Three kinds of interlayer polymer have been investigated: PVP with a surface energy of $44\,mN\,m^{-1}$, poly(methyl methacrylate) (PMMA) with a surface energy of $36\,mN\,m^{-1}$, and Teflon® with a surface energy of $17\,mN\,m^{-1}$. The adhesion of silver electrodes printed onto PVP increased from 0.4 to $1.5\,N\,mm^{-2}$ after sintering above the T_g of the polymers (Figure 4.9a), which is much higher than the adhesion of the electrodes onto a glass substrate ($0.3\,N\,mm^{-2}$). The adhesion is almost proportional to the surface energy of polymer interlayers (Figure 4.9b), indicating that the adhesion can be easily controlled by changing the internal polymer layers with appropriate surface energy and T_g. Cross-sectional transmission electron microscope (TEM) images revealed that interfused layers were formed between the printed silver and polymer interlayers, and that the thickness of the interfused layer depends on the surface energy of each underlayer (Figure 4.9c).

Using printed electrodes with high adhesion, no cracking/buckling of silver electrodes was observed even after outward bending with a bend radius of

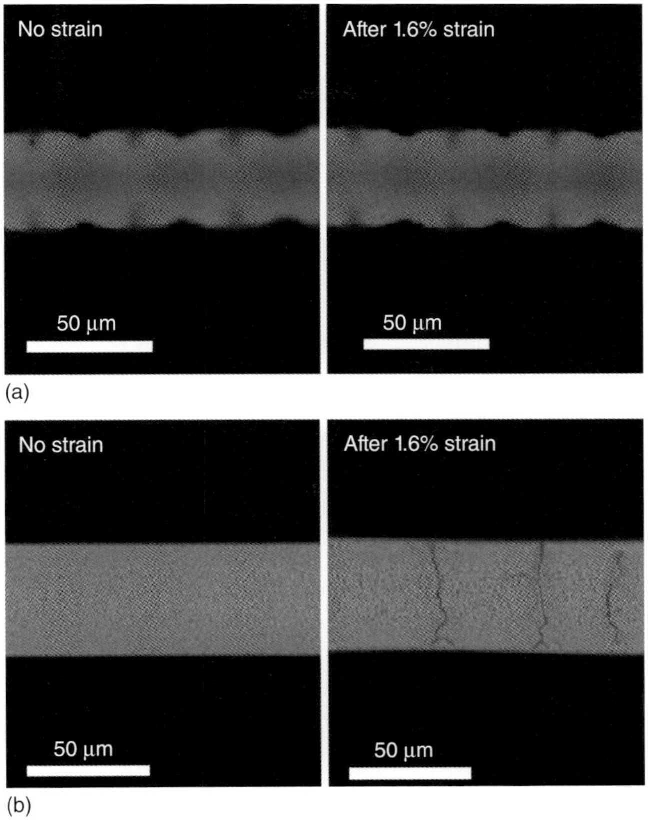

Figure 4.10 Photographs of printed silver source electrodes before (left) and after (right) the application of 1.6% tensile strain ($R = 4.0$ mm). (a) Silver electrodes with high adhesion and (b) with low adhesion. (Fukuda *et al.* 2013 [43]. Reproduced with permission of Nature Publishing Group.)

4 mm (1.6% tensile strain), and the electrodes exhibited almost the same surface after strong tensile strain (Figure 4.10a). In contrast, the silver electrodes with low adhesion exhibited cracking/buckling after the same strain (Figure 4.10b), decreasing the conductivity of the electrodes [43].

4.3.4 Printed Organic Transistors with Uniform Electrical Performance

Besides the high mobility, the uniformity of electrical performance is a key issue for printed electronic devices and systems to be used in practical applications. However, improvement of performance uniformity of printed TFTs is gathering less attention than improvement of high mobility. We proposed a simple technique for fabricating printed TFTs and circuits with uniform performances [44]. The combination of appropriate semiconducting materials with controlled growth of semiconducting films enables printed TFTs with excellent electrical uniformity. We used dithieno[2,3-d;2′,3′-d′]benzo[1,2-b;4,5-b′]dithiophene (DTBDT-C_6) as the organic semiconducting layer. A printed fluoropolymer layer was used as a confining bank layer, whereby the semiconducting layer was printed in the area defined by the bank layer using dispensing equipment. These printing techniques allowed accurate control of both the ink volume and the patterned area of the semiconducting solution. To avoid random generation of crystal grains, the dispensing point of the semiconducting ink solution was moved away from the center of the channel (Figure 4.11a). The resulting domain sizes of the semiconducting layer along the plane direction were more than 100 μm and the single-domain crystalline layers extended across the channel region between the source and drain electrodes (Figure 4.11b). The flow of the solution was constrained by the bank layer and *S*/*D* electrodes, allowing crystal growth to occur along the channel of the TFT devices.

Both the drop volume and layer area of small-molecule semiconducting solution can be controlled by the printing system, and this results in large single-domain crystalline grains that grow reproducibly along the channel. The organic TFT array with a 10 × 10 device layout on PEN film (Figure 4.11c) exhibited exceptionally uniform electrical characteristics, as well as almost 100% device yields (Figure 4.11d). The average carrier mobility obtained in this study was about 1.1 $cm^2\ V^{-1}\ s^{-1}$, which is higher than that of conventional amorphous silicon (a-Si) TFT devices. The average threshold voltage is -0.12 ± 0.09 V, which corresponds to a 0.4% spread in the operation voltage of 20 V (Figure 4.11e). This remarkable uniformity for our printed devices is comparable to evaporated TFT devices. Choosing an appropriate semiconducting material and developing appropriate printing techniques are both needed to make printed organic TFTs with superior electrical performance and uniformity.

4.3.5 Ultraflexible and Fully Printed Organic Circuits

Reducing the thickness of thin-film electronic devices is a primary goal in the field of flexible electronics, because it will improve both the flexibility and lightness of such devices. Recent progress has reduced the total thickness of flexible electronics to less than 1 μm [45], which makes electronic devices imperceptible and conformable to human bodies with little or no mounting stress. There has been a variety of applications using ultra-thin-film devices, such as integrated circuits [46–49], light emitting diodes (LEDs) [8, 50], solar cells [31, 51], magnetoelectronics [52], and sensors [45, 53–55].

The combination of such ultrathin properties and printing technology enables large-area, high-throughput manufacturing of imperceptible electronic applications. Although fabrication was originally based on the evaporation process, full printing processes have been adapted to make ultrathin- and large-area devices (Figure 4.12a) [47]. Printed ultrathin TFTs also possess high mechanical robustness; for instance, no discernible change was detected in the electrical characteristics of printed organic TFTs during the application of tensile strain with a bending radius of 140 μm, and the change in mobility was only 1.6% under this bending. When bent to a radius of 140 μm, the calculated strain was 0.5% [38], which caused a small change in the electrical performance of the TFTs.

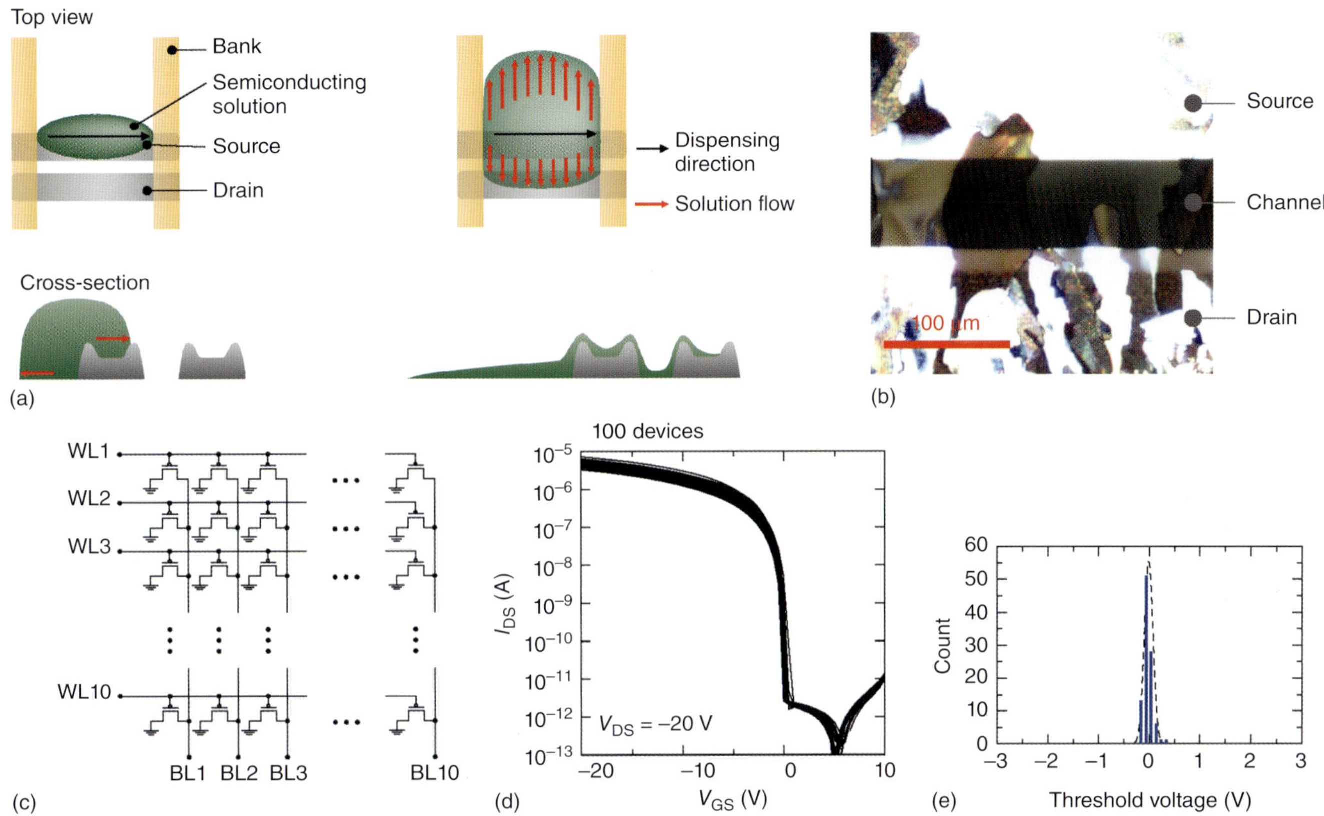

Figure 4.11 (a) Schematic illustration of flow of semiconducting solution. The dispensing point of the semiconducting ink solution was moved away from the center of the channel. Both bank layers and source/drain electrodes define the solution flow as shown by the red arrows in the figure. (b) Polarization microscope image of printed DTBDT-C_6 layer on parylene-C surface with source/drain electrodes. (c) Circuit diagram of the TFT array. (d) Transfer characteristics of 100 TFT devices in the array. (e) Distribution of threshold voltage as-measured results for 100 TFT devices in the array. (Fukuda *et al*. 2015 [44]. Reproduced with permission of John Wiley & Sons.)

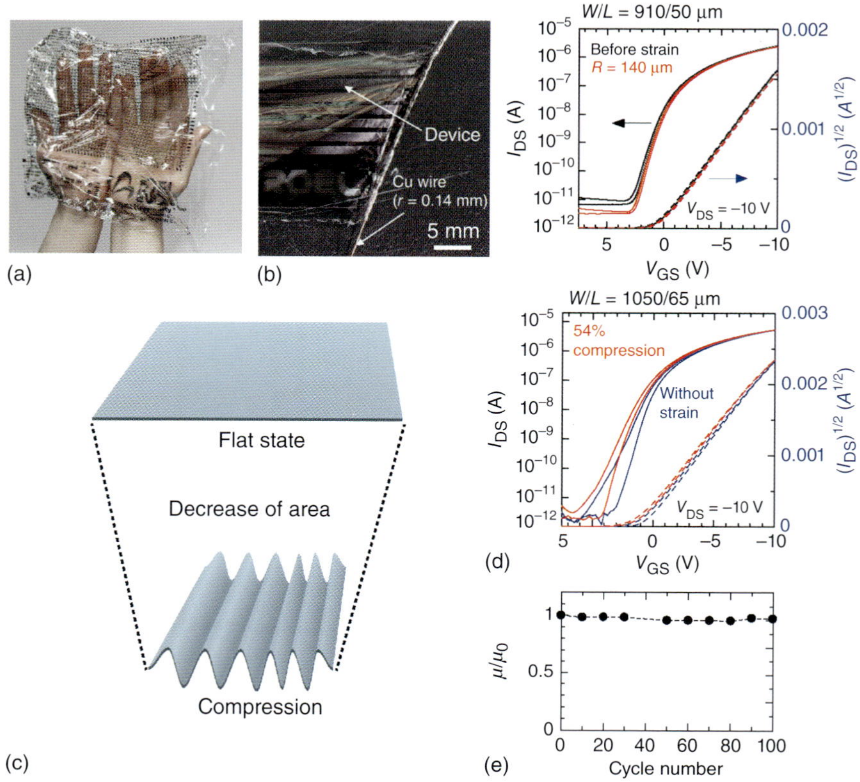

Figure 4.12 (a) Photograph of organic fully printed circuits fabricated on ultrathin films. (b) Photograph (left) and transfer characteristics (right) of TFTs wrapped around a copper wire with a radius of 140 μm. The TFT was measured in the bent and unbent states, with no discernible changes in the characteristics due to bending. (c) Schematic illustration of compression test. The compression forms out-of-plane wrinkles in the device, indicating the multiple bends with small bending radii of less than 10 μm. (d) Transfer characteristics of a TFT device operated under no strain (blue) and 54% compressive strain (red), demonstrating the mechanical stability of the fully printed TFT. (e) Mechanical durability during repeated compression and relaxation. The normalized mobility was plotted as a function of the number of cycles. (Fukuda *et al.* 2014 [47]. Reproduced with permission of Nature Publishing Group.)

Additionally, the printed circuits were fully functional and almost unchanged after 100 full cycles of 50% compression (Figure 4.13d).

Ultraflexible complementary *D* flip–flop circuits were also fabricated onto 1-μm-thick parylene film (Figure 4.13a and b) with a combination of newly developed printable n-type organic semiconducting material, benzobisthiadiazole-based material [56], and p-type material. The fabricated *D* flip-flop operated successfully at a voltage of 10 V, which clearly demonstrates the 100% yield of 40 TFTs composing each *D* flip-flop circuit including a buffer inverter (Figure 4.13c). The *D* flip-flop circuits functioned correctly at a clock frequency of 75 Hz, which corresponded to the estimated operating speed of the circuits in simulations.

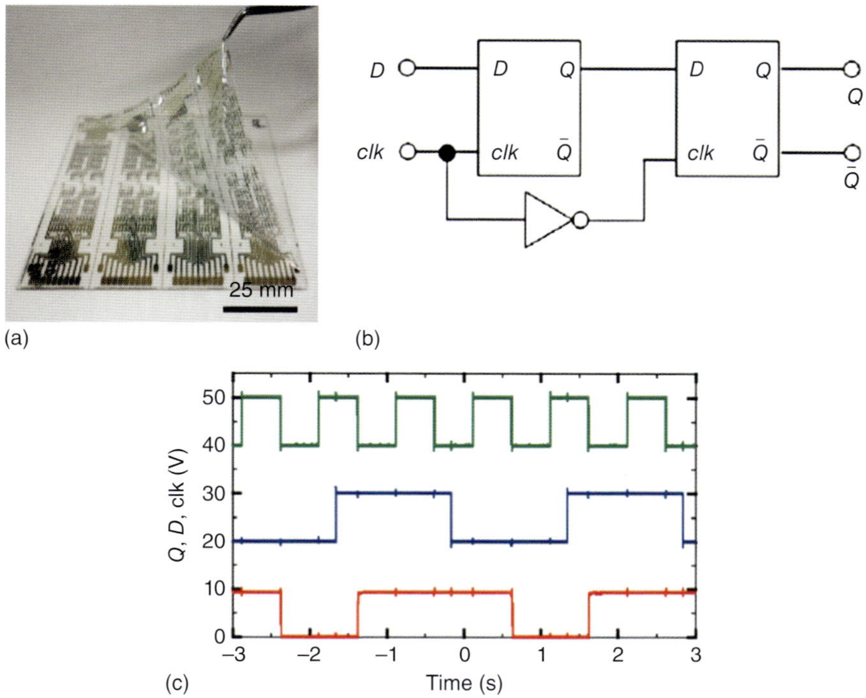

Figure 4.13 (a) Photograph of ultraflexible *D* flip–flop circuits. (b) Circuit diagram of a *D* flip–flop. (c) Dynamic characteristics with a clock frequency of 1 Hz and operating voltage of 10 V. (Takeda *et al.* 2016 [49]. Reproduced under CC BY 4.0; https://www.nature.com/articles/srep25714.)

4.4 Printed Biosensors

One of the most promising applications of printed TFT devices is in sensors requiring both high sensitivity and selectivity for use in healthcare [29]. Besides physical sensors, such as pressure or temperature sensors, chemical sensors that can detect specific materials in bodily fluids represent another important application for printed electronics. Creating low-cost electronic devices that monitor the health conditions of a patient has the potential to extend and improve their quality of life. Detection mechanisms for chemical species have been widely used, some of which are compatible with printing technologies [57].

For biosensor applications, we used extended-gate-type organic TFTs based on research work assuming that selective antibody detection is done in an aqueous solution using organic TFTs. In the designed device, the main TFT part is separated from the sensing site (the extended gate), enabling low voltage operation as well as preventing degradation by water. A gold (Au) thin film was employed as the extended-gate electrode, which easily allowed us to modify its surface with receptors. The detection of biological materials is based on an antigen–antibody reaction. A receptor can react to specific biological material (Figure 4.14). If the material has an electric charge, the reaction causes a change of electrical capacity

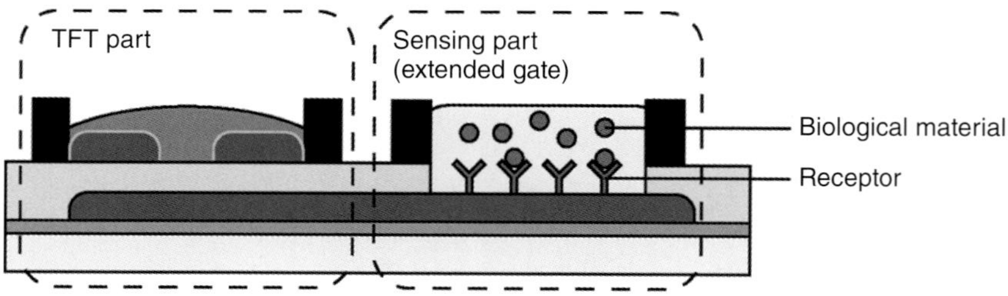

Figure 4.14 Schematic illustration of the organic TFTs with extended-gate electrodes.

between gate and source/drain electrodes then leads to a shift of threshold voltage of the TFTs. The shift of the threshold voltage or change of source/drain current has a correlation with the concentration of the target materials in the solution, so the biosensors have both selectivity and quantitative capabilities. Changing the types of receptors easily enables the sensors to work with different target materials. Several kinds of chemical species can be detected using printable organic TFTs with extended-gate electrodes, such as immunoglobulin G (IgG) [58, 59], glucose [60], cysteine [61], and Histamine [62].

To improve the sensitivity of the sensors, the amplifier circuit needs to suppress background noise and should augment only the small signals originating from the detection target. A differential amplifier is typically used for this purpose, and it requires the TFT devices to have uniform performance, because any nonuniformity will lead to a shift in the origin (zero-point) of the output signals. We fabricated a differential amplifier circuit consisting of two diode-load inverters (Figure 4.15a) using uniform printed organic TFTs mentioned in Section 3.4.2 [31]. The two inverter logic gates in the differential amplifier circuit had nearly the same input–output characteristics with reasonable small-signal gain values. For the biosensor application, the two inputs of the amplifier were connected to two extended gates (Figure 4.15b). Figure 4.15c shows the input–output characteristics of the differential amplifier with two extended gates. The switching voltage shifted from 0.57 to 1.16 V as the concentration of IgG on input A increased from 0 to 50 $\mu g\,mL^{-1}$. Figure 4.15d shows the relationship between the concentration of target IgG on input A and the change in differential output voltage, as calculated from the raw data. A positive shift in the input–output characteristics of the differential amplifier with increasing concentration in target IgG was clearly observed and a linear relationship was observed at low concentrations (<15 $\mu g\,mL^{-1}$). As the extended gate was not printed metal, this technique represents an alternative to printed metals, such as gold nanoparticle inks [63].

The development of both printing technologies and functional inks enables high performance and uniform printed circuits. The examples shown in this chapter exemplify that printed electronic devices have great potential for achieving novel applications that have particular properties such as disposability (low cost) and large size. The combination of printing technologies with flexible or stretchable substrates will open further novel electronic applications; the ultrathin and stretchy properties enable imperceptible sensing systems that attach softly onto human bodies and obtain biological information continuously.

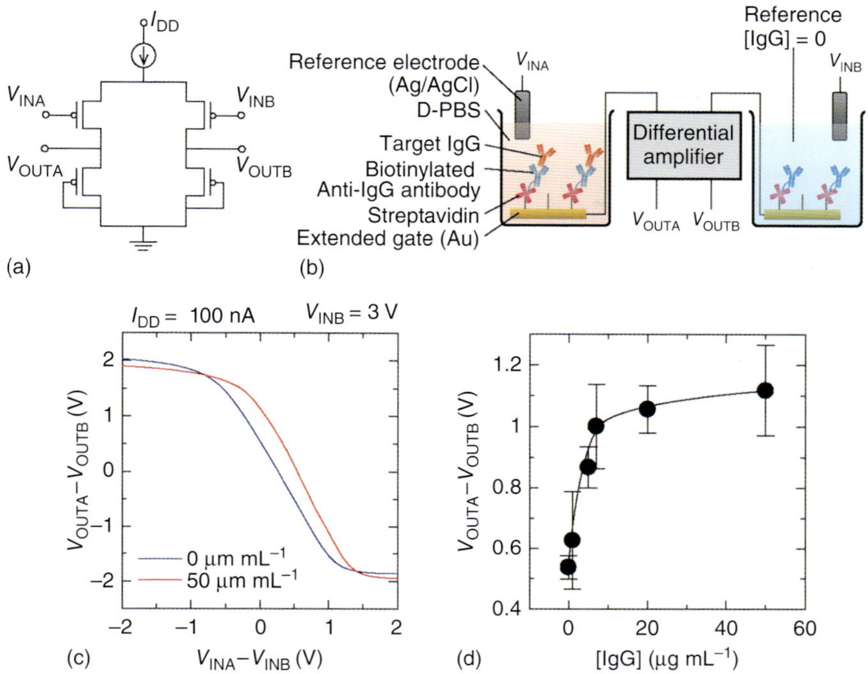

Figure 4.15 (a) Circuit diagram of fabricated differential amplifier. (b) Schematic illustration of the biosensor with differential amplifier. Two extended-gate electrodes (Au) were connected to each input of the differential amplifier. (c) Input–output characteristics of the differential amplifier upon titration with target IgG in a Dulbecco's phosphate-buffered saline (D-PBS) solution with 0.1 wt% bovine serum albumin (BSA). The blue line represents [target IgG] = 0 μg mL^{-1}, and the red line represents [target IgG] = 50 μg mL^{-1}. (d) Differential output voltage for the target IgG at various concentrations in a D-PBS solution with 0.1 wt% BSA. (Fukuda *et al.* 2015 [44]. Reproduced with permission of John Wiley & Sons.)

Further development of conductive inks and printing technologies will accelerate the industrialization of this new field of electronic applications.

References

1 Sekitani, T., Zschieschang, U., Klauk, H., and Someya, T. (2010) Flexible organic transistors and circuits with extreme bending stability. *Nat. Mater.*, **9**, 1015.

2 Minemawari, H., Yamada, T., Matsui, H., Tsutsumi, J., Haas, S., Chiba, R., Kumai, R., and Hasegawa, T. (2011) Inkjet printing of single-crystal films. *Nature*, **475**, 364.

3 Mizukami, M., Oku, S., Cho, S.-I., Tatetsu, M., Abiko, M., Mamada, M., Sakanoue, T., Suzuri, Y., Kido, J., and Tokito, S. (2015) A solution-processed organic thin-film transistor backplane for flexible multiphoton emission organic light-emitting diode displays. *IEEE Electron Device Lett.*, **36**, 1.

4 Myny, K., Steudel, S., Smout, S., Vicca, P., Furthner, F., van der Putten, B., Tripathi, A.K., Gelinck, G.H., Genoe, J., and Dehaene, W. (2010) Organic RFID transponder chip with data rate compatible with electronic product coding. *Org. Electron.*, **11**, 1176.
5 Yeom, C., Chen, K., Kiriya, D., Yu, Z., Cho, G., and Javey, A. (2015) Large-area compliant tactile sensors using printed carbon nanotube active-matrix backplanes. *Adv. Mater.*, **27**, 1561.
6 Matsuhisa, N., Kaltenbrunner, M., Yokota, T., Jinno, H., Kuribara, K., Sekitani, T., and Someya, T. (2015) Printable elastic conductors with a high conductivity for electronic textile applications. *Nat. Commun.*, **6**, 7461.
7 Yokota, T., Inoue, Y., Terakawa, Y., Reeder, J., Kaltenbrunner, M., Ware, T., Yang, K., Mabuchi, K., Murakawa, T., Sekino, M., Voit, W., Sekitani, T., and Someya, T. (2015) Ultraflexible, large-area, physiological temperature sensors for multipoint measurements. *Proc. Natl. Acad. Sci. U.S.A.*, **112**, 14533.
8 Yokota, T., Zalar, P., Kaltenbrunner, M., Jinno, H., Matsuhisa, N., Kitanosako, H., Tachibana, Y., Yukita, W., Koizumi, M., and Someya, T. (2016) Ultraflexible organic photonic skin. *Sci. Adv.*, **2**, e1501856.
9 Tee, B.C.-K., Chortos, A., Berndt, A., Nguyen, A.K., Tom, A., McGuire, A., Lin, Z.C., Tien, K., Bae, W.-G., Wang, H., Mei, P., Chou, H.-H., Cui, B., Deisseroth, K., Ng, T.N., and Bao, Z. (2015) A skin-inspired organic digital mechanoreceptor. *Science*, **350**, 313.
10 Suganuma, K. (2014) *Introduction to Printed Electronics*, Springer-Verlag, New York.
11 Kang, B., Lee, W.H., and Cho, K. (2013) Recent advances in organic transistor printing processes. *ACS Appl. Mater. Interfaces*, **5**, 2302.
12 Subramanian, V., Cen, J., de la Fuente Vornbrock, A., Grau, G., Kang, H., Kitsomboonloha, R., Soltman, D., and Tseng, H.-Y. (2015) High-speed printing of transistors: from inks to devices. *Proc. IEEE*, **103**, 567.
13 van der Bos, A., van der Meulen, M.-J., Driessen, T., van den Berg, M., Reinten, H., Wijshoff, H., Versluis, M., and Lohse, D. (2014) Profile inside piezoacoustic inkjet droplets in flight: comparison between experiment and numerical simulation. *Phys. Rev. Appl.*, **1**, 14004.
14 Martin, G.D., Hoath, S.D., and Hutchings, I.M. (2008) Inkjet printing – the physics of manipulating liquid jets and drops. *J. Phys. Conf. Ser.*, **105**, 12001.
15 Duineveld, P.C. (2003) The stability of ink-jet printed lines of liquid with zero receding contact angle on a homogeneous substrate. *J. Fluid Mech.*, **477**, 175.
16 Suzuki, K., Yutani, K., Nakashima, M., Onodera, A., Mizukami, S., Kato, M., Tano, T., and Tomono, H. (2011) Fabrication of all-printed organic TFT array on flexible substrate. *J. Photopolym. Sci. Technol.*, **24**, 565.
17 Zhang, H., Ramm, A., Lim, S., Xie, W., Ahn, B.Y., Xu, W., Mahajan, A., Suszynski, W.J., Kim, C., Lewis, J.A., Frisbie, C.D., and Francis, L.F. (2015) Wettability contrast gravure printing. *Adv. Mater.*, **27**, 7420.
18 Fukuda, K., Takeda, Y., Kobayashi, Y., Shimizu, M., Sekine, T., Kumaki, D., Kurihara, M., Sakamoto, M., and Tokito, S. (2013) Patterning method for silver nanoparticle electrodes in fully solution-processed organic thin-film transistors using selectively treated hydrophilic and hydrophobic surfaces. *Jpn. J. Appl. Phys.*, **52**, 50.

19 Sugano, R., Takeda, Y., Kobayashi, Y., Fukuda, K., Kumaki, D., and Tokito, S. (2014) Fine patterning method for silver nanoparticle electrodes using differential hydrophobic and hydrophilic surface properties. *Jpn. J. Appl. Phys.*, **53**, 04EK01.

20 Jung, M., Kim, J., Noh, J., Lim, N., Lim, C., Lee, G., Kim, J., Kang, H., Jung, K., Leonard, A.D., Tour, J.M., and Cho, G. (2010) All-printed and roll-to-roll-printable 13.56-MHz-operated 1-bit RF tag on plastic foils. *IEEE Trans. Electron Devices*, **57**, 571.

21 Jung, Y., Park, H., Park, J.-A., Noh, J., Choi, Y., Jung, M., Jung, K., Pyo, M., Chen, K., Javey, A., and Cho, G. (2015) Fully printed flexible and disposable wireless cyclic voltammetry tag. *Sci. Rep.*, **5**, 8105.

22 Hambsch, M., Reuter, K., Kempa, H., and Hübler, A.C. (2012) Comparison of fully printed unipolar and complementary organic logic gates. *Org. Electron. Phys. Mater. Appl.*, **13**, 1989.

23 Nguyen, H.A.D., Lee, C., Shin, K.-H., and Lee, D. (2015) An investigation of the ink-transfer mechanism during the printing phase of high-resolution roll-to-roll gravure printing. *IEEE Trans. Compon. Packag. Manuf. Technol.*, **5**, 1516.

24 Kitsomboonloha, R., Morris, S.J.S., Rong, X., and Subramanian, V. (2012) Femtoliter-scale patterning by high-speed, highly scaled inverse gravure printing—supporting information. *Langmuir*, **28**, 16711.

25 Hambsch, M., Reuter, K., Stanel, M., Schmidt, G., Kempa, H., Fügmann, U., Hahn, U., and Hübler, A.C. (2010) Uniformity of fully gravure printed organic field-effect transistors. *Mater. Sci. Eng. B*, **170**, 93.

26 Grau, G. and Subramanian, V. (2016) Fully high-speed gravure printed, low-variability, high-performance organic polymer transistors with sub-5 V operation. *Adv. Electron. Mater.*, **2**, 1500328.

27 Kang, H., Kitsomboonloha, R., Jang, J., and Subramanian, V. (2012) High-performance printed transistors realized using femtoliter gravure-printed sub-10 μm metallic nanoparticle patterns and highly uniform polymer dielectric and semiconductor layers. *Adv. Mater.*, **24**, 3065.

28 Fukuda, K., Yoshimura, Y., Okamoto, T., Takeda, Y., Kumaki, D., Katayama, Y., and Tokito, S. (2015) Reverse-offset printing optimized for scalable organic thin-film transistors with submicrometer channel lengths. *Adv. Electron. Mater.*, **1**, 1500145.

29 Kim, M., You, I.-K., Han, H., Jung, S.-W., Kim, T.-Y., Ju, B.-K., and Koo, J.B. (2011) Organic thin-film transistors with short channel length fabricated by reverse offset printing. *Electrochem. Solid-State Lett.*, **14**, H333.

30 Kusaka, Y., Koutake, M., and Ushijima, H. (2015) Fabrication of embedded electrodes by reverse offset printing. *J. Micromechanics Microengineering*, **25**, 045017.

31 Kaltenbrunner, M., White, M.S., Głowacki, E.D., Sekitani, T., Someya, T., Sariciftci, N.S., and Bauer, S. (2012) Ultrathin and lightweight organic solar cells with high flexibility. *Nat. Commun.*, **3**, 770.

32 Deegan, R.D., Bakajin, O., Dupont, T.F., Huber, G., Nagel, S.R., and Witten, T.A. (1997) Capillary flow as the cause of ring stains from dried liquid drops. *Nature*, **389**, 827.

33 Okuzono, T., Kobayashi, M., and Doi, M. (2009) Final shape of a drying thin film. *Phys. Rev. E: Stat. Nonlinear Soft Matter Phys.*, **80**. doi: 10.1103/physreve.80.021603
34 Fukuda, K., Sekine, T., Kumaki, D., and Tokito, S. (2013) Profile control of inkjet printed silver electrodes and their application to organic transistors. *ACS Appl. Mater. Interfaces*, **5**, 3916.
35 Kim, D.-H., Ahn, J.-H., Choi, W.M., Kim, H.-S., Kim, T.-H., Song, J., Huang, Y.Y., Liu, Z., Lu, C., and Rogers, J.A. (2008) Stretchable and foldable silicon integrated circuits. *Science*, **320**, 507.
36 Sekitani, T., Iba, S., Kato, Y., Noguchi, Y., Someya, T., and Sakurai, T. (2005) Ultraflexible organic field-effect transistors embedded at a neutral strain position. *Appl. Phys. Lett.*, **87**, 173502.
37 Sekitani, T., Kato, Y., Iba, S., Shinaoka, H., Someya, T., Sakurai, T., and Takagi, S. (2005) Bending experiment on pentacene field-effect transistors on plastic films. *Appl. Phys. Lett.*, **86**, 073511.
38 Gleskova, H., Wagner, S., Soboyejo, W., and Suo, Z. (2002) Electrical response of amorphous silicon thin-film transistors under mechanical strain. *J. Appl. Phys.*, **92**, 6224.
39 Shiyong, L., Ning, W., Wencai, X., and Yong, L. (2008) Preparation and rheological behavior of lead free silver conducting paste. *Mater. Chem. Phys.*, **111**, 20.
40 Takeda, Y., Yoshimura, Y., Kobayashi, Y., Kumaki, D., Fukuda, K., and Tokito, S. (2013) Integrated circuits using fully solution-processed organic TFT devices with printed silver electrodes. *Org. Electron.*, **14**, 3362.
41 Sekine, T., Ikeda, H., Kosakai, A., Fukuda, K., Kumaki, D., and Tokito, S. (2014) Improvement of mechanical durability on organic TFT with printed electrodes prepared from nanoparticle ink. *Appl. Surf. Sci.*, **294**, 20.
42 Sekine, T., Fukuda, K., Kumaki, D., and Tokito, S. (2015) Enhanced adhesion mechanisms between printed nano-silver electrodes and underlying polymer layers. *Nanotechnology*, **26**, 321001.
43 Fukuda, K., Hikichi, K., Sekine, T., Takeda, Y., Minamiki, T., Kumaki, D., and Tokito, S. (2013) Strain sensitivity and durability in p-type and n-type organic thin-film transistors with printed silver electrodes. *Sci. Rep.*, **3**. doi: 10.1038/srep02048
44 Fukuda, K., Minamiki, T., Minami, T., Watanabe, M., Fukuda, T., Kumaki, D., and Tokito, S. (2015) Printed organic transistors with uniform electrical performance and their application to amplifiers in biosensors. *Adv. Electron. Mater.*, **1**, 1400052.
45 Nawrocki, R.A., Matsuhisa, N., Yokota, T., and Someya, T. (2016) 300-nm imperceptible, ultraflexible, and biocompatible e-skin fit with tactile sensors and organic transistors. *Adv. Electron. Mater.*, **2**, 1500452.
46 Kaltenbrunner, M., Sekitani, T., Reeder, J., Yokota, T., Kuribara, K., Tokuhara, T., Drack, M., Schwödiauer, R., Graz, I., Bauer-Gogonea, S., Bauer, S., and Someya, T. (2013) An ultra-lightweight design for imperceptible plastic electronics. *Nature*, **499**, 458.
47 Fukuda, K., Takeda, Y., Yoshimura, Y., Shiwaku, R., Tran, L.T., Sekine, T., Mizukami, M., Kumaki, D., and Tokito, S. (2014) Fully-printed

high-performance organic thin-film transistors and circuitry on one-micron-thick polymer films. *Nat. Commun.*, **5**, 4147.

48 Bonfiglio, A., Mameli, F., and Sanna, O. (2003) A completely flexible organic transistor obtained by a one-mask photolithographic process. *Appl. Phys. Lett.*, **82**, 3550.

49 Takeda, Y., Hayasaka, K., Shiwaku, R., Yokosawa, K., Shiba, T., Mamada, M., Kumaki, D., Fukuda, K., and Tokito, S. (2016) Fabrication of ultra-thin printed organic TFT CMOS logic circuits optimized for low-voltage wearable sensor applications. *Sci. Rep.*, **6**, 25714.

50 White, M.S., Kaltenbrunner, M., Głowacki, E.D., Gutnichenko, K., Kettlgruber, G., Graz, I., Aazou, S., Ulbricht, C., Egbe, D.A.M., Miron, M.C., Major, Z., Scharber, M.C., Sekitani, T., Someya, T., Bauer, S., and Sariciftci, N.S. (2013) Ultrathin, highly flexible and stretchable PLEDs. *Nat. Photonics*, **7**, 811.

51 Kaltenbrunner, M., Adam, G., Głowacki, E.D., Drack, M., Schwödiauer, R., Leonat, L., Apaydin, D.H., Groiss, H., Scharber, M.C., White, M.S., Sariciftci, N.S., and Bauer, S. (2015) Flexible high power-per-weight perovskite solar cells with chromium oxide–metal contacts for improved stability in air. *Nat. Mater.*, **14**, 1032.

52 Melzer, M., Kaltenbrunner, M., Makarov, D., Karnaushenko, D., Karnaushenko, D., Sekitani, T., Someya, T., and Schmidt, O.G. (2015) Imperceptible magnetoelectronics. *Nat. Commun.*, **6**, 6080.

53 Khodagholy, D., Doublet, T., Quilichini, P., Gurfinkel, M., Leleux, P., Ghestem, A., Ismailova, E., Hervé, T., Sanaur, S., Bernard, C., and Malliaras, G.G. (2013) In vivo recordings of brain activity using organic transistors. *Nat. Commun.*, **4**, 1575.

54 Kim, D.-H., Lu, N., Ma, R., Kim, Y.-S., Kim, R.-H., Wang, S., Wu, J., Won, S.M., Tao, H., Islam, A., Yu, K.J., Kim, T., Chowdhury, R., Ying, M., Xu, L., Li, M., Chung, H.-J., Keum, H., McCormick, M., Liu, P., Zhang, Y., Omenetto, F.G., Huang, Y., Coleman, T., and Rogers, J.A. (2011) Epidermal electronics. *Science*, **333**, 838.

55 Lee, S., Reuveny, A., Reeder, J., Lee, S., Jin, H., Liu, Q., Yokota, T., Sekitani, T., Isoyama, T., Abe, Y., Suo, Z., and Someya, T. (2016) A transparent bending-insensitive pressure sensor. *Nat. Nanotechnol.*, **11**, 472.

56 Mamada, M., Shima, H., Yoneda, Y., Shimano, T., Yamada, N., Kakita, K., Machida, T., Tanaka, Y., Aotsuka, S., Kumaki, D., and Tokito, S. (2015) Unique solution-processable n-type semiconductor material design for high-performance organic field-effect transistors. *Chem. Mater.*, **27**, 141.

57 Magliulo, M., Manoli, K., Macchia, E., Palazzo, G., and Torsi, L. (2015) Tailoring functional interlayers in organic field-effect transistor biosensors. *Adv. Mater.*, **27**, 7528.

58 Minamiki, T., Minami, T., Kurita, R., Niwa, O., Wakida, S., Fukuda, K., Kumaki, D., and Tokito, S. (2014) Accurate and reproducible detection of proteins in water using an extended-gate type organic transistor biosensor. *Appl. Phys. Lett.*, **104**, 243703.

59 Minamiki, T., Minami, T., Kurita, R., Niwa, O., Wakida, S., Fukuda, K., Kumaki, D., and Tokito, S. (2014) A label-free immunosensor for IgG based

on an extended-gate type organic field effect transistor. *Materials (Basel)*, **7**, 6843.

60 Minami, T., Minamiki, T., Hashima, Y., Yokoyama, D., Sekine, T., Fukuda, K., Kumaki, D., and Tokito, S. (2014) An extended-gate type organic field effect transistor functionalised by phenylboronic acid for saccharide detection in water. *Chem. Commun.*, **50**, 15613.

61 Minami, T., Minamiki, T., Fukuda, K., Kumaki, D., and Tokito, S. (2015) Cysteine detection in water using an organic field-effect transistor with a gold extended-gate electrode. *Jpn. J. Appl. Phys.*, **54**, 04DK01.

62 Minamiki, T., Minami, T., Yokoyama, D., Fukuda, K., Kumaki, D., and Tokito, S. (2015) Extended-gate organic field-effect transistor for the detection of histamine in water. *Jpn. J. Appl. Phys.*, **54**, 04DK02.

63 Khan, Y., Pavinatto, F.J., Lin, M.C., Liao, A., Swisher, S.L., Mann, K., Subramanian, V., Maharbiz, M.M., and Arias, A.C. (2016) Inkjet-printed flexible gold electrode arrays for bioelectronic interfaces. *Adv. Funct. Mater.*, **26**, 1004.

5

Flexible Photovoltaic Systems

Lichen Zhao[1], Deying Luo[1], and Rui Zhu[1,2]

[1] *Peking University, Department of Physics, State Key Laboratory for Artificial Microstructure and Mesoscopic Physics, Chengfu Road 209, Beijing 100871, China*
[2] *Collaborative Innovation Center of Extreme Optics, Shanxi University, Taiyuan, Shanxi 030006, People's Republic of China*

5.1 Introduction

5.1.1 Introduction of Flexible Photovoltaics

Smart electronic devices, such as mobile phones, wristbands, and tablet computers, have become more and more popular worldwide. The increasing market demand and growing brand competition lead to constant product updates. One of the most essential challenges for these portable smart electronic devices is that posed by the battery. People need to recharge their mobile phones frequently due to the short-lasting batteries.

How to avoid frequent searching for an electric power supply, especially during the outdoor use of your portable electronics? The extra portable Li battery chargers are commonly used as the portable external power supply, particularly for outdoor use. Another promising solution for outdoor power supply is the portable photovoltaic devices, which may harvest the solar power and provide electricity for your smart electronics.

As portable power devices, the photovoltaic panels or solar cells in your pocket or backpack should have high sunlight-to-electricity conversion efficiency. They should also be foldable or bendable and be of light weight. The flexible photovoltaic (FPV) technology is the most promising candidate to fulfill these requirements. FPVs are also called flexible solar cells. They are a kind of thin-film solar cells that are made on flexible or bendable substrates, such as plastic plates or metallic foils. They possess several advantages:

1) *Flexible*: The mechanical flexibility of FPVs leads to superior compatibility with other elements of various shapes and sizes.
2) *Light-weight*: The thin and flexible substrates make FPVs suitable for the integrations and applications where weight is important.
3) *Printable*: "Roll-to-roll" printing technology allows for the low-cost production of FPV modules with various sizes and shapes.

Flexible and Stretchable Medical Devices, First Edition. Edited by Kuniharu Takei.

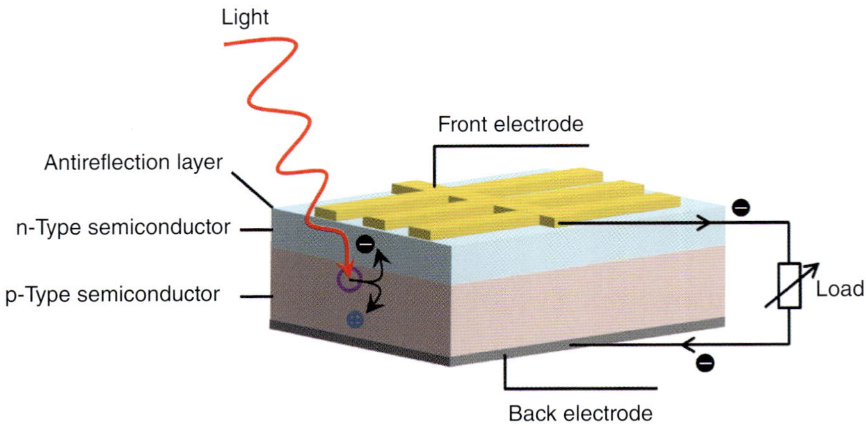

Figure 5.1 Schematic illustration of a typical solar cell.

In this chapter, we mainly focus on the advances of FPV systems. Some basics of solar cells are also briefly introduced. FPV systems based on varied materials are reviewed, including the inorganic, organic, and organic–inorganic hybrid FPV systems. The potential applications of these FPVs are also discussed.

5.1.2 Principles of Photovoltaics

Photovoltaics, as the name suggests, convert solar energy to electricity (direct current and voltage). The typical photovoltaic device is a solar cell, which consists of two layers of semiconductors with opposite polarity, as shown in Figure 5.1. One is a positive (p-type) layer and the other is a negative (n-type) layer. When the two semiconductor layers exist independently, they show electric neutrality. When the two layers are combined together with close contact, a p–n junction will be formed. At the contact interface in a p–n junction, electrons in the n-type semiconductor layer will diffuse into the p-type semiconductor layer, as shown in Figure 5.2a. The negative charge region is generated around the boundary in the p-type semiconductor. Similarly, the positive charge region is also generated around the boundary in the n-type semiconductor side (see Figure 5.2b). This charge diffusion behavior will generate the space charge area, and establish the build-in internal electric filed, with the direction pointing from the n-type semiconductor to the p-type semiconductor. The space charge area is also described as the depletion region, which will eventually inhibit the further charge diffusion behavior at the interface.

When a solar cell is irradiated by sunlight, electrons in the valence band of the semiconductor photoactive layer will absorb the energy $h\nu$ of incident photons. If the energy of incident photons is larger than the bandgap of the semiconductor, electrons in the valence band will have sufficient energy to jump into the conduction band; meanwhile, holes are left in the valence band, as shown in Figure 5.2c. The photo-generated electrons near the p–n junction will access to the corresponding side along the opposite orientation of the build-in internal electric field.

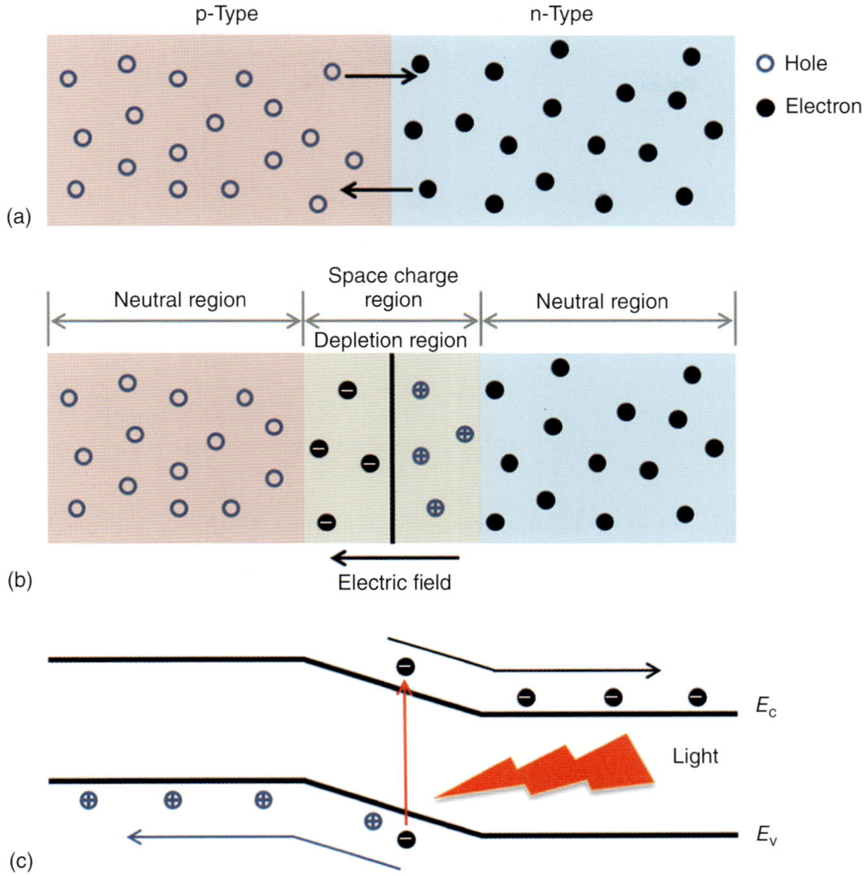

Figure 5.2 The photovoltaic effect of the p–n junction.

Subsequently, the equilibrium between the build-in internal electric field and the photo-generated electric field formed by photovoltaic effect results in the stable photocurrent. The photo-generated electrons will then flow into the external circuit to power a load. After their work, the electrons will finally return to the opposite electrode and recombine with holes generated in the valence band. This is the complete process of photovoltaic effect.

The relationship between the above-mentioned photocurrent and voltage is shown in the *current–voltage (I–V) characteristics* (Figure 5.3a). A solar cell can provide constant current if the illumination intensity is stable. The photocurrent is positively correlated with the incident light intensity.

From the I–V characteristic of a solar cell, several parameters can be extracted to evaluate its performance. Figure 5.3b indicates some important points in the J–V characteristic curve for the parameter calculation [1].

1) *Open-circuit voltage* (V_{oc}). V_{oc} for a solar cell is the voltage measured under the open-circuit condition where the device terminals are isolated. It is the intersection of I–V characteristic curve with the axe $I = 0$.

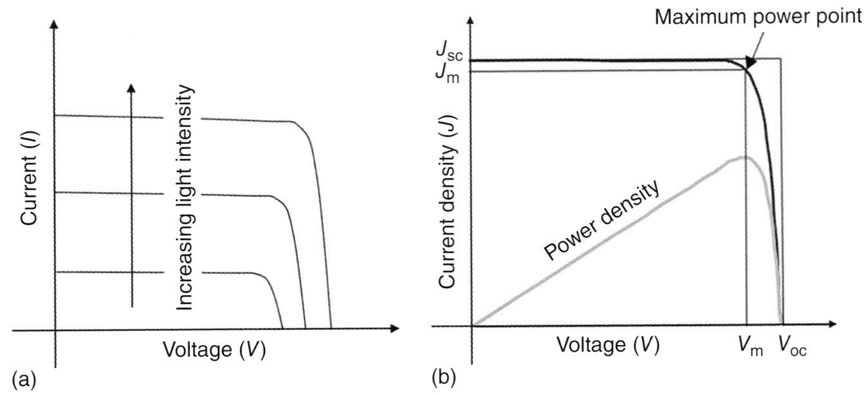

Figure 5.3 (a) Current–voltage curves of a solar cell under different levels of illumination. (b) The current density-voltage (black) and power density-voltage (gray) characteristics of an ideal solar cell.

2) *Short-circuit current* (I_{sc}) is the current measured under the condition where the device terminals are connected directly. On account of the roughly proportional relationship between the current and the effective illuminated area, the I_{sc} is often replaced by the *short-circuit current density* (J_{sc}) which is the intersection of J–V characteristic with the axe $V = 0$.
The J_{sc} has a very close relationship with the incident spectrum as described in the following equation:

$$J_{sc} = q \int f_{ph}(\lambda) \text{QE}(\lambda)\, d\lambda \tag{5.1}$$

where q is the electron charge ($q = 1.6 \times 10^{-19}$ C); $f_{ph}(\lambda)$ is the incident spectral photon flux density, that is, the number of the incident photons at a certain wavelength (λ) in unit time and on unit area; and QE(λ) is *quantum efficiency*, namely the probability that a photon of energy $E = hc/\lambda$ can drive an electron into the external circuit.
The QE(λ) of a material for a solar cell depends on four factors other than the incident spectrum:
   a) The absorption capacity of the material.
   b) The charge diffusion efficiency.
   c) The charge separation efficiency.
   d) The charge collection efficiency of the device.
3) *Power density* (P) of the cell is

$$P = JV \tag{5.2}$$

When P reaches the maximum (*maximum power*, P_m) at the maximum power point of the cell, the *maximum operating voltage* (V_m) is delivered with a corresponding *maximum current density* (J_m). As shown in Figure 5.3b, the area of the smaller inner rectangle represents $P_m = J_m \cdot V_m$, and the larger outer rectangle has an area of $J_{sc} \cdot V_{oc}$.

4) *Fill factor* (FF) is thus defined as the ratio of these two areas:

$$FF = \frac{J_m \cdot V_m}{J_{sc} \cdot V_{oc}} \tag{5.3}$$

5) *Power conversion efficiency* (*PCE*, η) is the specific value of P_m and the incident light power density (P_s):

$$\eta = \frac{P_m}{P_s} \tag{5.4}$$

Then η has a relationship with J_{sc} and V_{oc} through FF:

$$\eta = \frac{J_{sc} \cdot V_{oc} \cdot FF}{P_s} \tag{5.5}$$

Herein, these four parameters (J_{sc}, V_{oc}, FF, and η) are able to describe the performance characteristics of a solar cell comprehensively.

From Eq. (5.5), it can be seen that η is closely related to P_s. In order to make the efficiencies of different solar cells to be effectively comparable, it is necessary to express a fixed P_s under standard solar illumination conditions. The prevailing standard test condition (STC) for solar cells is described further.

Photovoltaic modules, regardless of materials, structure, and design, are commonly measured under the Air Mass 1.5 spectrum (AM 1.5G), an incident power density $P_s = 100\ \mathrm{mW\ cm^{-2}}$, and at an ambient temperature $T = 25 \pm 1\,°\mathrm{C}$.

5.1.3 The Flexible Substrates

To realize large-scale and low-cost "roll-to-roll" production, the flexible substrate materials are essential to the FPVs. They usually need to possess the following characteristics: (i) low cost and widely available raw materials, (ii) sufficient strength to withstand the tension stress during the preparation process, (iii) high thermal stability to adapt to the heating process, and (iv) thermal expansion coefficient matching with the photovoltaic materials.

Currently, there are mainly two kinds of substrate materials for flexible solar cells and metals as well as for alloys and polymers [2].

5.1.3.1 Metals and the Alloys

Using flexible metal and alloy materials as the substrates for thin-film solar cells allows high substrate temperature to deposit thin-film photovoltaic materials. Some examples of the metal substrates are stainless steel, titanium, aluminum, nickel, zinc, molybdenum, chromium, Inconel alloy (61% Ni, 22% Cr, 9% Mo, and 5% Fe), and so on. Among these candidates, stainless steel has been widely used as the substrate material for the flexible thin-film solar cells due to its advantages, such as high temperature resistance, corrosion resistance, superior conductivity, and malleability. Stainless steel substrates are also beneficial to the low-cost "roll-to-roll" fabrication processes, and great economic value can be realized from the large-area and continuous "roll-to-roll" production of solar cells.

5.1.3.2 Polymers

Most organic polymer film materials have small densities and high-impact resistance. Generally, they are lightweight, flexible, and portable. These are compatible with the high-yield and low-cost "roll-to-roll" printing technology. Polymer substrates, such as polyethylene terephthalate (PET), polyethylene naphtalate (PEN), and polyimide (PI), are commonly used as the flexible substrates. Even paper can be considered as a flexible substrate as well. With comparison to the fragile glass substrates, polymeric flexible substrates could present the smaller strain during the film fabrication process because of their flexibility. They also exhibit the comparable light transmittance with the conventional glass substrates. Although these flexible polymeric materials could replace glass substrates to some extent, they could not survive high temperatures due to their relatively low glass-transition temperature (T_g). Working at the temperature above T_g, the polymeric materials will transit from the glassy and hard state to the rubbery and soft state. Thus, the film-forming temperature of the photovoltaic materials needs to be lower enough to ensure their depositions on the polymeric flexible substrates.

5.1.4 The Types of Flexible Photovoltaic Systems

To date, four generations of solar cell technologies have been developed [3]. As it is widely known, the first generation solar cells, which are made of bulk crystalline silicon, are dominating the current photovoltaic market. The second generation solar cells are based on the inorganic thin-film photovoltaic materials. Examples include amorphous silicon solar cells, copper indium gallium selenide (CIGS) solar cells and cadmium telluride (CdTe) solar cells. The third generation solar cells involve a number of organic semiconducting materials and are described as organic solar cells. The fourth generation solar cells are developed based on the organic–inorganic hybrid material system. A representative example of the fourth generation is perovskite solar cell (PerSC), which is currently leading a new wave of solar cell research due to its high efficiency and low production cost. At present, the first and second generation solar cell technologies have been matured for commercial applications, while the third and fourth generation solar cells are still experiencing the vigorous development phase. All of these photovoltaic technologies can be utilized to generate FPV devices. More details will be presented in the following sections.

5.2 Flexible Inorganic Photovoltaic Systems

5.2.1 Flexible Silicon Photovoltaics

Silicon solar cells are widely used because of their excellent and convincing reliability. As there is a thorough understanding about their physical characteristics and principles, silicon solar cells are rather mature to be the mainstay in the solar energy industry [4].

There are three types of silicon wafers: monocrystalline silicon (m-Si), polycrystalline silicon (p-Si), and amorphous silicon (a-Si) [5]. The conventional crystalline silicon solar cells based on bulk m-Si and p-Si often suffer from high consumption of direct and indirect materials, shortages of silicon supplies and laborious processing steps. Then, the thin-film silicon solar cells based on a-Si have emerged to meet the critical requirements for low material dosage and simplified process technology. The a-Si wafer is much thinner than the bulk crystalline silicon (m-Si and p-Si) wafers, which results in that the thickness of the a-Si thin-film solar cell can be 300 times less than that of a traditional crystalline silicon counterpart [6]. In addition, the a-Si thin-film solar cells require only half as many process steps as the ones based on crystalline silicon. More importantly, the a-Si solar cells can make far more effective use of solar light than the crystalline silicon-based counterparts. These advantages could translate into reduced cost, light weight, and compatibility with automated processing technique. All the considerations mentioned above also therefore offer promising opportunities for flexible Si-based thin-film solar cells with broad applications such as embedding into walls, roofs, and windows.

For the flexible a-Si solar cells, a triple-junction device structure design has been a breakthrough because of the stability and high power conversion efficiency [7]. The structure of a typical flexible multijunction a-Si solar cell is shown in Figure 5.4. The metal/zinc oxide (metal/ZnO) back reflection layer is deposited on the flexible stainless steel or plastic substrate, followed by a triple junction (a-Si/a-SiGe/a-SiGe), then the indium tin oxide (ITO) electrode and conductive grids are deposited on the top.

Within this triple-junction structure, three cells with different bandgaps are stacked layer by layer. The top cell takes advantage of a-Si alloy with a bandgap of ~1.8 eV as the intrinsic (i) layer to absorb blue photons. The amorphous

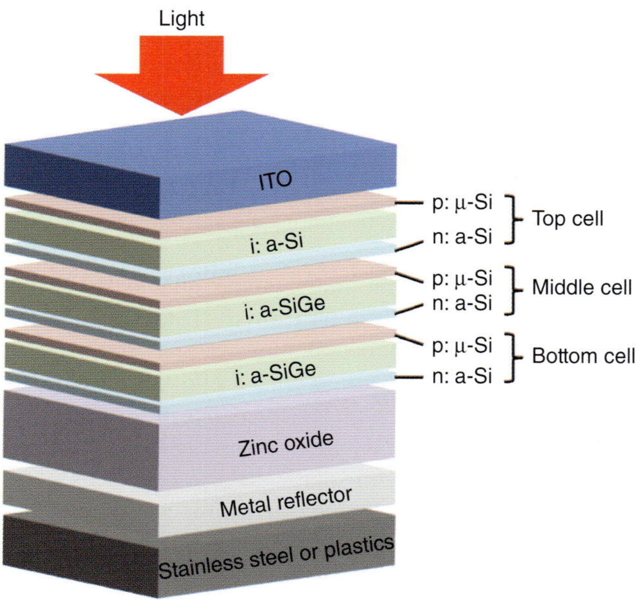

Figure 5.4 Schematic illustration of a flexible triple-junction silicon solar cell, where μ-Si represents microcrystalline silicon.

silicongermanium (a-SiGe) (Ge content: 10-15%) middle cell with an optical gap of ~1.6 eV is used to capture green photons. Another a-SiGe (~1.4 eV) intrinsic layer with a high Ge content (about 40-50%) is ideally suited for the bottom cell to absorb red and infrared photons. When the solar light is irradiated from the ITO side of the cell, it runs through the three semiconductor absorption layers within the triple-junction in sequence. Some photons still cannot be absorbed, which will be reflected by the metal/ZnO back reflector and reabsorbed by this triple-junction structure. Thus, the flexible a-Si solar cells could capture the incident photons more efficiently, leading to the enhanced photon-to-electron conversion efficiencies and improved power outputs. It is also reported that the hydrogenation treatment for the amorphous Si materials is crucial to improve the performances of the a-Si- or a-SiGe-based multijunction solar cells [8]. Based on a similar device design shown in Figure 5.4, hydrogenated a-Si (a-Si:H), hydrogenated a-SiGe (a-SiGe:H), and hydrogenated nanocrystalline Si (n-Si:H) layers have been stacked together onto the flexible substrates to deliver enhanced device efficiency.

To fabricate flexible a-Si solar cells, the most commonly used process is based on the low-temperature chemical vapor deposition (CVD), which could be incorporated with the "roll-to-roll" technology to realize the continuous production [9]. In this "roll-to-roll" production, rolls of stainless steel with fixed width are used as the substrates to deposit solar cells. The production line comprises four machines to achieve the continuous device fabrication: (i) the washing machine to clean the roll of stainless steel; (ii) the sputtering system to deposit the back conducting and reflection layer (metal/ZnO) on the cleaned stainless steel rolls; (iii) the CVD equipment for the depositions of stacked a-Si and a-SiGe alloy layers; and (iv) the antireflection coating machine for depositing the ITO transparent conducting film on the top of the stacked photoactive layers.

After being connected to the suitable electrode grids, the flexible solar cells are then encapsulated with the high-stability, UV-resistant, and weather-defying polymer films. In brief, a fluorine-containing polymer is coated on the top and a polyester material as adhesive is placed at the bottom side of the resulting device. After lamination and encapsulation, these finished solar cells benefiting from flexibility and light weight can be broadly used to charge storage batteries or even combined to the large-scale grid-connected systems.

In comparison with the conventional monocrystalline silicon cells, the above-mentioned flexible a-Si solar cells often suffer from the tradeoffs between performance and robustness. Although monocrystalline wafer is too rigid to achieve the flexible purpose, there are still some reported efforts that demonstrated the flexible function based on the high performance m-Si cells. For example, a research team led by Prof. John A. Rogers has developed a novel design to fabricate flexible arrays of tiny silicon solar cells (see Figure 5.5) [10]. These flexible modules incorporate the assembled arrays of interconnected microcells, and thus do not come with the tradeoff issues. An incorporation of etching and transfer-printing technique was utilized to fabricate this kind of flexible m-Si solar modules. The resulting arrays have sustained a comparable efficiency as the conventional cells although their thickness is only one-tenth that of conventional counterparts.

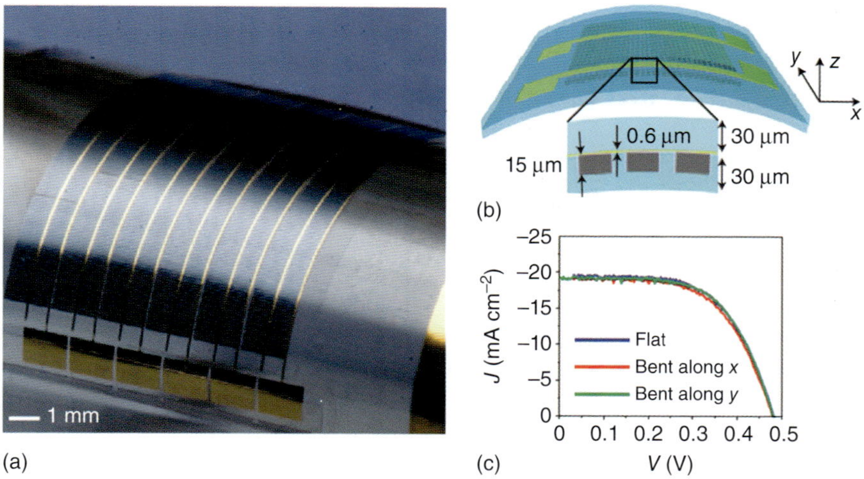

Figure 5.5 (a) Optical image, (b) schematic illustration, and (c) photovoltaic performance of mechanically flexible modules that incorporate arrays of interconnected microcells. (Yoon *et al.* 2008 [10]. Reproduced with permission of Nature Publishing Group.)

5.2.2 Flexible Copper Indium Gallium Selenide Photovoltaics

CIGS thin-film solar cells emerged in the mid-1970s, including copper indium selenide (CIS), CIGS, copper gallium selenide (CGS), and copper indium gallium selenide sulfur (CIGSS). They have rapidly moved to the forefront of thin-film solar cells due to their excellent conversion efficiency. CIGS, a kind of direct bandgap solid-solution semiconductor, belongs to the chalcopyrite crystal structure. By adjusting the Ga content, the energy gap of CIGS materials can be tuned between ~1.04 eV for pure CIS and ~1.68 eV for pure CGS. CIGS has been regarded as the most promising photovoltaic material because of its superior optical absorption coefficient [11].

Compared with a-Si, there are much fewer internal defects in the CIGS thin films. Hence, the solar cells based on CIGS film show better device stability, with a lifetime of up to 25 years. In fact, the migration of copper ions within the CIGS film can fix defects through a self-healing mechanism during actual operation of solar cells [12]. Thus, the performance of the CIGS module will gradually increase with time. This interesting phenomenon is quite different from the light-induced degradation [13] or Staebler–Wronski effect for a-Si solar cells [14].

Furthermore, the CIGS thin films can also be available on the flexible substrates to manufacture flexible solar modules [15, 16]. Figure 5.6 shows the structure of a typical flexible CIGS thin-film solar cell. A flexible CIGS solar cell usually consists of the following parts: substrates (metal foils or plastics), back contact (Mo), light-absorbing semiconductor layer (CIGS), buffer layer (CdS), and transparent conducting window layer (ZnO/ITO).

Dating back to 1993 [17], small-area flexible CIGS solar cells were already fabricated on the molybdenum foils and titanium foils. The CIGS thin films can be deposited on the flexible substrates with various approaches including the co-vapor deposition method, sequential sputtering process, nonvacuum

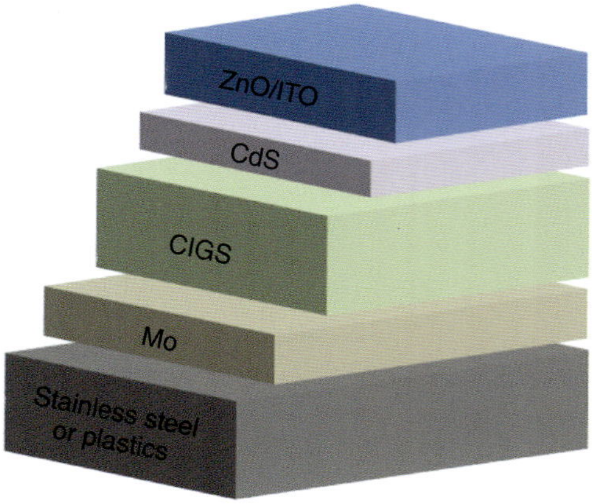

Figure 5.6 Schematic illustration of a typical flexible CIGS thin-film solar cell.

printing/spraying of metal oxides, and electrodeposition technology, followed by the selenium process. Subsequently, a report in 2000 comprehensively reviewed that there were considerable obstacles on the road to the commercially available and large-scale production of CIGS-based solar cells [18]. The most important issue was "the complexity of the material and the manufacturing processes."

Actually, researchers all over the world continue to explore the simple wet chemical solution method with lower manufacturing cost for CIGS thin films. This is also what a company named *Nanosolar* located in California, United States, has done [19]. In 2007, they first realized the commercialization of the flexible CIGS thin-film solar cells based on ink printing technology. They have developed a kind of nanostructured CIGS printing ink recipe and utilized the simple inkjet printing approach combined with "roll-to-roll" technology to fabricate highly efficient flexible CIGS devices on aluminum foils. From a technological perspective, one of the core challenges is in the use of homogeneous and stable printing ink. As shown in Figure 5.7, this new nanoink is a kind of polymer suspension containing a uniform mixture of CIGS nanoparticles. In large-scale printing, four kinds of atoms (Cu, In, Ga, and Se) will be deposited on the substrates with fixed element proportion if the nanoink remains chemically stable. It is more advantageous than the vacuum deposition technique used before since the latter needs a real-time adjustment for the proportion of each element used. Through this inkjet printing approach combined with "roll-to-roll"

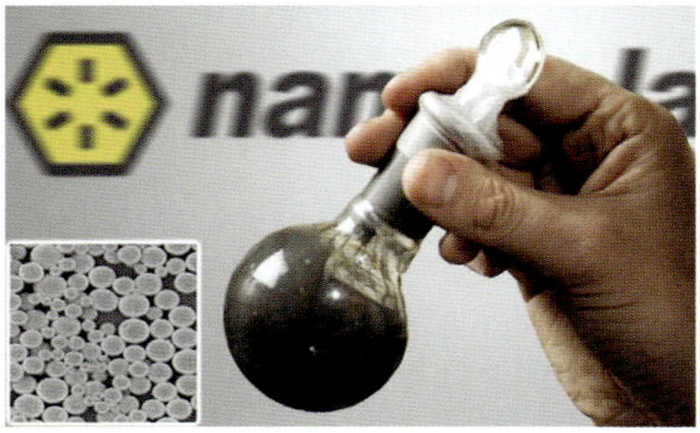

Figure 5.7 The CIGS nanoink of *Nanosolar*. (Photocourtesy: Nanosolar Corporation.)

technology, uniform, stable, and flexible CIGS solar cells have been processed with a highly efficient output.

5.3 Flexible Organic Photovoltaic Systems

Organic photovoltaics (OPVs), as the third generation solar cells, are usually formed by sandwiching organic active layers between two different electrodes with different work functions. The organic active layer is composed of conjugated organic donor materials blending with acceptor materials, and therefore, OPVs are also called "plastic solar cells." OPV devices have a potential advantage of low-cost fabrication using spin-coating or roll-to-roll printing. More importantly, they are compatible with the large-scaled flexible and stretchable substrates, and conjugated polymers are nontoxic. In the following text, we will briefly introduce the fundamental properties of organic semiconductors, the architecture, and the working mechanisms of OPV devices, as well as flexible OPV.

5.3.1 Fundamental Properties of OPV Materials

Prior to the 1970s, traditional polymers have been normally regarded as insulators resulting from the only σ-bonds formed between the neighboring carbon atoms [20]. Subsequently, a significant research breakthrough on the conducting and semiconducting nature of polymers has been achieved by the doping process [21]. Then, exploiting its optoelectronic properties the photovoltaic community throughout the world started to focus on exploiting its optoelectronic properties rapidly. Semiconducting properties of the emerging organic materials or polymers mainly depend on these molecules with conjugated chains of carbon (see Figure 5.8a,b), that is, molecules with alternative single- and double-bonds. For the conjugated organic molecules, each carbon atom enables to bind only three adjacent atoms, leaving one electron per carbon atom in the p_z orbital. The mutual overlapping between these p_z orbitals forms π-bonds along the conjugated backbone; thereby the resulting π electrons within the organic molecules are delocalized within the conjugated system. The delocalized π electrons fill up the whole energy band in the solids as shown in Figure 5.8c, conjugated polymers are thus intrinsic semiconductors. The filled π band is called the highest occupied molecular orbital (HOMO) and the empty π^* band is called the lowest unoccupied molecular orbital (LUMO).

Compared with the traditional inorganic semiconductors, a major difference is the presence of weak interaction between organic molecules in organic solids, leading to the delocalized electrons in organic solids with hopping transport (not energy-band transport). This makes the optoelectronic properties of organic semiconductors different from inorganic semiconductors [21], such as absorption, transport gaps, charge carrier separation, and transport. Typically, the photo-generated "electron-hole" pairs in organic materials are totally different from those in inorganic semiconductors. There is a large electrostatic force between these "electron–hole" pairs because of the low dielectric constant of organic materials [21], and therefore these neutral electron–hole pairs are not always freely mobile before dissociating under external electrical fields.

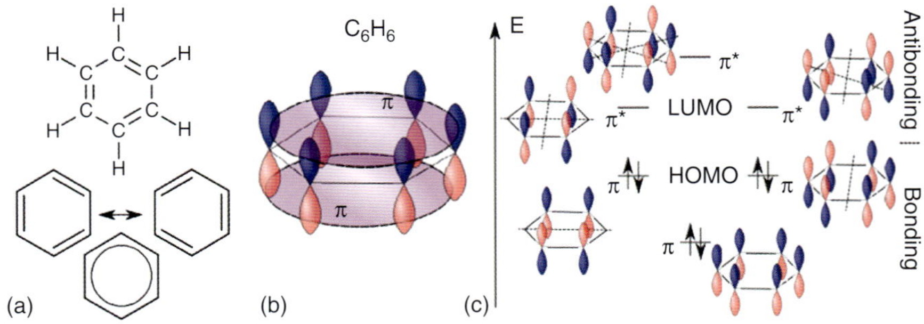

Figure 5.8 Benzene: (a) Kekulé structure, consisting of two resonance (mesomerism) structures. (b) Visualization of the location of the lowest bonding π-orbital. (c) The position of the six energy levels resulting from the overlap of the six p_z orbitals. The more nodes found in the wave function, the higher is the energy. (Reproduced from Ref. [20], with permission.)

5.3.2 Device Structure and Working Mechanisms

The first OPV device was made by sandwiching a single organic layer between two electrodes with different work functions [21], but the device efficiency is very low due to the lack of an effective heterojunction interface for the "electron-hole" pair (i.e., excitons) dissociation. Thus, the early OPV device has drawn little attention. As a milestone in 1986, Tang have proposed a bilayer planar heterojunction OPV device based on the p-type copper phthalocyanine (CuPc) and the n-type perylene tetracarboxylic derivative (PTCD) [22]. In this structure, the CuPc layer plays an electron-donating role while the PTCD layer serves as an acceptor, and ultimately a *PCE* of about 1% was achieved under the simulated AM 2 illuminations (691 $W\,m^{-2}$). In the double-layer structured OPV devices, "electron–hole" pairs will be photo-generated within the layers of CuPc donor and PTCD acceptor. These excited "electron–hole" pairs may lose their energy via radiative and nonradiative recombination. When the excited "electron–hole" pairs diffuse to the donor/acceptor interface before their energy loss, they are likely to be dissociated and then collected by the corresponding electrodes. As a consequence, the heterojunction interface between the donor and acceptor plays a very important role in governing ultimate device performance. The underlying reason for this is that excitons have a short lifetime and low mobility in the organic solid film, resulting in the short diffusion length of just ~10 nm [23]. Therefore, it is necessary to improve the charge carrier dissociation efficiency by increasing the contact interfaces between the donor and the acceptor.

To address this issue, in 1995, Prof. Alan J. Heeger and coworkers firstly reported bulk heterojunction-based organic photovoltaics (BHJ-OPVs) [24]. In their report, simply blending the electron donor (p-type) with electron acceptor (n-type) in the solution produced the thin film with bi-continuous and interconnecting network after post-annealing treatment. This condensed thin solid film, namely "bulk heterojunction" as shown in Figure 5.9a, could offer sufficient charge transfer pathways and achieve a *PCE* of over 3% [24] at that time. The attractive solution indeed improves the charge transfer from donor to acceptor within the organic active layer (i.e., a blending layer of donor and

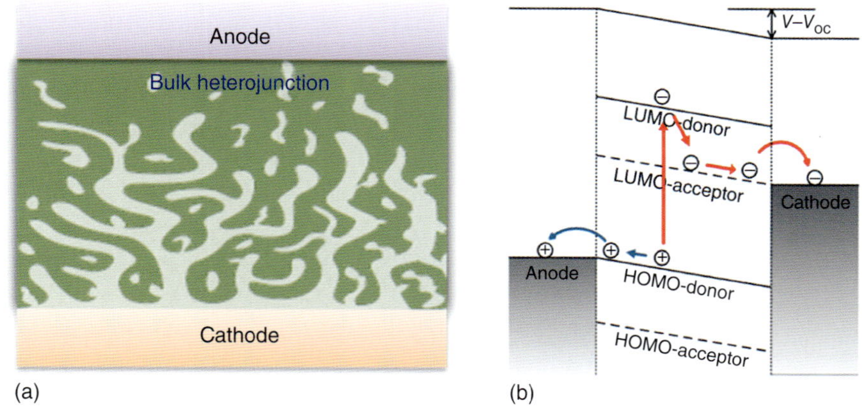

Figure 5.9 (a) Illustration of bulk heterojunction with bi-continuous interpenetration network of polymer and acceptor. (b) Schematic energy level diagram of a bulk heterojunction organic photovoltaic under a bias voltage. Red arrows indicate the transfer direction of the electrons and blue arrows point in the transfer direction of the holes.

acceptor, hereafter called organic active layer). However, a new challenge is that the photo-generated "electron–hole" pairs are required to migrate to their respective electrodes before recombination through the organic active layer. This suggests that the structure and morphology control of organic active layers are of significant importance to enhance photo-generated "electron–hole" pairs' transport and collection [24]. In order to get a better understanding on why the optimized device architecture and morphological control can improve device efficiency, the working mechanisms of the BHJ-OPV would be introduced first, as shown in Figure 5.9b.

A major process for the BHJ-OPV device involves the creation of free carriers from incident sunlight. The commonly accepted mechanism of charge generation in an organic active layer is that incident sunlight is absorbed by organic active layer to generate "electron-hole" pairs (also known as excitons), mostly by the donor materials [25]. Excitons need to diffuse to the interfaces between the donor and the acceptor materials, where the charges transfer from the LUMO level of the donor materials to the LUMO level of the acceptors if the energy level offset between these two LUMO levels is equal to or over 0.3 eV [25]. This process is also called "exciton dissociation" or "charge carrier generation." Subsequently, driven by an internal electric field, electrons or holes as charge carriers are transported toward the cathode or the anode, where they are extracted. Another possible mechanism involves a Förster resonance energy transfer (FRET) from the donor to the acceptor. In this mechanism, excitons are generated in the acceptor instead of the donor, followed by exciton dissociation via hole transfer to donor.

V_{oc}, J_{sc}, and FF, are critical device parameters that are closely correlated with the working mechanisms mentioned earlier [26]. The V_{oc} is directly linked to the energy difference between the LUMO level of the acceptor and the HOMO level of the donor. This energy difference provides the primary driving forces for charge separation. The J_{sc} critically depends on the light absorption, charge carrier transport and collection. Utilizing a broader solar spectrum and enlarging the energy level difference between the HOMO level of the donor and the LUMO level of the acceptor are the most promising strategies to deliver high values of J_{sc} and V_{oc} [27], respectively. A high FF is advantageous and indicates that a fairly strong photocurrent can be extracted close to the V_{oc} [25]. In this range, the internal field in the device assisting the charge separation and transport is fairly small. Consequently, a high FF can be obtained when the balanced charge transport could be realized.

5.3.3 Materials and Methods for OPV

Conjugated organic materials are one of the most important factors to govern the conversion efficiency of solar energy to electricity for flexible OPV devices. The commonly used organic polymers in the flexible OPV devices are identical to conventional materials used in the nonflexible ones. In general, a BHJ active layer in OPV is composed of a conjugated polymer as electron donor and an organic compound as electron acceptor. At present, the OPV devices are usually fabricated by a solution-processed method or a thermal evaporation process. Compared with the thermal evaporation process, the simple solution-processed protocol has attracted more attention because the solution-based process exhibits great potentials for low-cost device fabrication and is compatible with the printing process for flexible devices.

Among the solution-processed conjugated donor polymers, poly[2-methoxy-5-(2′-ethylhexyloxy)-*p*-phenylenevinylene] (MEH-PPV) was the earliest electron-donating material. By combining with fullerene derivative acceptors, such as phenyl-C_{61}-butyric acid methyl ester ($PC_{61}BM$), the MEH-PPV:fullerene blend could be used as the photoactive layer and generate the solution-processed BHJ-OPV devices, but the device efficiencies based on MEH-PPV were not high [26]. Later, poly(3-hexyl)thiophene (P3HT) became another commonly used donor material. The highest *PCE* of 4.0-5.0% [28, 29] was achieved for the OPV based on P3HT:$PC_{61}BM$ blend, but the V_{oc} is only 0.6 V. As mentioned, in the OPV with a BHJ structure, V_{oc} is directly proportional to the energy level difference between the HOMO level of the donor and the LUMO level of the acceptor. This means that an increase in the energy difference between donor and acceptor materials might have enhanced the V_{oc} for the device. Introducing a low density of alky side chain into the P3HT backbone (i.e., P3HTDTT) can significantly lower the HOMO level to −5.2 eV and result in the V_{oc} increasing to 0.82 V [30], as shown in Figure 5.10. By replacing alkyl groups with alkyl ester groups, the electron-withdrawing ability of ester substituents could lead to a HOMO level of −5.10 eV and a V_{oc} of 0.78 V without sacrificing the bandgap and absorption spectrum [31]. Recently, a novel PTCD with one alkyl ester substituent for every two thiophene units has been synthesized [32], and the function of stronger electron-withdrawing has further decreased the HOMO level to −5.26 eV. The ultimate V_{oc} of 0.91 V is among the highest values for the OPV devices based on P3HT derivatives.

To improve the *PCEs* of the BHJ-OPV, one approach is to increase V_{oc} by tuning the energy difference of two energy levels between donor and acceptor.

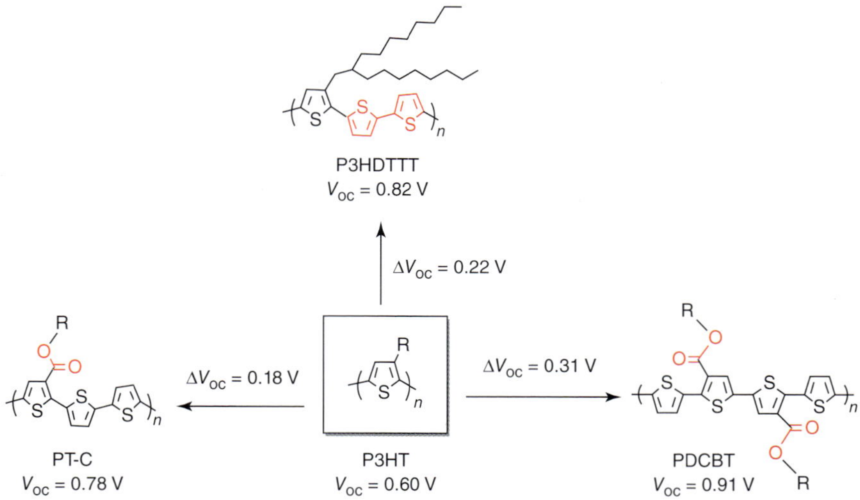

Figure 5.10 Examples for introducing functional substituents to increase V_{oc} of the OPV based on conventional P3HT donors [30–32].

The other approach is to broaden the light absorption to the infrared region of the solar spectrum. This means that the light absorbing materials should have a smaller bandgap to utilize more sunlight. Therefore, tremendous efforts have been devoted to improve device efficiency by designing new polymers with low bandgap and high absorption coefficient. For example, a new low band-gap polymer, named poly[2,6-(4,4-bis-(2-ethylhexyl)-4*H*-cyclopenta[2,1-*b*;3,4-*b*′]dithiophene)-*alt*-4,7-(2,1,3-benzothiadiazole)] (PCPDTBT), has shown to broaden the absorption to 900 nm [33]. Similarly, thieno[3,4-*b*]-thiophene (TT) and benzodithiophene (BDT) alternating units were successfully introduced into the polymers and a *PCE* of over 7% has been realized by using this polymer system [32]. Also, acceptors with broader light absorption range have been extensively studied, such as [6,6]-phenyl C_{71} butyric acid methyl ester ($PC_{71}BM$), which is the derivative of C_{70} fullerene and possesses higher absorption coefficient in comparison with $PC_{61}BM$ [26]. In addition to the fullerene derivative acceptors, nonfullerene acceptor materials have also attracted increasing attention. One of the representative examples is 3,9-bis(2-methylene-(3-(1,1-dicyanomethylene)-indanone)) (ITIC), which was developed by Prof. Zhan at Peking University [34]. A *PCE* of over 11% has been achieved based on the ITIC acceptor system [35].

5.3.4 Recent Advances in Flexible OPV

Currently, the OPVs are deemed to be one of the most promising flexible photovoltaic devices because they are nontoxic and are compatible with garments and textiles [36]. At present, the typical device configuration for flexible OPV devices is ITO-coated PET/PEDOT:PSS/organic active layer/Ca or LiF or BCP or Bphen/Al, in which the organic active layer varies from traditional P3HT:$PC_{61}BM$ blend to a highly efficient PTB7-Th:$PC_{71}BM$ blend [33]. As a photovoltaic device for flexible or bendable application, it is necessary to consider not only the flexibility but also the stretchability of the devices. Stretchable OPV devices have been fabricated directly on prestretched 200-500-μm-thick polydimethylsiloxane (PDMS) substrate, which can then obtain 27% strain reversibly [37].

For both the stretchable and flexible OPV devices, the actual OPV device layers only constitute < 0.25% of the total device thickness. Therefore, achieving stretchable and flexible OPV on the ultrathin and lightweight substrates is still a challenge. Very recently, Bauer *et al.* have presented ultrathin, light, flexible, and compliant OPV devices on only 1.4-μm-thick PET substrates [37] (Figure 5.11a,b), where the total thickness of the device is less than a typical thread of spider silk. Figure 5.11c shows the flexible OPV device on a 100-μm-thick prestretched 3 M VHB 4905 elastomer. More importantly, as the compressive strain of the elastomer is progressively increased to 30%, it is found that the device becomes wrinkled. The flexible OPV is to be stretched back to

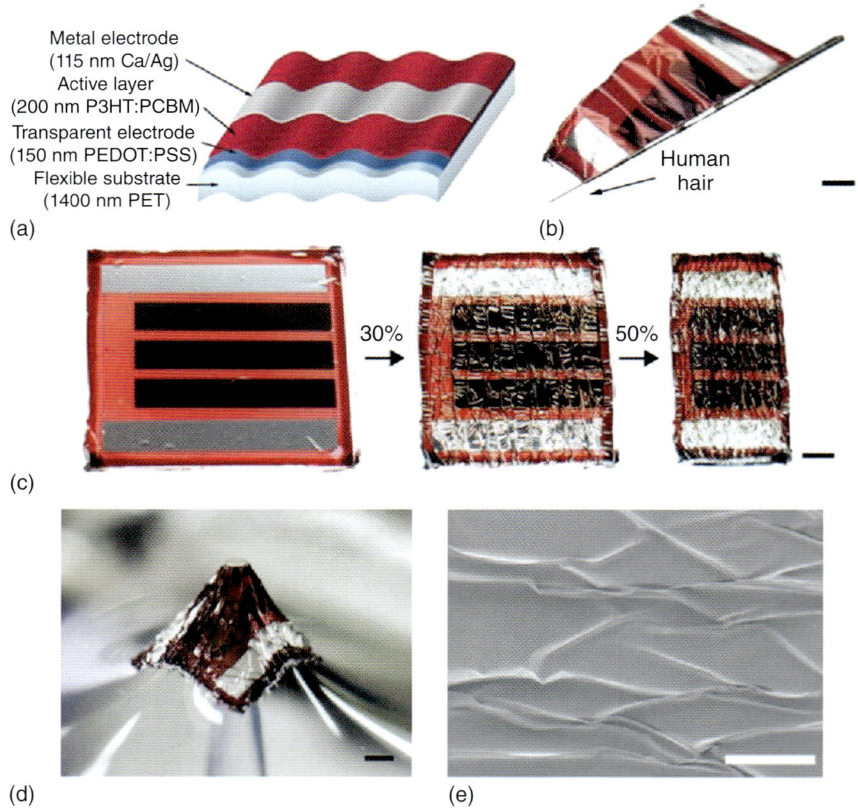

Figure 5.11 (a) Scheme of the ultralight and flexible organic solar cell. (b) Extreme bending flexibility demonstrated by wrapping a solar cell around a 35-μm-radius human hair. Scale bar is (also in c,d) 2 mm. (c) Stretchable solar cells made by attaching the ultrathin solar cell to a prestretched elastomer. (d) The device attached to the elastomeric support, under three-dimensional deformation by pressure from a 1.5 mm-diameter plastic tube. (e) SEM image of the PET surface of the solar cell in compressed state. (Kaltenbrunner *et al.* 2012 [37]. Reproduced with permission of Nature Publishing Group.)

the prestrain defined by the elastomer. The test of the extreme conformability of an ultrathin flexible OPV is presented by deforming the OPV on an elastomeric substrate with a plastic tube of 1.5 mm tip diameter in Figure 5.11d. Scanning electron microscopy (SEM) image (in Figure 5.11e) of the compressed OPV device highlights the random wrinkles with extremely small bending radii.

Flexibility and stretchability of the flexible OPV devices not only depend on substrates, but also are influenced by organic active layers due to the brittle crystalline feature of the fullerenes. All-polymer or nonfullerene OPV devices, consisting of polymer-donor and organic/polymer-acceptor materials, both possess many advantages over polymer-fullerene counterparts, including tunable chemical and electronic properties as well as enhanced stabilities. In recent years, many efforts have been devoted to developing optimal combinations of polymer-donor and polymer-acceptor materials with well-defined heterojunction morphologies. Among the nonfullerene acceptors, naphthalene diimide (NDI)-based copolymers have been the most successful polymer acceptors with low LUMO level and high electron mobility in the flexible OPV devices.

In order to compare the differences between the mechanical properties of $PC_{61}BM$-based OPVs and all-polymer OPV devices, the tensile characteristics of PBDTTTPD:$PC_{61}BM$ and PBDTTTPD:P(NDI2HD-T), mixing films have been tested by Kim *et al.* [38]. In their work, they first compared a quantitative difference of the mechanical properties of these two films. Figure 5.12a shows the stress–strain curves of the PBDTTTPD:$PC_{61}BM$ and PBDTTTPD:P(NDI2HD-T) blend films. Here, they mainly determined the elastic modulus and the elongation at break of the PBDTTTPD:$PC_{61}BM$ (1 : 1.5 w/w) blend films, which reached 1.76 GPa and 0.12%, respectively. The mixing PBDTTTPD:$PC_{61}BM$ organic active layer with different blend ratios obtained a similar tensile modulus of 0.80 GPa and an elongation at break of 0.30%. Interestingly, as illustrated in Figure 5.12b, it was observed that there was a decrease in brittleness as the $PC_{61}BM$ content was lowered, which was consistent with previous reports and suggested that $PC_{61}BM$ acceptor is the performance-limiting factor [32]. Moreover, it is noted that the tensile modulus of the PBDTTTPD:P(NDI2HD-T) blend film was only 0.43 GPa, and

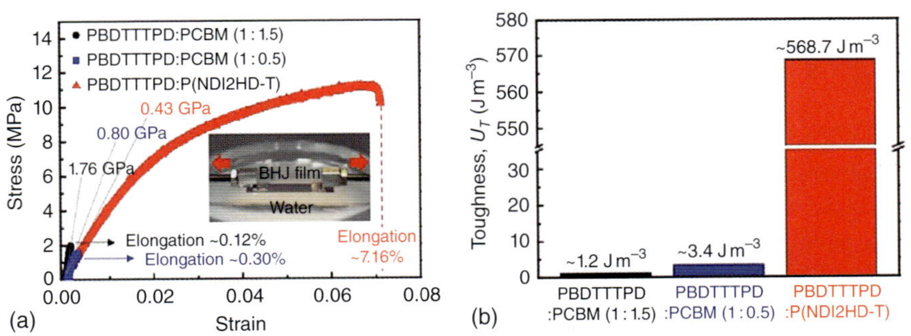

Figure 5.12 Tensile test of PBDTTTPD:$PC_{61}BM$ and PBDTTTPD:P(NDI2HD-T) blend films. (a) Strain–stress curves and (b) toughness of PBDTTTPD:PCBM and PBDTTTPD:P(NDI2HD-T) blend films. (Kim *et al.* 2015 [38], https://www.nature.com/articles/ncomms9547. Used under CC BY 4.0 https://creativecommons.org/licenses/by/4.0/.)

its elongation at break of PBDTTTPD:P(NDI2HD-T) mixing layer was 7.16%, which was a 60-fold enhancement over that of PBDTTTPD:PC_{61}BM.

Highly efficient and mechanically robust all-polymer flexible OPV devices have been fabricated by using poly[4,8-bis(5-(2-ethylhexyl) thiophen-2-yl) benzo[1,2-*b*:4,5-b_0]dithiophene-*alt*-1,3-bis(thiophen-2-yl)-5-(2-hexyldecyl)-4*H*-thieno[3,4-*c*]pyrrole-4,6(5*H*)-dione] (PBDTTTPD) as the electron donor and poly[[*N*,N_0-bis (2-hexyldecyl)-naphthalene-1,4,5,8-bis(dicarboximide)-2,6-diyl]-*alt*-5,50-thiophene] (P(NDI2HD-T)) as the electron acceptor. The all-polymer OPV based on this donor/acceptor pair of PBDTTTPD and P(NDI2HD-T) has exhibited a *PCE* of 6.64%, which is higher than that of PBDTTTPD:PCBM-based BHJ-OPVs (*PCE* of 6.12%) [38]. The better performance was attributed to the high V_{oc} of 1.06 V and the optimized BHJ active layers of polymer donor and acceptor with favorable interfacial interactions. Compared with fullerene-based blend films, all-polymer blend films offer superior flexibility, stretching, and bending properties.

In addition to the active layer, the investment in the electrodes is also important to achieve the improved flexibility for OPV devices. The commonly used conductive electrode is the ITO substrate which is brittle and not perfectly compatible with the flexible devices [36]. A promising replacement for the rigid ITO electrode is the silver nanowire-based electrode [39, 40], which has shown much better mechanical properties with similar optical and electrical properties. Moreover, the silver nanowire-based transparent electrode could also be used as both the bottom and top electrodes for OPV devices [40]. This may deliver the semi-transparent flexible OPVs, which might open the door for more applications than can be envisioned.

Overall, the most critical challenges for the flexible OPV arise from the relatively low device efficiency and the tolerance for large mechanical stress in bending tests. The enhancements in both the device efficiency and the mechanical properties will be the focus of future research and can be expected by optimizing device architecture or developing new materials (interface, photoactive or electrode materials).

5.4 Flexible Organic–Inorganic Hybrid Photovoltaic Systems

After silicon solar cells (the first generation), CIGS thin-film solar cells (the second generation), organic thin-film and dye-sensitized solar cells (DSSCs) (the third generation), a new type of solar cells based on hybrid organic–inorganic halide perovskite, namely PerSCs, have emerged as the next-generation photovoltaics. The first attempt to use perovskite as a sensitizer in the liquid electrolyte DSSCs can be tracked back to 2009, and an initial efficiency of 3.8% was reported by Miyasaka and his colleagues [41]. But it has drawn little attention due to poor device stability and since 2012, several impressive works on the solid-state PerSCs have been established [42–44], which have successfully addressed the degradation issue for hybrid perovskite materials in the liquid electrolyte. Since then, researches on PerSCs have experienced an unprecedented rapid development and have rapidly risen to the forefront of the emerging photovoltaic systems.

Based on their amazing progress, the development of PerSCs has been elected as one of the 10 breakthroughs by *Science* in 2013 [45]. In less than 7 years, the record certified efficiency for PerSCs has reached as high as 22.1% [46]. Such developing rates are far more beyond that of the rest of the solar cells in the photovoltaic community. The fast development of PerSCs is attributed to several superiorities in the organic–inorganic hybrid perovskite materials [47]. For example, the materials possess high absorption coefficient across the visible spectrum and ensure the efficient capture of visible photons; the low exciton-binding energy in the perovskite materials enables long electron–hole diffusion length and facilitates the efficient charge extraction. Moreover, both the wet solution process and low temperature treatment in the device fabrication have provided the PerSCs with great potential for the FPVs [48].

5.4.1 Fundamental Properties of Perovskites

Perovskite [47] is a generic term for a type of compound whose crystal structures are the same as that of calcium titanium oxide ($CaTiO_3$). The general formula of these compounds can be expressed as ABX_3 as shown in Figure 5.13. Specifically, the sites of "A," "B," and "X" stand for different elements in the hybrid organic–inorganic halide perovskites. The larger "A" cation represents organic cations, such as methylammonium ($CH_3NH_3^+$, MA^+) and formamidinium ($CH(NH_2)_2^+$, FA^+). "X" anion is halogen, generally iodine, although bromine and chlorine are also commonly used. "B" is divalent metal cation, such as Pb^{2+} and Sn^{2+}. For these highly efficient PerSCs, Pb^{2+} is preferred. The lead halide perovskites can be obtained through the chemical reaction between halogenated amines (AX) and the lead precursors. A typical perovskite is thus $MAPbX_3$,

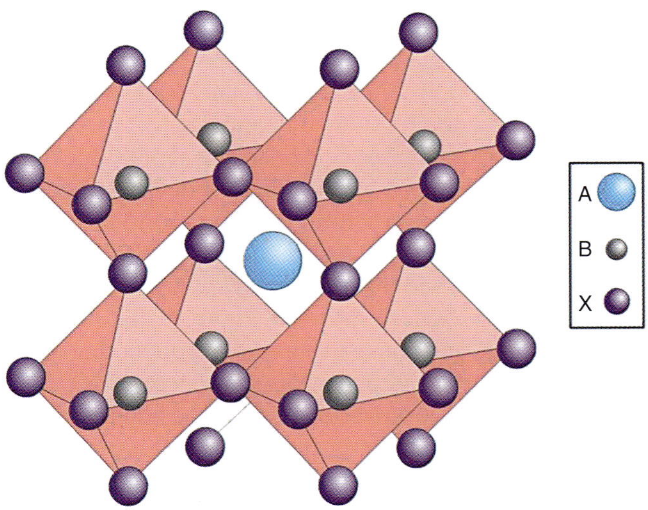

Figure 5.13 Structural representation of an organic–inorganic perovskite. (Green *et al.* 2014 [47]. Reproduced with permission of Nature Publishing Group.)

with $FAPbX_3$, the mixed-halide $MAPbI_{3-x}Cl_x$ and $MAPbI_{3-x}Br_x$, and the mixed-cation $(MA)_{1-x}(FA)_xPbI_3$ being equally important. Taking $CH_3NH_3PbI_3$ as an example, the larger $CH_3NH_3^+$ occupies a cubo-octahedral site shared with 12 I^- anions, whereas the smaller Pb^{2+} cation is stabilized in an octahedral site shared with six I^- anions. A regular octahedron structure is established. The band-gap of $CH_3NH_3PbI_3$ is 1.55 eV [42], with an absorption spectrum covering the whole visible light range.

As the absorber materials, perovskites have two exceptional benefits including excellent optoelectronic properties and low energy loss of charge separation. In particular, perovskite materials are direct-gap semiconductors. They have narrow bandgaps, high extinction coefficients over the whole visible spectrum, long carrier lifetimes, and high carrier motilities [42, 49]. The extinction coefficients are about 10 times higher than the conventional dye N719 in DSSCs. Snaith *et al.* have demonstrated that the diffusion lengths of the electrons and holes generated in the $CH_3NH_3PbI_3Cl_x$ material have both exceeded 1 μm [49]. Their carrier diffusion lengths and lifetimes are 10 times longer than common organic semiconductors. Meanwhile, Sum *et al.* have also suggested that the long-range balanced electron-hole transport can be achieved within the hybrid perovskite [50]. What is more, the energy loss of the charge separation for perovskite materials is small enough to realize a theoretical maximum V_{oc} of 1.3 V. In practice, V_{oc} approaching 1.2 V has already been obtained in a broad range of device architectures. Furthermore, the PerSCs devices can be manufactured with solution-based process, which will potentially reduce the cost for the solar panels. Thereby, motivations have been driven by the use of mature all-solution-processes and the spray-coating method in industrial application. All these are the reasons for the fast development of PerSCs. The solution-processed PerSCs also meet the needs of scalable roll-to-roll printing process. This will deliver the all-solid-state and flexible solar cell rolls, which will have great potential for broader applications.

5.4.2 Device Structure and Working Mechanisms

The initial PerSCs evolved from DSSCs, where solid-state perovskites with better conductivity were used to replace the traditional organic or metal complex dyes [41, 43]. Thus, the device structure of PerSC is relatively simple and similar to the solid-state DSSCs. Generally, there are two kinds of device structures for PerSCs: one is regular structure (n-i-p structure) evolving from DSSCs and the other is inverted structure (p-i-n structure) evolving from OPVs. [48] Both of the two architectures are compatible with flexible substrates and can be used for making PerSCs. In the regular PerSCs, as shown in Figure 5.14a, the electron transport layer (ETL) is first deposited on the transparent conducting oxide (TCO) substrate, followed by the coatings of perovskite photoactive layer, hole transport layer (HTL), and the anode. In the inverted PerSCs, the functional layers are coated on the TCO substrate following a reversed order: HTL, perovskite photoactive layer, ETL, and the cathode. (see Figure 5.14b)

The working mechanisms in PerSCs will be illustrated by taking an n-i-p structure as an example [47]. Under solar irradiation, the perovskite photoactive layer absorbs photons to generate excitons (electron–hole pairs). Perovskite materials

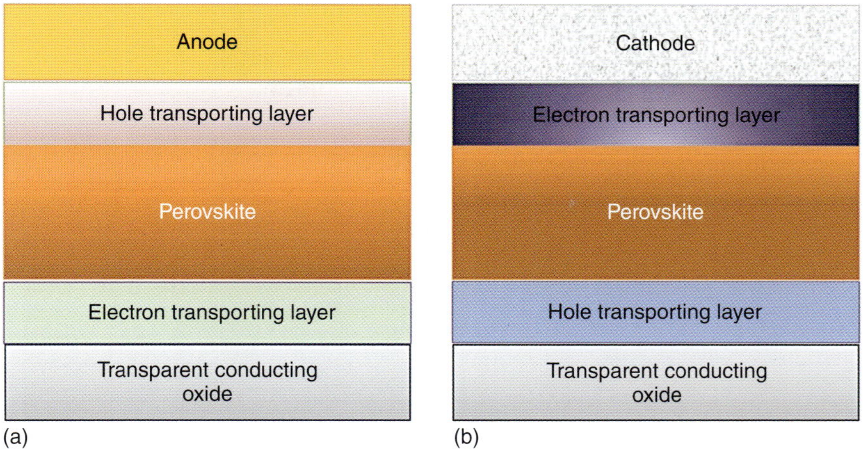

Figure 5.14 (a) Schematic diagram of regular planar structure; (b) schematic diagram of inverted planar structure. (Liu *et al.* 2016 [51]. Reproduced with permission of John Wiley & Sons.)

have low exciton binding energy, thus these excitons can dissociate into free charge carriers (free electrons and holes) to generate current or to recombine into excitons (dark reaction). Then, these photo-generated free electrons and holes are extracted by the ETL and HTL, respectively. The electrons transfer to the ETL from the perovskite layer to be collected by the TCO layer, the holes transfer to the HTL to be collected by the counter electrode. (see Figure 5.15) The photocurrent is produced when the electrons go through the external circuit from the TCO to the counter electrode to recombine with the holes at last.

5.4.3 Materials and Methods for Flexible PerSCs

For a flexible PerSC device, the flexible substrates usually involve TCO-coated plastics and silver nanowire-coated plastics. Metals such as Au, Ag, and Al, are commonly used as the counter electrodes. Moreover, carbon and graphene are also attractive electrode materials for the flexible PerSCs. Besides, interfacial layers are important to the performance and stability of the PerSCs [52]. TiO_2 and PCBM are the most commonly used ETLs in the regular structure and inverted structure, respectively. p-Type-doped 2,2′,7,7′-tetrakis[*N*,*N*-di(4-methoxyphenyl)-amino]-9,9′-spirobifluorene (spiro-OMeTAD), poly(3,4-ethylenedioxythiophene):poly(styrenesulfonate) (PEDOT:PSS), polytriarylamine (PTAA), and NiO are the most popular candidates for HTLs. Figure 5.16 gives a brief summary of different interface materials and their energy-level alignments with the perovskites.

High performances of PerSCs are critically determined by the excellent photoelectric properties of perovskite photoactive layer itself. Thus, achieving high-quality perovskite photoactive layers with the morphologies of smooth, large-grained as well as pinhole-free, is of significant importance to improve the device efficiency and stability. There are a variety of processing methods [53, 54] for the perovskite photoactive layers as summarized in Figure 5.17. "One-step"

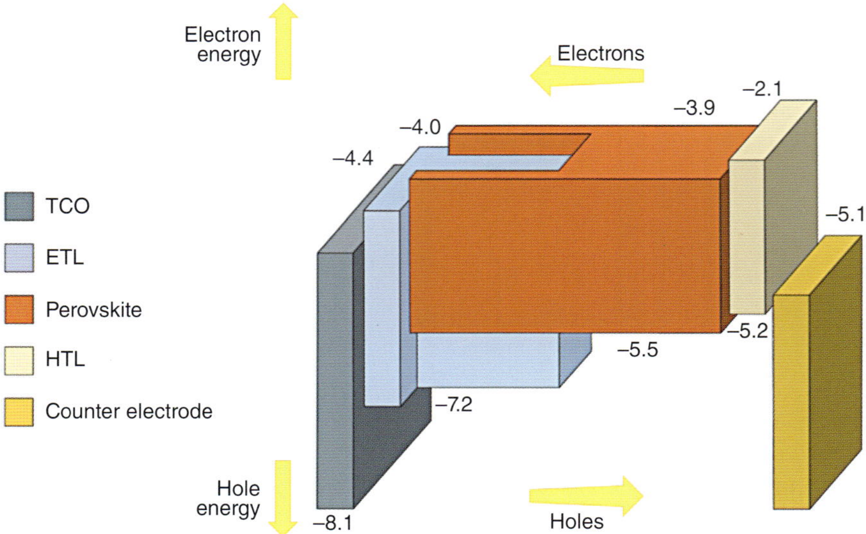

Figure 5.15 The schematic diagram of the working mechanism for perovskite solar cells with n–i–p structure. (Green *et al.* 2014 [47]. Reproduced with permission of Nature Publishing Group.)

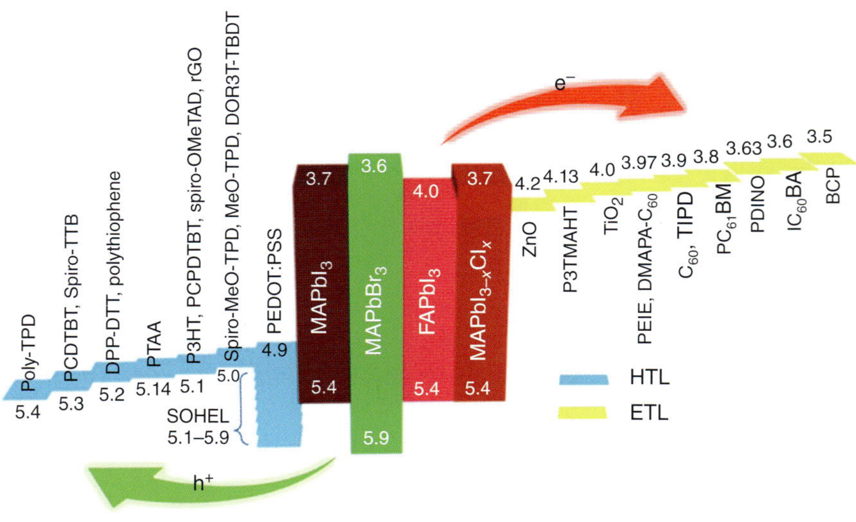

Figure 5.16 Energy level diagram of HTLs (left) and ETLs (right) used in PerSCs and perovskite light absorbers (middle). The unit for each value is (eV) but omitted. (Kim *et al.* 2016 [52]. Reproduced with permission of Royal Society of Chemistry.)

solution process is the earliest method demonstrated by Snaith *et al.* [42] for fabricating $CH_3NH_3PbI_3$ on the TiO_2 surface[42]. The perovskite precursor solution consisting of ammonium halide and lead sources in proper solvent is deposited onto the substrate directly. In 2013, Grätzel *et al.* have evolutionally developed a sequential deposition process which is also called the "two-step" method [55]. In this process, PbI_2 was first introduced from solution into a nanoporous TiO_2 film and subsequently exposed to a solution of CH_3NH_3I to

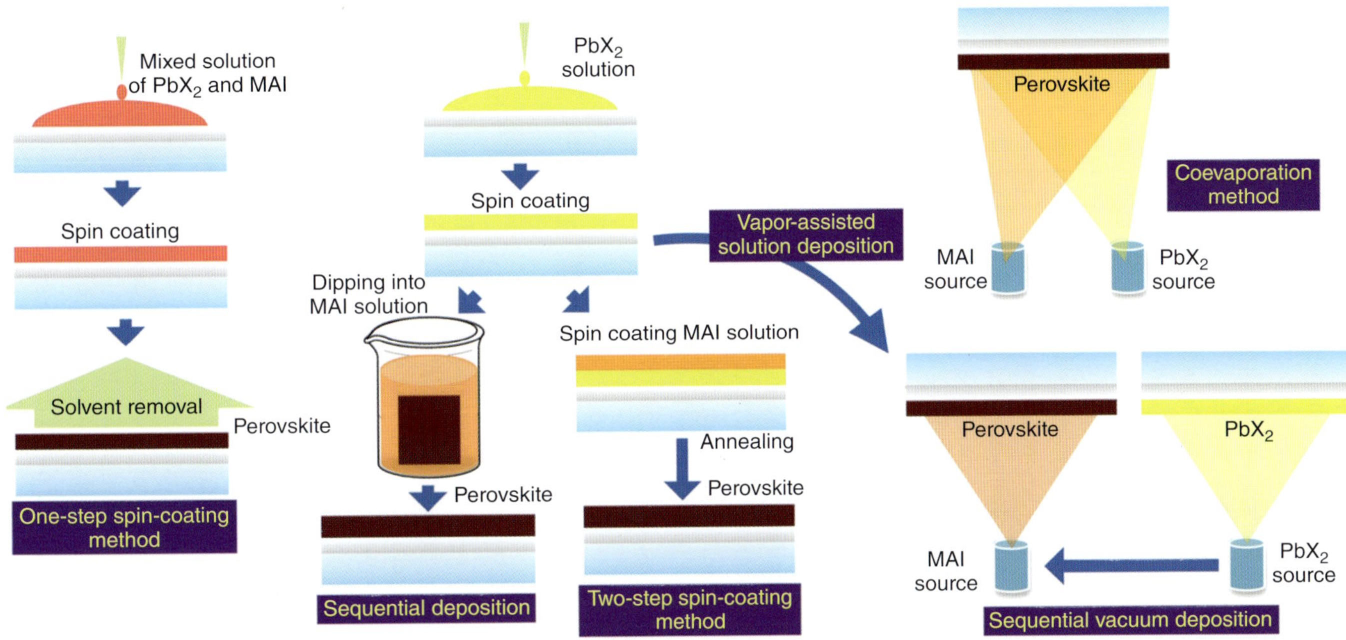

Figure 5.17 Schematic procedure for different preparation methods for perovskite films. (Zheng *et al*. 2015 [54]. Reproduced with permission of Royal Society of Chemistry.)

transform into the high-quality perovskite. In order to improve the film quality of the perovskite active layers, tremendous efforts have been made. For example, Snaith *et al.* have subsequently adopted a double source evaporation method to obtain the dense, uniform, and thickness-tunable perovskite films [56]. The precursor materials are thermally evaporated simultaneously, and the perovskite film is produced on the substrate through chemical reaction of precursors. Cheng *et al.* have reported a facile gas-assisted "one-step" solution processing technique [57]. They have introduced Ar gas flow on the top of the substrate during the spin coating, resulting in uniform perovskite thin films consisting of densely packed single crystalline grains. Antisolvent-assisted compositional engineering is representative of "one-step" solution process [58, 59]. During the spinning of the substrate, an antisolvent was dropped onto the film for fast removing of the host solvent. The resulting smooth, large-grained and pinhole-free perovskite thin films make this antisolvent-assisted method to be widely accepted for the fabrication of high-quality photoactive layers. More surprisingly, some very recent works have pointed out that the perovskite photoactive layers with the large-grained compact microstructures and smooth surfaces without involving any antisolvent process, have been achieved via introducing the "acetate route" by replacing the conventional lead halides ($PbCl_2$ or PbI_2) with lead acetate ($PbAc_2$) as the lead source [60, 61]. This method employs $PbAc_2$ as a lead source in the precursor solution, and obtains the smooth perovskite thin films by simple "one-step" solution process. It is notable that the film annealing time in the $PbAc_2$-based method is much shorter in comparison with the methods based on conventional lead halides ($PbCl_2$ or PbI_2). This is obviously superior to other methodologies, especially for the roll-to-roll printing fabrication for flexible PerSCs.

5.4.4 Recent Advances for Flexible PerSCs

As promising candidates for photovoltaics, PerSCs can be fabricated under low temperature with solution-based methods, which makes them compatible with the flexible substrates to deliver efficient flexible solar cells. Therefore, researches have been conducted to investigate the flexible PerSCs and explore their potential applications. Herein, some representative examples of flexible PerSCs are presented.

Kim *et al.* have fabricated highly bendable (up to 1 mm bending radius) PerSCs based on ITO-coated PEN flexible substrates and achieved an excellent *PCE* of 12.2% [62]. A cross-sectional SEM image and an image of the bendable device are shown in Figure 5.18b,c. As illustrated in Figure 5.18d,e, the power conversion efficiency of this flexible solar cell remained at 95% after 1000 cycles of bending tests with a bending radius of 10 mm. This shows the superior mechanical endurance properties of the devices. It is noteworthy that the n-type TiO_x compact interface layer was deposited via a plasma-enhanced ALD (PEALD) technique. This ALD coating method was believed to be crucial for the high performance of the flexible devices. The highly efficient and bendable PerSCs could potentially be used for the power solution for future wearable devices as demonstrated in Figure 5.18a.

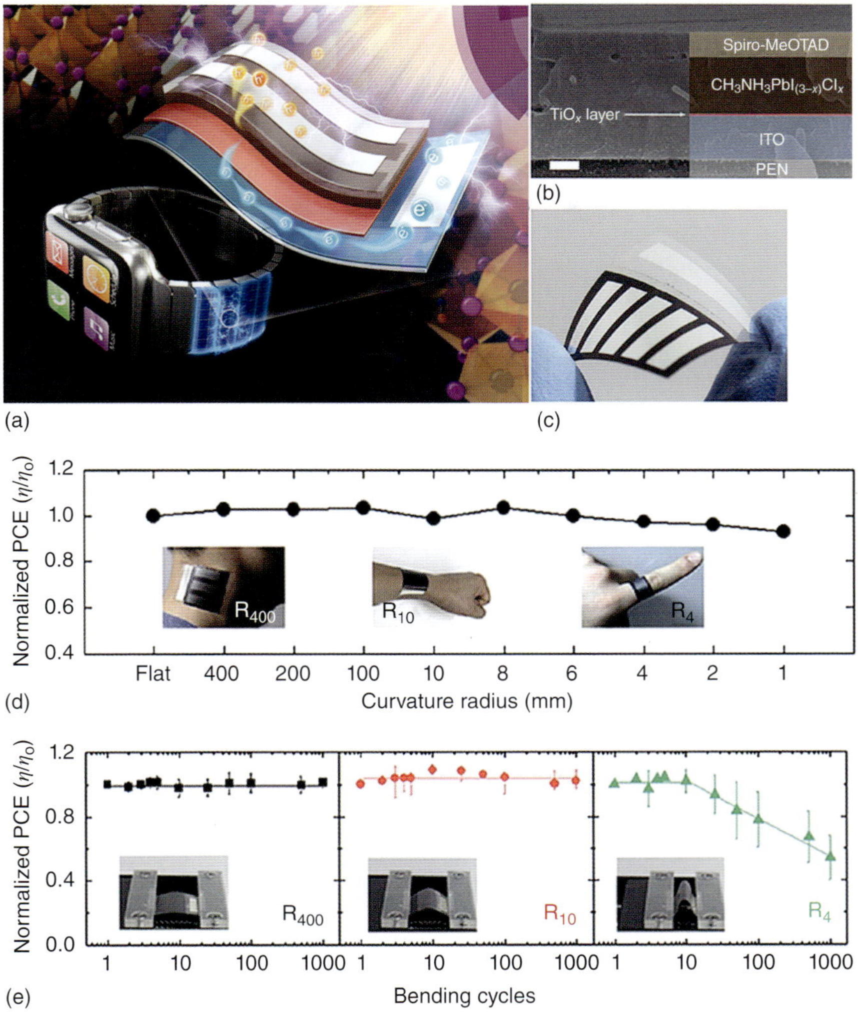

Figure 5.18 (a) Conceptual schematic diagram of a smart watch integrated with a flexible perovskite solar cell. (b) Cross-sectional SEM image of the inorganic–organic halide perovskite planar heterojunction flexible solar cell and schematic of the flexible device structure. Scale bar: 200 nm. (c) An actual bent image of a flexible perovskite solar cell. (d) Normalized *PCE* measured after bending the substrate within a specified radius of 400–1 mm. The inset shows the real images attached on the human neck, wrist, and finger corresponding to 400, 10, and 4 nm bending radii, respectively. The error bar represents standard deviation from 4 devices. (e) Normalized *PCE* of flexible perovskite devices as a function of bending cycles with different radii of 400, 10, and 4 mm. The inset shows the real images taken during the bending tests. The error bar represents the standard deviation from four devices. (Kim *et al*. 2015 [62]. Reproduced with permission of Royal Society of Chemistry.)

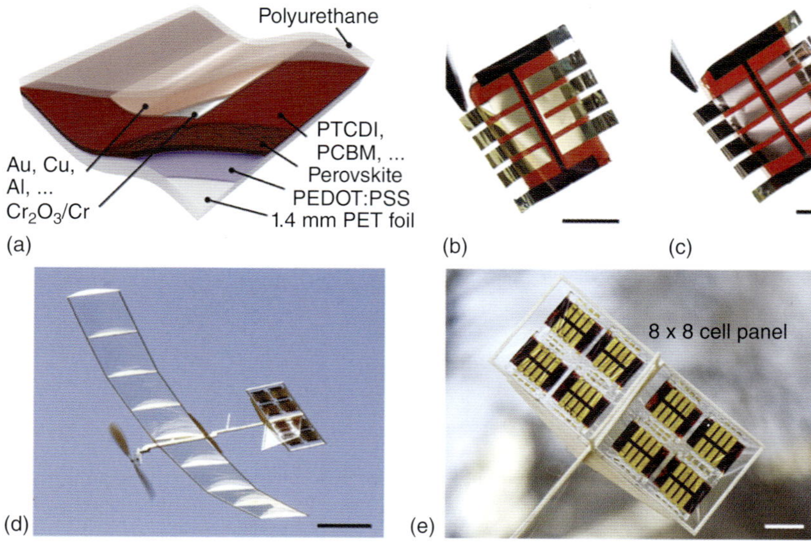

Figure 5.19 Ultrathin and light perovskite solar cells. (a) Schematic of the solar cell stack. (b) Free-standing 3-μm-thick solar cells with gold top metal. Scale bar, 1 cm. (c) Perovskite solar foil with low-cost copper back contacts. Scale bar, 1 cm. (d) Snapshot of the model plane during solar-powered outdoor flight. Scale bar, 10 cm. (e) Close-up photograph of the horizontal stabilizer with integrated solar panel. Scale bar, 2 cm. (Kaltenbrunner *et al.* 2015 [63]. Reproduced with permission of Nature Publishing Group.)

Kaltenbrunner *et al.* have constructed the PerSCs on the ultrathin PET foils. The finished highly flexible device with a total thickness of only 3 μm has delivered a stabilized efficiency of 12% [63]. High efficiency and low weight ($5.2\,\mathrm{g\,m^{-2}}$) lead to a very impressive power-to-weight ratio of $23\,\mathrm{W\,g^{-1}}$, and this ratio is used to evaluate the energy density for ultrathin flexible solar cells. As shown in Figure 5.19a–c, the PEDOT:PSS has not only been employed as the HTL but also as the electrode, eliminating the commonly used TCO electrodes. To facilitate air-stable operation of the flexible devices, they have introduced a thin chromium oxide-chromium interlayer between the ETL and the top electrode. Cr_2O_3 has great robustness against the aggressive oxidants, and this Cr_2O_3/Cr interlayer could effectively prevent the metal top contact from the chemical reactions with the perovskite photoactive layer. Thus the un-encapsulated devices with a Cr_2O_3/Cr interlayer remain functional after four days in air under continuous illumination. The viability of these ultrathin perovskite solar foils for laboratory-scale aeronautic applications was also demonstrated. They have fabricated two 4×8 solar modules based on 64 individual ultralightweight solar cells. The two solar modules were successfully integrated onto the horizontal stabilizers of a model airplane and used to power a direct current motor with propeller of the aviation models as shown in Figure 5.19d,e. These results revealed the potential of the flexible PerSCs for future applications.

Owing to their superior processibility, PerSCs can also be prepared on varied conducting substrates to realize the flexible function. Stainless steel fibers, silver-mesh/conducting polymer substrates, and titanium foils have been used as

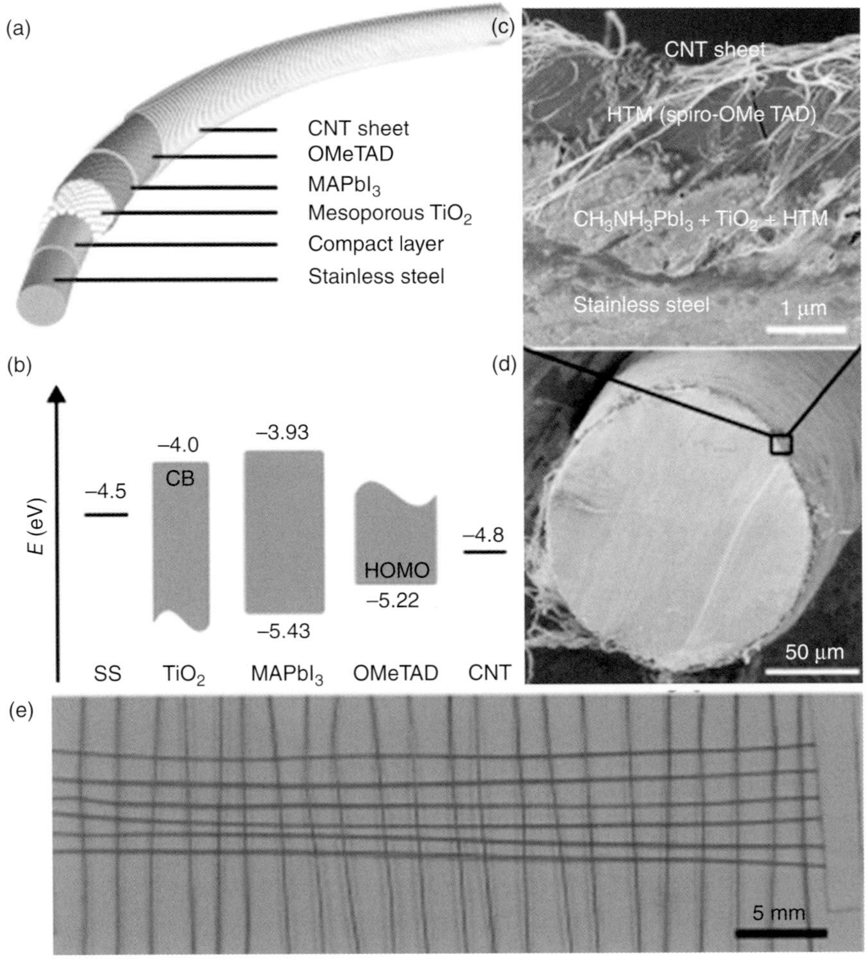

Figure 5.20 (a) Schematic, (b) energy level diagram (c,d) cross-sectional SEM images of the fiber-shaped perovskite solar cell. (e) Photograph of a textile. (Qiu *et al.* 2014 [64]. Reproduced with permission of John Wiley & Sons.)

the conducting substrates for flexible PerSCs. For example, Peng *et al.* [64] have used stainless steel fiber with a diameter of 127 mm as a substrate to prepare a coaxial fiber-shaped PerSC, as shown in Figure 5.20a–d. The device delivered a power conversion efficiency of 3.3%. It is also noteworthy that these coaxial fiber-shaped PerSCs were highly flexible and can be bent into various shapes without fatigue, and their energy conversion efficiencies maintained 95% of the initial *PCE* after bending for 50 cycles. This coaxial fiber-shaped PerSCs could potentially be woven into solar textiles for applications in wearable electronics as shown in Figure 5.20e.

Further, Li *et al.* [65] have demonstrated high-performance flexible PerSCs constructed on highly flexible and ultrathin silver-mesh/conducting polymer substrates as shown in Figure 5.21a. The device efficiency reached 14.0%, which is

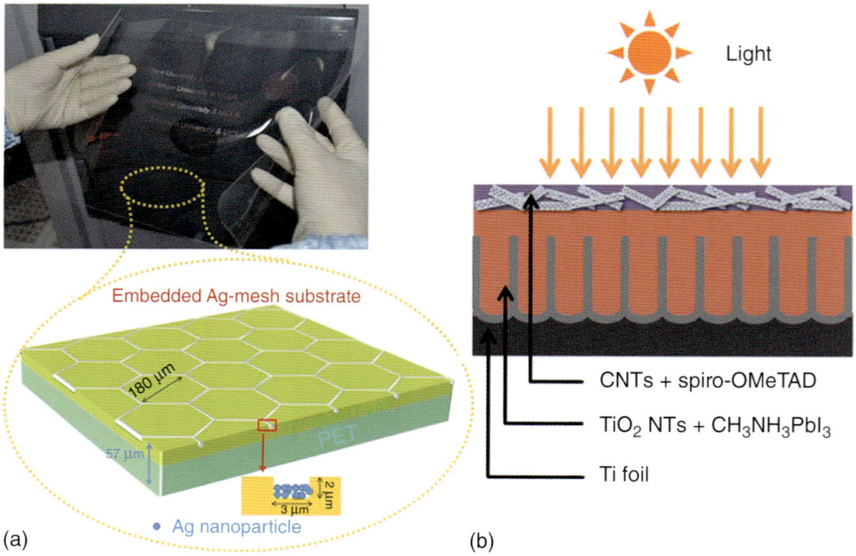

Figure 5.21 (a) Image and structure of a flexible PET substrate with embedded Ag-mesh with detail parameters. (Reproduced from Ref. [65], CC-BY-4.0.) (b) Schematic of a solid-state perovskite solar cell based on Ti foil/TiO_2 nanotubes and carbon nanotubes. (Wang *et al.* 2015 [66]. Reproduced with permission of Elsevier.)

among the best results for the flexible PerSCs. Wong *et al.* [66] reported the flexible perovskite based on titanium (Ti) foil/TiO_2 nanotubes (NTs), as shown in Figure 5.21b. Transparent conductive carbon nanotube network was laminated on top of perovskite and served as the hole collector as well as the transparent electrode for light illumination. This is a typical example of top-illuminated flexible PerSCs and efficiency of 8.31% was achieved. The device also demonstrated good flexibility and 100 mechanical bending cycles showed little deterioration to the device performance.

With all these efforts on the substrate materials, interface materials, and photoactive layer, the flexible PerSCs have been intensively explored. Both the device efficiencies and mechanical properties have been significantly enhanced. Along with the fast development of PerSCs, it can be expected that the flexible PerSC will be much more efficient and reliable for a wide range of applications.

5.5 Summary and Conclusion

This chapter reviewed the advances of some FPV candidates covering flexible Si solar cells, CIGS solar cells, organic solar cells, and PerSCs. We have discussed the fundamentals of converting light into electricity, the properties of photovoltaic materials, the operation mechanism of different solar cells, and the current status of different flexible solar cells and their potential applications. With the tremendous efforts from all over the world, particularly on some novel photovoltaic technologies, the flexible solar cells are being intensively explored.

Low-cost, compact, and efficient flexible solar cells are intended to impact all kinds of energy applications. Their future applications can be expected in a wide range of areas, providing energy solutions for many electronic devices, such as personal electronic devices, outdoor power stations, medical and health care devices, unmanned aircrafts and weather balloons for environmental and industrial monitoring, and even military security applications.

References

1 Nelson, J. (2003) *The Physics of Solar Cells*, World Scientific, London.

2 Mathew, X., Enriquez, J.P., Romeo, A., and Tiwari, A.N. (2004) CdTe/CdS solar cells on flexible substrates. *Sol. Energy*, **77** (6), 831–838.

3 Polman, A., Knight, M., Garnett, E.C., Ehrler, B., and Sinke, W.C. (2016) Photovoltaic materials: present efficiencies and future challenges. *Science*, **352** (6283), aad4424.

4 Shah, A., Torres, P., Tscharner, R., Wyrsch, N., and Keppner, H. (1999) Photovoltaic technology: the case for thin-film solar cells. *Science*, **285** (5428), 692–698.

5 Green, M.A. (1982) *Solar Cells: Operating Principles, Technology, and System Applications*, Prentice Hall, Kensington.

6 Carlson, D.E. and Wronski, C.R. (1976) Amorphous silicon solar cell. *Appl. Phys. Lett.*, **28** (11), 671–673.

7 Yang, J., Banerjee, A., and Guha, S. (1997) Triple-junction amorphous silicon alloy solar cell with 14.6% initial and 13.0% stable conversion efficiencies. *Appl. Phys. Lett.*, **70** (22), 2975–2977.

8 Yang, J., Yan, B., and Guha, S. (2005) Amorphous and nanocrystalline silicon-based multi-junction solar cells. *Thin Solid Films*, **487** (1), 162–169.

9 Ichikawa, Y., Yoshida, T., Hama, T., Sakai, H., and Harashima, K. (2001) Production technology for amorphous silicon-based flexible solar cells. *Sol. Energy Mater. Sol. Cells*, **66** (1), 107–115.

10 Yoon, J., Baca, A.J., Park, S.-I., Elvikis, P., Geddes, J.B., Li, L., Kim, R.H., Xiao, J., Wang, S., and Kim, T.-H. (2008) Ultrathin silicon solar microcells for semitransparent, mechanically flexible and microconcentrator module designs. *Nat. Mater.*, **7** (11), 907–915.

11 Rau, U. and Schock, H.-W. (1999) Electronic properties of $Cu(In,Ga)Se_2$ heterojunction solar cells-recent achievements, current understanding, and future challenges. *Appl. Phys. A*, **69** (2), 131–147.

12 Guillemoles, J.-F., Rau, U., Kronik, L., Schock, H.-W., and Cahen, D. (1999) $Cu(In,Ga)Se_2$ solar cells: device stability based on chemical flexibility. *Adv. Mater.*, **11** (11), 957–961.

13 Carlson, D. (1986) Hydrogenated microvoids and light-induced degradation of amorphous-silicon solar cells. *Appl. Phys. A*, **41** (4), 305–309.

14 Crandall, R.S. (1991) Defect relaxation in amorphous silicon: stretched exponentials, the Meyer–Neldel rule, and the Staebler–Wronski effect. *Phys. Rev. B*, **43** (5), 4057–4070.

15 Kessler, F. and Rudmann, D. (2004) Technological aspects of flexible CIGS solar cells and modules. *Sol. Energy*, **77** (6), 685–695.

16 Chirilă, A., Buecheler, S., Pianezzi, F., Bloesch, P., Gretener, C., Uhl, A.R., Fella, C., Kranz, L., Perrenoud, J., and Seyrling, S. (2011) Highly efficient Cu(In,Ga)Se_2 solar cells grown on flexible polymer films. *Nat. Mater.*, **10** (11), 857–861.

17 Başol, B.M., Kapur, V.K., Halani, A., and Leidholm, C. (1993) Copper indium diselenide thin film solar cells fabricated on flexible foil substrates. *Sol. Energy Mater. Sol. Cells*, **29** (2), 163–173.

18 Schock, H.W. and Noufi, R. (2000) CIGS-based solar cells for the next millennium. *Prog. Photovoltaics Res. Appl.*, **8** (1), 151–160.

19 Van Duren, J., Robinson, M., and Leidholm, C. (2006) Photovoltaic devices printed from nanostructured particles. US Patent 20070163638 A1.

20 Tress, W. (2012) *Device Physics of Organic Solar Cells: Drift-Diffusion Simulation in Comparison with Experimental Data of Solar Cells Based on Small Molecules*, Technische Universität Dresden.

21 Janssen, R. (2005) *Introduction to Polymer Solar Cells (3Y280)*, Departments of Chemical Engineering & Chemistry and Applied Physics Eindhoven University of Technology, The Netherlands.

22 Tang, C.W. (1986) Two-layer organic photovoltaic cell. *Appl. Phys. Lett.*, **48** (2), 183–185.

23 He, Z., Zhong, C., Su, S., Xu, M., Wu, H., and Cao, Y. (2012) Enhanced power-conversion efficiency in polymer solar cells using an inverted device structure. *Nat. Photonics*, **6** (9), 593–597.

24 Yu, G., Gao, J., Hummelen, J.C., Wudl, F., and Heeger, A.J. (1995) Polymer photovoltiac cells: enhanced efficiencies via a network of internal donor–acceptor heterojunctions. *Science*, **270** (5243), 1789–1791.

25 Park, S.H., Roy, A., Beaupre, S., Cho, S., Coates, N., Moon, J.S., Moses, D., Leclerc, M., Lee, K., and Heeger, A.J. (2009) Bulk heterojunction solar cells with internal quantum efficiency approaching 100%. *Nat. Photonics*, **3** (5), 297–302.

26 Li, G., Zhu, R., and Yang, Y. (2012) Polymer solar cells. *Nat. Photonics*, **6** (3), 153–161.

27 Liang, Y., Xu, Z., Xia, J., Tsai, S.T., Wu, Y., Li, G., Ray, C., and Yu, L. (2010) For the bright future-bulk heterojunction polymer solar cells with power conversion efficiency of 7.4%. *Adv. Mater.*, **22** (20), E135–E138.

28 Ma, W., Yang, C., Gong, X., Lee, K., and Heeger, A.J. (2005) Thermally stable, efficient polymer solar cells with nanoscale control of the interpenetrating network morphology. *Adv. Funct. Mater.*, **15** (10), 1617–1622.

29 Li, G., Shrotriya, V., Huang, J., Yao, Y., Moriarty, T., Emery, K., and Yang, Y. (2005) High-efficiency solution processable polymer photovoltaic cells by self-organization of polymer blends. *Nat. Mater.*, **4** (11), 864–868.

30 Hou, J., Chen, T.L., Zhang, S., Huo, L., Sista, S., and Yang, Y. (2009) An easy and effective method to modulate molecular energy level of poly(3-alkylthiophene) for high-V_{oc} polymer solar cells. *Macromolecules*, **42** (23), 9217–9219.

31 Zhang, M., Guo, X., Yang, Y., Zhang, J., Zhang, Z.-G., and Li, Y. (2011) Downwards tuning the HOMO level of polythiophene by carboxylate substitution for high open-circuit-voltage polymer solar cells. *Polym. Chem.*, **2** (12), 2900.

32 Zhang, M., Guo, X., Ma, W., Ade, H., and Hou, J. (2014) A polythiophene derivative with superior properties for practical application in polymer solar cells. *Adv. Mater.*, **26** (33), 5880–5885.

33 Zhang, H., Ye, L., and Hou, J. (2015) Molecular design strategies for voltage modulation in highly efficient polymer solar cells. *Polym. Int.*, **64** (8), 957–962.

34 Lin, Y., Zhao, F., He, Q., Huo, L., Wu, Y., Parker, T.C., Ma, W., Sun, Y., Wang, C., Zhu, D., Heeger, A.J., Marder, S.R., and Zhan, X. (2016) High-performance electron acceptor with thienyl side chains for organic photovoltaics. *J. Am. Chem. Soc.*, **138** (14), 4955–4961.

35 Zhao, W., Qian, D., Zhang, S., Li, S., Inganas, O., Gao, F., and Hou, J. (2016) Fullerene-free polymer solar cells with over 11% efficiency and excellent thermal stability. *Adv. Mater.*, **28** (23), 4734–4739.

36 Na, S.-I., Kim, S.-S., Jo, J., and Kim, D.-Y. (2008) Efficient and flexible ITO-free organic solar cells using highly conductive polymer anodes. *Adv. Mater.*, **20** (21), 4061–4067.

37 Kaltenbrunner, M., White, M.S., Glowacki, E.D., Sekitani, T., Someya, T., Sariciftci, N.S., and Bauer, S. (2012) Ultrathin and lightweight organic solar cells with high flexibility. *Nat. Commun.*, **3**, 770.

38 Kim, T., Kim, J.H., Kang, T.E., Lee, C., Kang, H., Shin, M., Wang, C., Ma, B., Jeong, U., Kim, T.S., and Kim, B.J. (2015) Flexible, highly efficient all-polymer solar cells. *Nat. Commun.*, **6**, 8547.

39 Zhu, R., Chung, C.-H., Cha, K.C., Yang, W., Zheng, Y.B., Zhou, H., Song, T.-B., Chen, C.-C., Weiss, P.S., and Li, G. (2011) Fused silver nanowires with metal oxide nanoparticles and organic polymers for highly transparent conductors. *ACS Nano*, **5** (12), 9877–9882.

40 Chen, C.-C., Dou, L., Zhu, R., Chung, C.-H., Song, T.-B., Zheng, Y.B., Hawks, S., Li, G., Weiss, P.S., and Yang, Y. (2012) Visibly transparent polymer solar cells produced by solution processing. *ACS Nano*, **6** (8), 7185–7190.

41 Kojima, A., Teshima, K., Shirai, Y., and Miyasaka, T. (2009) Organometal halide perovskites as visible-light sensitizers for photovoltaic cells. *J. Am. Chem. Soc.*, **131** (17), 6050–6051.

42 Lee, M.M., Teuscher, J., Miyasaka, T., Murakami, T.N., and Snaith, H.J. (2012) Efficient hybrid solar cells based on meso-superstructured organometal halide perovskites. *Science*, **338** (6107), 643–647.

43 Kim, H.-S., Lee, C.-R., Im, J.-H., Lee, K.-B., Moehl, T., Marchioro, A., Moon, S.-J., Humphry-Baker, R., Yum, J.-H., and Moser, J.E. (2012) Lead iodide perovskite sensitized all-solid-state submicron thin film mesoscopic solar cell with efficiency exceeding 9%. *Sci. Rep.*, **2**, 591.

44 Etgar, L., Gao, P., Xue, Z., Peng, Q., Chandiran, A.K., Liu, B., Nazeeruddin, M.K., and Grätzel, M. (2012) Mesoscopic $CH_3NH_3PbI_3/TiO_2$ heterojunction solar cells. *J. Am. Chem. Soc.*, **134** (42), 17396–17399.

45 Coontz, R. http://www.sciencemag.org/news/2013/12/sciences-top-10-breakthroughs-2013 (accessed 19 December 2013).

46 NREL (2016) http://www.nrel.gov/ncpv/images/efficiency_chart.jpg (accessed 20 September 2017).

47 Green, M.A., Ho-Baillie, A., and Snaith, H.J. (2014) The emergence of perovskite solar cells. *Nat. Photonics*, **8** (7), 506–514.

48 Docampo, P., Ball, J.M., Darwich, M., Eperon, G.E., and Snaith, H.J. (2013) Efficient organometal trihalide perovskite planar-heterojunction solar cells on flexible polymer substrates. *Nat. Commun.*, **4**, 2761.

49 Stranks, S.D., Eperon, G.E., Grancini, G., Menelaou, C., Alcocer, M.J., Leijtens, T., Herz, L.M., Petrozza, A., and Snaith, H.J. (2013) Electron–hole diffusion lengths exceeding 1 micrometer in an organometal trihalide perovskite absorber. *Science*, **342** (6156), 341–344.

50 Xing, G., Mathews, N., Sun, S., Lim, S.S., Lam, Y.M., Grätzel, M., Mhaisalkar, S., and Sum, T.C. (2013) Long-range balanced electron-and hole-transport lengths in organic–inorganic $CH_3NH_3PbI_3$. *Science*, **342** (6156), 344–347.

51 Liu, T., Chen, K., Hu, Q., Zhu, R., and Gong, Q. (2016) Inverted perovskite solar cells: progresses and perspectives. *Adv. Energy Mater.*, **6**, 1600457.

52 Kim, H., Lim, K.-G., and Lee, T.-W. (2016) Planar heterojunction organometal halide perovskite solar cells: roles of interfacial layers. *Energy Environ. Sci.*, **9** (1), 12–30.

53 Zhao, Y. and Zhu, K. (2016) Organic–inorganic hybrid lead halide perovskites for optoelectronic and electronic applications. *Chem. Soc. Rev.*, **45** (3), 655–689.

54 Zheng, L., Zhang, D., Ma, Y., Lu, Z., Chen, Z., Wang, S., Xiao, L., and Gong, Q. (2015) Morphology control of the perovskite films for efficient solar cells. *Dalton Trans.*, **44** (23), 10582–10593.

55 Burschka, J., Pellet, N., Moon, S.-J., Humphry-Baker, R., Gao, P., Nazeeruddin, M.K., and Grätzel, M. (2013) Sequential deposition as a route to high-performance perovskite-sensitized solar cells. *Nature*, **499** (7458), 316–319.

56 Liu, M., Johnston, M.B., and Snaith, H.J. (2013) Efficient planar heterojunction perovskite solar cells by vapour deposition. *Nature*, **501** (7467), 395–398.

57 Huang, F., Dkhissi, Y., Huang, W., Xiao, M., Benesperi, I., Rubanov, S., Zhu, Y., Lin, X., Jiang, L., and Zhou, Y. (2014) Gas-assisted preparation of lead iodide perovskite films consisting of a monolayer of single crystalline grains for high efficiency planar solar cells. *Nano Energy*, **10**, 10–18.

58 Xiao, M., Huang, F., Huang, W., Dkhissi, Y., Zhu, Y., Etheridge, J., Gray-Weale, A., Bach, U., Cheng, Y.B., and Spiccia, L. (2014) A fast deposition-crystallization procedure for highly efficient lead iodide perovskite thin-film solar cells. *Angew. Chem. Int. Ed.*, **126** (37), 10056–10061.

59 Jeon, N.J., Noh, J.H., Kim, Y.C., Yang, W.S., Ryu, S., and Seok, S.I. (2014) Solvent engineering for high-performance inorganic–organic hybrid perovskite solar cells. *Nat. Mater.*, **13** (9), 897–903.

60 Zhang, W., Saliba, M., Moore, D.T., Pathak, S.K., Hörantner, M.T., Stergiopoulos, T., Stranks, S.D., Eperon, G.E., Alexander-Webber, J.A., and Abate, A. (2015) Ultrasmooth organic–inorganic perovskite thin-film formation and crystallization for efficient planar heterojunction solar cells. *Nat. Commun.*, **6**, 6142.

61 Zhao, L., Luo, D., Wu, J., Hu, Q., Zhang, W., Chen, K., Liu, T., Liu, Y., Zhang, Y., and Liu, F. (2016) High-performance inverted planar heterojunction perovskite solar cells based on lead acetate precursor with efficiency exceeding 18%. *Adv. Funct. Mater.*, **26** (20), 3508–3514.

62 Kim, B.J., Kim, D.H., Lee, Y.-Y., Shin, H.-W., Han, G.S., Hong, J.S., Mahmood, K., Ahn, T.K., Joo, Y.-C., and Hong, K.S. (2015) Highly efficient and bending durable perovskite solar cells: toward a wearable power source. *Energy Environ. Sci.*, **8** (3), 916–921.

63 Kaltenbrunner, M., Adam, G., Głowacki, E.D., Drack, M., Schwödiauer, R., Leonat, L., Apaydin, D.H., Groiss, H., Scharber, M.C., and White, M.S. (2015) Flexible high power-per-weight perovskite solar cells with chromium oxide-metal contacts for improved stability in air. *Nat. Mater.*, **14** (10), 1032–1039.

64 Qiu, L., Deng, J., Lu, X., Yang, Z., and Peng, H. (2014) Integrating perovskite solar cells into a flexible fiber. *Angew. Chem. Int. Ed.*, **53** (39), 10425–10428.

65 Li, Y., Meng, L., Yang, Y.M., Xu, G., Hong, Z., Chen, Q., You, J., Li, G., Yang, Y., and Li, Y. (2016) High-efficiency robust perovskite solar cells on ultrathin flexible substrates. *Nat. Commun.*, **7**, 10214.

66 Wang, X., Li, Z., Xu, W., Kulkarni, S.A., Batabyal, S.K., Zhang, S., Cao, A., and Wong, L.H. (2015) TiO_2 nanotube arrays based flexible perovskite solar cells with transparent carbon nanotube electrode. *Nano Energy*, **11**, 728–735.

6

Materials Design for Flexible Thermoelectric Power Generators

Yoshiyuki Nonoguchi

Nara Institute of Science and Technology (NAIST), Graduate School of Materials Science, 8916-5 Takayama, Ikoma, Nara 630-0192, Japan

6.1 Introduction

Some challenges in sustainable energy supply and powering remain to be solved in the near future. Owing to an increase in crude oil prices and the possible depletion of oil resources, emergent energy harvesting from solar energy and wind power is a high requirement. Since energy prices are increasing more and more there is interest and need in extracting seemingly trivial and unprofitable energy resources that have been so far ignored. Thermoelectrics is a technique that immediately converts temperature difference into electric potential difference. Unlike conventional turbine generators with high-pressure gases and large facilities, thermoelectric generators can produce power from small temperature differences and therefore can be widely applied in the recovery of waste heat from currently untapped sources such as commercial buildings and industrial plants. In addition, it can be expected that a lot of waste heat is potentially used as supplementary power for mobile vehicles (cars, buses, etc.) and information technology (IT) equipment including security and medical devices. In particular, the application of flexible and light-weight thermoelectric generators will be expanded in the above-mentioned applications. Importantly, for practical thermoelectric power conversion materials in a temperature range lower than 400 K, flexibility is crucial to cover and adhere closely to the heat sources that emit low thermal radiation.

For the construction of such flexible power modules, it is crucial to integrate various polymer and nanostructured materials as substrates, powering layers, and electrodes. Subsequently, a comprehensive and multifaceted understanding of various research topics ranging from materials chemistry to applied physics is highly required. Historically, thermoelectrics has been an important topic in quantum condensed matter physics and thermodynamics, and has been well summarized in many textbooks. In spite of these efforts however, the viewpoints from a physics and mechanics perspective remain difficult for the elementary-level beginners (i.e., chemists and applied physicists) to overview and understand. Additionally, these textbooks often contain a lot of concepts

Flexible and Stretchable Medical Devices, First Edition. Edited by Kuniharu Takei.

not always important for organic and emergent materials. The following section commences with the fundamental thermoelectric concepts extracted from basic condensed matter physics, useful for materials chemists and applied physicists [1]. Following from the general principles, a section on thermoelectric materials design outlines several important strategies for the development of polymer- and nanocarbon-based flexible thermoelectrics.

6.2 General Principles

6.2.1 The Basic Principles of Thermoelectricity

Let us start by defining the three classical factors controlling the thermoelectric properties of a material. If an electric field is applied to a material, you will observe an electric current. When no temperature gradient is present, the ratio of a current density to an electric field determines the electrical conductivity (σ) of the material. In contrast, when a temperature gradient is applied in a material you might measure heat flow. For insulating materials you might observe almost no electric current. Under these conditions, the ratio of heat flow per unit area to the temperature gradient determines the thermal conductivity (κ) of the material.

Additionally, you might apply a temperature difference along a material without applying any electric field, which corresponds to simply generating an energy flow and induces an electric current. The latter corresponds to a thermoelectric current. When you measure this thermoelectric current, it is necessary to construct a closed circuit composed of different materials. It is obvious that no net current can be measured in a symmetric circuit made of the same metals (Figure 6.1a). The same absolute amounts of thermoelectric currents flow in two circuit arms between temperatures at both ends (T, and $T + \Delta T$), and no substantial current is measured. If the circuit comprises two different materials or the same material in different states, you can measure the net thermoelectric current (Figure 6.1b). Note that the magnitude of this thermoelectric current

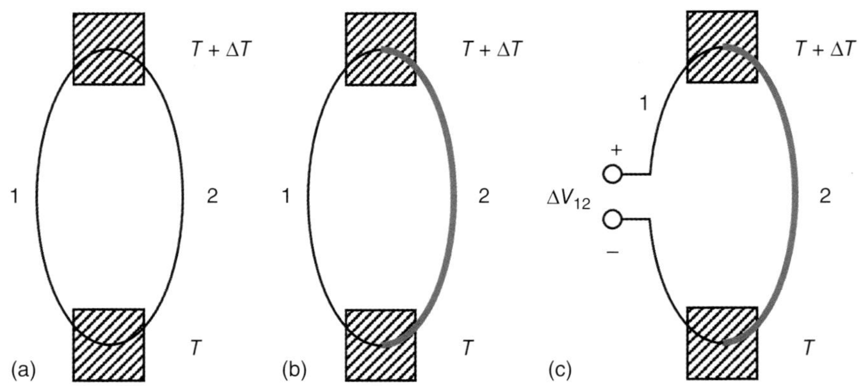

Figure 6.1 Basic thermoelectric circuits. (a) A closed circuit with two similar conductors. (b) A closed circuit with two different conductors. (c) An open circuit with two different conductors.

depends on the temperature difference and even on the shape and dimension of materials. Now, consider how to measure the thermoelectric properties of a given individual material concerned. An open circuit, currently known as a thermocouple (Figure 6.1c), is useful for evaluating the potential difference. Once the terminals (○) are set, a potential difference (ΔV_{12}) is determined only by the temperature difference. You can evaluate the absolute thermoelectric power of conductors that you are interested in by subtracting the known value of a reference (sample 1) from the measured total thermovoltage.

Let us now try to define the Seebeck coefficient using an intuitive and practical approach. As explained in the previous paragraph, once a temperature difference ΔT is applied between both edges of a material, you can observe a potential difference between the edges. This potential difference is proportional to the temperature gradient between both the ends. This phenomenon is called the Seebeck effect, and its proportionality constant, the Seebeck coefficient (α), is expressed as follows:

$$V = -\alpha \Delta T \tag{6.1}$$

Assume that a temperature gradient is applied between the hot end ($T + \Delta T$) and the cold end (T) of a given semiconductor or metal material where charged carriers can move. In this case, charged carriers are excited following the Boltzmann distribution at specific temperatures (T and $T + \Delta T$). As a result, since the density of charged carriers at the higher temperature end gets higher, charged carriers will flow from the hot side to the cold side, following the Fick's diffusion equation. Positively and negatively charged carriers in most semiconductors and metals possess their own different effective masses and diffusion coefficient. For example, negative charges will flow from a high temperature region to a low temperature region in the n-type materials that possess the larger diffusion coefficient of negatively charged carriers (Figure 6.2). The hot side is therefore positively charged and the cold side is negatively charged. p-Type materials, including most conducting polymers, show opposite charging. In most textbooks, the sign of the Seebeck coefficient is determined so that the α of p-type materials is positive as in Eq. (6.1). Practically, the sign of a measured voltage against an applied temperature gradient can define the polarity of a given material, where the positive and negative Seebeck coefficients indicate the p-type and n-type polarity, respectively.

6.2.2 Density of State and the Seebeck Coefficient

Since the Seebeck effect is controlled by the Boltzmann distribution, you might expect that the Seebeck coefficient is closely associated with the density of state (DOS) related comprehensively to the distribution and degeneracy of electronic states. Assuming some approximation for common metals and semiconductors, the Seebeck coefficient (α) is proportional to the gradient of density of state distribution (DOS(E)) function at the Fermi level ($E = E_F$) as follows:

$$\alpha \propto \left| \frac{\mathrm{dDOS}(E)}{\mathrm{d}E}_{@E=E_F} \right| \tag{6.2}$$

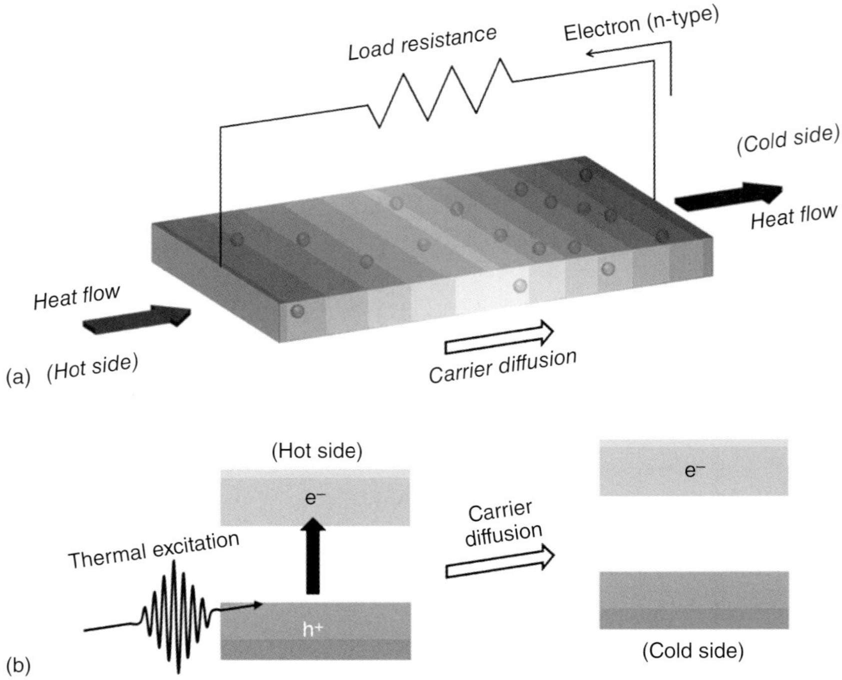

Figure 6.2 A practical view of thermoelectricity. (a) A schematic of, and (b) a band-based scheme for, carrier diffusion in a given n-type thermoelectric material.

Figure 6.3 shows the typical DOS with DOS on the horizontal axis and state energy on the vertical axis, for metals, one-dimensional semiconductors, and molecules. Following Eq. (6.2), you can obtain a large Seebeck coefficient of a given material when its DOS gradient is large at the Fermi energy (E_F). As shown in Figure 6.3, organic semiconductor materials including carbon nanotubes and conducting polymers possess low-dimensional structures, and then a sharp DOS around Fermi level. These facts might inspire one to obtain an excellent Seebeck coefficient and high-efficiency energy-to-electricity conversion. Owing to the presence of a sharp DOS shape, insulating materials with totally discrete electronic states should possess an extremely large Seebeck coefficient while their conductivity is quite low.

6.2.3 Energy Conversion Efficiency and Dimensionless Thermoelectric Figure of Merit *ZT*

Consider making a short circuit between the both ends of a given semiconductor material with a lead (conductor) with extremely low electrical resistivity (R) and thermal conductivity (Figure 6.2a). This is equivalent to the short circuit of a cell with a voltage of V ($=\alpha\Delta T$). Therefore, the steady current I of the given semiconductor and its maximum output power P_0 to an external circuit is calculated using the electrical conductivity (σ) as:

$$I = V/R \propto \alpha\sigma\Delta T \tag{6.3}$$

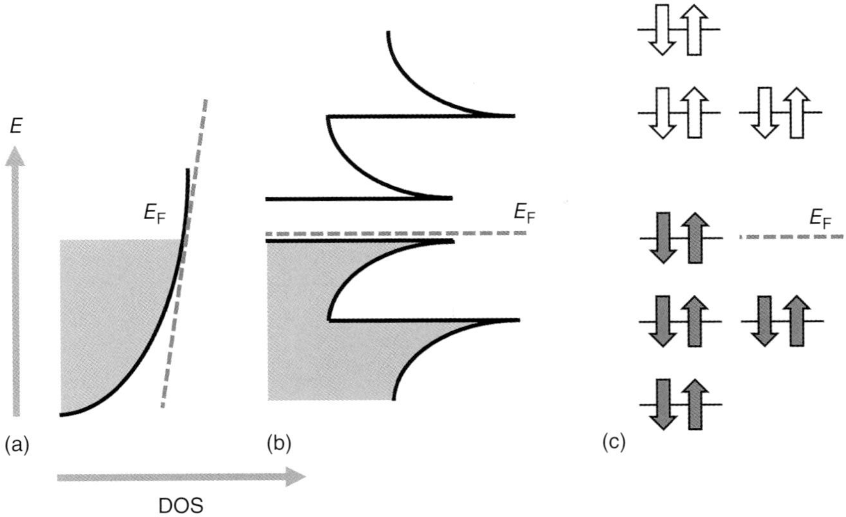

Figure 6.3 Typical density of state for (a) metals, (b) one-dimensional semiconductors, and (c) molecules and insulators. Dashed lines show the gradient at the Fermi level.

and

$$P_0 = IV \propto \alpha^2\sigma\Delta T^2 \tag{6.4}$$

Considering Eq. (6.4), the exploitation of a large $\alpha^2\sigma$ is preferred for the construction of high-performance thermoelectric materials. The term $\alpha^2\sigma$ is referred to as the thermoelectric power factor (PF). Insulating molecular crystals might exhibit an extremely large thermoelectric voltage, but cannot be used for the generation of electric energy since their σ, (i.e., P_0 and PF) is estimated as almost being zero.

Energy conversion efficiency (η) under a constant temperature gradient is determined by the ratio of output power calculated with the PF to thermal energy loss derived from spontaneous thermal conduction. Therefore, semiconductor materials with a large Z are advantageous for extracting excellent thermoelectric efficiency as follows:

$$Z = \frac{\alpha^2\sigma}{k} \tag{6.5}$$

where κ is thermal conductivity and is equivalent to the spontaneous energy loss due to thermal conduction. When the temperatures of materials at the hot and cold ends are T_H and T_L, respectively, and their average is T, heat-to-electricity conversion efficiency is given as

$$\eta_{max} = \frac{\Delta T}{T_H}\frac{(1+ZT)^{1/2}-1}{(1+ZT)^{1/2}+T_L/T_H} \tag{6.6}$$

ZT is widely used for the evaluation of the *figure of merit* of thermoelectric materials indicating the energy conversion efficiency. Figure 6.4 shows the relationship between ZT and η under the temperature gradient between 20 and 80 °C.

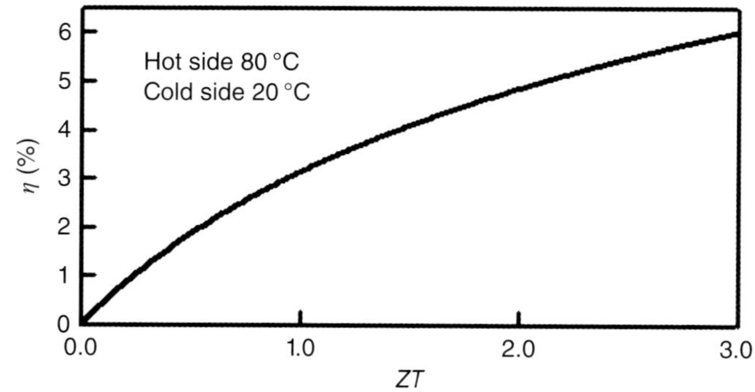

Figure 6.4 Heat-to-electricity conversion efficiency as a function of ZT between 80 and 20 °C.

For materials with ZT of a unity, you can calculate approximately 3% energy conversion efficiency. This value is often used as a standard in order to consider the feasibility of thermoelectric materials in many projects under development. It should be noted that one might pay attention to compare the thermoelectric properties of various materials since *figure of merit* ZT and conversion efficiency η depend heavily on temperature T and temperature gradient ΔT. Many high-performance inorganic materials showing $ZT > 2$ at raised temperatures have recently been reported [2], which might discourage organic chemists to consider conducting polymers as thermoelectric materials. It is true that these inorganic thermoelectric materials have an advantage over conducting polymers at temperatures above ~200 °C. However, organic materials showing moderate thermoelectric properties at lower temperatures are still attractive since most waste heat consists of low-grade energy below 100 °C.

6.2.4 A Classical Requirement for Efficient Module Design

Consider the practical thermoelectric modules. The basic structures of thermoelectric modules are simple; electric power generates when a thermoelectric material is sandwiched between hot and cold electrodes (Figure 6.5a). In this case, lead wires must be connected from electrodes at both hot and cold ends to a loading device at room temperature. If a metallic lead wire is used, most thermal energy is lost due to efficient thermal conduction through the wires. Consequently, such energy loss will lead to a dramatic decrease in energy conversion efficiency. The solution to this challenge requires a thermoelectric module consisting of both p-type and n-type thermoelectric materials sandwiched between, and connected in series to, the electrodes (Figure 6.5b). This module is called π-type. The energy conversion efficiency of π-type thermoelectric modules is also calculated using Eq. (6.6). Roughly speaking, one might use the lower electrical conductivity and higher thermal conductivity of either p-type or n-type thermoelectric materials to calculate ZT in Eq. (6.5). Therefore, not only high ZT for both p-type and n-type materials but also equivalent electrical and thermal conductivity are required. Considering these basic principles, the next section will discuss the materials design for organic and carbon thermoelectrics.

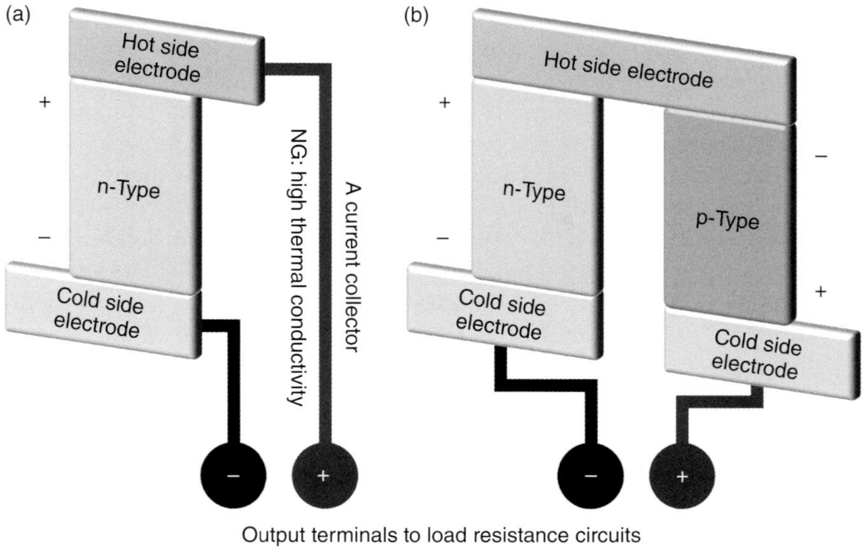

Figure 6.5 (a) Unipolar and (b) bipolar (π-type) thermoelectric modules.

6.3 Thermoelectric Materials Design

6.3.1 Organic Solids and Conducting Polymers

Since its discovery, the thermoelectricity of conducting polymers has long been examined for discriminating charge carrier polarity. In common, the conductivity of organic materials is limited by their conjugated structures and doping ability. Highly conducting organic materials include charge transfer complex crystals [3, 4], and conducting polymers [5, 6]. At least, *moderate* conductivity is required for appropriate measurements with *ordinary* (commercially available) electrometers. In this context, the thermoelectric properties of conducting polymers with tunable electrical conductivity (10^{-3}-10^{3} S cm^{-1}) can be easily examined. Additionally, the thermal conductivity of organic materials is substantially lower (<1 W m^{-1} K^{-1}) than that of most inorganic thermoelectric materials, irrespective of moderately high electrical conductivity. Therefore, strategies for high-performance organic thermoelectrics involve the elucidation of high PFs by tuning the Seebeck coefficient and electrical conductivity.

It is recognized that, from a microscopic point of view, the Seebeck coefficient in organic solids is governed by the lattice scattering of charge carriers [7]. In ideal organic semiconductor crystals with well-ordered lattices, charge carriers pass through the overlapped wavefunctions at neighboring molecules that induce a narrow, anisotropic band dispersion. In practical organic solids, in addition, electronic transport is controlled partly by the thermal perturbation of ordered molecules, modulating the carrier hopping integral and thus the bandwidth. The transport properties are also affected by the polarization of the electrons' environment. The strong interaction between the hopping charge carriers and the lattice and the induced phonon mode softening then results in an enhancement in the Seebeck coefficient. Such modulability in the Seebeck coefficient of soft organic solids is attractive to develop a new class of thermoelectric materials.

The thermoelectricity of various conducting polymers such as charge transfer complex crystals and doped polyaniline has long been examined. Toshima *et al.* reported in 1999 for the first time the complete thermoelectric properties (σ, α, and κ) of doped polyanilines [8]. They expanded their work to the thermoelectric properties of other conducting polymers and their stretched form. In 2007, they also demonstrated that the 310%-stretched, I_2-doped poly(*p*-phenylene vinylene) (PPV) derivative exhibits high electrical conductivity (350 S cm^{-1}) and low thermal conductivity (0.25 W m^{-1} K^{-1}) in addition to the moderate Seebeck coefficient (47 μV K^{-1}) [9]. Currently, this pioneering work with ZT of 0.1 remains highly stimulating within the research fields of organic electronics and materials science. Leclerc *et al.* also pioneered this field earlier in that decade [10, 11]. On the basis of their polymer chemistry background, they examined the excellent thermoelectric properties of synthetic carbazole-based polymers and their nanocarbon composites.

Poly(3,4-ethylenedioxythiophene) (PEDOT) derivatives are commercially available for many applications [12]. PEDOT:PSS, a typical conducting form, shows high conductivity (500–1000 S cm^{-1}) in the solid state with the aid of a small amount of dopants and structure-directing agents (dimethylsulfoxide (DMSO), ethyleneglycol (EG), etc.). Their high conductivity relies on various factors including planar PEDOT structures with the predominant S—O interaction, their polymerization degree, and doping stability (Figure 6.6). In 2011, Crispin *et al.* reported the high ZT thermoelectric properties of PEDOT doped with *p*-toluene sulfonate (Tos), and optimized by de-doping with tetrakis(dimethylamino)ethylene (TDAE) [13]. Wide-range thermopower measurements revealed that PEDOT:Tos exhibits the Seebeck coefficient of 40 μV K^{-1} at an oxidation level of 36% and 780 μV K^{-1} at the lowest considered oxidation level. The PF ($\sigma\alpha^2$) increased from 38 μW m^{-1} K^{-2} for the pristine doped polymer to 324 μW m^{-1} K^{-2} at the oxidation level of 22%. This report provided the first insight into tuning the thermoelectric properties of PEDOT derivatives by redox chemistry [14]. Excellent thermoelectric performance in PEDOT:Tos is reproduced by density functional theory (DFT) investigations on the doping control of PEDOT backbones and the consideration of charge carrier scattering [15].

Alternatively, PEDOT:PSS is highly sensitive to humidity, which can be used for modulating its thermoelectric effect in the solid state. Conducting polymers including PEDOT display an ionic thermoelectric effect in addition to the known electronic thermoelectric effect [16]. At a high humidity level, PEDOT derivatives present a thermo-induced voltage of up to several hundreds of microvolt per kelvin [17], which is identified as the ionic Seebeck effect. Ion currents themselves are also directly used for thermos-voltage generation. Single-ion conductors including silver Nafion (Ag-Nafion) and silver polystyrene-sulfonate (Ag-PSS) exhibit the thermogalvanic effect [18]. Through the generalized Soret effect, the concentration gradient of silver ions in Ag-Nafion and Ag-PSS formed, which generate an approximately millivolt voltage. Since this can be

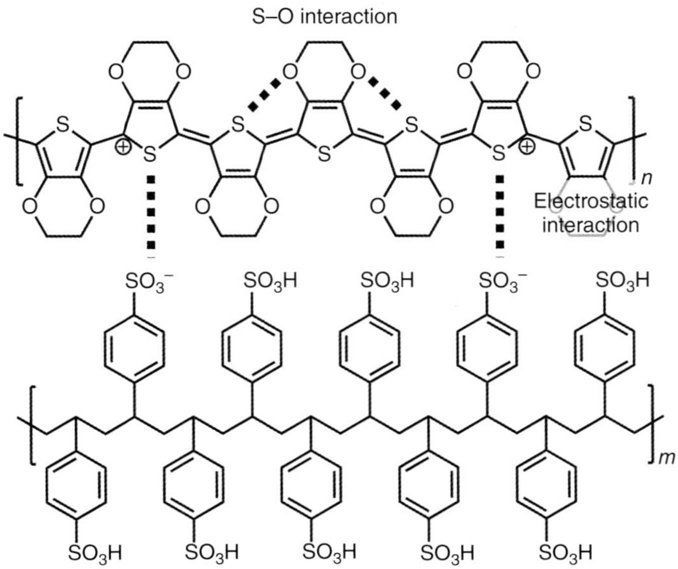

Figure 6.6 A typical molecular structure of PEDOT:PSS.

incorporated in the solid-state devices, such large-voltage generators might be preferred candidates for thermal sensor and capacitor materials.

The tuning of carrier concentration is required for thermoelectric power generation. In this context, doping processes for both p-type and n-type materials are necessary for PF optimization. Particularly, still missing is the stable n-type doping of conducting polymers. A rational strategy for stabilizing carboanions in n-type doped organic semiconductors is highly desirable. For this purpose, several molecular strategies for the backbones and n-type dopants are proposed (Figure 6.7). Electron-deficiency is the first criteria for high-performance n-type materials. Imide-functionalized backbones serve as highly electron-withdrawing units for relatively stable n-type materials. Naphthalene diimide (NDI)-based donor–acceptor polymers extrinsically doped with n-type dopant N-DMBI [19], and perylene diimide (PDI) derivatives self-doping with hydroxide side chains have been examined to generate moderate thermoelectric properties with PFs as high as 0.6 and 1.4 $\mu W\,m^{-1}\,K^{-2}$, respectively [20, 21]. It should be noted that hydride-releasing benzimidazol derivatives, such as N-DMBI, serve as an excellent n-type dopant not only for organic semiconductors but also for nanocarbon materials including fullerenes, carbon nanotubes, and graphenes [22, 23].

In addition to electron deficiency, molecular packing and planarity could influence the mobility and conductivity of organic solids. Benzodifurandione-based poly(*p*-phenylene vinylene) (BDPPV) derivatives with low-lying LUMO levels (below −4.0 eV) are highly electron-deficient via C=O groups and displays high electron mobility exceeding 1 $cm^2\,V^{-1}\,s^{-1}$ under ambient conditions [24]. A fluorinated BDPPV derivative forms the more planar molecular structure through dual C=O···H and C—F···H hydrogen-bonding interactions, showing

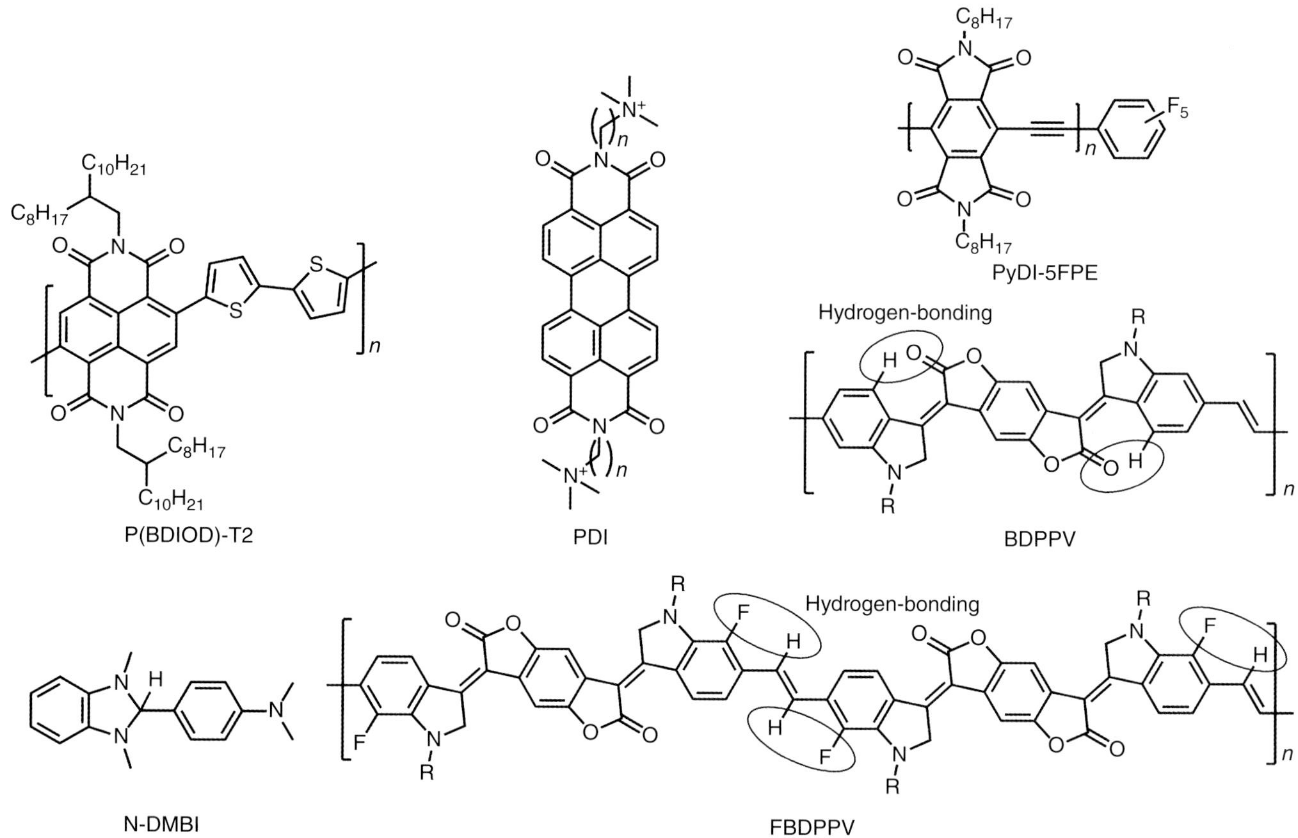

Figure 6.7 Typical n-type organic compounds (P(BDIOD-T2, PDI, PyDI-5FPE, BDPPV, and FBDPPV) and a dopant (N-DMBI).

electrical conductivities as high as $14\,\mathrm{S\,cm^{-1}}$ and PFs up to $28\,\mathrm{\mu W\,m^{-1}\,K^{-2}}$ through the modulation with a stable hydride-releasing n-type dopant N-DMBI. Weakly reducing inorganic reagents such as $SnCl_2$ was used to dope n-type polymers, enabling the exploitation of 0.1 *ZT* [25]. Doped fullerenes and powder-processed organometallic poly(Ni 1,1,2,2-ethenetetrathiolate) derivatives also showed highly conjugated and packed forms, and exhibited excellent n-type thermoelectric properties with electrical conductivities as high as 9 and $40\,\mathrm{S\,cm^{-1}}$ and PFs reaching 20 and $66\,\mathrm{\mu W\,m^{-1}\,K^{-2}}$, respectively [26, 27]. Organic semiconductors with high electron mobilities and their efficient and stable n-doping processes are being developed rapidly. As mentioned in Section 6.2.4, n-type thermoelectric polymers comparable to PEDOT derivatives are still in demand and further improvement in PF is under investigation.

6.3.2 Carbon Nanotubes and Related Matters

Carbon nanotubes are promising active thermoelectric materials owing to their narrow bandgap energy and high charge carrier mobility. Furthermore, they can be integrated into flexible thermoelectrics that can recover any waste heat [28, 29]. Indeed, single-walled carbon nanotubes (SWNTs) show relatively high thermopower at room temperature. A SWNT is a seamlessly patched cylinder-shaped graphene sheet. SWNTs possess a quantized and discrete electronic wave function along their circumference, and one-dimensional band structures in the axial direction. The band structures rely on how the single-layer graphitic sheets are rolled into graphene cylinders (Figure 6.8), where the order of graphene sheets in the cylinder is referred to as "chirality." Depending on the chirality, these graphitic cylinders are classified into two different electronic structures: semiconducting and metallic materials [30]. The bandgap of these materials is also determined by the chirality (Figure 6.9) [31].

Following the Mott equation (Eq. (6.2)), the Seebeck coefficient is proportional to the gradient of electronic DOS around the Fermi level. In one-dimensional materials such as SWNTs, the DOS diverges at the one-dimensional van Hove

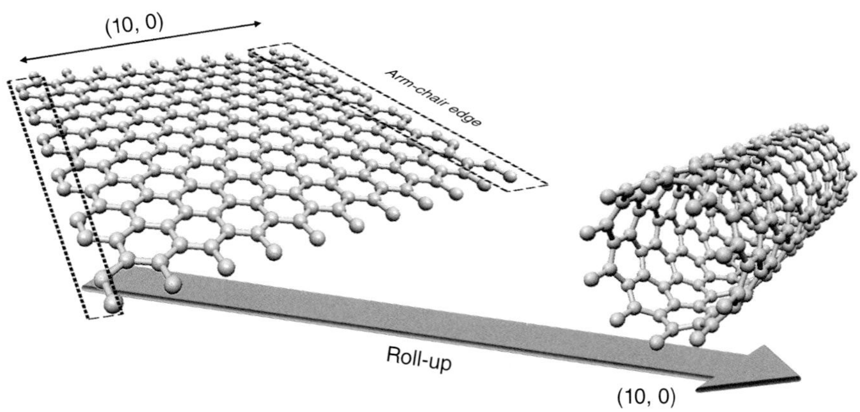

Figure 6.8 Representative schematic illustration of carbon nanotube formation from a 2D graphene sheet with two arm-chair edges.

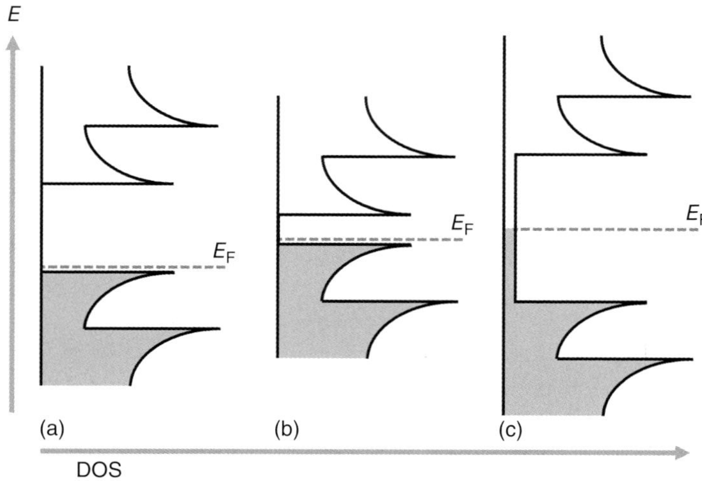

Figure 6.9 Representative schematic illustration of the DOS of semiconducting carbon nanotubes with (a) a smaller diameter and (b) a larger diameter, and (c) metallic carbon nanotubes.

singularity (DOS(E) d$E \propto E^{-1/2}$ dE). Considering SWNTs in air, oxygen molecules would adsorb on the SWNT surface, and SWNTs are hole-doped by the oxygen. Indeed, semiconductor-enriched SWNTs show the large Seebeck coefficient (>100 μV K^{-1}) because their Fermi level shifts to the valence band side, and in particular close to the DOS peak [32]. Metallic SWNTs usually exhibit lower thermopower since their Fermi level is far from the first DOS peak. Two- and three-dimensional materials do not show a similar effect since their DOS is proportional to a given constant, and $E^{1/2}$, respectively. It is then theoretically predicted that graphenes never show such excellent thermoelectric properties while pure (de-doped) fullerenes could exhibit the unexpectedly high Seebeck coefficient [33].

Since carrier conduction in SWNTs is ballistic, a net temperature gradient is highly dependent on the nature of resistive nanotube–nanotube junctions in the network films. Maniwa reported that thermally resistive junctions play an important role in the giant Seebeck effect of SWNT films [34]. They carefully measured the Seebeck coefficient as a function of the ratio of semiconducting (s) and metallic (m) SWNTs (Figure 6.10). They also simulated these results by first-principles transport simulations based on a simple SWNT junction model. Ferguson examined the thermoelectric properties of semiconductor-sorted SWNTs with various bandgaps ranging from 0.7 to 1.5 eV. Their experimental and theoretical studies revealed that moderate electrical conductivity and Seebeck coefficient coexist in ~1.4 nm diameter SWNTs that show a PF of >300 μW m^{-1} K^{-2} [35]. In order to obtain the large Seebeck coefficient, a carrier-energy filtering concept has been proposed. Designs for resistive nanotube–nanotube junctions with modular additives are important for enhancing the thermoelectric properties. The energy filtering of charged carriers has been realized using semiconductor nanoparticle junctions, and conjugated polymer-intercalated junctions [36, 37].

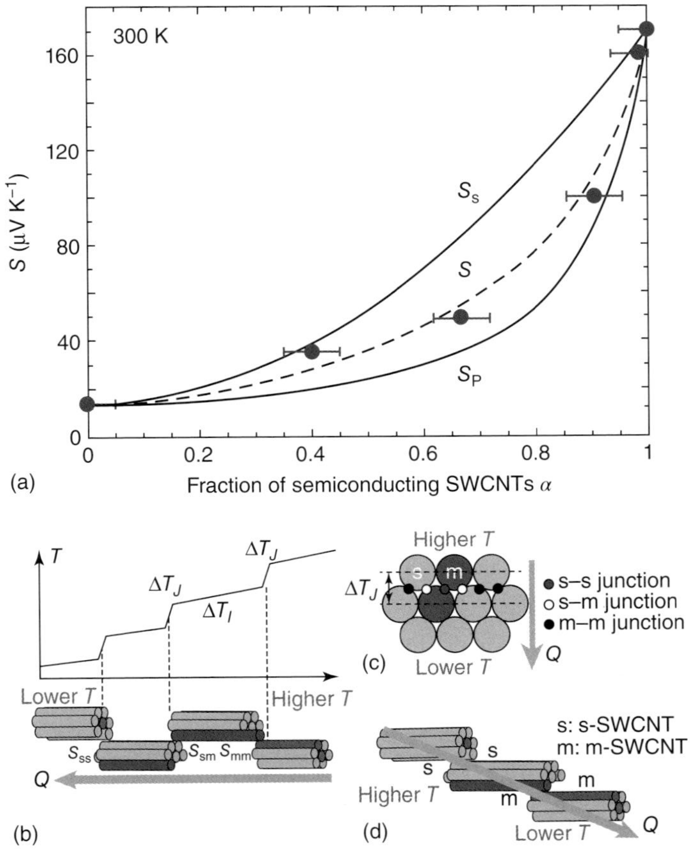

Figure 6.10 (a) Semiconducting fraction α dependence of Seebeck coefficient (S) at 300 K. (b) Schematic serial model for junction networks consisting of semiconducting (s) and metallic (m) SWCNTs, where temperature (T) varies along the series of SWCNT bundles. (Nakai *et al.* 2014 [34]. Reproduced with permission of The Japan Society of Applied Physics.)

As mentioned in Section 6.2.2, the control of carrier density (i.e., carrier doping) is crucial to optimizing the thermoelectric properties. Nanocarbons have an advantage in that the doping can modulate the electronic transport properties. Nanocarbon materials including fullerenes and carbon nanotubes are relatively air-stable in their p-type and n-type states. Similar to silicon (Si) technology, atom-exchange reactions from carbon to heteroatom in carbon frameworks is also effective for exploiting the doping level of SWNTs. Boron- and nitrogen-doped SWNTs show the positive and negative Seebeck coefficient, respectively, and have been utilized for the construction of bipolar thermoelectric modules [38].

Owing to the intrinsic nature of carboanions, negatively charged n-type organic semiconductors are seemingly unstable in air. Similarly, the stabilization of n-type SWNTs remains a challenge. Since weak electron-donating molecules such as polyethyleneimine (PEI) can alter the majority carrier in SWNTs, the construction of bipolar thermoelectric modules with SWNTs has been

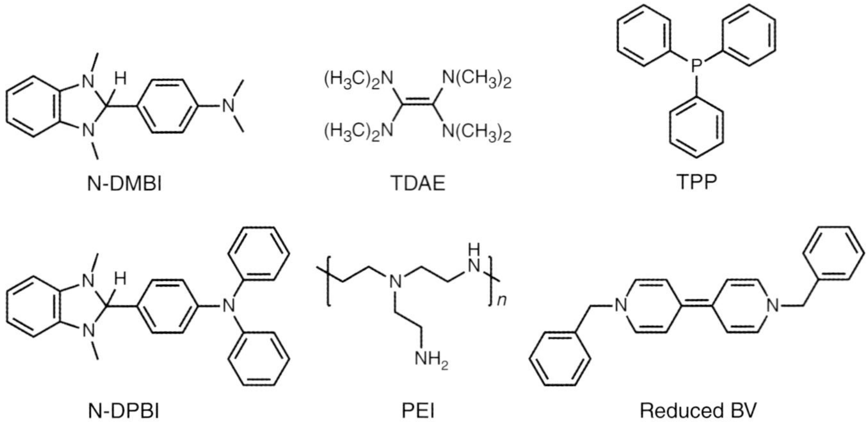

Figure 6.11 Typical organic n-type dopants.

demonstrated [39]. A number of weak electron donors have been examined to produce n-type SWNTs (Figure 6.11). However, the n-type states based on electron-doped SWNTs (i.e., carboanions) are highly reactive in air. Most reported n-type composites showed relatively slow degradation behavior in several days.

Considering the stability of chemical bonding and interaction, a balance between n-type SWNTs and their counter cations is important for improving stability in n-type characteristics of SWNTs (Figure 6.12). Indeed, small cations such as sodium ions are unlikely to stabilize large aromatic anions such as n-type fullerenes, carbon nanotubes, and graphenes. For this purpose, the charge density of sodium ions has been delocalized by complexing them with crown ether derivatives, which can be confirmed using the primary DFT calculation. Indeed, it has been successfully demonstrated that metal cation-crown ether complexes effectively stabilize n-type carbon nanotubes. The further delocalization of positive charges can be achieved using aryl-substituted crown ethers (Figure 6.13) [40]. This material demonstrates unprecedented durability in air

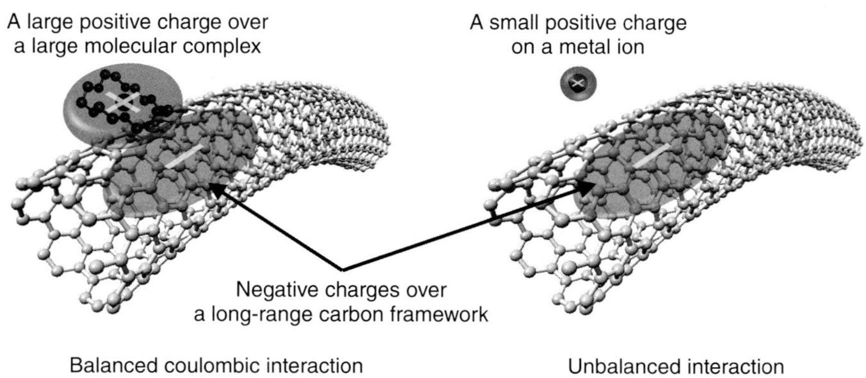

Figure 6.12 A schematic illustration of charge balanced n-type SWNT anion–metal cation complexes.

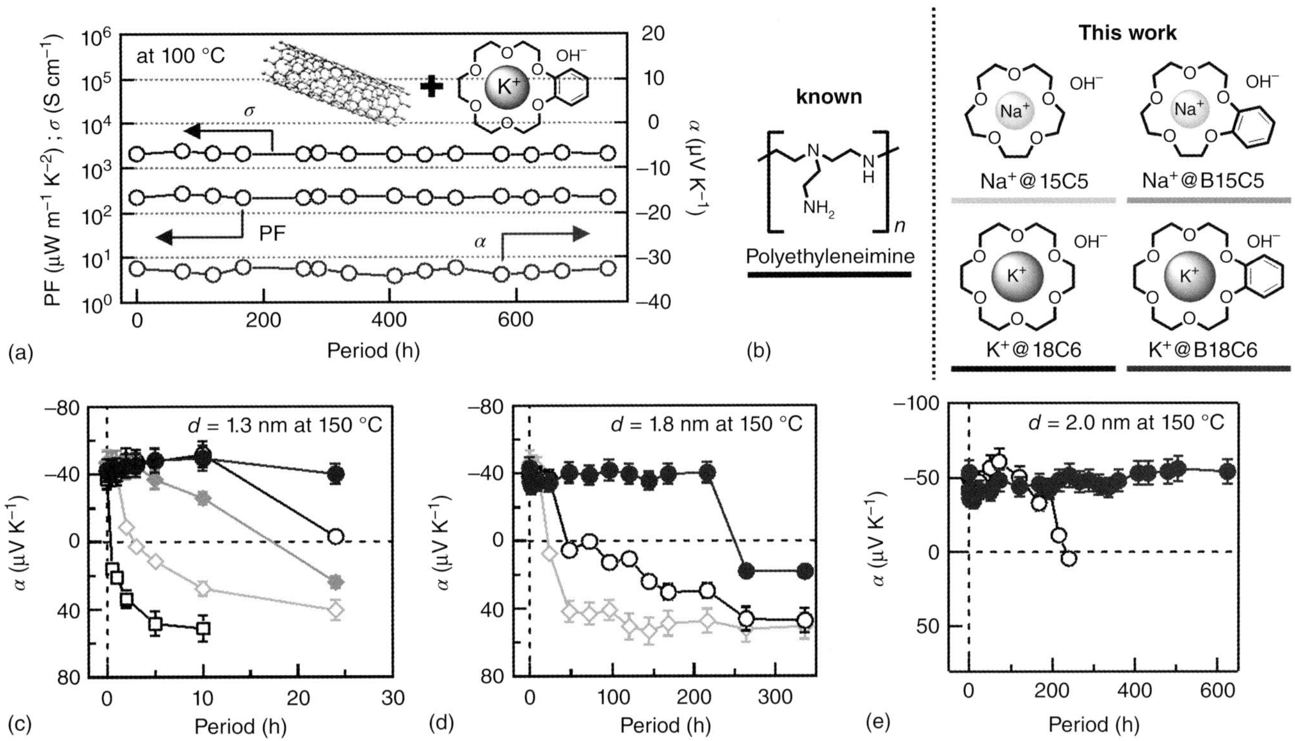

Figure 6.13 A thermal stability. (a) Temporal changes of the electrical conductivity, the Seebeck coefficient and power factor of n-type films derived from eDIPS-CNTs treated with KOH/benzo-18-crown ether at 100 °C. (b) Additives used in this study. Temporal changes of n-type films from (c) KH-CNTs 1.3 ± 0.2 nm in diameter; (d) Tuball-CNTs 1.8 ± 0.3 nm in diameter; (e) eDIPS-CNTs 2.0 ± 0.7 nm in diameter at 150 °C. Importantly, filled circles in (c–e) indicate the samples doped with KOH/benzo-18-crown ether. (Nonoguchi *et al.* 2016 [40]. Reproduced with permission of John Wiley & Sons.)

even at raised temperatures, which is an essential requirement in thermoelectric applications.

The crown ether-based cations ([M-crown]$^+$) behave as soft Lewis acids and efficiently stabilize soft bases under the classical hard and soft acids and bases (HSAB) concept. In the solid state, charge polarizability could also control cation–anion charge balance. Reynolds and co-workers have reported that n-type poly(3,4-ethylenedioxythiophene) (PEDOT) derivatives are specifically stabilized by inserting larger cations such as tetra-*n*-butylammonium (TBA$^+$), indicating the contribution of the HSAB theory. Similarly, the negative charges on n-type SWNTs seem to be delocalized over many aromatic units, which can be efficiently stabilized by soft Lewis acids such as [M-crown]$^+$. The positive charges in metal ion–benzocrown complexes are partly delocalized over the benzene ring supporting the further efficient stabilization of negatively charged SWNTs.

6.3.3 Useful Survey Methods for Discovering Efficient Thermoelectric Materials

Precise measurements in the highly resistive state of organic solids also provide a deep insight into their conducting nature. The Seebeck coefficient reflects the dynamics of thermally excited charge carriers and their entropy transfer. The transferred entropy is determined by the band structure of semiconducting materials and the scattering of charge carriers. Batlogg has demonstrated the field-effect-modulated Seebeck coefficient in organic semiconductors [7]. Carrier-density-dependent thermopower measurements in single crystals revealed that the Seebeck coefficient of organic semiconductors can be analyzed within the range of the electronic contribution in conventional inorganic semiconductors. Currently, this technique has been widely used to investigate and optimize the thermoelectric properties of various conducting polymers and carbon materials at a preferred doping level [41–43].

6.3.4 Prototype Thermoelectric Generators and Applications

This chapter has introduced the current aspects of thermoelectrics ranging from the basic principles to the development of flexible powering materials and devices. Prototype thermoelectric generators have been commercialized in 1990s, which was integrated in wristwatches [44]. A rapid increase in the need for portable power generators in various fields including plant management, medical application, and hobbies, is stimulating studies on energy harvesting techniques. For practical thermoelectric power conversion materials in a temperature range lower than 400 K, flexibility is crucial to cover and adhere closely to the heat sources emitting low thermal radiation. Therefore, flexible thermoelectric devices open up possibilities in emergent uses including medical cooling/heating devices and portable devices powered by the human body. Such flexible thermoelectric generators have recently been developed using

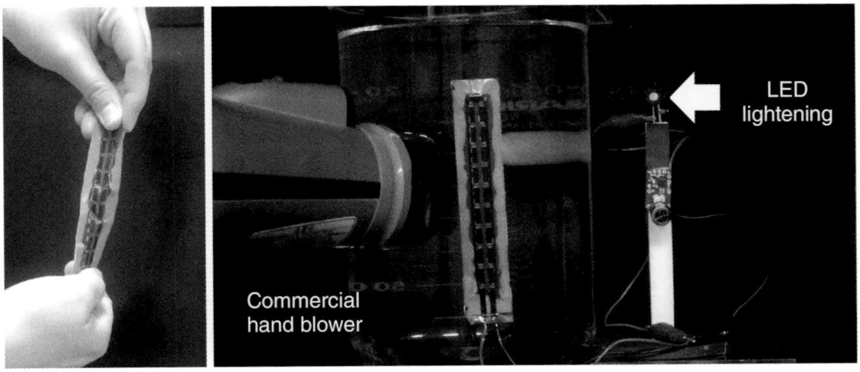

(a) (b)

Figure 6.14 (a) A flexible thermoelectric generator made of p-type and n-type carbon nanotubes as thermoelectric layers. (b) Power generation and LED lightening under a hot air blow with the thermoelectric generator. (The original pictures were supplied from Sekisui Chemical CO., LTD and Nara Institute of Science and Technology.)

the thin films of inorganic Bi_2Te_3-based semiconductors [45], organic-based coordination polymers, and SWNT-based materials [40]. In particular, this generator made of 20-leg p- and n-type SWNTs (Figure 6.14) can produce the electric power of microwatts-to-megawatts from ~50 K temperature difference. The device is stable under ambient conditions. Such high-performance generators with capacitors can power the LED devices using heat source (i.e., a commercial hand blower in Figure 6.14).

Also, these flexible thermoelectric modules may be used in the simultaneous detection of any other physical properties. Zhu *et al.* have developed self-powered devices that can simultaneously sense pressure and temperature, using organic thermoelectric materials (Figure 6.15) [46]. These thermoelectric power generators will be readily implanted in future smart electronic skin (*e-skin*) [47].

6.4 Outlook for Flexible Thermoelectric Generators

This chapter tries to provide an outlook on emergent medical devices that are proposed using flexible thermoelectric materials and devices. Such devices are in high demand for various physical/chemical sensing ranging from the self-powered, wireless healthcare monitoring [48], to the sensing-based system maintenance [49]. Additionally, self-powered robust devices could contribute to boost fundamental researches on monitoring the activities of animals [50]. It is expected that flexible thermoelectric generators will solve these current challenges through the materials design.

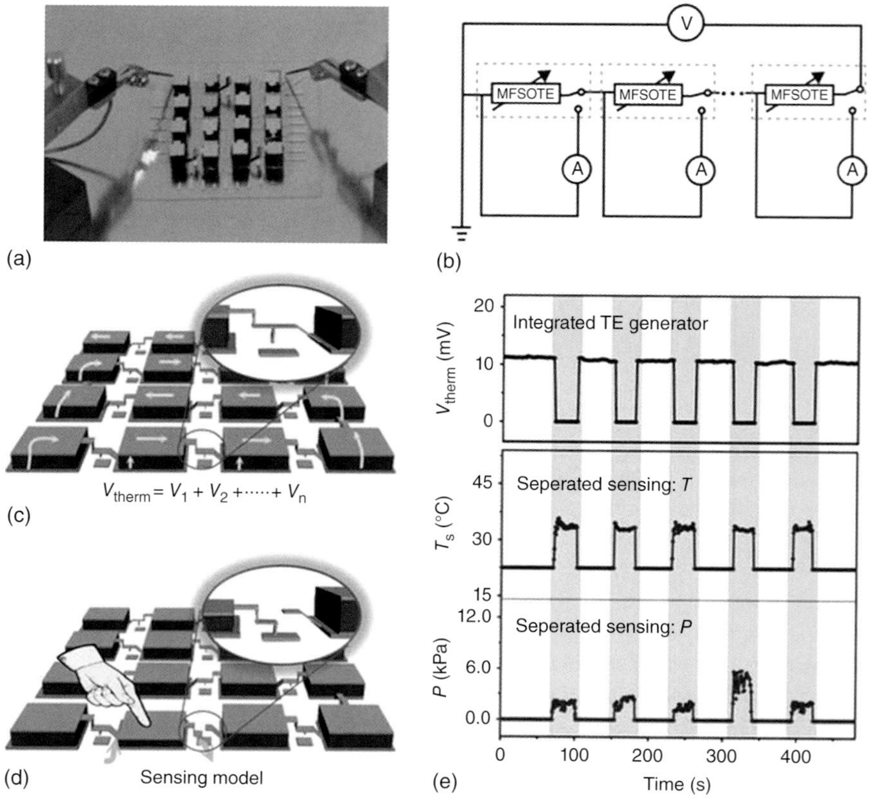

Figure 6.15 Multifunctional application of MFSOTE-based-sensing array. Graphs (a,b) show a photograph and circuit diagram, respectively, of an MFSOTE array with 4 × 4 pixels. Graphs (c,d) show schematic illustrations of the integrated array: (c) all the devices connected in series can be used as an electricity generator for harvesting energy. (d) The device switches to a self-powered dual-parameter sensor model when subjected to an external pressure. The insets in graph (c,d) show magnified views of the circuit connection between two pixels under unloading and loading conditions, respectively. (e) The thermoelectric voltage (top), temperature (middle), and pressure (bottom) responses of a MFSOTE array to five finger-touch cycles. The bottom surface of the MFSOTE array is heated with a Peltier element. (Zhang *et al.* 2015 [46], https://www.nature.com/articles/ncomms9356. Used under CC BY 4.0 https://creativecommons.org/licenses/by/4.0/.)

References

1 MacDonald, D.K.C. (1962) *Thermoelectricity: An Introduction to the Principles*, John Wiley & Sons, Inc., New York.

2 Zhao, L.D., Lo, S.H., Zhang, Y., Sun, H., Tan, G., Uher, C., Wolverton, C., Dravid, V.P., and Kanatzidis, M.G. (2014) Ultralow thermal conductivity and high thermoelectric figure of merit in SnSe crystals. *Nature*, **508**, 373–377.

3 Mori, T., Inokuchi, H., Kobayashi, A., Kato, R., and Kobayashi, H. (1988) Electrical conductivity, thermoelectric power, and ESR of a new family of

molecular conductors, dicyanoquinonediimine-metal [$(DCNQI)_2M$] compounds. *Phys. Rev. B*, **38**, 5913–5923.

4 Urayama, H., Yamochi, H., Saito, G., Sugano, T., Kinoshita, M., Inabe, T., Mori, T., Maruyama, Y., and Inokuchi, H. (1988) Valence state of copper atoms and transport property of an organic superconductor, $(BEDT\text{-}TTF)_2Cu(NCS)_2$, measured by ESCA, ESR, and thermoelectric power. *Chem. Lett.*, **17**, 1057–1060.

5 Park, Y.W., Denenstein, A., Chiang, C.K., Heeger, A.J., and MacDiarmid, A.G. (1979) Semiconductor–metal transition in doped $(CH)_x$: thermoelectric power. *Solid State Commun.*, **29**, 747–751.

6 Yoon, C.O., Reghu, M., Moses, D., Heeger, A.J., and Cao, Y. (1993) Counterion-induced processibility of polyaniline: thermoelectric power. *Phys. Rev. B*, **48**, 14080–14084.

7 Pernstich, K.P., Rössner, B., and Batlogg, B. (2007) Field-effect-modulated Seebeck coefficient in organic semiconductors. *Nat. Mater.*, **7**, 321–325.

8 Yan, H. and Toshima, N. (1999) Thermoelectric properties of alternatively layered films of polyaniline and (±)-10-camphorsulfonic acid-doped polyaniline. *Chem. Lett.*, **28**, 1217–1218.

9 Hiroshige, Y., Ookawa, M., and Toshima, N. (2007) Thermoelectric figure-of-merit of iodine-doped copolymer of phenylenevinylene with dialkoxyphenylenevinylene. *Synth. Met.*, **157**, 467–474.

10 Badrou Aïch, R., Blouin, N., Bouchard, A., and Leclerc, M. (2009) Electrical and thermoelectric properties of poly(2,7-carbazole) derivatives. *Chem. Mater.*, **21**, 751–757.

11 Dubey, N. and Leclerc, M. (2011) Conducting polymers: efficient thermoelectric materials. *J. Polym. Sci., Part B: Polym. Phys.*, **49**, 467–475.

12 Heywang, G. and Jonas, F. (1992) Poly(alkylenedioxythiophene)s—new, very stable conducting polymers. *Adv. Mater.*, **4**, 116–118.

13 Bubnova, O., Khan, Z.U., Malti, A., Braun, S., Fahlman, M., Berggren, M., and Crispin, X. (2011) Optimization of the thermoelectric figure of merit in the conducting polymer poly(3,4-ethylenedioxythiophene). *Nat. Mater.*, **10**, 429–433.

14 Bubnova, O., Berggren, M., and Crispin, X. (2012) Tuning the thermoelectric properties of conducting polymers in an electrochemical transistor. *J. Am. Chem. Soc.*, **134**, 16456–16459.

15 Shi, W., Zhao, T., Xi, J., Wang, D., and Shuai, Z. (2015) Unravelling doping effects on PEDOT at the molecular level: from geometry to thermoelectric transport properties. *J. Am. Chem. Soc.*, **137**, 12929–12938.

16 Wang, H., Ail, U., Gabrielsson, R., Berggren, M., and Crispin, X. (2015) Ionic Seebeck effect in conducting polymers. *Adv. Energy Mater.*, **5**, 1500044.

17 Wei, Q., Mukaida, M., Kirihara, K., Naito, Y., and Ishida, T. (2014) Thermoelectric power enhancement of PEDOT:PSS in high-humidity conditions. *Appl. Phys Express*, **7**, 031601.

18 Chang, W.B., Evans, C.M., Popere, B.C., Russ, B.M., Liu, J., Newman, J., and Segalman, L. (2016) Harvesting waste heat in unipolar ion conducting polymers. *ACS Macro Lett.*, **5**, 94–98.

19 N-DMBI is ((4-(1,3-dimethyl-2,3-dihydro-1*H*-benzoimidazol-2-yl)phenyl) dimethylamine). Wei, P., Oh, J.H., Dong, G., and Bao, Z. (2010) Use of a 1*H*-benzoimidazole derivative as an n-type dopant and to enable air-stable solution-processed n-channel organic thin-film transistors. *J. Am. Chem. Soc.*, **132**, 8852–8853.

20 Schlitz, R.A., Brunetti, F.G., Glaudell, A.M., Miller, P.L., Brady, M.A., Takacs, C.J., Hawker, C.J., and Chabinyc, M.L. (2014) Solubility-limited extrinsic n-type doping of a high electron mobility polymer for thermoelectric applications. *Adv. Mater.*, **26**, 2825–2830.

21 Russ, B., Robb, M.J., Brunetti, F.G., Miller, P.L., Perry, E.E., Patel, S.N., Ho, V., Chang, W.B., Urban, J.J., Chabinyc, M.L., Hawker, C.J., and Segalman, R.A. (2014) Power factor enhancement in solution-processed organic n-type thermoelectrics through molecular design. *Adv. Mater.*, **26**, 3473–3477.

22 Wang, H., Wei, P., Li, Y., Han, J., Lee, H.R., Naab, B.D., Liu, N., Wang, C., Adijanto, E., Tee, B.C.-K., Morishita, S., Li, Q., Gao, Y., Cui, Y., and Bao, Z. (2014) Tuning the threshold voltage of carbon nanotube transistors by n-type molecular doping for robust and flexible complementary circuits. *Proc. Natl. Acad. Sci. U.S.A.*, **111**, 4776–4781.

23 Xu, W., Lim, T.-S., Seo, H.-K., Min, S.-Y., Cho, H., Park, M.-H., Kim, Y.-H., and Lee, T.-W. (2014) N-doped graphene field-effect transistors with enhanced electron mobility and air-stability. *Small*, **10**, 1999–2005.

24 Shi, K., Zhang, F., Di, C.A., Yan, T.W., Zou, Y., Zhou, X., Zhu, D., Wang, J.Y., and Pei, J. (2015) Toward high performance n-type thermoelectric materials by rational modification of BDPPV backbones. *J. Am. Chem. Soc.*, **137**, 6979–6982.

25 Ireland, R.M., Liu, Y., Guo, X., Cheng, Y.-T., Kola, S., Wang, W., Jones, T., Yang, R., Falk, M.L., and Katz, H.E. (2015) $ZT > 0.1$ electron-carrying polymer thermoelectric composites with in situ $SnCl_2$ microstructure growth. *Adv. Sci.*, **2**. doi: 10.1002/advs.201500015

26 Sumino, M., Harada, K., Ikeda, M., Tanaka, S., Miyazaki, K., and Adachi, C. (2011) Thermoelectric properties of n-type C_{60} thin films and their application in organic thermovoltaic devices. *Appl. Phys. Lett.*, **99**, 093308.

27 Sun, Y., Sheng, P., Di, C., Jiao, F., Xu, W., Qiu, D., and Zhu, D. (2012) Organic thermoelectric materials and devices based on p- and n-type poly(metal 1,1,2,2-ethenetetrathiolate)s. *Adv. Mater.*, **24**, 932–937.

28 Hewitt, C.A., Kaiser, A.B., Roth, S., Craps, M., Czerw, R., and Carroll, D.L. (2012) Multilayered carbon nanotube/polymer composite based thermoelectric fabrics. *Nano Lett.*, **12**, 1307–1310.

29 Nonoguchi, Y., Ohashi, K., Kanazawa, R., Ashiba, K., Hata, K., Nakagawa, T., Adachi, C., Tanase, T., and Kawai, T. (2013) Systematic conversion of single walled carbon nanotubes into n-type thermoelectric materials by molecular dopants. *Sci. Rep.*, **3**. doi: 10.1038/srep03344

30 Odom, T.W., Huang, J.-L., Kim, P., and Lieber, C.M. (1998) Atomic structure and electronic properties of single-walled carbon nanotubes. *Nature*, **391**, 62–64.

31 Sato, K., Saito, R., Jiang, J., Dresselhaus, G., and Dresselhaus, M.S. (2007) Discontinuity in the family pattern of single-wall carbon nanotubes. *Phys. Rev. B*, **76**. doi: 10.1103/physrevb.76.195446

32 Yu, C., Shi, L., Yao, Z., Li, D., and Majundar, A. (2005) Thermal conductance and thermopower of an individual single-wall carbon nanotube. *Nano Lett.*, **5**, 1842–1846.

33 Kojima, H., Abe, R., Ito, M., Tomatsu, Y., Fujiwara, F., Matsubara, R., Yoshimoto, N., and Nakamura, M. (2015) Giant Seebeck effect in pure fullerene thin films. *Appl. Phys. Express*, **8**, 121301.

34 Nakai, Y., Honda, K., Yanagi, K., Kataura, H., Kato, T., Yamamoto, T., and Maniwa, Y. (2014) Giant Seebeck coefficient in semiconducting single-wall carbon nanotube film. *Appl. Phys Express*, **7**, 025103.

35 Avery, A.D., Zhou, B.H., Lee, J., Lee, E.-S., Miller, E.M., Ihly, R., Wesenberg, D., Mistry, K.S., Guillot, S.L., Zink, B.L., Kim, Y.-H., Blackburn, J.L., and Ferguson, A. (2016) Tailored semiconducting carbon nanotube networks with enhanced thermoelectric properties. *Nat. Energy*, **1**, 16033.

36 Ito, M., Okamoto, N., Abe, R., Kojima, H., Matsubara, R., Yamashita, I., and Nakamura, M. (2014) Enhancement of thermoelectric properties of carbon nanotube composites by inserting biomolecules at nanotube junctions. *Appl. Phys Express*, **7**, 065102.

37 Yao, Q., Wang, Q., Wang, L., Wang, Y., Sun, J., Zeng, H., Jin, Z., Huang, X., and Chen, L. (2014) The synergic regulation of conductivity and Seebeck coefficient in pure polyaniline by chemically changing the ordered degree of molecular chains. *J. Mater. Chem. A*, **2**, 2634–2640.

38 Dörling, B., Ryan, J.D., Craddock, J.D., Sorrentino, A., Basaty, A.E., Gomez, A., Garriga, M., Pereiro, E., Anthony, J.E., Weisenberger, M.C., Goñi, A.R., Müller, C., and Campoly-Quiles, M. (2016) Photoinduced p- to n-type switching in thermoelectric polymer-carbon nanotube composites. *Adv. Mater.*, **28**, 2782–2789.

39 Yu, C., Murali, A., Choi, K., and Ryu, Y. (2012) Air-stable fabric thermoelectric modules made of N- and P-type carbon nanotubes. *Energy Environ. Sci.*, **5**, 9481–9486.

40 Nonoguchi, Y., Nakano, M., Murayama, T., Hagino, H., Hama, S., Miyazaki, K., Matsubara, R., Nakamura, M., and Kawai, T. (2016) Simple salt-coordinated n-type nanocarbon materials stable in air. *Adv. Funct. Mater.*, **26**, 3021–3028.

41 Zhang, F., Zang, Y., Huang, D., Di, C.-A., Gao, X., Sirringhaus, H., and Zhu, D. (2015) Modulated thermoelectric properties of organic semiconductors using field-effect transistors. *Adv. Funct. Mater.*, **25**, 3004–3012.

42 Venkateshvaran, D., Nikolka, M., Sadhanala, A., Lemaur, V., Zelazny, M., Kepa, M., Hurhangee, M., Kronemeijer, A.J., Pecunia, V., Nasrallah, I., Romanov, I., Broch, K., McCulloch, I., Emin, D., Olivier, Y., Cornil, J., Beljonne, D., and Sirringhaus, H. (2014) Approaching disorder-free transport in high-mobility conjugated polymers. *Nature*, **515**, 384–388.

43 Yanagi, K., Kanda, S., Oshima, Y., Kitamura, Y., Kawai, H., Yamamoto, T., Takenobu, T., Nakai, Y., and Maniwa, Y. (2014) Tuning of the thermoelectric properties of one-dimensional material networks by electric double layer techniques using ionic liquids. *Nano Lett.*, **14**, 6437–6442.
44 Kishi, M., Nemoto, H., Hamao, T., Yamamoto, M., Sudou, S., Mandai M., and Yamamoto, S. (1999) Micro thermoelectric modules and their application to wristwatches as an energy source. 18th International Conference on Thermoelectrics, pp. 301–307.
45 Kato, K., Hatasako, Y., Uchino, M., Nakata, Y., Suzuki, Y., Hayakawa, T., Adachi, C., and Miyazaki, K. (2014) Flexible porous bismuth telluride thin films with enhanced figure of merit using micro-phase separation of block copolymer. *Adv. Mater. Interfaces*, **1**. doi: 10.1002/admi.201300015
46 Zhang, F.J., Zang, Y.P., Huang, D.Z., Di, C.A., and Zhu, D.B. (2015) Flexible and self-powered temperature–pressure dual-parameter sensors using microstructure-frame-supported organic thermoelectric materials. *Nat. Commun.*, **6**, 8356.
47 Someya, T., Sekitani, T., Iba, S., Kato, Y., Kawaguchi, H., and Sakurai, T. (2004) A large-area, flexible pressure sensor matrix with organic field-effect transistors for artificial skin applications. *Proc. Nat. Acad. Sci. U.S.A.*, **101**, 9966–9970.
48 Hande, A., Polk, T., Walker, W., and Bhatia, D. (2006) Self-powered wireless sensor networks for remote patient monitoring in hospitals. *Sensors*, **6**, 1102–1117.
49 Opasjumruskit, K., Thanthipwan, T., Sathusen, O., Sirinamarattana, P., Gadmanee, P., Pootarapan, E., Wongkomet, N., Thanachayanont, A., and Thamsirianunt, M. (2006) Self-powered wireless temperature sensors exploit RFID technology. *IEEE Pervasive Comput.*, **5**, 54–61.
50 Hayami, H., Takehara, H., Nagata, K., Haruta, M., Noda, T., Sasagawa, K., Tokuda, T., and Ohta, J. (2016) Wireless image-data transmission from an implanted image sensor through a living mouse brain by intra body communication. *Jpn. J. Appl. Phys.*, **55**, 04EM03.

7

Flexible Supercapacitors Based on Two-Dimensional Materials

Dianpeng Qi and Xiaodong Chen

Nanyang Technological University, School of Materials Science and Engineering, 50 Nanyang Avenue, Singapore 639798, Singapore

7.1 Introduction

Flexible devices have shown booming development in recent years, implying that flexible devices might lead the new revolution of electronics. Currently, flexible displays [1–5], artificial skins [6–13], flexible medical devices [14–17], and even bendable mobile phones have been produced. To satisfy the mechanical properties' requirement of flexible devices, energy storage devices are demanded to be flexible too. As a result, energy storage components and power sources, such as supercapacitors, thin-film Li ion batteries, and solar cells with mechanical properties of flexibility or even stretchability are being developed. It is required that these energy storage units can maintain high power and energy supply under consecutive mechanical deformation, such as twist, bend and even stretch. Furthermore, these energy storage devices are desired to possess remarkable mechanical strength to afford the numerous shape deformations resulting from the daily activities of human beings; this is especially important for the power source to power wearable healthcare and medical electronics.

Currently, portable and flexible electric devices mainly use rechargeable batteries as their power sources. Thin-film batteries or microbatteries have been commercially available and the market for such batteries has shown rapid expansion. Rechargeable batteries, particularly Li ion batteries, can provide high-energy density. However, the disadvantage is that they suffer from relatively slow charging/discharging rates, low power densities and short lifecycle. As an alternative to batteries, supercapacitors were created after capacitors had been developed for more than 100 years. Their power deliveries are superior to that of capacitors, which bridge the gap between capacitors and batteries, as shown in the Ragone plot (Figure 7.1) [18, 19]. Compared to batteries, supercapacitors (also named as ultracapacitors or electrochemical capacitors) can work for quite a long duration, usually millions (10^5–10^6) of charging/discharging cycles, without losing their electrochemical performances. Supercapacitors also possess much higher capacitance as compared to capacitors. Therefore, they are essential toward meeting increasing energy demands, for example, the electric

Flexible and Stretchable Medical Devices, First Edition. Edited by Kuniharu Takei.

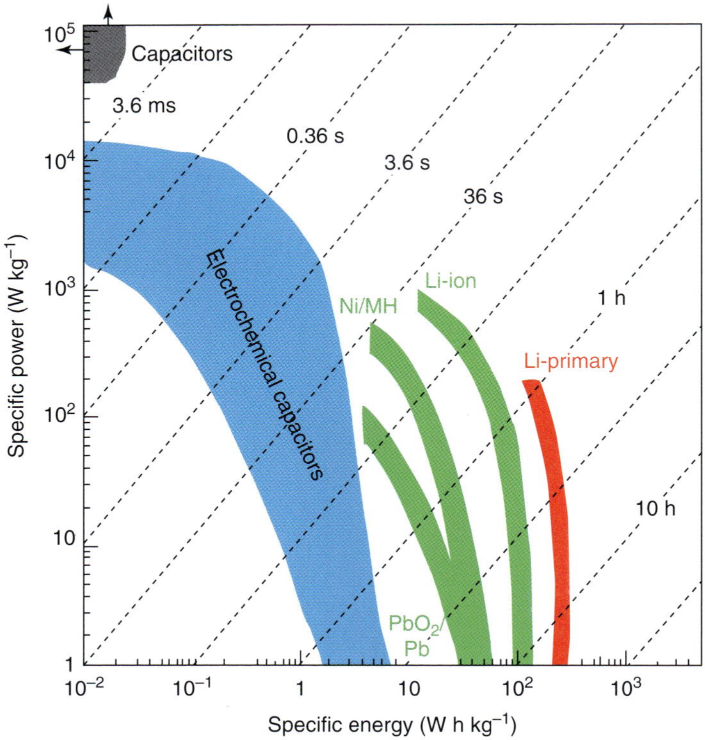

Figure 7.1 Ragone plot showing the specific power against specific energy for various electrical energy storage systems. (Simon and Gogotsi 2008 [18]. Reproduced with permission of Nature Publishing Group.)

vehicles that require high power delivery [20]. However, integrating with flexible electronic components has been proven to be cumbersome in the case of conventional supercapacitors (usually with rigid mechanical properties), which limits their widespread applications. Consequently, flexible supercapacitors that can maintain their performances while under mechanical deformation are developed to catch up with the booming rise of the requirement for flexible devices.

7.2 Flexible Supercapacitors Based on 2D Materials

Based on the different energy storage mechanisms, supercapacitors can be classified into three categories: (i) electric double-layer supercapacitors (EDLCs) that electrostatically store charges on the large-area electrode–electrolyte interface [21], normally, based on carbon materials [19, 22]. It is demonstrated that ions were distributed in two regions of the electrode–electrolyte interface (Figure 7.2): the Stern layer (the nearest layer to the electrode surface where ions are strongly adsorbed) and a diffuse layer (ions distributed in a relatively low concentration driven by the thermal motion). Therefore, the capacitance of EDLCs can be considered as originating from two parts, the capacitance of the

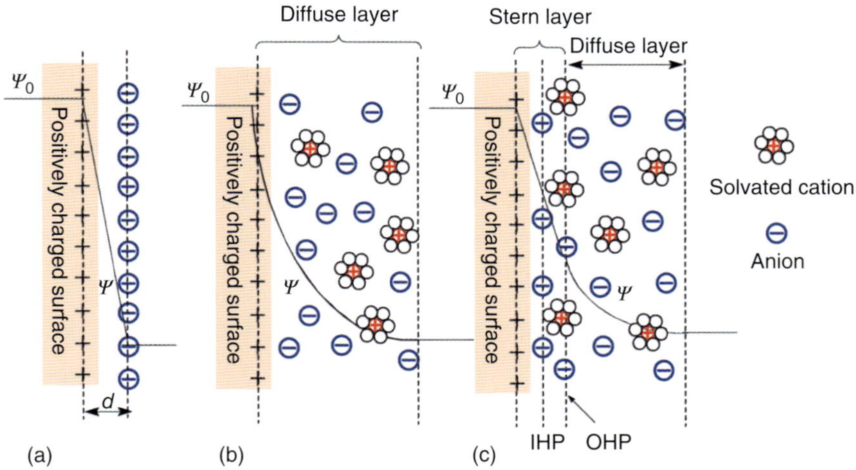

Figure 7.2 Models of the electrical double layer at a positively charged surface: (a) the Helmholtz model, (b) the Gouy–Chapman model, and (c) the Stern model, showing the inner Helmholtz lane (IHP) and outer Helmholtz plane (OHP). The IHP refers to the distance of closest approach of specifically adsorbed ions (generally anions) and OHP refers to that of the nonspecifically adsorbed ions. The OHP is also the plane where the diffuse layer begins. (d) the double layer distance described by the Helmholtz model. ψ_0 and ψ are the potentials at the electrode surface and the electrode/electrolyte interface, respectively. (Zhang and Zhao 2009 [19]. Reproduced with permission of Royal Society of Chemistry.)

Stern layer as well as the diffuse region; (ii) pseudosupercapacitors where the electrical energy is stored in an electrochemical way with electron transfer during reversible redox reactions. It is another type of capacitance, which is different from electric double-layer capacitance. This capacitance is not electrostatic in origin and comes into sight when a charge transferring process takes places in an electrochemical way at the surface of electrode materials, typically, based on metal oxides and conducting polymers; (iii) Hybrid supercapacitors, which are a combination of the two previous categories, since both the significant electric double-layer capacitance and the pseudocapacitance work together in this type of supercapacitor.

7.2.1 2D Electrode Materials for Flexible EDLCs

In EDLCs, the electrical energy is directly stored through an electrostatic way (known as non-faradaic electrical energy storage), as positive and negative charges store on the surface of two electrodes. In such energy storage systems, the electrons move to and from the capacitor electrodes during charging and discharging processes, and no chemical reactions occur. Since it is a non-faradaic charge storage process, ideally, no electron transfers from the electrodes into the electrolyte. Electrons only transport reversibly between the electrode via the external circuit, while cations and anions move in the electrolyte to the electrode–electrolyte interfaces. Therefore, the charging/discharging process of EDLCs is highly reversible, and such capacitors have a high degree of cycling stability (10^5–10^6 cycles).

Normally, for commercial supercapacitors, active carbon is the most widely used electrode-active material due to its chemical stability, high surface area, and low cost. However, the disadvantage of active carbon is its rigid mechanical property, which restricts the flexibility of supercapacitors. When the supercapacitors are employed for powering flexible systems, they have to suffer bend, twist, and even stretch [23, 24]. These mechanical deformations could easily result in cracking and peeling of the active carbons, which could decrease the electrochemical performance of the supercapacitors. To prevent the electrode-active materials from cracking and peeling off, polymer binders and conductive additives are added. The binders and conductive additives can enhance the electrical conductivity and improve the adhesion between the electrode materials and the substrates [25–28]. However, a disadvantage of using additives is that it could affect the electrochemical performance of the supercapacitors. For example, the capacitance would be decreased due to some aggregations resulting in "dead volume" caused in the electrode where the ions cannot penetrate. Simultaneously, compared with active electrode materials, the additives contribute a lower capacitance, and as a result, the specific capacitance will be decreased [29–34]. Therefore, to enable the flexible supercapacitors with synergic excellent energy storage as well as good flexibility is a great challenge. Generally, flexible supercapacitors require the electrode materials to be thin and highly flexible, so that they can be integrated into flexible substrates. The electrode materials are demanded to possess not only distinguished electrochemical performance, but also stable mechanical properties upon shape deformation (twist, bend, fold, and even stretch). Therefore, the selection of the electrode active materials of flexible supercapacitors is critical for realizing the required performance.

Recently, considerable attention has been drawn to the preparation of electrode materials for flexible supercapacitors based on numerous nanomaterials [22, 35–38]. A major feature that discriminates various types of nanostructures is their dimensionality. According to the dimensionality of the electrode active materials, they can be classified into zero-dimensional (0D), one-dimensional (1D), two-dimensional (2D), and three-dimensional (3D) materials [34]. Nanoparticles belong to the 0D category; they expose large active surface to the electrolyte, which can enhance the electrochemical energy storage. However, as discussed previously, when they are used as the electrode materials of flexible supercapacitors, they suffer from cracks and peeling off from the substrate, and therefore, polymer binders and conductive additives need to be added. Nanowires, nanotubes, and nanorods belong to the 1D category; nanosheets belong to the 2D category, while foam and network structure are described as belonging to the 3D category. In contrast to 0D materials, 1D, 2D, and 3D materials are of great advantage for the electrode materials of flexible supercapacitors, owing to their remarkable mechanical flexibility that results from the overlapping between each other during their stacking to form a thin film. Especially for the 2D materials, their thickness lies in several nanometers (single or several atomic layers), which bring synergic advantages of tunable electrical natures, large surface area, and distinguished electrochemical activities. In this chapter, we try to give an introduction to the flexible supercapacitors based on 2D materials.

Electrode materials are the key components of flexible EDLCs. They need to meet two critical requirements. Firstly, they are required to be active to store charge at the electrode–electrolyte interface, which contributes to the capacitance of the supercapacitor. Secondly, they are demanded to possess the ability to mechanically integrate on the flexible substrate, so that a high and stable energy delivery could be realized during their shape deformation process. One-dimensional materials, such as nanowires, nanotubes, and core-shell nanostructures have been widely investigated and reported to serve as active electrode materials for flexible supercapacitors, owing to their large length-to-diameter ratio to overlay with individuals to construct thin-film architectures possessing good mechanical stability [39–50]. Among these 1D nanomaterials, carbon-derived materials have got considerable attention to be used as active materials for EDLCs [51–62]. For example, using one-step aerosol synthesis method to produce thin single wall carbon nanotube (SWCNT) films and transferring them to different substrates by a dry press transfer technique, Kallio *et al.* successfully achieved flexible supercapacitors with an area-specific capacitance of $552\,\mu F\,cm^{-2}$ ($178\,F\,g^{-1}$ in mass) [63]. The as-prepared SWCNT thin film exhibits excellent mechanical strength, and the capacitance of the flexible supercapacitors does not degrade during 10 000 loading cycles. Moreover, helically coiled carbon nanotubes (HCNTs) can also work as the electrode materials for flexible supercapacitors. Kar *et al.*, via a catalytic chemical vapor deposition (CVD) process, synthesized free-standing mesoporous HCNTs on unidirectional carbon fiber to get hierarchical structures [64]. The as-prepared hierarchical HCNTs/carbon fiber structures was used as electrodes for the flexible supercapacitors and a highest gravimetric capacitance of $125.7\,F\,g^{-1}$ ($145.3\,mF\,cm^{-2}$ in area) at a current density of $0.28\,mA\,cm^{-2}$ was obtained. Here, the excellent specific capacitance is contributed by the high surface area, hierarchical electrode structures, and also the richness of the functional groups (oxygen-containing surface) of the HCNTs. Furthermore, owing to the helically coiled structure of the carbon nanotube (CNT), they can connect with each other more firmly, simultaneously; the carbon fiber which works as the depositing substrate as well as current collector is highly flexible. Therefore, the capacitance decrease of the as-prepared supercapacitors was not noted even under a 120° bend. Besides 1D nanomaterials (CNT), 1D micromaterials are also developed as electrode materials for flexible supercapacitors. One-dimensional nanomaterials (nanotube, nanowires, etc.) are always produced through an artificial synthesis process. Contrastingly, micromaterials with 1D structure (e.g., microwires) could be directly achieved from plants. Hence, the electrode materials fabrication process could be simplified; furthermore, the total cost of the flexible supercapacitors could be reduced. Motivated by such advantages, Tour *et al.* demonstrated the design and fabrication of a flexible microporous nitrogen-doped carbonized cotton by a facile template-free method [65]. Microporous structures are formed where NH_3 reacts with the carbon cotton during a thermal treatment process. The N doping increases the electronic conductivity and induces pseudocapacitive effects of carbon cotton. Furthermore, the N doping can also enhance the wettability of carbon cotton, which benefits the penetration of electrolyte into the inner part of electrode materials, leading to efficient usage of the internal surface of electrode materials. Therefore, the resulting flexible supercapacitors show a high specific capacitance of 207 F g^{-1} as well as an energy density of 7.2 W h kg^{-1} at the current density of 1 A g^{-1}. The device also exhibits good flexibility; it still maintains stable performance after 4000 bending times.

Since the discovery of graphene in 2004, as one of the widely investigated 2D materials, materials with two-dimensional structures have drawn more and more interest. With their high surface area and the ability to form thin film easily, 2D materials, such as graphene and metal oxide nanosheets are employed as a material's platform for electrode active materials for flexible supercapacitors [66–71]. The unique advantages of the 2D materials to work as electrode materials for flexible supercapacitors are that, firstly, the ultrathin structures (atomic level thickness) of 2D materials expose a large surface area to the electrolyte. Consequently, numerous active sites can be involved in the electrochemical process, which is very important for enhancing the capacitive behavior of supercapacitors. Secondly, the formation of thin-film electrode of 2D materials is enhanced by their overlapping connection: the large overlapping area between individual sheets contribute to the enhanced flexibility of the thin film electrode [66].

Among these 2D materials, graphene-based materials are widely explored as active materials of flexible supercapacitors, because of their unique properties, including large surface area (~2630 m^2 g^{-1}), high conductivity, wide potential windows, and excellent mechanical flexibility. Single-layer graphene is characterized to possess a specific areal capacitance of ~27 F cm^{-2} [72]. Therefore, theoretical capacitance (EDLCs) as large as ~550 F g^{-1} could be realized from graphene materials, which ideally obtain the maximum capacitive performance of carbon-based materials. The predominant electrochemical performance of graphene is impacted by the sheet's size and the amount of sheet layers as well as by the density of defects [73]. To date, several strategies have been adopted with regard to the synthesis of graphene. CVD has been demonstrated as an efficient method for graphene production [74–78]. Graphene synthesized by this method exhibits nearly perfect properties owing to few defects and big crystal domains in the sheets, which have contributed to enhancing the charge mobility for electronic applications. Nevertheless, because of the low yield and high cost of this technology, this technology is not considered to be competent to fordize electrode materials for energy storage devices. Besides the CVD strategy, two strategies were discovered for mass production of graphene with low cost and high output: liquid-phase exfoliation and reduction of graphene oxide (GO). During the liquid-phase exfoliation process, the van der Waals attraction between the graphene layers is weakened by dispersing pristine graphite particles in a solvent. Then ultrasonication [79], by electric field [80] or shearing [81], is employed to exfoliate the graphite into graphene sheets. In the second strategy, first, GO is synthesized by strong oxidation of pristine graphite, consequently, GO is further reduced though a chemical, thermal, or electrochemical processes to restore the π network. The quality of graphene produced by these two methods is not as high as that produced by the CVD process due to defects such as edges, deformations, and O–/H– containing groups. But these methods provide a way for the mass production of graphene

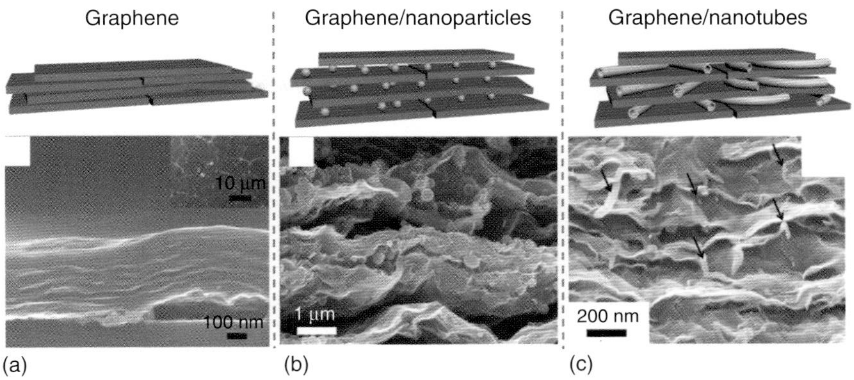

Figure 7.3 (a) Schematic drawing of stacking graphene film and cross-sectional SEM image of the reduced graphene oxide films (inset: SEM image of its surface). Qi *et al.* 2015 [87]. Reproduced with permission of John Wiley & Sons. (b) Schematic drawing of stacking graphene/nanoparticles film and cross-sectional SEM image of graphene/carbon nanosphere film. Lu *et al.* 2016 [95]. Reproduced with permission of Elsevier. (c) Schematic drawing of stacking graphene/nanotubes film and cross-sectional SEM image of graphene/carbon nanotubes film. (Lu *et al.* 2011 [96]. Reproduced with permission of Elsevier.)

materials with contained cost and are therefore, suitable technologies for the production of graphene materials for energy conversion and storage devices.

Apart from the high yield and low cost, excellent flexibility, good mechanical properties, large surface area, and good conductance also make graphene as promising active materials for flexible supercapacitors [82–85]. However, as the graphene sheets always lie in microscale, assembling these micro sheets into films to serve as the electrodes is a critical issue for graphene-based flexible supercapacitors. Recently, several methods have been successfully employed for the preparation of graphene films, such as synchronous reduction and assembly [86, 87], vacuum filtration [88, 89]. Spin-coating [90], Langmuir–Blodgeett process [91], electrophoresis [71], layer-by-layer deposition [92], and interfacial self-assembly [93]. Via a simple vacuum filtration strategy, graphene films were fabricated and employed as flexible electrode materials for supercapacitors [94]. It is notable that graphene sheets can be individually dispersed in the solution, and during the following vacuum filtration process, aggregation and restacking occur to the graphene sheets because of the strong van der Waals interactions among the graphene sheets (Figure 7.3a) [87]. Consequently, a much lower surface area of the graphene-based electrode than the theoretical value ($\sim$2630 $cm^2\ g^{-1}$) results and the penetration of electrolyte ions into the electrode is reduced [83]. As a result, the electrochemical performances (capacitance, power, and energy density) are lower than the expected values.

To prevent the graphene sheets from aggregation during the electrode film fabricating process, attention has been paid to many efforts and effective strategies have been developed including infrared laser reduction [97], adding spacers [98, 99], template-assisted growth [100], and crumpling method [101]. Irradiation of the GO film using the infrared laser can reduce the GO, and based on this principle GO films on flexible substrate were directly reduced to graphene by the laser from a commercial LightScribe DVD optical drive [97]. Simultaneously, the initially stacked GO films were converted into well-exfoliated reduced graphene oxide (rGO) films. The supercapacitors, employing the laser-reduced GO as electrode materials, show excellent performance among the flexible supercapacitors based graphene materials. In addition, adding 0D (nanoparticles) or 1D (nanotube or nanorod) materials into the interspace among the graphene sheets has proved to be an effective strategy to prevent stacking [98, 99]. Through a vacuum filtration strategy, Lian *et al.* used carbon black nanoparticles to restrict the stacking of graphene layers, resulting in high-active surface area of the electrode materials. Therefore, the carbon black nanoparticles incorporated graphene-based supercapacitors perform a remarkable capacitance. The mass specific capacitance is $138\,F\,g^{-1}$ (scan rate; $10\,mV\,s^{-1}$) and a negligible 3.85% capacitance degradation is obtained after 2000 charging/discharging cycles. Similarly, mesoporous carbon nanospheres are also employed as the spacer for reducing the stacking of graphene sheets in the fabricating procedure. In a typical experiment, the graphene papers inserted with mesoporous carbon nanospheres show a specific surface area of $584\,m^2\,g^{-1}$ that is higher than that of graphene papers ($37\,m^2\,g^{-1}$) without nanosphere insertion [95]. Cross-sectional scanning electron microscopy (SEM) images demonstrate that the stacking of graphene sheets has been effectively inhabited (Figure 7.3b), facilitating ions to access the surfaces of graphene in forming electric double layers. When the as-prepared graphene film inserted with carbon nanospheres was used as the electrode of supercapacitors (1 M KOH electrolyte), excellent electrochemical performance was obtained, including high specific capacitance ($211\,F\,g^{-1}$ at $0.2\,A\,g^{-1}$), excellent electrochemical stability (4% capacity loss after 5000 cycles), and good rate capability (61% capacity retention at $20\,A\,g^{-1}$). The utilization of 0D materials can effectively reduce the self-stacking of graphene sheets in the fabricating procedure, resulting in excellent electrochemical performance of the graphene-based flexible supercapacitors.

Besides the good electrochemical performance as flexible electrodes, the mechanical property of the graphene- based electrode is another crucial issue that needs to be addressed. It is supposed that the inserted nanoparticles would decrease the mechanical strength of the graphene film because the nanoparticles reduce the stacking of individual graphene sheets, resulting in the decrease of the overlaps among the graphene sheets. However, the influence of the inserted nanoparticles or nanospheres on the mechanical properties of the graphene films is still less investigated. Adding 1D materials (nanotube, nanofiber) instead of 0D materials is an alternative way to suppress the influence of spacer materials on the mechanical properties of graphene-based electrode. Similar to 0D spacers, 1D spacers could also result in decreasing the overlap among graphene sheets, but overlaps between the graphene sheets and spacers (nanotube or nanofiber) and overlaps between the spacers themselves will form, which could enhance the mechanical strength of the graphene films. Furthermore, the conductive 1D spacers can bridge the defects for electron transfer among the graphene sheets [102–105]. For example, CNT is employed to serve as the spacers in the graphene film for flexible supercapacitors. In a typical experiment, both GO and CNT were dispersed in water solution, after conducting a vacuum filtration strategy, and the graphene/CNT film was achieved [96]. In this design, the CNT not only efficiently decreases the stacking but also enhances the electron transfer among graphene sheets, resulting in a high electrolyte–electrode interfaces for the forming of electric double layers (Figure 7.3c). The supercapacitor based on graphene/CNT film possesses a specific capacitance of 265 F g^{-1} (0.1 A g^{-1}) as well as a good rate capability (49% capacity retention at 50 A g^{-1}). Moreover, 97% of the capacitance is retained after continuous charging/discharging of 2000 cycles. Recently, by employing vertically aligned CNTs to separate the parallel graphene layers, a novel 3D structure has been designed by a computational model. It reveals that this structure can possess good electrochemical performance [102]. Consequently, experimental fabrication of the graphene films with vertically aligned CNTs grown in between graphene sheets is realized via a CVD approach. The as-prepared graphene/CNT films have been successfully used as electrodes for flexible supercapacitors, and a maximum specific capacitance of 385 F g^{-1} (scan rate 10 mV s^{-1}) has been realized [103]. The capacitance of supercapacitors is significantly affected by the electrode–electrolyte interfaces. Apart from preventing the stacking of graphene sheets, the interfaces also can be increased by constructing the electrode materials with 3D porous structures, such as aerogels, sponges, frameworks, and foams. These 3D structures, possessing nanostructures, microstructures, even macroporous networks, can provide high electrode–electrolyte interface areas and benefit the electron/ion transport. For instance, graphene film with 3D macroporous bubbles is produced by using the assembled polymethyl methacrylate (PMMA) spheres as the sacrificial template. The porous diameter could be tailored by adjusting the diameter of the PMMA spheres. The prepared 3D macroporous graphene film as a "binder-free" supercapacitor electrode can afford quite a high-rate capability (1.0 V s^{-1}). In addition, polystyrene (PS) spheres can be used as the sacrificial template for the preparation of graphene macroporous structures. Additionally, by employing nickel foam as the template, graphene foam can be prepared via a synchronous reduction and assembly strategy or CVD process [106, 107]. The as-prepared graphene foams possess high surface areas. Compared with the graphene foam achieved via a synchronous reduction and assembly strategy, the graphene foam produced by a CVD strategy gives a higher conductivity due to few defects produced in the CVD process. As a result, it exhibits an excellent electrochemical performance, which serves as electrode active materials for flexible supercapacitors. The fabrication of 3D porous graphene materials could also be further simplified by a one-step fabricating method. For example, inspired by the leavening process, Chen *et al.* successfully transferred compact graphene films to fluffy films with 3D porous networks with a submicrometer to several micrometers pore sizes [108]. Employing the as-prepared 3D porous graphene film to serve as both the electrode and current collector, flexible supercapacitors are built up with a specific capacitance of 110 F g^{-1}. No obvious capacitance decrease is observed when the device was under bending, which demonstrates its excellent flexibility.

Another factor that limits the electrochemical performance of supercapacitors fabricated from graphene-based materials is their low conductivity, which limits electron transport in the electrodes and thus reduces the performance of supercapacitors. The reduction of GO by methane (CH_4) plasma treatment is demonstrated to be an efficient approach to increase the conductivity of graphene-based materials. During this treatment, the CH_4 plasma, rich as a carbon source (such as C^+, CH_n^+ and CH_n $n = 1–3$), would repair the defects in GO, thus a high C/O ratio (9.2) could be obtained and high electrical conductivity ($345\ S\ cm^{-1}$) resulted. A flexible supercapacitor based on CH_4-plasma-treated graphene was reported by the researchers in the Max-Planck-Institute [109]. After CH_4-plasma treatment, the maximum area and stack capacitance of their supercapacitor is $80.7\ \mu F\ cm^{-2}$ and $17.9\ F\ cm^{-3}$, respectively, which is much higher than that of the supercapacitor ($32.6\ \mu F\ cm^{-2}$ and $7.3\ F\ cm^{-3}$) fabricated from untreated graphene materials. This work demonstrates that the conductivity of electrode materials plays a vital role in the performance of flexible supercapacitors.

The advantages of 2D materials are even obvious when they are employed as the electrode materials for in-plane microsupercapacitors [66, 110]. Compared with the conventional supercapacitors with sandwiched structures, a particular metric of in-plane microsupercapacitors is the design of interdigitated microelectrode fingers. Particularly, the in-plane interdigitated architectures offer several advantages over the sandwiched architectures. Firstly, this design enables the electrodes to possess a high edge-to-area ratio and makes the open edges to be side-by-side. So, the electrode–electrolyte interfaces could be increased as the edges of the electrodes are exposed to electrolyte. As a result, excellent power density that is many orders larger than that of conventional supercapacitors and batteries can be achieved [66]. Secondly, due to the narrow interspace between electrode fingers as well as the elimination of the separators (necessary in supercapacitors with conventional sandwiched structures), the electrolyte ion transport resistance in the supercapacitors can be reduced and charging/discharging at high frequency can be achieved. This is crucial for future miniaturized portable electronics [111]. Thirdly, the unique in-plane architecture facilitates the microsupercapacitors to be flexible, especially, when 2D electrode materials are employed; the overlap between the sheets prevents the electrode film from fracture. Finally, the in-plane electrode architectures facilitate the integration of microsupercapacitors to on-chip integrated circuits [112–114]. Therefore, microsupercapacitors with in-plane architectures are suitable candidates for power supply and energy storage components of miniaturized healthy and medical electronics.

Taking graphene as a typical sample of 2D materials, the in-plane design of interdigitated electrode arrays is straight forward to efficiently utilize the surface of individual graphene layers for electric charge storage, since the open architecture and multilayer structure of graphene electrode films are very favorable to increase the electrode–electrolyte interfaces [115], as shown in Figure 7.4 [23]. An in-plane ultrathin microsupercapacitor fabricated from pristine graphene or multilayer rGO has been successfully demonstrated. Compared to conventional sandwich structured supercapacitors, a dramatic increase in capacitance of in-plane microsupercapacitors is achieved [115]. However, as discussed previously, for the electrode composed of graphene materials, the electrochemical performance is also hindered by the aggregation and restacking of graphene sheets during processing and the actual accessible surface area

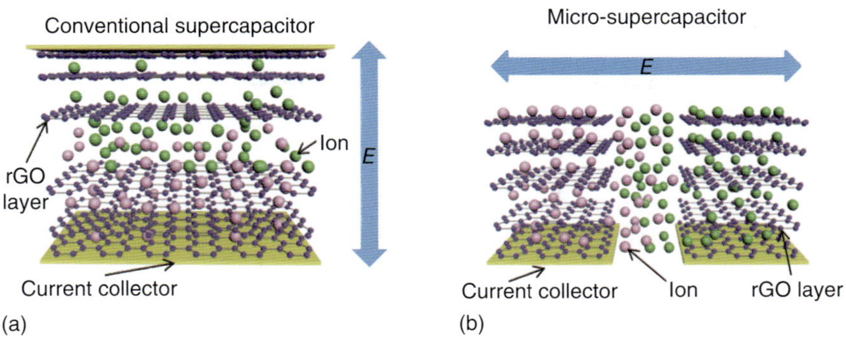

Figure 7.4 Schematic depiction of the operating principle of: (a) the stacked-geometry conventional supercapacitors, and (b) in-plane micro-supercapacitors. (Qi *et al.* 2016 [23]. Reproduced with permission of John Wiley & Sons.)

is much lower than the theoretical value (~2600 $m^2\,g^{-1}$). Therefore, spacers are added among graphene layers to prevent their restacking. For example, when using CNTs as the spacers, nanochannels form among graphene sheets and graphene stacking could be effectively reduced [116]. The nanochannels enlarge the surface area of the electrodes, and provide pathways for efficient ion transportation parallel to the graphene planes. Hence, the electrochemical performance of microsupercapacitors is enhanced [117].

The performance of flexible supercapacitors fabricated with graphene-based materials could be enhanced by constructing graphene into 3D structures, owing to the enlarged electrolyte accessible surface areas of 3D structures. Graphene hydrogels and aerogels consisting of 3D macrostructures have been successfully produced by one-step hydrothermal reduction process [118–122]. They are also successful in application as flexible electrodes for supercapacitors. For instance, Shi *et al.* reported a 3D-structured graphene hydrogel synthesized by reducing the GO dispersed aqueous solution with sodium ascorbate [119]. The resulting graphene hydrogel possess a well-defined and cross-linked 3D porous structures; simultaneously, the hydrogels are mechanically flexible and show a conductivity of 1 $S\,m^{-1}$, and therefore, they show remarkable electrochemical performances with a specific capacitance of 240 $F\,g^{-1}$ (1.2 $A\,g^{-1}$ in 1 M H_2SO_4 solution). Moreover, the conductivity of the graphene hydrogel could be improved by further reduction of the GO with hydrazine or hydroiodic acid [123]. After reduction, the graphene hydrogels exhibit a relatively high conductivity (1.3–3.2 $S\,m^{-1}$). Accordingly, when the graphene hydrogel is employed as electrodes of flexible supercapacitors, a specific capacitance of 220 $F\,g^{-1}$ at the current density of 1 $A\,g^{-1}$ can be achieved.

7.2.2 2D Materials for Pseudocapacitive Supercapacitors

The performance of EDLCs is based on the non-faradaic electrostatic attraction of ions in the electrode–electrolyte interface. High charging/discharging rate and high power density are the main features of EDLCs. Recently, graphene-based materials have been the most widely investigated electrode materials for flexible

EDLCs. Good conductivity, high surface area, excellent mechanical strength and flexibility, as well as chemical stability in aqueous and organic electrolyte are the advantages of graphene-based materials for this application. However, the capacitance and energy density is still low even when the stacking of graphene sheets is decreased by inserting spacers (carbon nanoparticles, CNTs). A great enhancement in capacitance and energy density can be obtained if a quick faradaic process takes place. In this case, the electrode process involves electrons transfer reversibly between electrode and ions or molecules in the electrolyte. This type of supercapacitor arises from some redox reactions at the electrode surfaces, which is different from that of the EDLCs. The capacitance presented by such systems is regarded as pseudocapacitance. It originates from the reversible process of electron transfer between an oxidized state and a reduced state, and when the redox reaction is some continuous function of the applied potential, the pseudocapacitance arises. In principle, this pseudocapacitance can be much larger (10–100 times) than those of electric double-layer systems in the same volume or weight. Thus, pseudocapacitive materials hold the potential of reaching the energy density level of a battery. Commonly, when conducting polymers (polypyrrole (PPy), polyaniline (PANI), polythiophenes (PTh) and their derivatives) [124–135], and transition metal oxides (RuO_2, IrO_2, MnO_2) [136–143] are used as the electrode materials of supercapacitors, the pseudocapacitance would be revealed.

Conducting polymers exhibit pseudocapacitance by storing and releasing charges via a redox process of the π-conjugated polymer chains [133–135, 144–151]. The following essential features define the electrochemical behavior of conductive polymers: (i) the sequential range of oxidized states that supervenes the applied potential and (ii) the reversibility of the redox reactions corresponding to charge withdrawal and reinjection in the surface of electrode materials. When oxidation occurs, ions transfer from electrolyte to the polymer backbone. Reversibly, when reduction takes place, ions are released back to the electrolyte. The process shows an almost mirror image of voltammograms in cyclic voltammetry that is typical of charging and discharging behavior, and also responsive current, which is corresponding to the sweep rate. Therefore, their energy storage behavior exhibits a battery-type, while, their electrical characteristics are those of a capacitor. Furthermore, conductive polymers can be fabricated into electrode films by a simple electrochemical process; they are good candidates of electrode materials for pseudocapacitive capacitors. Among the most extensively studied conducting polymers, PPy is currently widely employed as the electrode materials for the supercapacitors owing to its high conductivity as well as excellent stability [152, 153]. In addition, PPy also possesses good flexibility and mechanical strength after doping with appropriate molecule [124, 154]. Thus, PPy shows remarkable capability for flexible energy storage devices. For example, using PPy/Nafion as a flexible electrode, a flexible supercapacitor is demonstrated [133]. Specific capacitance of $380\,F\,g^{-1}$, power density of $15.50\,kW\,kg^{-1}$, and energy density of $56\,W\,h\,kg^{-1}$ are obtained. However, the insertion/de-insertion of counterions during the charging/discharging cycles causes volumetric changes of the electrode materials, accompanying progressive electrode degradation due to the swelling, breaking, and shrinkage, which could result in a conductivity loss of the electrode. On the other hand, the surface area of the conducting polymer film is not high, which limits the capacitance of as-prepared supercapacitors. Therefore, conductive carbon materials are introduced as the resilient and the surface-area-enlarging additives for enhancing the mechanical properties, simultaneously ensuring the good conductivity of the electrodes [22, 155–166]. Furthermore, combining PPy with polyimide is employed to enhance the energy storage capabilities of PPy based electrode materials, because the oxidative degradation of PPy can be protected by the polyimide matrix [167]. Since conducting polymers were utilized as electrode materials for supercapacitors in the mid-1990s, many efforts have been devoted to this area. However, the conducting-polymers-based 2D electrode materials for supercapacitors are still less reported, and the possible reason is that the synthesis of conducting polymers in 2D structures is not facile.

Additionally, supercapacitors that employ transition metal oxides to serve as electrode materials have been widely investigated during the past decades [168–179], because the metal oxide materials (RuO_2, IrO_2, MnO_2 NiO, Fe_3O_4) are accessible to faradaic behavior of oxidation and reduction. Among them, ruthenium oxide (RuO_2) has been widely studied since Trasatti and Buzzanca demonstrated its capacitive properties [180], owing to its electric conductance and three distinct oxidation states accessible within 1.2 V [98, 116]. Its pseudocapacitive behavior exhibits the following feature: fast reversible electron transfer accompanied with protons adsorbed on the RuO_2 surface, according to Eq. (7.1), resulting in the change of Ru oxidation states.

$$RuO_2 + xH^+ + xe^- = RuO_2 - x(OH)_x \tag{7.1}$$

The value of x ($0 \leq x \leq 2$) changes corresponding to the proton insertion or de-insertion that takes within a potential window of about 1.2 V. Considerable attention has been drawn for the development of high pseudocapacitive RuO_x-based electrode materials [181, 182]. For instance, a supercapacitor is fabricated through electro-deposition of mesoporous RuO_x, which gives a maximum specific capacitance of 12.6 mF cm^{-2} [181].

Although noble metal oxides (RuO_2, IrO_2) show excellent pseudocapacitive performance, the drawback is their relatively high cost. Consequently, people try to explore other low-cost alternatives. In recent years, base metal oxides, such as iron [183, 184], cobalt [185, 186], nickel [47, 187, 188], vanadium [189, 190], molybdenum [191], and manganese [192–194] have drawn much attention. Particularly, manganese oxide (MnO_2) has got maximum attention because of its outstanding pseudocapacitive behavior (1370 F g^{-1}), eco-friendly nature, easy to obtain, and low cost of raw material [195–200]. The energy storage of MnO_2 is contributed by the electrolyte cations (C^+) adsorbed on its surface as well as proton incorporation according to the Eq. (7.2):

$$MnO_2 + xC^+ + yH^+ + (x+y)e^- = MnOOC_xH_y \tag{7.2}$$

Its voltammogram is close to that of an electric double-layer capacitor due to the fast, reversible, and successive surface redox behavior. In recent decades, MnO_2 has been widely employed as the active material for flexible supercapacitors [201, 202]. It is notable that although it possesses a high theoretical specific capacitance (1370 F g^{-1}), the energy density of the supercapacitors based on pristine MnO_2 materials is still limited owing to its intrinsically poor conductivity (10^{-5}–10^{-6} S cm^{-1}). Therefore, conductive carbon-based additives, such as carbon nanoparticles [203], CNT [204], and graphene [205] are employed to enhance the conductivity, resulting in enhanced electrochemical performance of the devices. Another kind of conductive additive is derived from metals. For instance, nanoporous Au could work as highly conductive additives to support MnO_2 (Figure 7.5a,b) [28]. The nanoporous Au promotes the electrons to speedily transport through the MnO_2, greatly enhancing the ion transfer between MnO_2 and electrolytes, and consequently, a capacitance of 1145 F g^{-1} is realized. Additionally, the energy and power densities of the flexible supercapacitors (Figure 7.5c) fabricated from the hybrid Au/MnO_2 structures increase by adding the loading amount of MnO_2, and get to maximum of 57 W h kg^{-1} and 16 kW kg^{-1}, respectively. Generally, it is demonstrated that the electrodes based on hierarchical nanostructure assembled from 2D nanosheets can enhacne the electrochemical performance of supercapacitors, due to their enchanced electrode–electrolyte interfaces and electroactive sites [174, 206]. Recently, 3D MnO_2 nanosheets/$ZnCo_2O_4$ nanowired structures grown on carbon cotton have been employed as the electrode of supercapacitors. In this design, MnO_2 nanosheets were vertically synthesised on the surface of $ZnCo_2O_4$ nanowires, which dramtically enhanced the electrochemical active sites. The as-prepared electrode exhibits an area capacitance of 3.6 F cm^{-2} at a current density of 2 mA cm^{-2} and of 2.3 F cm^{-2} even at a current density of 100 mA cm^{-2}. Moreover, the electrode also exhibits an excellent cycling stability by retaining 95.5% of its capacitance after 5000 charging/discharging cycles, rendering the 3D $ZnCo_2O_4$ nanowired/MnO_2 nanosheet structures as good candidates of electrode material for high-performance flexible supercapacitors [207]. Furthermore, mixed transition metal oxides have been believed to hold great potential as advanced electrodes for supercapacitors, owing to their improved electronic conductivity as well as rich redox reactions [206, 208–210]. For example, $Na_2Ti_3O_7$ nanosheet arrays fabricated on carbon textiles are used as the electrode materials for enhancing the electrochemcial performance of flexible pseudocapacitors [210]. An energy density of 55 W h kg^{-1} and power density of 3000 W kg^{-1} are obtained. Additionally, the flexible device exhibits a stable electrochemical performance almost without losing any capacitance even under harsh mechanical deformation. Hierarchical $NiMoO_4$ structures consisted with uniformly aligned nanosheets grown on nickel foam are explored as the electrode materials [206]. In this design, two different metal materials are involved in the metal oxide (Figure 7.5d); as a result, a great number of redox reavtive sites and enhanced conductivity are obtained. These architectures with an extended voltage window of 0–1.7 V show excellent electrochemical performance. $NiMoO_4$ nanosheets (Figure 7.5e) as electrode materials for supercapacitors possess higher faradaic capacitance than that of $NiMoO_4$ nanorods. They give a high energy density of 60.9 W h kg^{-1} as well as a power density of 850 W kg^{-1}. Moreover, the device retains 85.7% of its initial specific capacitance after 10 000 charging/discharging cycles (Figure 7.5f). It is demonstrated that

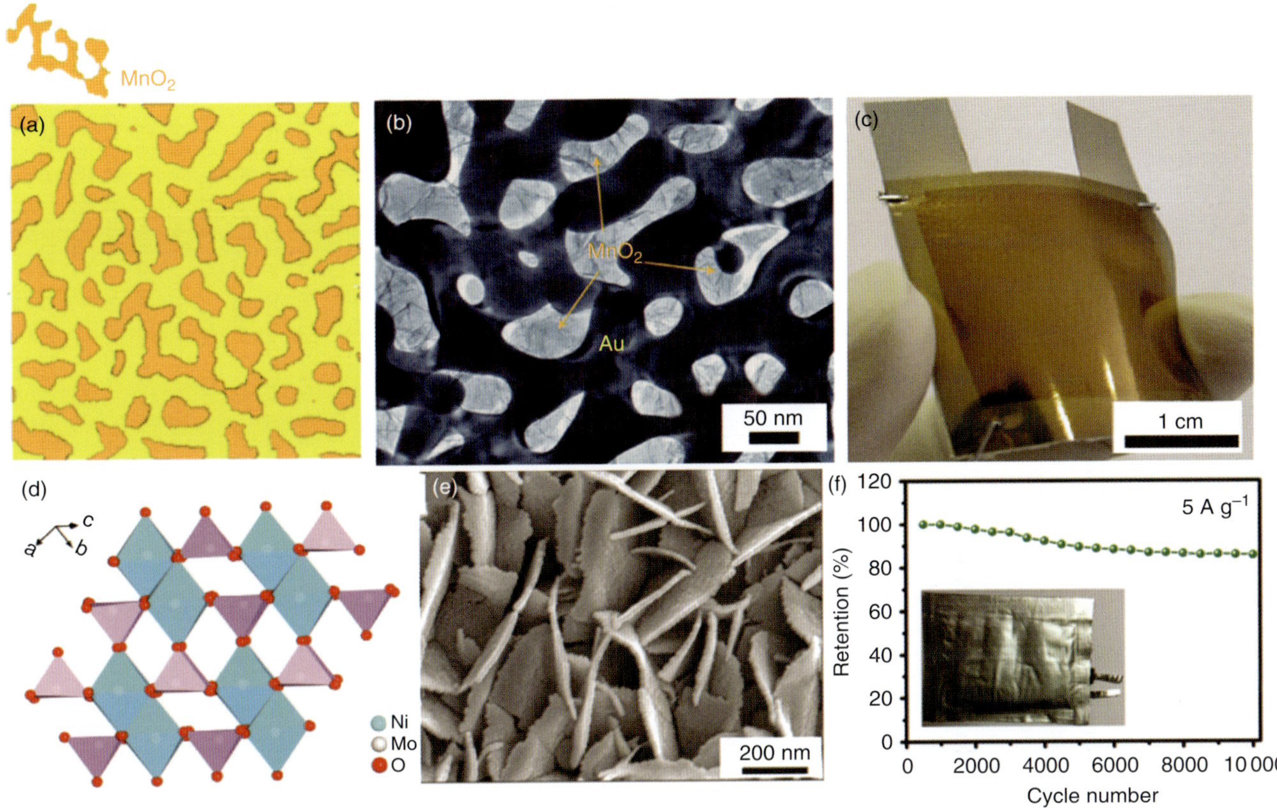

Figure 7.5 (a) Schematic showing the fabrication process for nanoporous gold/MnO_2 hybrid materials by directly growing MnO_2 (orange) onto nanoporous gold. (b) Bright-field TEM image of the nanoporous gold/MnO_2 hybrid nanostructure, which can be identified by the contrast between the bright MnO_2 filler and the dark gold skeleton. (c) Photograph of a nanoporous gold/MnO_2-based supercapacitor. (d) Crystal structure of $NiMoO_4$ (e) crystallized $NiMoO_4$ nanosheets arrays. (f) Cycling stability of $NiMoO_4$ at a current density of 5 A g^{-1} (the inset shows the photograph of the device). (a–c: Lang *et al*. 2011 [28]. Reproduced with permission of Nature Publishing Group; d–f: Peng *et al*. 2015 [206]. Reproduced with permission of John Wiley & Sons.)

these $NiMoO_4$-based nanomaterils can be fabricated on various conductive substrates (i.e., Ni foam, Ti foil, stainless-steel foil, and graphite paper), and therefore, can be used as the electrode materials for flexible supercapacitors.

As discussed previously, the advantages of 2D materials for supercapacitors become even obvious when they are employed in the in-plane microsupercapacitors, because the open edges of the in-plane electrode fingers provide a path for electrolyte ion diffusion. As a result, the ions can penetrate deeply into the inside of active materials and enlarge the electrode–electrolyte interfaces, whereby the specific capacitance could be dramatically enhanced. Recently, vanadium disulfide (VS_2) thin films were successfully produced for constructing electrode fingers of in-plane microsupercapacitors [211]. Here, the VS_2 films are assembled from VS_2 nanosheets that are exfoliated from bulk VS_2 flakes. Owing to the layered structure formed from the stacking of conducting S-V-S layers by weak van der Waals interactions, VS_2 offers an ideal material candidate for the flexible supercapacitors due to its synergic metallic nature and 2D-structured characteristics. The as-prepared microsupercapacitors possess a specific capacitance of 4.76 mF cm^{-2}.

7.2.3 2D Electrode Materials for Hybrid Flexible Supercapacitors

For practical application, it is crucial to develop flexible supercapacitors with higher energy density, high power density and excellent cycling stability. EDLCs can deliver a high power density but possess a low energy density, since the charge only stores at the electrode–electrolyte interfaces via a non-faradaic process. In contrast, pseudocapacitors can achieve high energy density contributed by the faradaic redox reactions that happens on the electrode surface; however, their power-delivering ability and cycling stability are limited too. Hybrid systems, combining the advantages of EDLCs and pseudocapacitors, provide a choice for enabling the supercapacitors with high energy density as well as high power density. One strategy to obtain hybrid materials for supercapacitors is to mix electric double-layer capacitive materials (i.e., carbon, CNT, graphene) with pseudocapacitive materials (i.e., PPy, PANI, MnO_2) [204, 205, 212–217]. For example, a structure where MnO_2 nanosheets electrodeposited on CNT textile is fabricated serves as the hybrid materials for supercapacitors [204]. This nanostructure could effectively reduce the ion diffusion and electron transport resistance in the electrode. Furthermore, compared with metal substrates, a stronger binding is achieved between the MnO_2 and CNT textile fibers, which can enhance the stability of cycling performance. For a certain areal mass loading, the thickness of MnO_2 deposited on textile fibers is much smaller than that on the metal substrate. So this structure could provide a greater number of electrochemical active sites for charge store, which contributes to an excellent areal capacitance of 2.8 F cm^{-2} (0.05 mV s^{-1}). Full cells are successfully fabricated, where the MnO_2/CNT/textile is employed as the positive electrode, while reduced MnO_2/CNT/textile is employed as the negative electrode. The as-prepared pseudocapacitor proves a suitable candidate as an economical energy storage and wearable power unit. Furthermore, when the 2D active materials of electrode are used to construct 3D structures for electrodes, the surface of 2D materials could be efficiently utilized. Consequently, high electrochemical performances could be achieved. For example, 3D graphene networks are employed as the supporter for MnO_2 deposition. These 3D structures permit a large mass (9.8 mg cm^{-2}) loading of MnO_2 which is almost 92.9% of the mass of whole electrode, giving a high area capacitance of 1.42 F cm^{-2} at a scan rate of 2 mV s^{-1}. After optimizing, a maximum capacitance of 130 F g^{-1} can be realized. Finally, flexible supercapacitors are obtained by encapsulating the supercapacitors by polyethylene terephthalate (PET) films [218]. Similarly, the 3D graphene structures are also used to support conductive polymer materials for the fabrication of hybrid materials for electrodes [219].

Another strategy to obtain electrodes with hybrid materials is to fabricate the electrodes with alternating stacked electric double-layer capacitive materials and pseudocapacitive materials. In this design, the layers of electric double-layer capacitive materials provide a pathway for the electron transport during the charging/discharging processes, while the pseudocapacitive materials contribute to the high faradaic capacitance; the overall performance is therefore improved.

The advantage of such an alternating structure is more obvious for the in-plane microsupercapacitors, where the open edges of the electrode fingers facilitate the penetration of electrolyte into the inner parts of electrodes. In a typical work, alternating stacked graphene/PANI hybrid structures are fabricated to serve as the electrode materials of in-plane microsupercapacitors [220]. A specific areal capacitance of 210 mF cm^{-2} at a scan rate of 10 mV s^{-1} is achieved. The super performance results from (i) an additional capacitance that is contributed by the easily accessible channels with the porous graphene-coupled PANI nanosheets; (ii) the flexible graphene layers that not only serve as the capacitive layer for charge storage and offer an electron pathway in the electrodes, but also provide an elastic spatial confinement effect to buffer the large volume changes of the redox PANI nanosheets during the charging/discharging process.

Besides the hybrid materials, the other strategy that combines the advantages of EDLCs and pseudocapacitors lies in the asymmetric supercapacitors, which are constitutive of pseudocapacitive materials in one electrode and electric double-layer capacitive materials in the other electrode [221–229]. Such hybrid architectures yield an enlarged operating voltage window for high energy density contributed by a synergistic effect of high energy delivered electrode and high power capable electrode with different working voltage. A crucial aspect to be considered when designing asymmetric supercapacitors is the balance of mass ratio between the two electrodes [230]. The amount of charge stored in each electrode is demanded to be as close as possible to maximize the total capacitance. The optimal mass ratio of positive electrode over the negative electrode (m_+/m_-) can be calculated by the following Eq. (7.3): [231, 232]

$$\frac{m_+}{m_-} = \frac{c_- v_-}{c_+ v_+} \tag{7.3}$$

According to the optimal mass loading for asymmetric architectures, the mass of electric double-layer capacitive materials (i.e., carbon-based materials,

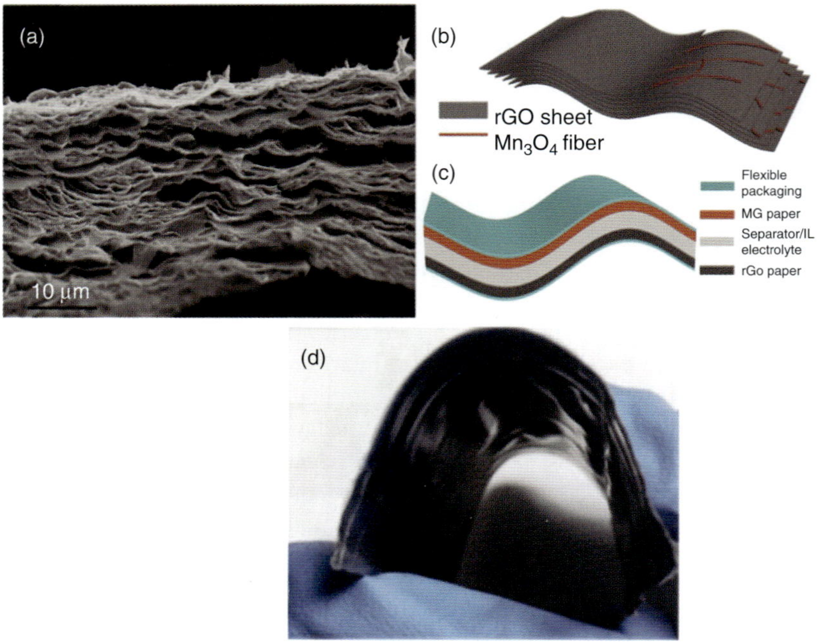

Figure 7.6 (a) Cross-sectional SEM image of the MnO_x/graphene oxide nanohybrid paper. (b) Schematic diagram showing how MnO_x nanofibers are embedded among reduced graphene oxide sheets. (c) Schematic illustration of the flexible asymmetric supercapacitor based on MnO_x/graphene oxide nanohybrid paper as the positive electrode and reduced graphene paper as the negative electrode in a diluted ionic liquid (1 M $EMIMBF_4$ in acetone nitrile) electrolyte, wrapped in a flexible packaging. (d) Photo of the freely bended asymmetric supercapacitor device. (Hu *et al.* 2015 [229]. Reproduced with permission of John Wiley & Sons.)

such as CNT, graphene) is generally greater than that of pseudocapacitive materials (conducting polymers or metal oxides). At the initial stage, activated carbon is chosen as the negative electrode of asymmetric supercapacitors [233]. Subsequently, carbon nanomaterials are developed as a replacement for activated carbon for fast power delivery and long cycle stability. For instance, by combining gel formation and electrochemical reduction processes, Mn_3O_4 nanofibers are successfully deposited onto 2D rGO paper (Figure 7.6a,b) [229]. The electrical conductivity of this Mn_3O_4/rGO nanohybrid paper is enhanced by conducting an electrochemical reduction process, while maintaining its mechanical strength. When incorporated with an electrochemically reduced rGO paper as the anode, a flexible asymmetric supercapacitor, based on the Mn_3O_4/rGO nanohybrid architecture as the cathode, is assembled (Figure 7.6c,d). It demonstrates excellent electrochemical performances: a volumetric capacitance of $54.6\,F\,cm^{-3}$ ($546.05\,mF\,cm^{-2}$), and remarkable volumetric energy and power density ($5.5\times10^{-3}\,W\,h\,cm^{-3}$ and $10.95\,W\,cm^{-3}$) are realized. This kind of nanohybrid paper promises great enhancement for flexible energy devices in terms of electrochemical performances and mechanical properties.

7.3 Conclusions

Flexible supercapacitors are drawing tremendous attention and research interest due to the increasing requirement for flexible/wearable energy storage devices. Numerous materials (from 0D to 3D) have been developed as electrode materials of flexible supercapacitors. In this chapter, we have tried to summarize the recent developments in flexible supercapacitors using nanomaterials of different morphologies. Special emphasis has been given to 2D materials, because 2D materials possess the advantages of high surface areas and excellent mechanical properties, providing an ideal platform for the preparation of thin film electrodes, which is crucial for the fabrication of flexible supercapacitors. In this regard, it is demonstrated that (i) to realize efficient utilization of the surface area of 2D materials, the stacking of the nanosheets should be avoided, especially for graphene-based materials. An effective way to prevent the 2D materials from stacking is to add spacers (i.e., carbon nanoparticles and CNT) among the 2D nanosheets; (ii) 2D materials possess redox active behaviors displaying better electrochemical performance but they suffer from low conductivity; therefore, methods such as doping the metal oxide materials with another metal or adding conductive additives (CNT) are employed to improve the conductivity; (iii) the advantages of 2D materials are particularly evident when they are employed as the electrode materials of in-plane microsupercapacitors; the in-plane interdigitated design of electrode fingers provide a high edge-to-area ratio, thus the open edges benefit the penetration of electrolyte into the electrode materials. Finally, an excellent electrochemical performance can be achieved. To sum up, 2D materials open a new gate for the development of flexible supercapacitors with enhanced electrochemical and mechanical performances.

Although considerable development has been achieved in the development of flexible supercapacitors, including the discovery of new electrode materials and rational design of the electrode structure as well as the improvement of fabricating technology, there are still obstacles to be surmounted for their practical applications. Future flexible supercapacitors are expected to come close to current Li ion batteries in energy density while maintaining their high speed power delivery capability. It is expected that the flexible supercapacitors could be produced in an effective and efficient technological process to satisfy industry receptacles. In order to realize this goal, the following several crucial issues need to be considered. Firstly, the development of an electrolyte with a large operating voltage window could enhance the energy density of the flexible supercapacitors, because the energy density is positively related to the square of the operating voltage. Furthermore, in order to avoid leakage of the electrolyte, the development of all-solid-state electrolytes with excellent ion-transporting properties and a high voltage window is desired. Secondly, developing 2D materials with both excellent pseudocapacitance and good electric conductivity is still a challenge. Most of the metal oxide materials with pseudocapacitive behavior are not conductive or semiconductive, which limits the electrochemical performance due to the low capability of electron and ion transporting in the electrochemical process. Thirdly, the development of simple, low-cost and time-saving manufacturing technologies is required to boost the application of flexible supercapacitors in flexible/wearable devices. More attention is needed on how to effectively assemble the 2D electrode materials on a flexible substrate with good ohmic contact. Last but not the least, compared with conventional flexible supercapacitors with sandwiched constructions, the in-plane interdigitated electrodes design of microsupercapacitors promises more efficient utilization of the 2D materials, owing to the open edges. This design also benefits the integration of supercapacitors with on-chip electronics. Recently, significant work on flexible microsupercapacitors has been demonstrated [71, 109, 110, 116]. Moreover, besides flexibility, stretchability is another important issue for portable electronics, especially for wearable medical devices, where stretching is inevitable. In recent years, stretchable in-plane microsupercapacitors have been obtained by introducing stretchable serpentine interconnections between microsupercapacitor arrays [234–237]. In such a design, the stretchability is contributed by stretchable interconnections, while

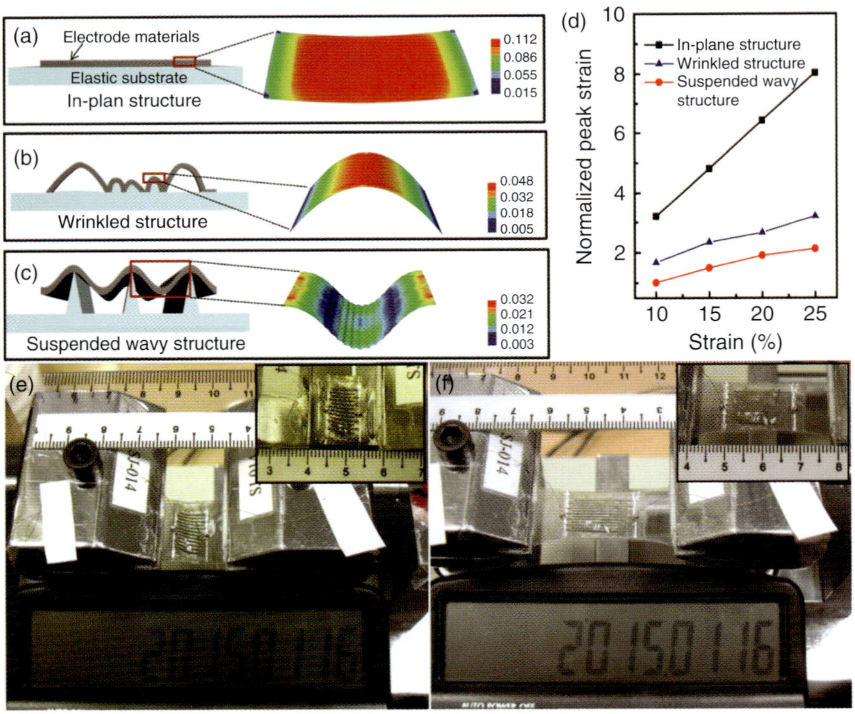

Figure 7.7 Schematic drawing of the different electrode arrays and their relevant strain distribution by the finite element modeling analysis for (a) in-plane structure, (b) wrinkled structure, and (c) suspended wavy structure. (d) The peak strain comparison of in-plane structure, wrinkled structure, and suspended wavy structure, respectively. Liquid-crystal display (LCD) lit by the stretchable micro-supercapacitors under (e) 0 strain and (f) 100% strains (insets show the distance). (Qi *et al.* 2015 [87]. Reproduced with permission of John Wiley & Sons.)

the supercapacitor devices themselves are rigid. A novel strategy to fabricate stretchable in-plane microsupercapacitors based on 2D materials is to design an out-of-plane sinusoidal-like structure of electrode fingers, as shown in Figure 7.7 [87]. Such architecture could decrease the stress induced in the electrode fingers; therefore, excellent electrochemical performance during the stretching/relaxing processes are realized. To date, microsupercapacitors, which themselves possess stretchability, are still less investigated. Therefore, in the future, more attention needs to be paid to the fabrication of stretchable microsupercapacitors, which can retain good electrochemical performance under stretching and can be integrated into wearable medical devices as an energy storage unit. In addition, the encapsulation of flexible supercapacitors deserves more efforts, as encapsulation could prevent the leakage of liquid electrolyte and protect the all-solid-state electrolyte and electrode materials from being exposed to air, thereby inhibiting their degradation.

References

1 Sher, C.W., Chen, K.J., Lin, C.C., Han, H.V., Lin, H.Y., Tu, Z.Y., Tu, H.H., Honjo, K., Jiang, H.Y., Ou, S.L., Horng, R.H., Li, X.L., Fu, C.C., and Kuo, H.C. (2015) Uniform white light led source on a flexible substrate. *Opt. Express*, **23**, A1167.

2 Gossler, C., Bierbrauer, C., Moser, R., Kunzer, M., Holc, K., Pletschen, W., Kohler, K., Wagner, J., Schwaerzle, M., Ruther, P., Paul, O., Neef, J., Keppeler, D., Hoch, G., Moser, T., and Schwarz, U.T. (2014) Gan-based micro-LED arrays on flexible substrates for optical cochlear implants. *J. Phys. D: Appl. Phys.*, **47**, 205401.

3 Zhang, Q., Di, Y.F., Huard, C.M., Guo, L.J., Wei, J., and Guo, J.B. (2015) Highly stable and stretchable graphene-polymer processed silver nanowires hybrid electrodes for flexible displays. *J. Mater. Chem. C*, **3**, 1528.

4 Donaldson, L. (2013) Stretchable and foldable electronic displays. *Mater. Today*, **16**, 416.

5 Sekitani, T., Nakajima, H., Maeda, H., Fukushima, T., Aida, T., Hata, K., and Someya, T. (2009) Stretchable active-matrix organic light-emitting diode display using printable elastic conductors. *Nat. Mater.*, **8**, 494.

6 Wang, H., Zhu, B.W., Wang, H., Ma, X.H., Hao, Y., and Chen, X.D. (2016) Ultra-lightweight resistive switching memory devices based on silk fibroin. *Small*, **12**, 3360.

7 Zhu, B.W., Wang, H., Leow, W.R., Cai, Y.R., Loh, X.J., Han, M.Y., and Chen, X.D. (2016) Silk fibroin for flexible electronic devices. *Adv. Mater.*, **28**, 4250.

8 Zhu, B.W., Wang, H., Liu, Y.Q., Qi, D.P., Liu, Z.Y., Wang, H., Yu, J.C., Sherburne, M., Wang, Z.H., and Chen, X.D. (2016) Skin-inspired haptic memory arrays with an electrically reconfigurable architecture. *Adv. Mater.*, **28**, 1559.

9 Zhu, B.W., Niu, Z.Q., Wang, H., Leow, W.R., Wang, H., Li, Y.G., Zheng, L.Y., Wei, J., Huo, F.W., and Chen, X.D. (2014) Microstructured graphene arrays for highly sensitive flexible tactile sensors. *Small*, **10**, 3625.

10 Ge, J., Sun, L., Zhang, F.R., Zhang, Y., Shi, L.A., Zhao, H.Y., Zhu, H.W., Jiang, H.L., and Yu, S.H. (2016) A stretchable electronic fabric artificial skin with pressure-, lateral strain-, and flexion-sensitive properties. *Adv. Mater.*, **28**, 722.

11 Chortos, A., Liu, J., and Bao, Z.A. (2016) Pursuing prosthetic electronic skin. *Nat. Mater.*, **15**, 937.

12 Boutry, C.M., Nguyen, A., Lawal, Q.O., Chortos, A., Rondeau-Gagne, S., and Bao, Z.N. (2015) A sensitive and biodegradable pressure sensor array for cardiovascular monitoring. *Adv. Mater.*, **27**, 6954.

13 Liu, Z.Y., Qi, D.P., Guo, P.Z., Liu, Y., Zhu, B.W., Yang, H., Liu, Y.Q., Li, B., Zhang, C.G., Yu, J.C., Liedberg, B., and Chen, X.D. (2015) Thickness-gradient films for high gauge factor stretchable strain sensors. *Adv. Mater.*, **27**, 6230.

14 Qi, D.P., Liu, Z.Y., Yu, M., Liu, Y., Tang, Y.X., Lv, J.H., Li, Y.C., Wei, J., Bo, L., Yu, Z., and Chen, X.D. (2015) Highly stretchable gold nanobelts with sinusoidal structures for recording electrocorticograms. *Adv. Mater.*, **27**, 3145.

15 Khan, Y., Ostfeld, A.E., Lochner, C.M., Pierre, A., and Arias, A.C. (2016) Monitoring of vital signs with flexible and wearable medical devices. *Adv. Mater.*, **28**, 4373.

16 Lu, J.S. and Kowalewski, T.M. (2015) Flexible, stretchable skin sensors for two-dimensional position tracking in medical simulators. *J. Med. Devices*, **9**, 020927.

17 Pu, Z.H., Wang, R.D., Wu, J.W., Yu, H.X., Xu, K.X., and Li, D.C. (2016) A flexible electrochemical glucose sensor with composite nanostructured surface of the working electrode. *Sens. Actuators, B*, **230**, 801.

18 Simon, P. and Gogotsi, Y. (2008) Materials for electrochemical capacitors. *Nat. Mater.*, **7**, 845.

19 Zhang, L.L. and Zhao, X.S. (2009) Carbon-based materials as supercapacitor electrodes. *Chem. Soc. Rev.*, **38**, 2520.

20 Al Sakka, M., Gualous, H., Van Mierlo, J., and Culcu, H. (2009) Thermal modeling and heat management of supercapacitor modules for vehicle applications. *J. Power Sources*, **194**, 581.

21 Zhang, H., Cao, G.P., Yang, Y.S., Xu, B., and Zhang, W.F. (2008) Novel carbon materials for electrochemical double layer capacitors and their applications. *Prog. Chem.*, **20**, 1495.

22 Bose, S., Kuila, T., Mishra, A.K., Rajasekar, R., Kim, N.H., and Lee, J.H. (2012) Carbon-based nanostructured materials and their composites as supercapacitor electrodes. *J. Mater. Chem.*, **22**, 767.

23 Qi, D.P., Liu, Y., Liu, Z.Y., Zhang, L., and Chen, X.D. (2016) Design of architectures and materials in in-plane micro-supercapacitors: current status and future challenges. *Adv. Mater.* doi: 10.1002/adma.201602802

24 Niu, Z.Q., Dong, H.B., Zhu, B.W., Li, J.Z., Hng, H.H., Zhou, W.Y., Chen, X.D., and Xie, S.S. (2013) Highly stretchable, integrated supercapacitors based on single-walled carbon nanotube films with continuous reticulate architecture. *Adv. Mater.*, **25**, 1058.

25 Naoi, K., Naoi, W., Aoyagi, S., Miyamoto, J., and Kamino, T. (2013) New generation "nanohybrid supercapacitor". *Acc. Chem. Res.*, **46**, 1075.

26 Zhang, H.G., Yu, X.D., and Braun, P.V. (2011) Three-dimensional bicontinuous ultrafast-charge and -discharge bulk battery electrodes. *Nat. Nanotechnol.*, **6**, 277.

27 Taberna, L., Mitra, S., Poizot, P., Simon, P., and Tarascon, J.M. (2006) High rate capabilities Fe_3O_4-based Cu nano-architectured electrodes for lithium-ion battery applications. *Nat. Mater.*, **5**, 567.

28 Lang, X.Y., Hirata, A., Fujita, T., and Chen, M.W. (2011) Nanoporous metal/oxide hybrid electrodes for electrochemical supercapacitors. *Nat. Nanotechnol.*, **6**, 232.

29 Tang, Y.X., Zhang, Y.Y., Deng, J.Y., Qi, D.P., Leow, W.R., Wei, J.Q., Yin, S.Y., Dong, Z.L., Yazami, R., Chen, Z., and Chen, X.D. (2014) Unravelling the correlation between the aspect ratio of nanotubular structures and their electrochemical performance to achieve high-rate and long-life lithium-ion batteries. *Angew. Chem. Int. Ed.*, **53**, 13488.

30 Chung, S.Y., Bloking, J.T., and Chiang, Y.M. (2002) Electronically conductive phospho-olivines as lithium storage electrodes. *Nat. Mater.*, **1**, 123.

31 Chen, Z., Zhang, D.Q., Wang, X.L., Jia, X.L., Wei, F., Li, H.X., and Lu, Y.F. (2012) High-performance energy-storage architectures from carbon nanotubes and nanocrystal building blocks. *Adv. Mater.*, **24**, 2030.

32 Faraji, S. and Ani, F.N. (2015) The development supercapacitor from activated carbon by electroless plating-a review. *Renewable Sustainable Energy Rev.*, **42**, 823.

33 Divyashree, A. and Hegde, G. (2015) Activated carbon nanospheres derived from bio-waste materials for supercapacitor applications - a review. *RSC Adv.*, **5**, 88339.

34 Yu, Z.N., Tetard, L., Zhai, L., and Thomas, J. (2015) Supercapacitor electrode materials: nanostructures from 0 to 3 dimensions. *Energy Environ. Sci.*, **8**, 702.

35 Zhang, X., Zhang, H.T., Li, C., Wang, K., Sun, X.Z., and Ma, Y.W. (2014) Recent advances in porous graphene materials for supercapacitor applications. *RSC Adv.*, **4**, 45862.

36 Wei, W.F., Cui, X.W., Chen, W.X., and Ivey, D.G. (2011) Manganese oxide-based materials as electrochemical supercapacitor electrodes. *Chem. Soc. Rev.*, **40**, 1697.

37 He, D., Xing, S.X., Sun, B.N., Cai, H., Suo, H., and Zhao, C. (2016) Design and construction of three-dimensional flower-like Cuo hierarchical nanostructures on copper foam for high performance supercapacitor. *Electrochim. Acta*, **210**, 639.

38 Singh, A.K., Sarkar, D., Karmakar, K., Mandal, K., and Khan, G.G. (2016) High-performance supercapacitor electrode based on cobalt oxide-manganese dioxide-nickel oxide ternary 1d hybrid nanotubes. *ACS Appl. Mater. Interfaces*, **8**, 20786.

39 Li, L.M., Zhang, X.M., Wu, G.S., Peng, X., Huo, K.F., and Chu, P.K. (2015) Supercapacitor electrodes based on hierarchical mesoporous Mnox/nitrided TiO_2 nanorod arrays on carbon fiber paper. *Adv. Mater. Interfaces*, **2**, 1400446.

40 Li, H.L., He, Y., Pavlinek, V., Cheng, Q.L., Saha, P., and Li, C.Z. (2015) MnO_2 nanoflake/polyaniline nanorod hybrid nanostructures on graphene paper for high-performance flexible supercapacitor electrodes. *J. Mater. Chem. A*, **3**, 17165.

41 Wu, H., Lou, Z., Yang, H., and Shen, G.Z. (2015) A flexible spiral-type supercapacitor based on $ZnCo_2O_4$ nanorod electrodes. *Nanoscale*, **7**, 1921.

42 Li, S.Z., Wen, J., Mo, X.M., Long, H., Wang, H.N., Wang, J.B., and Fang, G.J. (2014) Three-dimensional MnO_2 nanowire/ZnO nanorod arrays hybrid nanostructure for high-performance and flexible supercapacitor electrode. *J. Power Sources*, **256**, 206.

43 Miao, F.J., Shao, C.L., Li, X.H., Wang, K.X., and Liu, Y.C. (2016) Flexible solid-state supercapacitors based on freestanding nitrogen-doped porous carbon nanofibers derived from electrospun polyacrylonitrile@polyaniline nanofibers. *J. Mater. Chem. A*, **4**, 4180.

44 Zhang, J., Yi, X.B., Wang, X.C., Ma, J., Liu, S., and Wang, X.J. (2015) Nickel oxide grown on carbon nanotubes/carbon fiber paper by electrodeposition as flexible electrode for high-performance supercapacitors. *J. Mater. Sci. Mater. Electron.*, **26**, 7901.

45 Kong, D.Z., Ren, W.N., Cheng, C.W., Wang, Y., Huang, Z.X., and Yang, H.Y. (2015) Three-dimensional $NicCo_2O_4$@polypyrrole coaxial nanowire arrays on carbon textiles for high-performance flexible asymmetric solid-state supercapacitor. *ACS Appl. Mater. Interfaces*, **7**, 21334.

46 Cheng, Y.L., Huang, L., Xiao, X., Yao, B., Yuan, L.Y., Li, T.Q., Hu, Z.M., Wang, B., Wan, J., and Zhou, J. (2015) Flexible and cross-linked N-doped carbon nanofiber network for high performance freestanding supercapacitor electrode. *Nano Energy*, **15**, 66.

47 Dong, X.L., Guo, Z.Y., Song, Y.F., Hou, M.Y., Wang, J.Q., Wang, Y.G., and Xia, Y.Y. (2014) Flexible and wire-shaped micro-supercapacitor based on $Ni(OH)_2$-nanowire and ordered mesoporous carbon electrodes. *Adv. Funct. Mater.*, **24**, 3405.

48 Zhao, J.W., Chen, J., Xu, S.M., Shao, M.F., Zhang, Q., Wei, F., Ma, J., Wei, M., Evans, D.G., and Duan, X. (2014) Hierarchical nimn layered double hydroxide/carbon nanotubes architecture with superb energy density for flexible supercapacitors. *Adv. Funct. Mater.*, **24**, 2938.

49 Chen, L.F., Huang, Z.H., Liang, H.W., Yao, W.T., Yu, Z.Y., and Yu, S.H. (2013) Flexible all-solid-state high-power supercapacitor fabricated with nitrogen-doped carbon nanofiber electrode material derived from bacterial cellulose. *Energy Environ. Sci.*, **6**, 3331.

50 Niu, Z.Q., Du, J.J., Cao, X.B., Sun, Y.H., Zhou, W.Y., Hng, H.H., Ma, J., Chen, X.D., and Xie, S.S. (2012) Electrophoretic build-up of alternately multilayered films and micropatterns based on graphene sheets and nanoparticles and their applications in flexible supercapacitors. *Small*, **8**, 3201.

51 Li, W.C., Mak, C.L., Kan, C.W., and Hui, C.Y. (2014) Enhancing the capacitive performance of a textile-based Cnt supercapacitor. *RSC Adv.*, **4**, 64890.

52 Zhu, Y.G., Wang, Y., Shi, Y.M., Wong, J.I., and Yang, H.Y. (2014) Coo nanoflowers woven by Cnt network for high energy density flexible micro-supercapacitor. *Nano Energy*, **3**, 46.

53 Kang, Y.J., Chung, H., Kim, M.S., and Kim, W. (2015) Enhancement of CNT/PET film adhesion by nano-scale modification for flexible all-solid-state supercapacitors. *Appl. Surf. Sci.*, **355**, 160.

54 Huang, S.H., Zhao, C.S., Pan, W., Cui, Y., and Wu, H. (2015) Direct writing of half-meter long CNT based fiber for flexible electronics. *Nano Lett.*, **15**, 1609.

55 Sun, P., Deng, Z.W., Yang, P.H., Yu, X., Chen, Y.L., Liang, Z.M., Meng, H., Xie, W.G., Tan, S.Z., and Mai, W.J. (2015) Freestanding CNT-WO_3 hybrid electrodes for flexible asymmetric supercapacitors. *J. Mater. Chem. A*, **3**, 12076.

56 Xiao, X., Peng, X., Jin, H.Y., Li, T.Q., Zhang, C.C., Gao, B., Hu, B., Huo, K.F., and Zhou, J. (2013) Freestanding mesoporous Vn/CNT hybrid electrodes for flexible all-solid-state supercapacitors. *Adv. Mater.*, **25**, 5091.

57 Jin, Y., Chen, H.Y., Chen, M.H., Liu, N., and Li, Q.W. (2013) Graphene-patched CNT/MnO_2 nanocomposite papers for the electrode of high-performance flexible asymmetric supercapacitors. *ACS Appl. Mater. Interfaces*, **5**, 3408.

58 Kang, Y.J., Kim, B., Chung, H., and Kim, W. (2010) Fabrication and characterization of flexible and high capacitance supercapacitors based on MnO_2/CNT/papers. *Synth. Met.*, **160**, 2510.

59 Ujjain, S.K., Ahuja, P., Bhatia, R., and Attri, P. (2016) Printable multi-walled carbon nanotubes thin film for high performance all solid state flexible supercapacitors. *Mater. Res. Bull.*, **83**, 167.

60 Fan, L., Yang, L., Ni, X.Y., Han, J., Guo, R., and Zhang, C.F. (2016) Nitrogen-enriched meso-macroporous carbon fiber network as a binder-free flexible electrode for supercapacitors. *Carbon*, **107**, 629.

61 Senthilkumar, S.T., Fu, N.Q., Liu, Y., Wang, Y., Zhou, L.M., and Huang, H.T. (2016) Flexible fiber hybrid supercapacitor with $NiCo_2O_4$ nanograss@carbon fiber and bio-waste derived high surface area porous carbon. *Electrochim. Acta*, **211**, 411.

62 Iqbal, N., Wang, X.F., Babar, A.A., Yu, J.Y., and Ding, B. (2016) Highly flexible $NiCo_2O_4$/CNTs doped carbon nanofibers for CO_2 adsorption and supercapacitor electrodes. *J. Colloid Interface Sci.*, **476**, 87.

63 Kanninen, P., Luong, N.D., Sinh, L.H., Anoshkin, I.V., Tsapenko, A., Seppala, J., Nasibulin, A.G., and Kallio, T. (2016) Transparent and flexible high-performance supercapacitors based on single-walled carbon nanotube films. *Nanotechnology*, **27**, 235403.

64 Cherusseri, J., Sharma, R., and Kar, K.K. (2016) Helically coiled carbon nanotube electrodes for flexible supercapacitors. *Carbon*, **105**, 113.

65 Li, L., Zhong, Q.F., Kim, N.D., Ruan, G.D., Yang, Y., Gao, C.T., Fei, H.L., Li, Y.L., Ji, Y.S., and Tour, J.M. (2016) Nitrogen-doped carbonized cotton for highly flexible supercapacitors. *Carbon*, **105**, 260.

66 Peng, X., Peng, L.L., Wu, C.Z., and Xie, Y. (2014) Two dimensional nanomaterials for flexible supercapacitors. *Chem. Soc. Rev.*, **43**, 3303.

67 Shao, Y.L., El-Kady, M.F., Wang, L.J., Zhang, Q.H., Li, Y.G., Wang, H.Z., Mousavi, M.F., and Kaner, R.B. (2015) Graphene-based materials for flexible supercapacitors. *Chem. Soc. Rev.*, **44**, 3639.

68 Kim, B.C., Hong, J.Y., Wallace, G.G., and Park, H.S. (2015) Recent progress in flexible electrochemical capacitors: electrode materials, device configuration, and functions. *Adv. Energy Mater.*, **5**, 1500959.

69 Chee, W.K., Lim, H.N., Zainal, Z., Huang, N.M., Harrison, I., and Andou, Y. (2016) Flexible graphene-based supercapacitors: a review. *J. Phys. Chem. C*, **120**, 4153.

70 Liu, L.L., Niu, Z.Q., Zhang, L., Zhou, W.Y., Chen, X.D., and Xie, S.S. (2014) Nanostructured graphene composite papers for highly flexible and foldable supercapacitors. *Adv. Mater.*, **26**, 4855.

71 Niu, Z.Q., Zhang, L., Liu, L., Zhu, B.W., Dong, H.B., and Chen, X.D. (2013) All-solid-state flexible ultrathin micro-supercapacitors based on graphene. *Adv. Mater.*, **25**, 4035.

72 Xia, J.L., Chen, F., Li, J.H., and Tao, N.J. (2009) Measurement of the quantum capacitance of graphene. *Nat. Nanotechnol.*, **4**, 505.

73 Raccichini, R., Varzi, A., Passerini, S., and Scrosati, B. (2015) The role of graphene for electrochemical energy storage. *Nat. Mater.*, **14**, 271.

74 Dong, X.C., Shi, Y.M., Huang, W., Chen, P., and Li, L.J. (2010) Electrical detection of DNA hybridization with single-base specificity using transistors based on Cvd-grown graphene sheets. *Adv. Mater.*, **22**, 1649.

75 Losurdo, M., Giangregorio, M.M., Capezzuto, P., and Bruno, G. (2011) Graphene Cvd growth on copper and nickel: role of hydrogen in kinetics and structure. *Phys. Chem. Chem. Phys.*, **13**, 20836.

76 Wang, Y., Zheng, Y., Xu, X.F., Dubuisson, E., Bao, Q.L., Lu, J., and Loh, K.P. (2011) Electrochemical delamination of CVD-grown graphene film: toward the recyclable use of copper catalyst. *ACS Nano*, **5**, 9927.

77 Suk, J.W., Kitt, A., Magnuson, C.W., Hao, Y.F., Ahmed, S., An, J.H., Swan, A.K., Goldberg, B.B., and Ruoff, R.S. (2011) Transfer of CVD-grown monolayer graphene onto arbitrary substrates. *ACS Nano*, **5**, 6916.

78 Sun, Z.H., Liu, Z.K., Li, J.H., Tai, G.A., Lau, S.P., and Yan, F. (2012) Infrared photodetectors based on CVD-grown graphene and PbS quantum dots with ultrahigh responsivity. *Adv. Mater.*, **24**, 5878.

79 Cai, M.Z., Thorpe, D., Adamson, D.H., and Schniepp, H.C. (2012) Methods of graphite exfoliation. *J. Mater. Chem.*, **22**, 24992.

80 Wei, D., Grande, L., Chundi, V., White, R., Bower, C., Andrew, P., and Ryhanen, T. (2012) Graphene from electrochemical exfoliation and its direct applications in enhanced energy storage devices. *Chem. Commun.*, **48**, 1239.

81 Paton, K.R., Varrla, E., Backes, C., Smith, R.J., Khan, U., O'Neill, A., Boland, C., Lotya, M., Istrate, O.M., King, P., Higgins, T., Barwich, S., May, P., Puczkarski, P., Ahmed, I., Moebius, M., Pettersson, H., Long, E., Coelho, J., O'Brien, S.E., McGuire, E.K., Sanchez, B.M., Duesberg, G.S., McEvoy, N., Pennycook, T.J., Downing, C., Crossley, A., Nicolosi, V., and Coleman, J.N. (2014) Scalable production of large quantities of defect-free few-layer graphene by shear exfoliation in liquids. *Nat. Mater.*, **13**, 624.

82 Stoller, M.D. and Ruoff, R.S. (2010) Best practice methods for determining an electrode material's performance for ultracapacitors. *Energy Environ. Sci.*, **3**, 1294.

83 Stoller, M.D., Park, S.J., Zhu, Y.W., An, J.H., and Ruoff, R.S. (2008) Graphene-based ultracapacitors. *Nano Lett.*, **8**, 3498.

84 Huang, Y., Liang, J.J., and Chen, Y.S. (2012) An overview of the applications of graphene-based materials in supercapacitors. *Small*, **8**, 1805.

85 Li, D. and Kaner, R.B. (2008) Materials science - graphene-based materials. *Science*, **320**, 1170.

86 Cao, X.B., Qi, D.P., Yin, S.Y., Bu, J., Li, F.J., Goh, C.F., Zhang, S., and Chen, X.D. (2013) Ambient fabrication of large-area graphene films via a synchronous reduction and assembly strategy. *Adv. Mater.*, **25**, 2957.

87 Qi, D.P., Liu, Z.Y., Liu, Y., Leow, W.R., Zhu, B.W., Yang, H., Yu, J.C., Wang, W., Wang, H., Yin, S.Y., and Chen, X.D. (2015) Suspended wavy graphene microribbons for highly stretchable microsupercapacitors. *Adv. Mater.*, **27**, 5559.

88 Dikin, D.A., Stankovich, S., Zimney, E.J., Piner, R.D., Dommett, G.H.B., Evmenenko, G., Nguyen, S.T., and Ruoff, R.S. (2007) Preparation and characterization of graphene oxide paper. *Nature*, **448**, 457.

89 Li, D., Muller, M.B., Gilje, S., Kaner, R.B., and Wallace, G.G. (2008) Processable aqueous dispersions of graphene nanosheets. *Nat. Nanotechnol.*, **3**, 101.

90 Becerril, H.A., Mao, J., Liu, Z., Stoltenberg, R.M., Bao, Z., and Chen, Y. (2008) Evaluation of solution-processed reduced graphene oxide films as transparent conductors. *ACS Nano*, **2**, 463.

91 Li, X.L., Zhang, G.Y., Bai, X.D., Sun, X.M., Wang, X.R., Wang, E., and Dai, H.J. (2008) Highly conducting graphene sheets and Langmuir-Blodgett films. *Nat. Nanotechnol.*, **3**, 538.

92 Gunes, F., Shin, H.J., Biswas, C., Han, G.H., Kim, E.S., Chae, S.J., Choi, J.Y., and Lee, Y.H. (2010) Layer-by-layer doping of few-layer graphene film. *ACS Nano*, **4**, 4595.

93 Gan, S.Y., Zhong, L.J., Wu, T.S., Han, D.X., Zhang, J.D., Ulstrup, J., Chi, Q.J., and Niu, L. (2012) Spontaneous and fast growth of large-area graphene nanofilms facilitated by oil/water interfaces. *Adv. Mater.*, **24**, 3958.

94 Yu, A.P., Roes, I., Davies, A., and Chen, Z.W. (2010) Ultrathin, transparent, and flexible graphene films for supercapacitor application. *Appl. Phys. Lett.*, **96**. doi: 10.1063/1.3455879

95 Lu, X.J., Dou, H., and Zhang, X.G. (2016) Mesoporous carbon nanospheres inserting into graphene sheets for flexible supercapacitor film electrode. *Mater. Lett.*, **178**, 304.

96 Lu, X.J., Dou, H., Gao, B., Yuan, C.Z., Yang, S.D., Hao, L., Shen, L.F., and Zhang, X.G. (2011) A flexible graphene/multiwalled carbon nanotube film as a high performance electrode material for supercapacitors. *Electrochim. Acta*, **56**, 5115.

97 El-Kady, M.F., Strong, V., Dubin, S., and Kaner, R.B. (2012) Laser scribing of high-performance and flexible graphene-based electrochemical capacitors. *Science*, **335**, 1326.

98 Wang, G.K., Sun, X., Lu, F.Y., Sun, H.T., Yu, M.P., Jiang, W.L., Liu, C.S., and Lian, J. (2012) Flexible pillared graphene-paper electrodes for high-performance electrochemical supercapacitors. *Small*, **8**, 452.

99 Qiu, L., Yang, X.W., Gou, X.L., Yang, W.R., Ma, Z.F., Wallace, G.G., and Li, D. (2010) Dispersing carbon nanotubes with graphene oxide in water and synergistic effects between graphene derivatives. *Chem. Eur. J.*, **16**, 10653.

100 Vickery, J.L., Patil, A.J., and Mann, S. (2009) Fabrication of graphene-polymer nanocomposites with higher-order three-dimensional architectures. *Adv. Mater.*, **21**, 2180.

101 Liu, C.G., Yu, Z.N., Neff, D., Zhamu, A., and Jang, B.Z. (2010) Graphene-based supercapacitor with an ultrahigh energy density. *Nano Lett.*, **10**, 4863.

102 Yoo, E., Kim, J., Hosono, E., Zhou, H., Kudo, T., and Honma, I. (2008) Large reversible Li storage of graphene nanosheet families for use in rechargeable lithium ion batteries. *Nano Lett.*, **8**, 2277.

103 Fan, Z.J., Yan, J., Zhi, L.J., Zhang, Q., Wei, T., Feng, J., Zhang, M.L., Qian, W.Z., and Wei, F. (2010) A three-dimensional carbon nanotube/graphene sandwich and its application as electrode in supercapacitors. *Adv. Mater.*, **22**, 3723.

104 Kim, Y.K. and Min, D.H. (2009) Durable large-area thin films of graphene/carbon nanotube double layers as a transparent electrode. *Langmuir*, **25**, 11302.

105 Yu, D.S. and Dai, L.M. (2010) Self-assembled graphene/carbon nanotube hybrid films for supercapacitors. *J. Phys. Chem. Lett.*, **1**, 467.

106 Yin, S.Y., Wu, Y.L., Hu, B.H., Wang, Y., Cai, P.Q., Tan, C.K., Qi, D.P., Zheng, L.Y., Leow, W.R., Tan, N.S., Wang, S.T., and Chen, X.D. (2014) Three-dimensional graphene composite macroscopic structures for capture of cancer cells. *Adv. Mater. Interfaces*, **1**, 1300043.

107 Chen, Z.P., Ren, W.C., Gao, L.B., Liu, B.L., Pei, S.F., and Cheng, H.M. (2011) Three-dimensional flexible and conductive interconnected graphene networks grown by chemical vapour deposition. *Nat. Mater.*, **10**, 424.

108 Niu, Z.Q., Chen, J., Hng, H.H., Ma, J., and Chen, X.D. (2012) A leavening strategy to prepare reduced graphene oxide foams. *Adv. Mater.*, **24**, 4144.

109 Wu, Z.S., Parvez, K., Feng, X.L., and Mullen, K. (2013) Graphene-based in-plane micro-supercapacitors with high power and energy densities. *Nat. Commun.*, **4**. doi: 10.1038/ncomms3487

110 Beidaghi, M. and Gogotsi, Y. (2014) Capacitive energy storage in micro-scale devices: recent advances in design and fabrication of micro-supercapacitors. *Energy Environ. Sci.*, **7**, 867.

111 Meng, C.Z., Maeng, J., John, S.W.M., and Irazoqui, P.P. (2014) Ultrasmall integrated 3D micro-supercapacitors solve energy storage for miniature devices. *Adv. Energy Mater.*, **4**, 1301269.

112 Huang, P., Lethien, C., Pinaud, S., Brousse, K., Laloo, R., Turq, V., Respaud, M., Demortiere, A., Daffos, B., Taberna, P.L., Chaudret, B., Gogotsi, Y., and Simon, P. (2016) On-chip and freestanding elastic carbon films for micro-supercapacitors. *Science*, **351**, 691.

113 Huang, P.H., Pech, D., Lin, R.Y., McDonough, J.K., Brunet, M., Taberna, P.L., Gogotsi, Y., and Simon, P. (2013) On-chip micro-supercapacitors for operation in a wide temperature range. *Electrochem. Commun.*, **36**, 53.

114 Gu, S.S., Lou, Z., Li, L.D., Chen, Z.J., Ma, X.D., and Shen, G.Z. (2016) Fabrication of flexible reduced graphene oxide/Fe_2O_3 hollow nanospheres based on-chip micro-supercapacitors for integrated photodetecting applications. *Nano Res.*, **9**, 424.

115 Yoo, J.J., Balakrishnan, K., Huang, J.S., Meunier, V., Sumpter, B.G., Srivastava, A., Conway, M., Reddy, A.L.M., Yu, J., Vajtai, R., and Ajayan, P.M. (2011) Ultrathin planar graphene supercapacitors. *Nano Lett.*, **11**, 1423.

116 Beidaghi, M. and Wang, C.L. (2012) Micro-supercapacitors based on interdigital electrodes of reduced graphene oxide and carbon nanotube composites with ultrahigh power handling performance. *Adv. Funct. Mater.*, **22**, 4501.

117 Chang, J., Adhikari, S., Lee, T.H., Li, B., Yao, F., Pham, D.T., Le, V.T., and Lee, Y.H. (2015) Leaf vein-inspired nanochanneled graphene film for highly efficient micro-supercapacitors. *Adv. Energy Mater.*, **5**, 1500003.

118 Wu, Z.S., Winter, A., Chen, L., Sun, Y., Turchanin, A., Feng, X.L., and Mullen, K. (2012) Three-dimensional nitrogen and boron Co-doped graphene for high-performance all-solid-state supercapacitors. *Adv. Mater.*, **24**, 5130.

119 Xu, Y.X., Sheng, K.X., Li, C., and Shi, G.Q. (2010) Self-assembled graphene hydrogel via a one-step hydrothermal process. *ACS Nano*, **4**, 4324.

120 Li, C. and Shi, G.Q. (2012) Three-dimensional graphene architectures. *Nanoscale*, **4**, 5549.

121 Chen, W.F. and Yan, L.F. (2011) In situ self-assembly of mild chemical reduction graphene for three-dimensional architectures. *Nanoscale*, **3**, 3132.

122 Xu, Y.X., Lin, Z.Y., Zhong, X., Huang, X.Q., Weiss, N.O., Huang, Y., and Duan, X.F. (2014) Holey graphene frameworks for highly efficient capacitive energy storage. *Nat. Commun.*, **5**, 4554.

123 Zhang, L. and Shi, G.Q. (2011) Preparation of highly conductive graphene hydrogels for fabricating supercapacitors with high rate capability. *J. Phys. Chem. C*, **115**, 17206.

124 Li, Z.Y., Cai, J., Cizek, P., Niu, H.T., Dua, Y., and Lin, T. (2015) A self-supported, flexible, binder-free pseudo-supercapacitor electrode material with high capacitance and cycling stability from hollow, capsular polypyrrole fibers. *J. Mater. Chem. A*, **3**, 16162.

125 Huang, X.H., Kim, M., Suh, H., and Kim, I. (2016) Hierarchically nanostructured carbon-supported manganese oxide for high-performance pseudo-capacitors. *Korean J. Chem. Eng.*, **33**, 2228.

126 Choi, B.N., Chun, W.W., Qian, A., Lee, S.J., and Chung, C.H. (2015) Dendritic Ni(Cu)- polypyrrole hybrid films for a pseudo-capacitor. *Nanoscale*, **7**, 18561.

127 Ni, W., Cheng, J.L., Li, X.D., Gu, G.F., Huang, L., Guan, Q., Yuan, D.M., and Wang, B. (2015) Polymeric cathode materials of electroactive conducting poly(triphenylamine) with optimized structures for potential organic pseudo-capacitors with higher cut-off voltage and energy density. *RSC Adv.*, **5**, 9221.

128 Mohamoud, M.A. (2014) Unexpected redox enhancement and electrochemical pseudo-capacitance performance of polyaniline/poly(vinyl alcohol) (Pan/Pva) composite films. *Electrochim. Acta*, **139**, 201.

129 Cui, Z.M., Guo, C.X., Yuan, W.Y., and Li, C.M. (2012) In situ synthesized heteropoly acid/polyaniline/graphene nanocomposites to simultaneously boost both double layer- and pseudo-capacitance for supercapacitors. *Phys. Chem. Chem. Phys.*, **14**, 12823.

130 Noh, K.A., Kim, D.W., Jin, C.S., Shin, K.H., Kim, J.H., and Ko, J.M. (2003) Synthesis and pseudo-capacitance of chemically-prepared polypyrrole powder. *J. Power Sources*, **124**, 593.

131 Zhou, H.B., Han, G.Y., Chang, Y.Z., Fu, D.Y., and Xiao, Y.M. (2015) Highly stable multi-wall carbon nanotubes@poly(3,4-ethylenedioxythiophene)/poly (styrene sulfonate) core-shell composites with three-dimensional porous nano-network for electrochemical capacitors. *J. Power Sources*, **274**, 229.

132 Pandey, G.P. and Rastogi, A.C. (2013) Synthesis and characterization of pulsed polymerized poly(3,4-ethylenedioxythiophene) electrodes for high-performance electrochemical capacitors. *Electrochim. Acta*, **87**, 158.

133 Kim, B.C., Too, C.O., Kwon, J.S., Bo, J.M., and Wallace, G.G. (2011) A flexible capacitor based on conducting polymer electrodes. *Synth. Met.*, **161**, 1130.

134 Ryu, K.S., Lee, Y.G., Kim, K.M., Park, Y.J., Hong, Y.S., Wu, X.L., Kang, M.G., Park, N.G., Song, R.Y., and Ko, J.M. (2005) Electrochemical capacitor with chemically polymerized conducting polymer based on activated carbon as hybrid electrodes. *Synth. Met.*, **153**, 89.

135 Hong, J.I., Yeo, I.H., and Paik, W.K. (2001) Conducting polymer with metal oxide for electrochemical capacitor - poly(3,4-ethylenedioxythiophene) RuO_x electrode. *J. Electrochem. Soc.*, **148**, A156.

136 Ullah, S., Khan, I.A., Choucair, M., Badshah, A., Khan, I., and Nadeem, M.A. (2015) A novel Cr_2O_3-carbon composite as a high performance pseudo-capacitor electrode material. *Electrochim. Acta*, **171**, 142.

137 Zhang, C., Qian, L.H., Zhang, K., Yuan, S.L., Xiao, J.W., and Wang, S. (2015) Hierarchical porous Ni/Nio core-shells with superior conductivity for electrochemical pseudo-capacitors and glucose sensors. *J. Mater. Chem. A*, **3**, 10519.

138 Cheng, S., Yang, L.F., Chen, D.C., Ji, X., Jiang, Z.J., Ding, D., and Liu, M.L. (2014) Phase evolution of an alpha MnO_2-based electrode for pseudo-capacitors probed by in operando Raman spectroscopy. *Nano Energy*, **9**, 161.

139 Zhang, Y.Q., Li, L., Shi, S.J., Xiong, Q.Q., Zhao, X.Y., Wang, X.L., Gu, C.D., and Tu, J.P. (2014) Synthesis of porous Co_3O_4 nanoflake array and its temperature behavior as pseudo-capacitor electrode. *J. Power Sources*, **256**, 200.

140 Cheng, S., Yang, L., Liu, Y., Lin, W., Huang, L., Chen, D.C., Wong, C.P., and Liu, M.L. (2013) Carbon fiber paper supported hybrid nanonet/nanoflower nickel oxide electrodes for high-performance pseudo-capacitors. *J. Mater. Chem. A*, **1**, 7709.

141 Wang, X.F., Ruan, D.B., Wang, P., and Lu, Y.Q. (2008) Pseudo-capacitance of ruthenium oxide/carbon black composites for electrochemical capacitors. *J. Univ. Sci. Technol. B*, **15**, 816.

142 Deng, M.J., Chang, J.K., Wang, C.C., Chen, K.W., Lin, C.M., Tang, M.T., Chen, J.M., and Lu, K.T. (2011) High-performance electrochemical pseudo-capacitor based on MnO_2 nanowires/Ni foam as electrode with a novel Li-ion quasi-ionic liquid as electrolyte. *Energy Environ. Sci.*, **4**, 3942.
143 Porto, R.L., Frappier, R., Ducros, J.B., Aucher, C., Mosqueda, H., Chenu, S., Chavillon, B., Tessier, F., Chevire, F., and Brousse, T. (2012) Titanium and vanadium oxynitride powders as pseudo-capacitive materials for electrochemical capacitors. *Electrochim. Acta*, **82**, 257.
144 Zhu, H.H., Peng, S.J., and Jiang, W.J. (2013) Electrochemical properties of pani as single electrode of electrochemical capacitors in acid electrolytes. *Sci. World J.*, **2013**, 940153.
145 Li, H.L., Wang, J.X., Chu, Q.X., Wang, Z., Zhang, F.B., and Wang, S.C. (2009) Theoretical and experimental specific capacitance of polyaniline in sulfuric acid. *J. Power Sources*, **190**, 578.
146 Mcmanus, P.M., Cushman, R.J., and Yang, S.C. (1987) Influence of oxidation and protonation on the electrical-conductivity of polyaniline. *J. Phys. Chem.*, **91**, 744.
147 Snook, G.A., Kao, P., and Best, A.S. (2011) Conducting-polymer-based supercapacitor devices and electrodes. *J. Power Sources*, **196**, 1.
148 Ma, X.P., Wang, X.Y., Li, M.X., Chen, T.N., Zhang, H., and Cheng, Q. (2016) Improved performances of solid tantalum electrolytic capacitors using Eg-treated pedot: Pss conducting polymer as cathode electrodes. *Chem. Lett.*, **45**, 717.
149 Wang, F.X., Liu, Z.C., Wang, X.W., Yuan, X.H., Wu, X.W., Zhu, Y.S., Fu, L.J., and Wu, Y.P. (2016) A conductive polymer coated MoO_3 anode enables an Al-ion capacitor with high performance. *J. Mater. Chem. A*, **4**, 5115.
150 Lim, Y.G., Park, M.S., Kim, K.J., Jung, K.S., Kim, J.H., Shahabuddin, M., Byun, D., and Yu, J.S. (2015) Incorporation of conductive polymer into soft carbon electrodes for lithium ion capacitors. *J. Power Sources*, **299**, 49.
151 Kawakubo, T. (2004) Recent development of capacitor technology - capacitor technology for practical use - 4. high voltage capacitor using conductive polymer. *Electrochemistry*, **72**, 767.
152 Hung, S.L., Wen, T.C., and Gopalan, A. (2002) Application of statistical design strategies to optimize the conductivity of electro synthesized polypyrrole. *Mater. Lett.*, **55**, 165.
153 Naoi, K., Oura, Y., Maeda, M., and Nakamura, S. (1995) Electrochemistry of surfactant-doped polypyrrole film(I) - formation of columnar structure by electropolymerization. *J. Electrochem. Soc.*, **142**, 417.
154 Wang, J.Z., Too, C.O., and Wallace, G.G. (2005) A highly flexible polymer fibre battery. *J. Power Sources*, **150**, 223.
155 An, K.H., Jeon, K.K., Heo, J.K., Lim, S.C., Bae, D.J., and Lee, Y.H. (2002) Capacitance supercapacitor using a nanocomposite electrode of single-walled carbon nanotube and polypyrrole. *J. Electrochem. Soc.*, **149**, A1058.
156 Arbizzani, C., Mastragostino, M., Meneghello, L., and Paraventi, R. (1996) Electronically conducting polymers and activated carbon: electrode materials in supercapacitor technology. *Adv. Mater.*, **8**, 331.

157 Chen, G.Z., Shaffer, M.S.P., Coleby, D., Dixon, G., Zhou, W.Z., Fray, D.J., and Windle, A.H. (2000) Carbon nanotube and polypyrrole composites: coating and doping. *Adv. Mater.*, **12**, 522.

158 Wang, J., Xu, Y.L., Zhu, J.B., Bai, Y., Mao, S.C., and Xiong, L.L. (2016) Capacitive characteristics of nanocomposites of conducting polypyrrole and functionalized carbon nanotubes: pulse current synthesis and tailoring. *J. Solid State Electrochem.*, **20**, 1413.

159 Hui, N., Chai, F.L., Lin, P.P., Song, Z.L., Sun, X.T., Li, Y.N., Niu, S.Y., and Luo, X.L. (2016) Electrodeposited conducting polyaniline nanowire arrays aligned on carbon nanotubes network for high performance supercapacitors and sensors. *Electrochim. Acta*, **199**, 234.

160 Cai, X.Y., Lim, S.H., Poh, C.K., Lai, L.F., Lin, J.Y., and Shen, Z.X. (2015) High-performance asymmetric pseudocapacitor cell based on cobalt hydroxide/graphene and polypyrrole/graphene electrodes. *J. Power Sources*, **275**, 298.

161 Liew, S.Y., Thielemans, W., and Walsh, D.A. (2014) Polyaniline- and poly(ethylenedioxythiophene)-cellulose nanocomposite electrodes for supercapacitors. *J. Solid State Electrochem.*, **18**, 3307.

162 Bai, X.X., Hu, X.J., Zhou, S.Y., Yan, J., Sun, C.H., Chen, P., and Li, L.F. (2013) In situ polymerization and characterization of grafted poly (3,4-ethylenedioxythiophene)/multiwalled carbon nanotubes composite with high electrochemical performances. *Electrochim. Acta*, **87**, 394.

163 Zhang, D., Dong, Q.Q., Wang, X., Yan, W., Deng, W., and Shi, L.Y. (2013) Preparation of a three-dimensional ordered macroporous carbon nanotube/polypyrrole composite for supercapacitors and diffusion modeling. *J. Phys. Chem. C*, **117**, 20446.

164 Rosario-Canales, M.R., Deria, P., Therien, M.J., and Santiago-Aviles, J.J. (2012) Composite electronic materials based on poly(3,4-propylenedioxythiophene) and highly charged poly(aryleneethynylene)-wrapped carbon nanotubes for supercapacitors. *ACS Appl. Mater. Interfaces*, **4**, 102.

165 Nagaraja, M., Mahesh, H.M., Manjanna, J., Rajanna, K., Kurian, M.Z., and Lokesh, S.V. (2012) Effect of multiwall carbon nanotubes on electrical and structural properties of polyaniline. *J. Electron. Mater.*, **41**, 1882.

166 Sun, X.F., Xu, Y.L., and Wang, J. (2012) Electropolymerized composite film of polypyrrole and functionalized multi-walled carbon nanotubes: effect of functionalization time on capacitive performance. *J. Solid State Electrochem.*, **16**, 1781.

167 Iroh, J.O. and Levine, K. (2003) Capacitance of the polypyrrole/polyimide composite by electrochemical impedance spectroscopy. *J. Power Sources*, **117**, 267.

168 Hu, C.C. and Chen, W.C. (2004) Effects of substrates on the capacitive performance of RuO_x center dot $Nh_{(2)}O$ and activated carbon-RuO_x electrodes for supercapacitors. *Electrochim. Acta*, **49**, 3469.

169 Lin, P., She, Q.J., Hong, B.L., Liu, X.A.J., Shi, Y.N., Shi, Z., Zheng, M.S., and Dong, Q.F. (2010) The nickel oxide/CNT composites with high capacitance for supercapacitor. *J. Electrochem. Soc.*, **157**, A818.

170 Yang, G.W., Xu, C.L., and Li, H.L. (2008) Electrodeposited nickel hydroxide on nickel foam with ultrahigh capacitance. *Chem. Commun.*, 6537.

171 Cao, L., Xu, F., Liang, Y.Y., and Li, H.L. (2004) Preparation of the novel nanocomposite $Co(OH)_2$/ultra-stable Y zeolite and its application as a supercapacitor with high energy density. *Adv. Mater.*, **16**, 1853.

172 Meng, F.L., Fang, Z.G., Li, Z.X., Xu, W.W., Wang, M.J., Liu, Y.P., Zhang, J., Wang, W.R., Zhao, D.Y., and Guo, X.H. (2013) Porous Co_3O_4 materials prepared by solid-state thermolysis of a novel Co-MOF crystal and their superior energy storage performances for supercapacitors. *J. Mater. Chem. A*, **1**, 7235.

173 Kolathodi, M.S., Rao, S.N.H., Natarajan, T.S., and Singh, G. (2016) Beaded manganese oxide (Mn_2O_3) nanofibers: preparation and application for capacitive energy storage. *J. Mater. Chem. A*, **4**, 7883.

174 Huang, Z.Y., Zhang, Z., Qi, X., Ren, X.H., Xu, G.H., Wan, P.B., Sun, X.M., and Zhang, H. (2016) Wall-like hierarchical metal oxide nanosheet arrays grown on carbon cloth for excellent supercapacitor electrodes. *Nanoscale*, **8**, 13273.

175 Tung, M.T., Thuy, H.T.B., and Hang, L.T.T. (2015) Metal doped manganese oxide thin films for supercapacitor application. *J. Nanosci. Nanotechnol.*, **15**, 6949.

176 Zhi, J., Deng, S., Wang, Y.F., and Hu, A.G. (2015) Highly ordered metal oxide nanorods inside mesoporous silica supported carbon nanomembranes: high performance electrode materials for symmetrical supercapacitor devices. *J. Phys. Chem. C*, **119**, 8530.

177 Liu, W.J., Liu, N.S., Shi, Y.L., Chen, Y., Yang, C.X., Tao, J.Y., Wang, S.L., Wang, Y.M., Su, J., Li, L.Y., and Gao, Y.H. (2015) A wire-shaped flexible asymmetric supercapacitor based on carbon fiber coated with a metal oxide and a polymer. *J. Mater. Chem. A*, **3**, 13461.

178 Jiang, H., Ma, J., and Li, C.Z. (2012) Mesoporous carbon incorporated metal oxide nanomaterials as supercapacitor electrodes. *Adv. Mater.*, **24**, 4197.

179 Wang, X.F., You, Z., and Ruan, D.B. (2006) A hybrid metal oxide supercapacitor in aqueous Koh electrolyte. *Chin. J. Chem.*, **24**, 1126.

180 Trasatti, S. and Buzzanca, G. (1971) Ruthenium dioxide - new interesting electrode material - solid state structure and electrochemical behaviour. *J. Electroanal. Chem.*, **29**, A1.

181 Makino, S., Yamauchi, Y., and Sugimoto, W. (2013) Synthesis of electrodeposited ordered mesoporous RuO_x using lyotropic liquid crystal and application toward micro-supercapacitors. *J. Power Sources*, **227**, 153.

182 Wu, X., Xiong, W., Chen, Y.Y., Lan, D.N., Pu, X.L., Zeng, Y., Gao, H.R., Chen, J.S., Tong, H., and Zhu, Z.H. (2015) High-rate supercapacitor utilizing hydrous ruthenium dioxide nanotubes. *J. Power Sources*, **294**, 88.

183 Jiao, Y., Liu, Y., Yin, B.S., Zhang, S.W., Qu, F.Y., and Wu, X. (2014) Hybrid alpha-Fe_2O_3@NiO heterostructures for flexible and high performance supercapacitor electrodes and visible light driven photocatalysts. *Nano Energy*, **10**, 90.

184 Li, R.Z., Wang, Y.M., Zhou, C., Wang, C., Ba, X., Li, Y.Y., Huang, X.T., and Liu, J.P. (2015) Carbon-stabilized high-capacity ferroferric oxide nanorod

array for flexible solid-state alkaline battery-supercapacitor hybrid device with high environmental suitability. *Adv. Funct. Mater.*, **25**, 5384.

185 Wang, Y.C., Zhou, T., Jiang, K., Da, P.M., Peng, Z., Tang, J., Kong, B.A., Cai, W.B., Yang, Z.Q., and Zheng, G.F. (2014) Reduced mesoporous Co_3O_4 nanowires as efficient water oxidation electrocatalysts and supercapacitor electrodes. *Adv. Energy Mater.*, **4**, 1400696.

186 Ghosh, D., Mandal, M., and Das, C.K. (2015) Solid state flexible asymmetric supercapacitor based on carbon fiber supported hierarchical $Co(OH)_XCO_3$ and $Ni(OH)_2$. *Langmuir*, **31**, 7835.

187 Qiu, H.J., Peng, L., Li, X., and Wang, Y. (2015) Enhanced supercapacitor performance by fabricating hierarchical nanoporous nickel/nickel hydroxide structure. *Mater. Lett.*, **158**, 366.

188 Yao, M.M., Hu, Z.H., Liu, Y.F., Liu, P.P., Ai, Z.H., and Rudolf, O. (2015) 3D hierarchical mesoporous roselike NiO nanosheets for high-performance supercapacitor electrodes. *J. Alloys Compd.*, **648**, 414.

189 Zhai, T., Lu, X.H., Ling, Y.C., Yu, M.H., Wang, G.M., Liu, T.Y., Liang, C.L., Tong, Y.X., and Li, Y. (2014) A new benchmark capacitance for supercapacitor anodes by mixed-valence sulfur-doped V_6O_{13-X}. *Adv. Mater.*, **26**, 5869.

190 Foo, C.Y., Sumboja, A., Tan, D.J.H., Wang, J.X., and Lee, P.S. (2014) Flexible and highly scalable V_2O_5-rGO electrodes in an organic electrolyte for supercapacitor devices. *Adv. Energy Mater.*, **4**, 1400236.

191 Firmiano, E.G.D., Rabelo, A.C., Dalmaschio, C.J., Pinheiro, A.N., Pereira, E.C., Schreiner, W.H., and Leite, E.R. (2014) Supercapacitor electrodes obtained by directly bonding 2D MoS_2 on reduced graphene oxide. *Adv. Energy Mater.*, **4**, 1301380.

192 Wang, H.L., Xu, Z.W., Li, Z., Cui, K., Ding, J., Kohandehghan, A., Tan, X.H., Zahiri, B., Olsen, B.C., Holt, C.M.B., and Mitlin, D. (2014) Hybrid device employing three-dimensional arrays of MnO in carbon nanosheets bridges battery-supercapacitor divide. *Nano Lett.*, **14**, 1987.

193 Chen, L.F., Huang, Z.H., Liang, H.W., Guan, Q.F., and Yu, S.H. (2013) Bacterial-cellulose-derived carbon nanofiber@MnO_2 and nitrogen-doped carbon nanofiber electrode materials: an asymmetric supercapacitor with high energy and power density. *Adv. Mater.*, **25**, 4746.

194 Lee, E., Lee, T., and Kim, B.S. (2014) Electrospun nanofiber of hybrid manganese oxides for supercapacitor: relevance to mixed inorganic interfaces. *J. Power Sources*, **255**, 335.

195 Gambou-Bosca, A. and Belanger, D. (2016) Electrochemical accessibility of porous submicron MnO_2 spheres as active electrode materials for electrochemical capacitors. *Electrochim. Acta*, **201**, 20.

196 Lu, S.Q., Yan, D.L., Chen, L., Zhu, G.S., Xu, H.R., and Yu, A.B. (2016) One-pot fabrication of hierarchical Ag/MnO_2 nanoflowers for electrochemical capacitor electrodes. *Mater. Lett.*, **168**, 40.

197 Hsieh, C.T., Tzou, D.Y., Lee, W.Y., and Hsu, J.P. (2016) Deposition of MnO_2 nanoneedles on carbon nanotubes and graphene nanosheets as electrode materials for electrochemical capacitor. *J. Alloys Compd.*, **660**, 99.

198 Jia, Z., Wang, J., Wang, Y., Li, B.Y., Wang, B.G., Qi, T., and Wang, X. (2016) Interfacial synthesis of delta-MnO_2 nano-sheets with a large surface area and their application in electrochemical capacitors. *J. Mater. Sci. Technol.*, **32**, 147.

199 Hu, Y., Wang, J., Jiang, X.H., Zheng, Y.F., and Chen, Z.X. (2013) Facile chemical synthesis of nanoporous layered delta-MnO_2 thin film for high-performance flexible electrochemical capacitors. *Appl. Surf. Sci.*, **271**, 193.

200 Wang, Q.F., Xu, J., Wang, X.F., Liu, B., Hou, X.J., Yu, G., Wang, P., Chen, D., and Shen, G.Z. (2014) Core-shell $CuCo_2O_4$@MnO_2 nanowires on carbon fabrics as high-performance materials for flexible, all-solid-state, electrochemical capacitors. *ChemElectroChem*, **1**, 559.

201 Yu, M.H., Zhai, T., Lu, X.H., Chen, X.J., Xie, S.L., Li, W., Liang, C.L., Zhao, W.X., Zhang, L.P., and Tong, Y.X. (2013) Manganese dioxide nanorod arrays on carbon fabric for flexible solid-state supercapacitors. *J. Power Sources*, **239**, 64.

202 Chen, Y.C., Hsu, Y.K., Lin, Y.G., Lin, Y.K., Horng, Y.Y., Chen, L.C., and Chen, K.H. (2011) Highly flexible supercapacitors with manganese oxide nanosheet/carbon cloth electrode. *Electrochim. Acta*, **56**, 7124.

203 Yuan, L.Y., Lu, X.H., Xiao, X., Zhai, T., Dai, J.J., Zhang, F.C., Hu, B., Wang, X., Gong, L., Chen, J., Hu, C.G., Tong, Y.X., Zhou, J., and Wang, Z.L. (2012) Flexible solid-state supercapacitors based on carbon nanoparticles/MnO_2 nanorods hybrid structure. *ACS Nano*, **6**, 656.

204 Hu, L.B., Chen, W., Xie, X., Liu, N.A., Yang, Y., Wu, H., Yao, Y., Pasta, M., Alshareef, H.N., and Cui, Y. (2011) Symmetrical MnO_2-carbon nanotube-textile nanostructures for wearable pseudocapacitors with high mass loading. *ACS Nano*, **5**, 8904.

205 Cheng, Y.W., Lu, S.T., Zhang, H.B., Varanasi, C.V., and Liu, J. (2012) Synergistic effects from graphene and carbon nanotubes enable flexible and robust electrodes for high-performance supercapacitors. *Nano Lett.*, **12**, 4206.

206 Peng, S.J., Li, L.L., Wu, H.B., Madhavi, S., and Lou, X.W. (2015) Controlled growth of $NiMoO_4$ nanosheet and nanorod arrays on various conductive substrates as advanced electrodes for asymmetric supercapacitors. *Adv. Energy Mater.*, **5**, 1401172.

207 Liu, B., Zhang, J., Wang, X.F., Chen, G., Chen, D., Zhou, C.W., and Shen, G.Z. (2012) Hierarchical three-dimensional $ZnCo_2O_4$ nanowire arrays/carbon cloth anodes for a novel class of high-performance flexible lithium-ion batteries. *Nano Lett.*, **12**, 3005.

208 Wu, H.B., Pang, H., and Lou, X.W. (2013) Facile synthesis of mesoporous $Ni_{0.3}Co_{2.7}O_4$ hierarchical structures for high-performance supercapacitors. *Energy Environ. Sci.*, **6**, 3619.

209 Liang, Y.Y., Wang, H.L., Zhou, J.G., Li, Y.G., Wang, J., Regier, T., and Dai, H.J. (2012) Covalent hybrid of spinel manganese-cobalt oxide and graphene as advanced oxygen reduction electrocatalysts. *J. Am. Chem. Soc.*, **134**, 3517.

210 Dong, S.Y., Shen, L.F., Li, H.S., Pang, G., Dou, H., and Zhang, X.G. (2016) Flexible sodium-ion pseudocapacitors based on 3D $Na_2Ti_3O_7$ nanosheet arrays/carbon textiles anodes. *Adv. Funct. Mater.*, **26**, 3703.

211 Feng, J., Sun, X., Wu, C.Z., Peng, L.L., Lin, C.W., Hu, S.L., Yang, J.L., and Xie, Y. (2011) Metallic few-layered VS_2 ultrathin nanosheets: high two-dimensional conductivity for in-plane supercapacitors. *J. Am. Chem. Soc.*, **133**, 17832.

212 Li, L., Li, R.M., Gai, S.L., Ding, S.J., He, F., Zhang, M.L., and Yang, P.P. (2015) Nanosheets grown on nitrogen-doped hollow carbon shells as a high-performance electrode for asymmetric supercapacitors. *Chem. Eur. J.*, **21**, 7119.

213 Sun, S.M., Li, S.D., Wang, S., Li, Y.N., Han, L.F., Kong, H.J., and Wang, P.Y. (2016) Fabrication of hollow $NiCo_2O_4$ nanoparticle/graphene composite for supercapacitor electrode. *Mater. Lett.*, **182**, 23.

214 Zhou, H.H. and Zhai, H.J. (2016) A highly flexible solid-state supercapacitor based on the carbon nanotube doped graphene oxide/polypyrrole composites with superior electrochemical performances. *Org. Electron.*, **37**, 197.

215 Singu, B.S., Palaniappan, S., and Yoon, K.R. (2016) Polyaniline-nickel oxide nanocomposites for supercapacitor. *J. Appl. Electrochem.*, **46**, 1039.

216 Liu, Y., Cai, X.Y., Luo, B.F., Yan, M., Jiang, J.H., and Shi, W.D. (2016) MnO_2 decorated on carbon sphere intercalated graphene film for high-performance supercapacitor electrodes. *Carbon*, **107**, 426.

217 Sun, Y.M., Cheng, Y.B., He, K., Zhou, A.J., and Duan, H.W. (2015) One-step synthesis of three-dimensional porous ionic liquid-carbon nanotube-graphene gel and MnO_2-graphene gel as freestanding electrodes for asymmetric supercapacitors. *RSC Adv.*, **5**, 10178.

218 He, Y.M., Chen, W.J., Li, X.D., Zhang, Z.X., Fu, J.C., Zhao, C.H., and Xie, E.Q. (2013) Freestanding three-dimensional graphene/MnO_2 composite networks as ultra light and flexible supercapacitor electrodes. *ACS Nano*, **7**, 174.

219 Chi, K., Zhang, Z.Y., Xi, J.B., Huang, Y.A., Xiao, F., Wang, S., and Liu, Y.Q. (2014) Freestanding graphene paper supported three-dimensional porous graphene-polyaniline nanoconnposite synthesized by inkjet printing and in flexible all-solid-state supercapacitor. *ACS Appl. Mater. Interfaces*, **6**, 16312.

220 Wu, Z.S., Parvez, K., Li, S., Yang, S., Liu, Z.Y., Liu, S.H., Feng, X.L., and Muellen, K. (2015) Alternating stacked graphene-conducting polymer compact films with ultrahigh areal and volumetric capacitances for high-energy micro-supercapacitors. *Adv. Mater.*, **27**, 4054.

221 Goubard-Bretesche, N., Crosnier, O., Buvat, G., Favier, F., and Brousse, T. (2016) Electrochemical study of aqueous asymmetric $FeWO_4/MnO_2$ supercapacitor. *J. Power Sources*, **326**, 695.

222 Mu, X.M., Zhang, Y.X., Wang, H., Huang, B.Y., Sun, P.B., Chen, T., Zhou, J.Y., Xie, E.Q., and Zhang, Z.X. (2016) A high energy density asymmetric supercapacitor from ultrathin manganese molybdate nanosheets. *Electrochim. Acta*, **211**, 217.

223 Nagamuthu, S., Vijayakumar, S., and Ryu, K.S. (2016) Synthesis of Ag anchored Ag_3VO_4 stacked nanosheets: toward a negative electrode material for high-performance asymmetric supercapacitor devices. *J. Phys. Chem. C*, **120**, 18963.

224 Wang, X.Z., Xiao, Y.H., Su, D.C., Xu, S.G., Zhou, L.M., Wu, S.D., Han, L.F., Fang, S.M., and Cao, S.K. (2016) Hierarchical porous cobalt monoxide nanosheet@ultrathin manganese dioxide nanosheet core-shell arrays for high-performance asymmetric supercapacitor. *Int. J. Hydrogen Energy*, **41**, 13540.

225 Wen, P., Fan, M.J., Yang, D.S., Wang, Y., Cheng, H.L., and Wang, J.Q. (2016) An asymmetric supercapacitor with ultrahigh energy density based on nickle cobalt sulfide nanocluster anchoring multi-wall carbon nanotubes hybrid. *J. Power Sources*, **320**, 28.

226 Zhou, G.Y., Xiong, T.R., He, S.J., Li, Y.H., Zhu, Y.M., and Hou, H.Q. (2016) Asymmetric supercapacitor based on flexible TiC/CNF felt supported interwoven nickel-cobalt binary hydroxide nanosheets. *J. Power Sources*, **317**, 57.

227 Khalid, S., Cao, C.B., Wang, L., Zhu, Y.Q., and Wu, Y. (2016) A high performance solid state asymmetric supercapacitor device based upon $NiCo_2O_4$ nanosheets//MnO_2 microspheres. *RSC Adv.*, **6**, 70292.

228 An, C.H., Wang, Y.J., Jiao, L.F., and Yuan, H.T. (2016) Mesoporous Ni@C hybrids for a high energy aqueous asymmetric supercapacitor device. *J. Mater. Chem. A*, **4**, 9670.

229 Hu, Y.T., Guan, C., Feng, G.X., Ke, Q.Q., Huang, X.L., and Wang, J. (2015) Flexible asymmetric supercapacitor based on structure-optimized Mn_3O_4/reduced graphene oxide nanohybrid paper with high energy and power density. *Adv. Funct. Mater.*, **25**, 7291.

230 Li, J.L. and Gao, F. (2009) Analysis of electrodes matching for asymmetric electrochemical capacitor. *J. Power Sources*, **194**, 1184.

231 Khomenko, V., Raymundo-Pinero, E., and Beguin, F. (2006) Optimisation of an asymmetric manganese oxide/activated carbon capacitor working at 2 V in aqueous medium. *J. Power Sources*, **153**, 183.

232 Chen, P.C., Shen, G.Z., Shi, Y., Chen, H.T., and Zhou, C.W. (2010) Preparation and characterization of flexible asymmetric supercapacitors based on transition-metal-oxide nanowire/single-walled carbon nanotube hybrid thin-film electrodes. *ACS Nano*, **4**, 4403.

233 Xu, C.J., Du, H.D., Li, B.H., Kang, F.Y., and Zeng, Y.Q. (2009) Asymmetric activated carbon-manganese dioxide capacitors in mild aqueous electrolytes containing alkaline-earth cations. *J. Electrochem. Soc.*, **156**, A435.

234 Hong, S.Y., Yoon, J., Jin, S.W., Lim, Y., Lee, S.J., Zi, G., and Ha, J.S. (2014) High-density, stretchable, all-solid-state microsupercapacitor arrays. *ACS Nano*, **8**, 8844.

235 Kim, D., Shin, G., Kang, Y.J., Kim, W., and Ha, J.S. (2013) Fabrication of a stretchable solid-state micro-supercapacitor array. *ACS Nano*, **7**, 7975.

236 Lim, B.Y., Yoon, J., Yun, J., Kim, D., Hong, S.Y., Lee, S.J., Zi, G., and Ha, J.S. (2014) Biaxially stretchable, integrated array of high performance microsupercapacitors. *ACS Nano*, **8**, 11639.

237 Lim, Y., Yoon, J., Yun, J., Kim, D., Hong, S.Y., Lee, S.J., Zi, G., and Ha, J.S. (2015) Biaxially stretchable, integrated array of high performance microsupercapacitors. *ACS Nano*, **9**, 6634.

8

Organometal Halide Perovskites for Next Generation Fully Printed and Flexible LEDs and Displays

Thomas Geske[1,2,3], *Sri Ganesh R. Bade*[1,2], *Matt Worden*[1,2], *Xin Shan*[1,2], *Junqiang Li*[1,2], *and Zhibin Yu*[1,2,3]

[1] *Florida State University, Department of Industrial and Manufacturing Engineering,, Tallahassee FL 32310, USA*
[2] *Florida State University, High Performance Materials Institute, 2005 Levy Avenue, Rm. 243,, Tallahassee FL 32310, USA*
[3] *Florida State University, Department of Materials Science and Engineering, Tallahassee, FL 32306, USA*

8.1 Introduction

During the past decades, the size of microchips has continued to shrink following the Moore's law. This has led to more and more powerful and functional consumer electronics that has drastically improved the convenience of our daily life. Along with the advancement in rechargeable batteries that exhibit increased energy density, a number of the electronic devices now have the characteristics of small size and light weight to fit into our pockets, which has resulted in greatly enhanced portability.

In contrast, the size of information displays has been seen to grow larger: having a larger screen reduces the need to scroll through a document and can greatly increase productivity. Large external displays, such as projectors, can now connect to laptop and notepad computers for daily office work. However, carrying these large displays for travel is currently not practical given their large size and heavy weight. An ideal solution is to develop new displays that are light weight and highly flexible or even stretchable. Thus, they could be rolled up or folded into small sizes for easy portability and unfolded into large screens to plug into other small size portable electronics such as cell phones, smart watches, fitness trackers, and Google glasses. In addition to enhanced portability, such displays could also conformally cover uneven surfaces and cope with body movement, or resemble the mechanic properties of human skin, which would enable new applications of wearable electronics for real-time health monitoring and diagnosis (Figure 8.1).

Liquid crystal display (LCD) technology is currently the dominant technology for various display applications. However, LCD displays contain encapsulated liquid cells, and inventing a highly flexible or stretchable LCD display would be quite challenging without the risk of liquid spilling. Active-matrix light-emitting diode (LED) displays have been envisioned as LCD replacements due to the advantages

Flexible and Stretchable Medical Devices, First Edition. Edited by Kuniharu Takei.

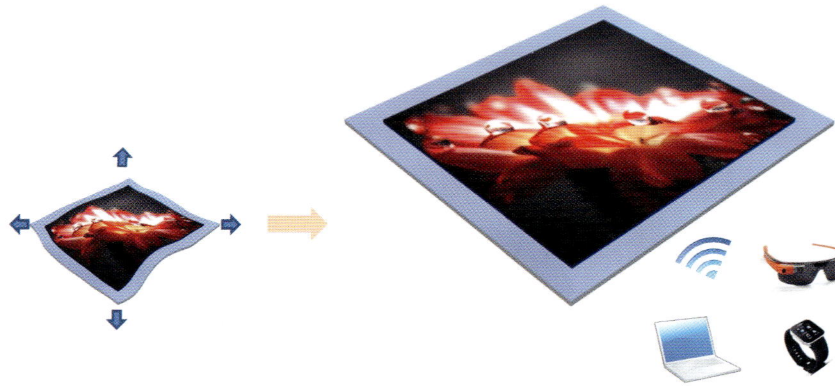

Figure 8.1 One potential application for stretchable OLED displays, which are light weight and can be stretchable from a small stowed volume into large-size displays for various portable electronics and next generation wearable medical devices.

of having high energy efficiency, high brightness, large contrast ratios, and the light weight of LED displays. The essential components in an active-matrix LED display include an array of thin film transistors (TFTs) as the backplane, an array of patterned LED lighting pixels, and conductive lines to connect individual LEDs to the backplane. Significant progress has been made in developing new materials and adopting new device architectures enabling high performance flexible backplanes and interconnections, and a number of seminal review articles have been published [1, 2]. The focus of this chapter will be to introduce new technologies for realizing highly flexible LEDs and displays.

8.1.1 General Background for LEDs

Modern LED research began in the mid-1950s with the advent of advanced semiconductor synthesis and processing techniques. The first reported LEDs were composed of III–V compound semiconductors (InP, GaAs, GaSb) [3]. By the 1970s, these compounds had produced high-efficiency light in red, yellow, and green spectra; however, high quality blue light emission remained elusive until 1994 when Nakamura *et al.* demonstrated the first high-efficiency blue LED based on InGaN [4, 5]. With this discovery, LEDs now have the ability to produce red, green, and blue light which caused LEDs to grow to be a dominant technology used in display and lighting technologies.

In recent years, the III–V semiconductor LED technology has further matured, and despite their complex processing they have become increasingly adapted in the lighting market [6]. However, their applications are limited to static systems due to the brittleness exhibited by the III–V compounds. Owing to these limitations, researchers have been seeking new materials to use for LEDs in flexible applications. Materials that are to be considered for flexible LEDs should have high efficiency, facile processing, and color tunability, and should be able to be processed on flexible substrates.

Organic light-emitting diodes (OLEDs) have been at the forefront of the flexible display research effort for the last few decades. These are LEDs that are based on polymeric semiconductors, or small molecular organic dyes, and have been shown promise for application in flexible displays [7, 8]. While the efficiency and brightness of those devices have met most application needs, the used materials do come with some drawbacks. The first is that these materials have yet to realize, a highly efficient blue emission material with lifetime stability [8]. This limits their application, as blue light is necessary for full color display and white light sources. The second drawback is that these materials are highly susceptible to moisture damage, meaning these materials have to rely on encapsulation techniques to prevent them from degrading, and adds unnecessary costs to the fabrication process [9]. The third is that they still use relatively expensive fabrication techniques, and have a complicated multilayer device structure [9]. Owing to these drawbacks OLEDs leave something to be desired for flexible display applications.

Quantum dot LEDs have also received much attention in recent years for application in flexible LED displays [10, 11]. They show some promise for LED applications, due to their ability to produce a wider range of colors than previously mentioned LED technologies. However, they have a lower upper limit on efficiency compared to other technologies likely due to the high surface area of quantum dots [11]. The high surface areas cause a large amount of surface defect states, which increases nonradiative decay for excitons. This is a major limitation, as it puts a low upper bound on their efficiency [11]. In addition, they still have not been produced on an industrial scale, raising some concerns of the scalability of this technology.

Organometal halide perovskite materials have emerged in the past 2 years as new emissive materials for use in LED displays. This is due to their rapidly increasing efficiencies and brightness [12–14]. In addition, they exhibit other desirable properties such as color tunability and solution processability [14]. They were first considered for LED applications in 2014 when it was recognized that halide perovskite materials exhibited nearly 100% internal quantum efficiency in solar-cell applications [15]. It has been shown that an excellent solar cell material must also be an excellent light-emitting material; thus, this sparked interest in perovskites for use in light-emitting applications [16, 17]. In this chapter, we will review the evolution of perovskites for use in LEDs since their discovery, and discuss their future use in the area of large-scale flexible displays for next generation portable and wearable electronics.

8.1.2 Fundamentals of Halide Perovskites

Halide perovskites are characterized by their ABX_3 structure where A is a +1 cation such as methylammonium ($CH_3NH_3^+$) or Cs^+, B is a +2 cation such as lead or tin, and X is a −1 anion such chlorine, bromine, or iodine as seen in Figure 8.2a. Depending on the ions present in the perovskite it will exhibit different crystal structures at room temperature, which leads to perovskites having a wide variety of morphologies, structural properties, and optical properties [18, 19].

One of the most attractive properties of perovskites for use in LED applications is their exceptional optoelectronic properties. The first of these is color tunability through halide substitution. Xing *et al.* showed that through substitution of the halide ions, the color emission of halide perovskite materials could be

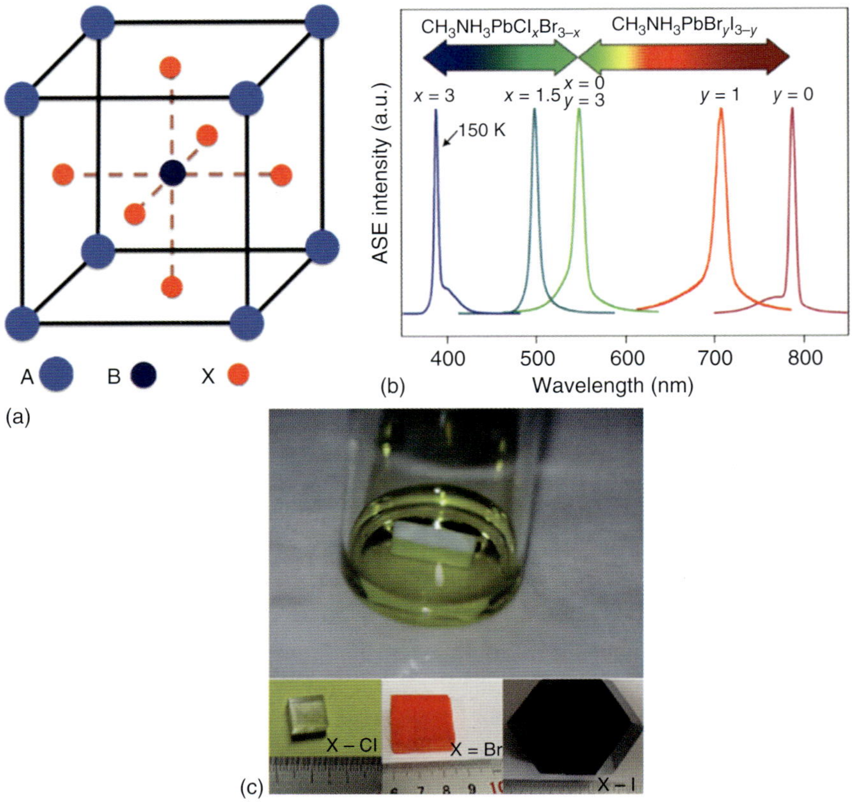

Figure 8.2 (a) The atomic structure of perovskite, A is a +1 cation, B is a +2 cation, and X is a −1 halide ion. (b) The emission wavelength as a function of halide composition. (c) Perovskite containing solution, and bulk crystals grown using solution processing.

controlled between about 400 nm (using $CH_3NH_3PbCl_3$) to about 785 nm (using $CH_3NH_3PbI_3$) and could cover the entire CIE 1931 color space [20]. Further studies showed that the emission wavelengths could be calculated using rule of mixture calculations using bandgap energies and volume fractions of halide ions with some fractions demonstrated in Figure 8.2b. Another exceptional property of perovskites is that their crystals have a very low internal defect concentration when formed, which limits the amount of nonradiative recombination that happens in the material [21]. The final favorable property perovskites exhibit is a low exciton binding energy of 20–50 meV per pair [22], and a large exciton mobility between 1 and 10 $cm^2 V^{-1} s^{-1}$ [23], which means that resistive losses in the emissive layer have the possibility to be small compared to those found in OLEDs and quantum dot LEDs.

Another property of halide perovskites that is highly desirable is that they are solution processable in organic solvents as seen in Figure 8.2c. Single crystals up to 2 in. dimension have been successfully grown by evaporating the dissolving solvents [24]. It has been shown that perovskites are soluble in large variety of solvents including: Dimethyl sulfoxide (DMSO), Dimethylformamide (DMF), and γ-Butyrolactone (GBL) [24]. This wide range of solvents allows for considerable flexibility in the manufacturing process as well as for allowing the perovskites to be composited with a variety of polymers. In addition, perovskites have a relatively low processing temperature of about 100–200° C compared to inorganic LED technologies that use high temperature to decompose the precursors and initiate the epitaxial thin film growth [24]. This low processing temperature is quite desirable, as it allows for significant energy saving in the manufacturing process and becomes compatible to low-cost glass or plastic substrates.

8.1.3 Multilayer Perovskite LEDs

Owing to the wide variety of perovskite structures, and the solution processability there are many different methods for preparing perovskite LEDs, and many different architectures for perovskite LEDs. Most of these architectures are based on a multilayer approach similar to that seen in OLEDs.

Era *et al.* made the first perovskite LED in 1994 [25]. Their device produced an emission peak at 520 nm with a narrow half-width of 10 nm. They measured a luminance of 10 000 cd m^2 at a current density of 2 A cm^{-2}. However, the high performance of these devices was only stable below 200 K. The device used an electron transport layer oxadiazole (OXD7), MgAg cathode, and an indium tin oxide (ITO) anode in a multilayer structure. In these first generations devices the organic cation used was $C_6H_5C_2H_4NH_3$, which is much larger than the ones used currently. Two years later, Hattori *et al.* made two new devices by replacing the organic cation with $C_6H_9C_2H_4NH_3$ and $C_6H_5C_4H_8NH_3$. They measured an external quantum efficiency (EQE) of 2.8% in these devices and a luminance above 4000 cd m^{-2} with a current density of 50 mA cm^{-2} at 24 V [26]. Although these devices had a much better efficiency the new organic cations did not solve the problem of thermal quenching that occurred above low temperatures. In 1999, Mitzi *et al.* designed a new molecule, $H_3NC_2H_4C_{16}H_8S_4C_2H_4NH_3$ to be used as the organic cation [27]. They achieved a perovskite structure device that was able to operate at room temperature. However, the power conversion efficiency was only 0.11% and the luminance was only 0.1 lm W^{-1} at 8 V and 0.24 mA, all of which were much lower than other LED technologies at the time.

Work on halide perovskite LEDs was resumed by Tan *et al.* in 2014; due to the intense interest in methylammonium-based perovskites in the area of solar cells [15]. This group incorporated the three-dimensional hybrid metal halide perovskites to achieve electroluminescence in the near-infrared, green and red regions by altering the halide composition. The infrared device was fabricated by incorporating a thin layer of $CH_3NH_3PbI_{3-x}Cl_x$ and green-light-emitting device was achieved with $CH_3NH_3PbBr_3$ (Br-Pero) both sandwiched between electron transporting and hole injecting layers. The device architecture for each of the devices can be seen in Figure 8.3.

The fabrication of these LEDs used atomic layer deposition for the TiO_2 layer; spin coating for the perovskite, poly(9,9-dicotylfluorene)(F8), poly(3,4-ethylenedioxythiophene) polystyrene sulfonate (PEDOT:PSS) layers; and vacuum-assisted thermal evaporation for the MoO_3, Ca, and Ag layers. This report demonstrated the possibility of using perovskite materials as

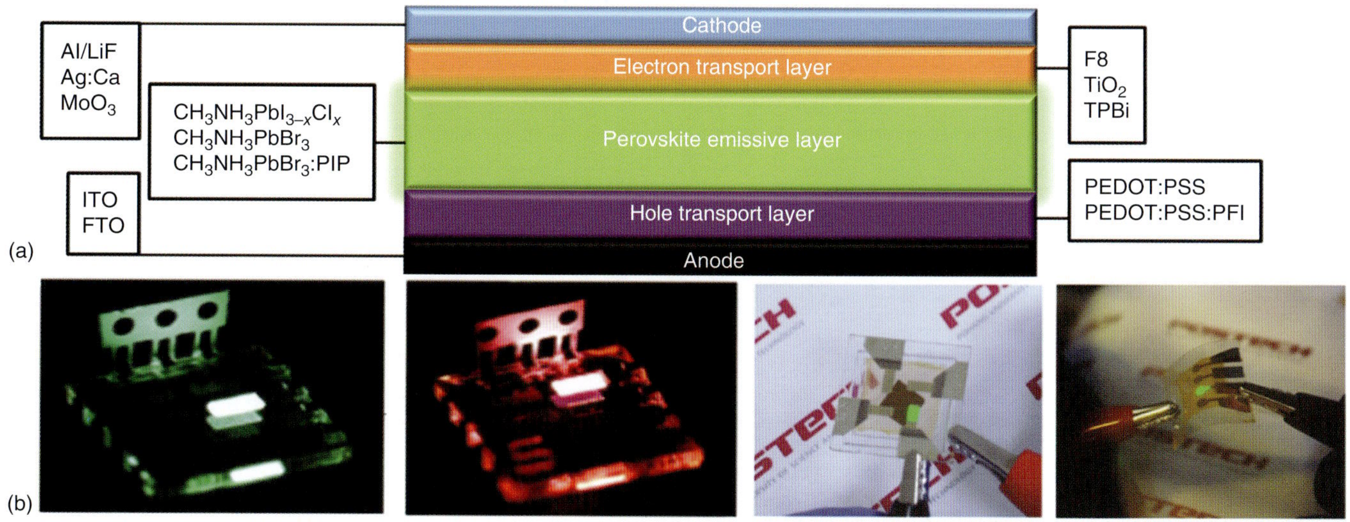

Figure 8.3 (a) The multilayer architecture commonly found in perovskite solar cells. Different layers have been labeled with common materials used in that layer. When a forward bias is applied, electrons are injected from the cathode side and holes are injected from the anode side into the perovskite emissive layer. Light emission is generated when the electrons and holes meet and combine radiatively. The use of the electron transportation layer and the hole transportation layer is to lower the energy barriers between the perovskite and the electrodes, assuring that both can be injected at a sufficiently low voltage. (b) Different multilayer devices illuminated; the far right shows perovskite LEDs in flexible applications.

light-emitting materials, and making use of traditional LED architecture by using F8 as an electron injection layer (EIL) and PEDOT:PSS as a hole injection layer (HIL).

Li *et al.* also fabricated perovskite LEDs using a similar sandwich architecture outlined earlier [28]. However, they embedded Br-Pero nanocrystals in a thin matrix of dielectric polyimide precursor (PIP) forming a perovskite nanocrystal–PIP polymer composite. The transparent and electrically insulating PIP helped in the formation of pin hole free thin film, which served as a charge-blocking layer and also provided much needed material stability. The perovskite nanocrystals were uniformly distributed in the thin-film matrix of PIP by *in situ* formation, which was achieved by blending perovskite precursor solution and commercially available aromatic PIP prior to spin coating. The devices had the following architecture: ITO/PEDOT: PSS/Perovskite–PIP composite/F8/Ca/Ag and the device layers were deposited by spin coating and vacuum deposition techniques. Different weight ratios of PIP were employed while blending the perovskite and polymer solutions and it was observed that the size and area occupied by the perovskite crystals decreased with an increase in PIP–perovskite ratio. The best performing devices had a PIP–perovskite ratio between 1 : 2 and 1 : 1. The polymer also helped in clean color emission from the devices and also effectively prevented shorting between the F8 and PEDOT:PSS. The best performing devices had an EQE of 1.2%

Another progress in using perovskite in flexible applications came from Kim *et al.* [29]. They used a device architecture similar to that found in OLEDs, but fabricated the devices on a flexible substrate composed of polyethylene terephthalate (PET). Br-Pero was used as the active light-emitting layer with a self-organized buffer composed of PEDOT:PSS and a perfluorinated polymeric acid (PFI) that acted as the HIL, and 2,2′,2″-(1,3,5-Benzinetriyl)-tris(1-phenyl-1-H-benzimidazole) (TPBi) that acted as the EIL. The utilization of a high work function buffer-HIL was to overcome the high hole injection barrier caused by the conventional PEDOT: PSS polymer thereby reducing the luminescence quenching that occurs at HIL/emitting layer. The green-light-emitting device employing the buffer-HIL had a current efficiency of 0.577 cd A^{-1}, an EQE of 0.125% and a maximum luminance of 417 cd m^{-2} which was a modest improvement over the devices that employed only PEDOT:PSS as HIL.

The most efficient multilayer perovskite LED reported to date is by Cho *et al.* [30]. This device used the multilayer structure with a bottom electrode and HIL composed of self-organized PEDOT:PSS and a perfluorinated polymeric acid (PFI). The perovskite emission layer was then deposited via a spin coating process, and using solvent engineering techniques the film was made nanocrystalline with an average grain diameter of about 100 nm and a film thickness of 400 nm. The EIL and top electrode were composed of TPBi and LiF/Al, respectively. The best reported devices had a current efficiency of 42.9 cd A^{-1}, an EQE of 8.53%, and a maximum luminance of ~15 000 cd m^{-2}. This is the highest efficiency reported to date for multilayer perovskite LEDs and represents a large increase over other reported devices. This group also reported device fabrication on flexible substrates, but the efficiency, luminance, and strain values were not reported for their flexible devices.

The main drawback of all the devices thus far is that they employ a multilayer device architecture, analogous to traditional LEDS, OLEDs, and quantum dot LEDs which greatly increases manufacturing complexity. In addition, all these devices use one or more high vacuum deposition techniques, which greatly hinder the scalability of device fabrication as well as lowering throughput of production. Some of the layers present are also highly susceptible to moisture damage and would make processing require highly controlled environments further adding to the costs of production, and the complexity of the devices.

8.2 Single Layer Perovskite LEDs

Recently, a novel process was seen in perovskites for flexible applications and was demonstrated by Li *et al.* [31] They fabricated a device that employed polymer blending similar to the process outlined by Li *et al.* [28]. Their device was notable because it used a single layer architecture as opposed to a multilayer structure seen in other LED technologies. The structure constituted a Br-Pero/PEO composite active layer with an ITO anode, and an indium gallium (In-Ga) eutectic for the top electrode. The best-performing devices had a current efficiency of $0.74\ \mathrm{cd\ A^{-1}}$, an EQE of 0.165% and a maximum luminance of $4064\ \mathrm{cd\ m^{-2}}$, which represented a small increase in the efficiency of perovskite LEDs and a modest increase in maximum luminance at the time their paper was published. If this structure could be matured to have efficiencies and brightness similar to current OLED and quantum dot LED technologies this would represent a large improvement over current LED technologies due to an immense drop in processing costs. Various colors have been obtained by tuning the composition of the perovskite emissive materials as seen in Figure 8.4b. The LEDs can also be made flexible by using constructing the devices on a flexible PET/ITO substrate.

The authors hypothesized that this architecture was made possible due to the ionic conducting abilities of the PEO polymer and the loose binding of the methylammonium ion in the perovskite lattice. These two phenomena allowed for the methylammonium ions to migrate toward the cathode when a bias was applied and caused a highly doped n-region near the cathode while a high doped p-region was seen near the anode due to lack of methylammonium and then a graded area was present in between that could be characterized as mostly intrinsic. This structure can be seen in Figure 8.4a with the band structure of the regions seen in Figure 8.4c. This hypothesis was strengthened by the recent work done by Xiao *et al.* who demonstrated that large ionic movement could be seen in perovskite materials under applied biases [32]. These highly doped regions then caused an extreme bending in the bands as seen in Figure 8.4c and greatly reduced the contact resistance between the emissive layer and the electrodes.

This group also extended their work in a subsequent paper that used the same single layer architecture, but used different electrode materials and substrates [33]. In addition, this paper outlined a screen printing process that

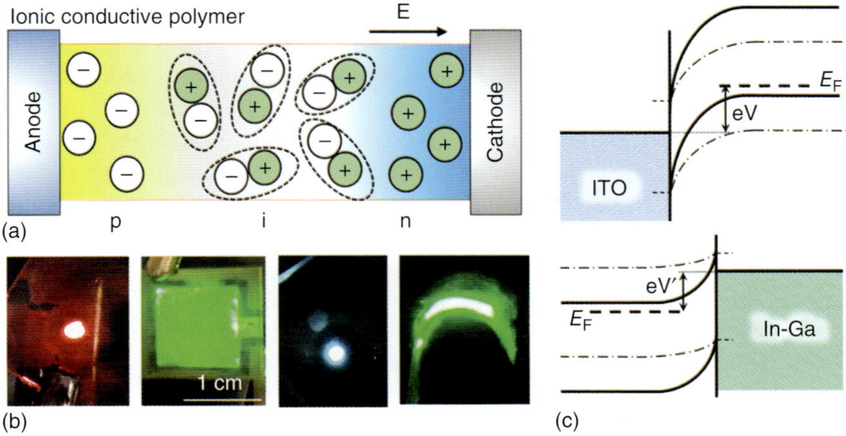

Figure 8.4 (a) The p–i–n junction formation formed in single layer perovskite LEDs. (b) Multiple color devices fabricated using the single layer approach, on the right is a flexible device (c) the band structure of the p–i–n junction. The high levels of ion accumulation near the electrodes allow for a tunnel junction to form.

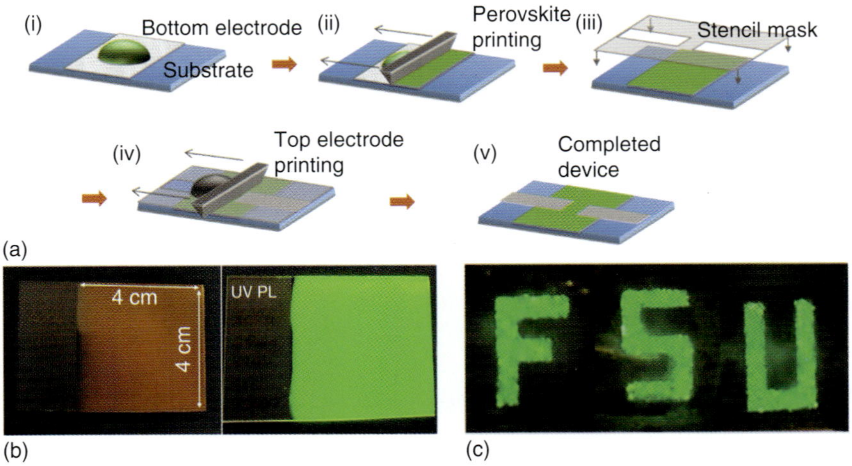

Figure 8.5 (a) The printing process outlined as a five-step process (b) large area covered via the printing process, under UV illumination it is apparent that it is extremely uniform. (c) Letter fabrication via mask patterning in the top electrode printing step.

could promise roll-to-roll printing of LEDs, which would allow for a scalable process and high-volume manufacturing. At the time of writing, the authors had demonstrated a 4 cm × 4 cm perovskite device that had been printed using this process (Figure 8.5b), which is one of the largest emissive layers that have been fabricated to day for perovskite LEDs.

Bade *et al.* [33] presented two different printed devices both employing the PEO/Br-Pero composite emission layer outlined above applied via a screen printing process that can be seen in Figure 8.5a. The first device was printed on top of an ITO/glass substrate and utilized silver nanowires as the top electrode and can be seen in Figure 8.5c. This device had a current efficiency of 4.91 cd A^{-1}, an EQE of 1.1%, and a maximum luminance of 21 014 cd m^{-2}, which is the brightest perovskite LED achieved at the time of writing this paper. In addition, this device was 1 cm by 1 cm in area, which is one of the largest active areas to date. The second device presented was printed on a polyacrylate substrate and used carbon nanotubes as the bottom substrate and silver nanowires for the top electrode. The best performing device had a current efficiency of 0.6 cd A^{-1}, an EQE of 0.14%, a maximum luminance of 360 cd m^{-2}, and remained operational with over 2% applied strain. Although this device had relatively low efficiencies and brightness it is the first flexible device with reported strain values. The authors also noted that the efficiency may possibly be increased by optimizing the CNT electrode, which possessed a large sheet resistance.

One final point of interest that was present by Bade *et al.* [33] was that their printing process was carried out completely in ambient air. This is in contrast to other processes outlined in the multilayer architecture section, which all required one or more vacuum processing steps during fabrication as well as a controlled humidity environment. The authors hypothesized that this was possible because the PEO polymer protected the perovskite material from moisture damage. This finding is significant as it allows the costs of manufacturing perovskite LEDs to be reduced even further. The material and processing concepts proposed by this work are of interest because they could be used for scalable manufacturing of flexible Pero-based optoelectronic devices. In their conclusion, the authors described devices that would be light weight and flexible and could be folded into small sizes for easy portability and unfolded into large screens to plug into a number of small size portable electronics for use as a large size, external screen. The displays could also cover uneven surfaces and cope with body movement, thus making them wearable, for example, in human clothing which has been a recent goal for the display community.

8.3 Current Challenges

The most substantial challenges currently facing perovskite LEDs is their stability in ambient air and their operational lifetime. Initially, it was believed that moisture had detrimental effects on methylammonium halide perovskite material in terms of damaging the crystallinity of the material. Stoumpos *et al.* showed that degradation occurred in air citing that lead containing perovskites degraded after a few weeks in humid environment, while tin containing perovskites degraded in a matter of hours [34]. The authors also postulated that the stability of perovskites may be strongly linked to their atomic and molecular composition, and that stability issues may be solved by substituting different ions in the lattice. Cho *et al.* [30] also saw a degradation when devices were exposed to air and postulated that moisture and oxygen are able to diffuse along grain boundaries, and react with the crystal to form metallic lead. This caused the breakdown of the PbX_6 tetrahedrons in the crystal structure, and allowed for nonradiative trap states on the crystal's surface, which in turn decreased the luminance.

However, as of late, there have been several conflicting reports demonstrating that the atmospheric humidity actually helped in improving the quality and efficiency of the perovskite films. Bass *et al.* [35] compared the properties and structures of air-exposed and nonair-exposed methylammonium lead iodide and methylammonium lead bromide perovskites. It was observed that moisture facilitated crystallization in these materials and also showed long luminescence lifetime when exposed or prepared in air. Bade *et al.* [33] also reported a large increase in luminance and EQE when devices were processed in ambient air with a 484% increase in luminance and 256% increase in EQE when compared with a control sample fabricated in dry nitrogen. The group also compared the microstructures of the two processes, and did not observe any notable degradation in the microstructure of the moisture exposed samples. You *et al.* [36] also reported a moisture-assisted growth process for solar cell fabrication where the precursor film was annealed in a humid environment. They showed that the morphology of the films processed in ambient air was superior to those that were prepared either in oxygen or in nitrogen environments. However, they did note that a relatively high humidity (>80%) actually caused a degradation in device performance supporting the hypothesis that perovskites are moisture unstable. Overall, more research needs to be performed in the area of perovskite moisture stability, and the degradation mechanism seen at high humidity levels needs to be accurately identified. In addition to moisture stability issues, perovskites still need additional studies in the area of thermal stability and lifetime stability as there have been few studies in this significant area that needs to be addressed prior to commercialization.

Another considerable challenge is to replace the lead ion in perovskite LEDs due to the toxicological issues associated with lead. There has been some research in this area, with some groups exploring the use of tin ions to replace the lead in solar cell applications [34, 37]. Very recently, Hong *et al.* [38] reported near-infrared (~950 nm) LEDs based on cesium tin triiodide. The devices emitted 40 $W\,Sr^{-1}\,m^{-2}$ at a current density of 364.3 $mA\,cm^{-2}$, and a maximum EQE of 3.8% at 4.5 V. The result was encouraging. However, the tin substitution is much less stable when compared to lead ions as noted above, and the efficiency optimization and operation stability have to be both examined in the near future. Another potential solution to the lead toxicity problem would be to implement an extensive recycling initiative, similar to what is currently in place for compact fluorescent lights that use mercury vapors.

A final issue that perovskite-based LEDs face is their relatively low efficiencies, and brightness compared to other more mature LED technologies. Currently, the best-performing OLEDs operate with an EQE of roughly 30% and a brightness of around 100 000 $cd\,m^{-2}$, while quantum dot LEDs have achieved an EQE of around 20% with a brightness of roughly 70 000 $cd\,m^{-2}$ [14]. However, perovskite LEDs are analogous to perovskite solar cells and have seen a large increase in efficiency

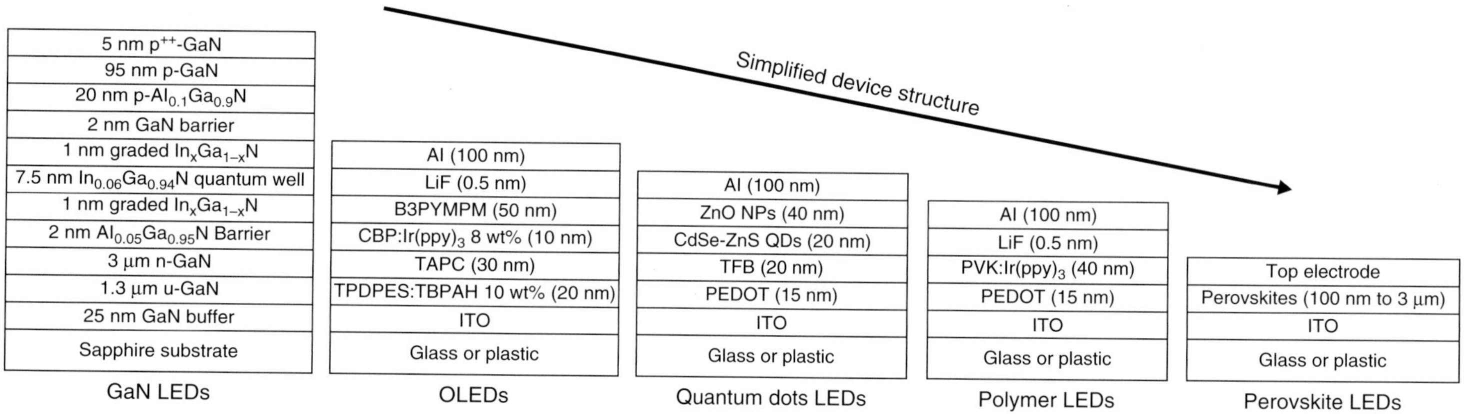

Figure 8.6 The device structures of various LED technologies. Perovskites have proven to have the simplest device structure to date containing only one layer between the electrodes.

in the past 2 years of study suggesting that they may surpass other technologies in coming years if the current rates of improvement continue.

8.4 Conclusions and Outlook

The remarkable optoelectronic properties seen in perovskite LEDs have garnered much attention in the research community in the past few years. Their color tunability, solution processability and simple device structure (Figure 8.6) are extremely promising toward achieving the goal of fabricating large-area flexible displays at a low cost.

However, for these devices to be commercialized, significant steps would need to be taken to overcome the challenges that have been presented thus far. Overall, the large advances seen in perovskite LEDs in such a short time span is evidence that significant interest has been evinced in the research of these materials , and may one day become the basis for large-area flexible and stretchable displays.

Acknowledgments

The authors are thankful for the financial support from Air Force Office of Scientific Research under Award FA9550-16-1-0124 and the support from National Science Foundation under Award ECCS-1609032.

References

1 Wang, C., Takei, K., Takahashi, T., and Javey, A. (2013) Carbon nanotube electronics – moving forward. *Chem. Soc. Rev.*, **42** (7), 2592–2609.
2 Cai, L. and Wang, C. (2015) Carbon nanotube flexible and stretchable electronics. *Nanoscale Res. Lett.*, **10**, 320.
3 Braunstein, R. (1955) Radiative transitions in semiconductors. *Phys. Rev.*, **99** (6), 1892–1893.
4 Schubert, E.F. (2006) *Light-Emitting Diodes*, 2nd edn, Cambridge University Press.
5 Nakamura, S., Mukai, T., and Senoh, M. (1994) Candela-class high-brightness InGaN/AlGaN double-heterostructure blue-light-emitting diodes. *Appl. Phys. Lett.*, **64** (13), 1687–1689.
6 Comstock, O. and Jarzomski, K. (2014) *LED Bulb Efficiency Expected to Continue Improving as Cost Declines – Today in Energy*, U.S. Energy Information Administration (EIA) [Online], https://www.eia.gov/todayinenergy/detail.cfm?id=15471 (accessed 01 July 2016).
7 Kamtekar, K.T., Monkman, A.P., and Bryce, M.R. (2010) Recent advances in white organic light-emitting materials and devices (WOLEDs). *Adv. Mater.*, **22** (5), 572–582.

8 Mikami, A., Koshiyama, T., and Tsubokawa, T. (2005) High-efficiency color and white organic light-emitting devices prepared on flexible plastic substrates. *Jpn. J. Appl. Phys.*, **44** (1B), 608–612.

9 Ouyang, M. (2005) OLED structures with strain relief, antireflection and barrier layers. US20050093437 A1, 05 May 2005.

10 Yang, Y., Zheng, Y., Cao, W., Titov, A., Hyvonen, J., Manders, J.R., Xue, J., Holloway, P.H., and Qian, L. (2015) High-efficiency light-emitting devices based on quantum dots with tailored nanostructures. *Nat. Photonics*, **9** (4), 259–266.

11 Mashford, B.S., Stevenson, M., Popovic, Z., Hamilton, C., Zhou, Z., Breen, C., Steckel, J., Bulovic, V., Bawendi, M., Coe-Sullivan, S., and Kazlas, P.T. (2013) High-efficiency quantum-dot light-emitting devices with enhanced charge injection. *Nat. Photonics*, **7** (5), 407–412.

12 12. Stranks, S.D. and Snaith, H.J. (2015) Metal-halide perovskites for photovoltaic and light-emitting devices. *Nat. Nano*, **10** (5), 391–402.

13 Veldhuis, S.A., Boix, P.P., Yantara, N., Li, M., Sum, T.C., Mathews, N., and Mhaisalkar, S.G. (2016) Perovskite materials for light-emitting diodes and lasers. *Adv. Mater.*, **28** (32), 6804–6834.

14 Yin, W.-J., Yang, J.-H., Kang, J., Yan, Y., and Wei, S.-H. (2015) Halide perovskite materials for solar cells: a theoretical review. *J. Mater. Chem. A*, **3** (17), 8926–8942.

15 Tan, Z.-K., Moghaddam, R.S., Lai, M.L., Docampo, P., Higler, R., Deschler, F., Price, M., Sadhanala, A., Pazos, L.M., Credgington, D., Hanusch, F., Bein, T., Snaith, H.J., and Friend, R.H. (2014) Bright light-emitting diodes based on organometal halide perovskite. *Nat. Nanotechnol.*, **9** (9), 687–692.

16 Miller, O.D., Yablonovitch, E., and Kurtz, S.R. (2012) Strong internal and external luminescence as solar cells approach the Shockley–Queisser limit. *IEEE J. Photovoltaics*, **2** (3), 303–311.

17 Green, M.A. (2012) Radiative efficiency of state-of-the-art photovoltaic cells. *Prog. Photovoltaics Res. Appl.*, **20** (4), 472–476.

18 Oku, T. (2015) Crystal structures of $CH_3NH_3PbI_3$ and related perovskite compounds used for solar cells, in *Solar Cells – New Approaches and Reviews* (ed. L.A. Kosyachenko), InTech, pp. 78–98.

19 Heidrich, K., Schäfer, W., Schreiber, M., Söchtig, J., Trendel, G., Treusch, J., Grandke, T., and Stolz, H.J. (1981) Electronic structure, photoemission spectra, and vacuum-ultraviolet optical spectra of $CsPbCl_3$ and $CsPbBr_3$. *Phys. Rev. B*, **24** (10), 5642–5649.

20 Xing, G., Mathews, N., Lim, S.S., Yantara, N., Liu, X., Sabba, D., Grätzel, M., Mhaisalkar, S., and Sum, T.C. (2014) Low-temperature solution-processed wavelength-tunable perovskites for lasing. *Nat. Mater.*, **13** (5), 476–480.

21 Shi, D., Adinolfi, V., Comin, R., Yuan, M., Alarousu, E., Buin, A., Chen, Y., Hoogland, S., Rothenberger, A., Katsiev, K., Losovyj, Y., Zhang, X., Dowben, P.A., Mohammed, O.F., Sargent, E.H., and Bakr, O.M. (2015) Low trap-state density and long carrier diffusion in organolead trihalide perovskite single crystals. *Science*, **347** (6221), 519–522.

22 Priante, D., Dursun, I., Alias, M.S., Shi, D., Melnikov, V.A., Ng, T.K., Mohammed, O.F., Bakr, O.M., and Ooi, B.S. (2015) The recombination

mechanisms leading to amplified spontaneous emission at the true-green wavelength in $CH_3NH_3PbBr_3$ perovskites. *Appl. Phys. Lett.*, **106** (8), 081902.
23 Motta, C., El-Mellouhi, F., and Sanvito, S. (2015) Charge carrier mobility in hybrid halide perovskites. *Sci. Rep.*, **5**, 12746.
24 Yucheng, L., Zhou, Y., Dong, C., Xiaodong, R., Jiankun, S., Xiaojing, L., Jingru, Z., Qingbo, W., Haibo, F., and Frank, L. (2015) Two-inch-sized perovskite $CH_3NH_3PbX_3$(X=Cl, Br, I) crystals: growth and characterization. *Adv. Mater.*, **27** (35), 5176–5183.
25 Era, M., Morimoto, S., Tsutsui, T., and Saito, S. (1994) Organic–inorganic heterostructure electroluminescent device using a layered perovskite semiconductor $(C_6H_5C_2H_4NH_3)_2PbI_4$. *Appl. Phys. Lett.*, **65** (6), 676–678.
26 Hattori, T., Taira, T., Era, M., Tsutsui, T., and Saito, S. (1996) Highly efficient electroluminescence from a heterostructure device combined with emissive layered-perovskite and an electron-transporting organic compound. *Chem. Phys. Lett.*, **254** (1–2), 103–108.
27 Chondroudis, K. and Mitzi, D.B. (1999) Electroluminescence from an organic–inorganic perovskite incorporating a quaterthiophene dye within lead halide perovskite layers. *Chem. Mater.*, **11** (11), 3028–3030.
28 Li, G., Tan, Z.-K., Di, D., Lai, M.L., Jiang, L., Lim, J.H.-W., Friend, R.H., and Greenham, N.C. (2015) Efficient light-emitting diodes based on nanocrystalline perovskite in a dielectric polymer matrix. *Nano Lett.*, **15** (4), 2640–2644.
29 Kim, Y.-H., Cho, H., Heo, J.H., Kim, T.-S., Myoung, N., Lee, C.-L., Im, S.H., and Lee, T.-W. (2015) Multicolored organic/inorganic hybrid perovskite light-emitting diodes. *Adv. Mater.*, **27** (7), 1248–1254.
30 Cho, H., Jeong, S.-H., Park, M.-H., Kim, Y.-H., Wolf, C., Lee, C.-L., Heo, J.H., Sadhanala, A., Myoung, N., Yoo, S., Im, S.H., Friend, R.H., and Lee, T.-W. (2015) Overcoming the electroluminescence efficiency limitations of perovskite light-emitting diodes. *Science*, **350** (6265), 1222–1225.
31 Li, J., Bade, S.G.R., Shan, X., and Yu, Z. (2015) Single-layer light-emitting diodes using organometal halide perovskite/poly(ethylene oxide) composite thin films. *Adv. Mater.*, **27** (35), 5196–5202.
32 Xiao, Z., Yuan, Y., Shao, Y., Wang, Q., Dong, Q., Bi, C., Sharma, P., Gruverman, A., and Huang, J. (2015) Giant switchable photovoltaic effect in organometal trihalide perovskite devices. *Nat. Mater.*, **14** (2), 193–198.
33 Bade, S.G.R., Li, J., Shan, X., Ling, Y., Tian, Y., Dilbeck, T., Besara, T., Geske, T., Gao, H., Ma, B., Hanson, K., Siegrist, T., Xu, C., and Yu, Z. (2016) Fully printed halide perovskite light-emitting diodes with silver nanowire electrodes. *ACS Nano*, **10** (2), 1795–1801.
34 Stoumpos, C.C., Malliakas, C.D., and Kanatzidis, M.G. (2013) Semiconducting tin and lead iodide perovskites with organic cations: phase transitions, high mobilities, and near-infrared photoluminescent properties. *Inorg. Chem.*, **52** (15), 9019–9038.
35 Bass, K.K., McAnally, R.E., Zhou, S., Djurovich, P.I., Thompson, M.E., and Melot, B.C. (2014) Influence of moisture on the preparation, crystal structure, and photophysical properties of organohalide perovskites. *Chem. Commun.*, **50** (99), 15819–15822.

36 You, J., (Michael) Yang, Y., Hong, Z., Song, T.-B., Meng, L., Liu, Y., Jiang, C., Zhou, H., Chang, W.-H., Li, G., and Yang, Y. (2014) Moisture assisted perovskite film growth for high performance solar cells. *Appl. Phys. Lett.*, **105** (18), 183902.
37 Hao, F., Stoumpos, C.C., Cao, D.H., Chang, R.P.H., and Kanatzidis, M.G. (2014) Lead-free solid-state organic–inorganic halide perovskite solar cells. *Nat. Photonics*, **8** (6), 489–494.
38 Hong, W.-L., Huang, Y.-C., Chang, C.-Y., Zhang, Z.-C., Tsai, H.-R., Chang, N.-Y., and Chao, Y.-C. (2016) Efficient low-temperature solution-processed lead-free perovskite infrared light-emitting diodes. *Adv. Mater.*, **28** (36), 8029–8036.

9

Flexible Floating Gate Memory

Ye Zhou[1,2]*, Su-Ting Han*[1,3]*, and Arul Lenus Roy Vellaisamy*[1]

[1] *City University of Hong Kong, Department of Materials Science and Engineering, College of Science and Engineering, Tat Chee Avenue, Kowloon, Hong Kong, SAR, P.R. China*
[2] *Shenzhen University, Division of Physics, Institute for Advanced Study, Nanhai Avenue, 3688, Shenzhen, Guangdong, P.R. China*
[3] *Shenzhen University, College of Electronic Science and Technology, Department of Microelectronics, Nanhai Avenue, 3688, Shenzhen, Guangdong, P.R. China*

9.1 Introduction

In modern era, electronic devices such as sensors, displays, and actuators are migrating toward thin and lightweight. As essential components required in various electronic devices, memories are more and more desirable in flexible or wearable devices. It is crucial to have flexible nonvolatile memory devices that possess high density, high speed, and low power consumption. Despite considerable achievements in flexible electronic devices, including integrated circuits (ICs), organic light-emitting diodes (OLEDs), and sensors, nonvolatile memories remain under-exploited [1]. Nowadays, flash memory devices are basically constructed by field effect transistors (FETs) with floating gate design. FET structure has several merits compared with capacitor or resistor memory structures. It is compatible with IC such as NAND and NOR and also the current complementary metal–oxide–semiconductor (CMOS) process. It can be also used for single transistor realization and nondestructive read-out [2–4]. The floating gate structure is widely used in the electronic market nowadays due to their excellent retention performance, capability for multibit storage, and suitability for ICs with various functions [5].

This chapter focuses on the flexible floating gate memories. We begin with the fundamentals of electronic memories and then describe the basics and the theory of floating gate memory followed by the operating principles of floating gate memory. Next, an overview of the state-of-the-art floating gate memory will be presented. We will also discuss how to analyze the mechanical properties of the floating gate memory on flexible substrates.

Flexible and Stretchable Medical Devices, First Edition. Edited by Kuniharu Takei.

9.2 Device Operation of Floating Gate Memory

Figure 9.1a shows the device structure of a typical FET with a bottom gate electrode. On top of the gate electrode, there is an insulating layer, a semiconductor layer, and top source and drain electrodes. The gate voltage can control the current flow in the semiconductor channel [6]. The typical transfer curve of FET is shown in Figure 9.1b. In this curve, the threshold voltage (V_{th}) can be determined by extrapolating a plot of $(I_{DS\,sat})^{1/2}$ versus V_{GS} to I_{DS} equal to 0 is fixed at constant V_{DS}.

$$I_{DS\,sat} = \frac{W}{2L}\mu C_i(V_{GS} - V_{th})^2$$

where $I_{DS\,sat}$ is the source-drain current in the saturation region, W is the channel width of the FET, L is the channel length, μ is the mobility of the semiconductor material, C_i is the capacitance per unit area of the insulating layer, V_{GS} is the source-gate voltage, and V_{th} is the threshold voltage. within contrast to the transistor structure, as depicted in Figure 9.1c, the floating gate memory has a floating gate sandwiched between the blocking dielectric layer and tunneling dielectric layer. The blocking dielectric layer is thick and can prevent the charge carriers from transferring to the gate electrode when the memory devices are under programming and erasing operation [7]. The tunneling dielectric layer is relatively thin, which can stop the charge transfer from the floating gate to the semiconductor layer. When designing the memory device based on the floating gate structure, we need to strictly consider the thickness of the tunneling dielectric layer and the speed of program/erase, and retention property should be optimized together.

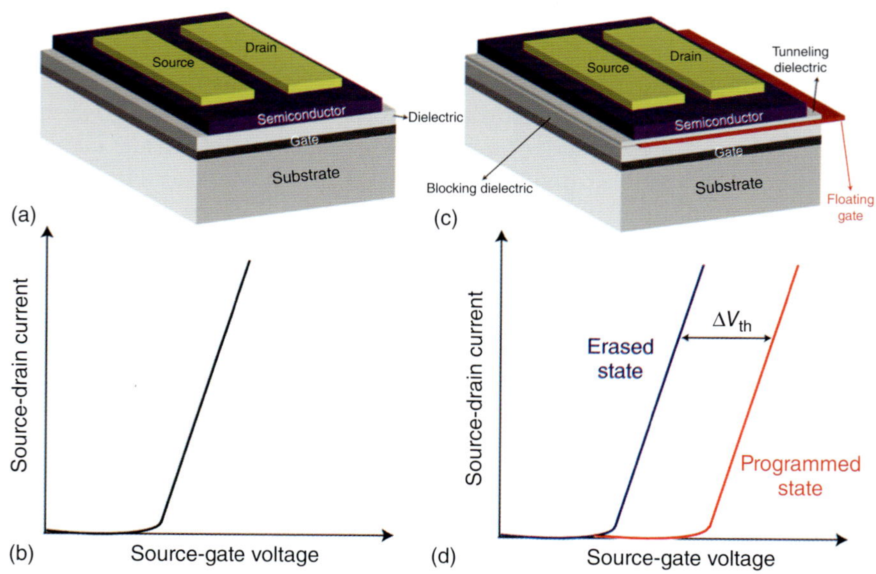

Figure 9.1 (a) Schematic diagram of the FET structure. (b) Typical transfer curve of FET. (c) Schematic diagram of the floating gate memory structure. (d) Typical transfer curve of the floating gate memory.

The charge carriers from the semiconductor can be injected and trapped in the floating gate when a gate bias is applied, and this process is called "program" operation. The charge carriers that are trapped in the floating gate can move back to the semiconductor layer during "erase" operation by applying a reverse bias at the gate electrode [5]. The memory effect of floating gate memory is achieved by trapping and de-trapping the charge carriers in the floating gate layer. When we have a look at the transfer curve, V_{th} can be controlled because the channel conductance changes when the charge carriers are trapped and de-trapped in the floating gate. The programmed state and erased state of floating gate memory device could be confirmed by comparing the V_{th} or I_{DS} after the "program" operation and "erase" operation. The typical transfer curve of floating gate memory at programmed and erased state is demonstrated in Figure 9.1d. The transfer curve shifts direction is different when the floating gate performs as hole or electron storage element. During the memory operation, the erased state and programmed state can be recognized as ON state and OFF state, respectively.

9.3 Charge Injection Mechanism in Floating Gate Memory

9.3.1 The Hot-electron Injection Mechanism

In the floating gate memory, if we apply a lateral electrical field between the source electrode and drain electrode, the hot-electron injection happens. The electrons can transfer from the source electrode to the drain electrode. During this process, the energy of electrons is received from the lateral electrical field and lost due to the lattice vibrations. At the low electrical field, the dynamic equilibrium will be broken until the electrical field strength reaches $100\,\text{kV cm}^{-1}$ [8]. If the electrical field exceeds that value, the electrons will heated by the lateral electric field. The electrons will have enough energy to cross the energy barrier and transfer from the semiconductor layer to the floating gate layer. Under the vertical electrical field, the electrons can be trapped in the floating gate. If the electrons need to overcome the potential barrier, the following conditions must be fulfilled: (i) the potential energy barrier in the tunneling dielectric layer should be lower than the kinetic energy of the electrons; (ii) charge carriers should be injected in the same direction of the energy barrier; and (iii) the electrons should be collected by the electrical field at the tunneling dielectric layer [9].

People often use the "lucky electron" model to describe and simulate the hot-electron injection. For the tunneled electrons, three independence probabilities can be hypnotized: [10] (i) driven by the lateral electric field, the electrons are lucky enough to get sufficient energy to cross the tunneling dielectric, after the collision, enough energy should be reserved to redirect the electron on the way to the semiconductor/dielectric interface; (ii) the electrons move to the semiconductor/dielectric interface without any collision; and (iii) in the tunneling dielectric layer, the electrons could surmount the tunneling energy barrier and reach the floating gate without any energy-robbing collision. In conclusion, if the electrons can fulfill all the above conditions, they are able to be injected and trapped into the floating gate.

However, the commonly used flexible semiconductors usually have low drift velocity; on the other hand, irregular injection of the electrons may induce worthless "program" operation and increase the power consumption. Therefore, instead of the hot-electron injection, Fowler–Nordheim (F-N) tunneling and direct tunneling are proposed to be the favorable approaches in flexible floating gate memory [11].

9.3.2 Fowler–Nordheim (F-N) Tunneling Mechanism

F–N tunneling is the process where the electrons tunnel through a barrier under a high electric field. This quantum mechanical tunneling process is a significant mechanism for thin barriers [12]. This mechanism is highly applicable in flexible floating gate memory when the charge carriers tunnel through the thin dielectric layer. The energy diagram of the floating gate memory with p-type semiconductor is shown in Figure 9.2a, and negative gate bias is applied in the "program" operation. Several parameters such as the energy level and the energy barrier may influence the tunneling probability of the charge carriers. The width of the energy barrier decreases extensively after applying a voltage on the gate electrode. The current density of the tunneling charge carriers can be estimated from Wentzel–Kramers–Brillouin (WKB) approximation [13, 14]:

$$J = \frac{q^3F^2}{16\pi^2h^2\Phi_B}\exp\left[-4(2m_{ox}^*)^{\frac{1}{2}}\Phi_B{}^{\frac{3}{2}}/3hqF\right]$$

where Φ_B is the height of the energy barrier, q is the fundamental unit of charge, h is the Plank's constant, m_{ox}^* is the effective mass of the charge carrier in the forbidden gap of the dielectric layer, and F is the electric field through the tunneling dielectric layer. From the equation, we can find that the current density of the tunneling charge carriers has exponential dependence on the applied electrical field. Therefore, the design of the tunneling barrier is crucial for the "program" and "erase" operation. We also have the assumption that charge carriers can be treated as a three-dimensional gas of free particles in the classical theory and these particles are with Boltzmann distribution of energy. Nevertheless, they are limited to a narrow potential well if the semiconductor is accumulated or depleted. In this condition, the quantization of motion perpendicular to the interface is required. Therefore, the correct treatment of the charge carriers is with a two-dimensional quantum mechanical gas [15]. With this treatment, we can find that the barrier height is voltage dependent which is lower than the classic one. Furthermore, the electrical field across the tunneling dielectric layer is also lower than the classic one since much greater voltage has dropped in the semiconductor layer [16]. The above equation can be rewritten in the following simple form:

$$J = AF^2\exp\left[-\frac{B}{F}\right]$$

where A and B are the functions of electric field including the quantum effects [17]. The F–N tunneling mechanism is used to describe the "program" and "erase" process owing to the low power consumption during the device operation and the high tunneling efficiency of charge carriers. The F–N tunneling

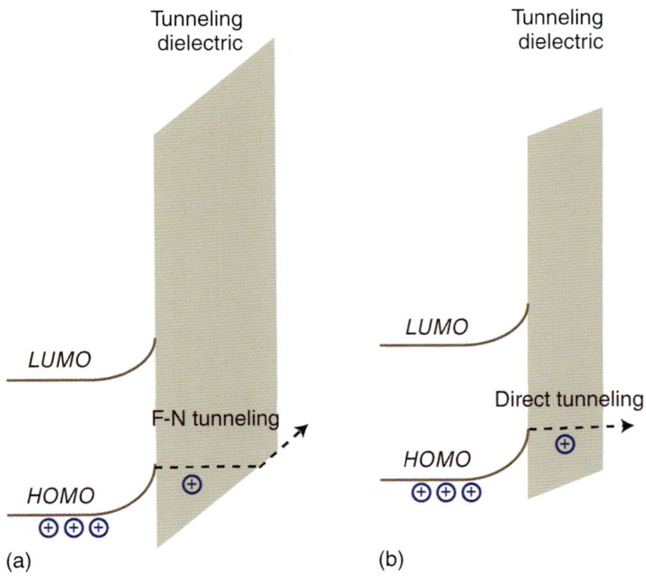

Figure 9.2 (a) Schematic diagram of F–N tunneling in the floating gate memory; (b) Schematic diagram of direct tunneling in the floating gate memory.

mechanism also has some limitations such as the use of high applied electrical field and long access time.

9.3.3 Direct Tunneling Mechanism

The thickness of the tunneling dielectric layer needs to be decreased when the single cell size of the floating gate memory decreases, and this can keep away from the short channel effect. In the direct tunneling process, the charge carriers can cross the tunneling dielectric layer when the thickness of the tunneling dielectric layer is thin enough. Figure 9.2b shows the energy diagram of the direct tunneling mechanism of the floating gate memory. The direct tunneling current depends on many parameters including the external electrical field. Its mechanism is much more complicated when comparing with F–N tunneling in memory operation. Fast program speed and low applying voltage are the major advantages of the direct tunneling process; however, the much thinner thickness of the tunneling dielectric layer may influence the data retention property.

9.4 Flexible Nanofloating Gate Memory

The idea of using a floating gate to obtain nonvolatile storage was suggested by Kahng and Sze in 1967 [18]. After that, the floating gate memory has developed rapidly and has been commercialized in the electronic device market. Recently, researchers focus on device engineering and new material application in the flexible memories. Someya *et al.* demonstrated a flexible floating gate memory in which aluminum served as the floating gate and chemically modified aluminum oxide served as the tunneling and blocking dielectric layer [19]. It is easy to fabricate a metal layer between two dielectric layers using a thermal evaporation method. However, the high vacuum deposition process is not desirable for low-cost and large-area flexible electronics. On the other hand, the metal floating gate has some intrinsic limitations when scaling down the device size owing to decreased coupling ratio, increased current leakage, and poor data retention property [20, 21]. In order to manipulate the trap sites and trap levels, using the nanofloating gate is an alternative way as the density and work function of nanoparticles can both be modulated [5, 22].

Nanofloating gate memory devices using nanomaterials such as metal nanoparticles as floating gate have received a lot of interest owing to the simple device fabrication process and controlled floating gate density. Noble metal nanoparticles are excellent candidates for the floating gate structure due to their chemical stability, easy processability, and high work function [23]. The metal nanoparticles floating gate can be formed by several approaches such as the thermal evaporation process [24, 25], electrostatic self-assembly [26–28], and block copolymer method [21, 29]. For the thermal evaporation method, metal nanoparticles can be easily deposited on the flexible substrate. During the deposition process, noble metal atoms can penetrate into the polymer layer because the penetration depth of metal atom is inversely proportional to the reactivity of metal [30]. Therefore, thicker tunneling dielectric layer in top-gate bottom-contact transistor structure or thicker blocking dielectric layer in bottom-gate top-contact transistor structure is needed to prevent noble metal atom penetration, which may influence the device performance. But this method has drawbacks since thicker dielectric layer is not conducive for scaling down of the nanodevice. In contrast, electrostatic self-assembled metal nanoparticles can be used in flexible floating gate memory without the need of thick dielectric layer. The advantages of self-assembled metal nanoparticles method are solution-processable, controllable nanoparticle size, and low temperature process, which are compatible with the commonly used bendable or stretchable substrate. Generally, the solution-synthesized metal nanoparticles have negative surface charges. The repulsive force between them can make each nanoparticle well dispersed on the desired surface of the insulator. Similar to self-assembled nanoparticles, solution-processed block copolymer wrapped nanoparticles monolayer can also be used in flexible floating gate memory. Incorporation of metal nanoparticles in polymer matrix can bring us exceptional properties of the polymer as well as the nanoparticles. This floating gate layer could be fabricated in the device using the spin-coating process. The successful use of block copolymer method generally requires controlling over the distribution as well as loading the nanoparticles in the polymer matrix. The preparation of well-ordered polymer-nanoparticle composites which contain sufficient concentration of nanoparticles is a big challenge.

The above mentioned nanofloating gate fabrication approaches have several drawbacks. The thermal evaporation method cannot enhance the density of metal nanoparticles since the metal nanoparticles become bigger via Ostwald ripening with the growing of film thickness [25]. The electrostatic and block copolymer methods suffer from poor order and comparatively low density of the nanoparticles. Therefore, in order to optimize the performance of floating gate memory, metal nanoparticles with high nanoparticle density and uniform size distribution are highly needed.

Recently, novel 2D nanomaterials have also been investigated and applied in floating gate memories. Graphene is a potential candidate for advanced electronic devices owing to its high electrical conductivity, unique optical property, outstanding mechanical flexibility, and stiffness [31–40]. Graphene can be produced by chemical vapor deposition (CVD) or physical exfoliation. Nevertheless, the two methods are not compatible with low-cost and high-yield mass production. Solution procesability should be a key issue when considering the floating gate candidates. Although the electrical properties of chemically reduced graphene oxide (rGO) degrade slightly due to lattice defects, rGO have been investigated a lot in floating gate memory architectures by scientists [33].

9.5 Characterization of Floating Gate Memory

The electrical performance of the floating gate memory can be measured using a semiconductor parameter analyzer. In the p-type transistor based floating gate memory, when the charge carriers of p-type semiconductor are trapped by the floating gate with negative gate bias, this operation is called "program". In contrast, if the trapped charge carriers are moved back to the semiconductor from the floating gate by applying positive gate bias, this operation is called "erase". The memory window ΔV_{th} is defined as V_{th} (erased)—V_{th} (programmed). For measuring the data retention properties, the programmed/erased states will be obtained by programming/erasing operation, and then the V_{th} will be measured as a function of elapsed time. The "program" and "erase" operations will be repeated for the number of times required to determine the memory endurance properties. The V_{th} of the memory devices will be recorded with respect to the number of "program" and "erase" cycles.

Figure 9.3 shows an example of electrical characterization of flexible floating gate memory. In this structure, microcontact printable (μCP) ultrahigh-density alkanethiol-protected Au nanoparticles array has been used in flexible floating gate memory [3]. Following evaporation of the solvent, the closely packed Au nanoparticles array is formed on the surface of water. To fabricate the nanofloating gate, the Au monolayer was transferred to the poly(dimethysiloxane) (PDMS) stamp pad by the Langmuir–Schaefer method. Then the Au nanopartciles can be transferred to the desired flexible substrate by the stamp as shown in Figure 9.3a. The optical image of the flexible floating gate memories is illustrated in Figure 9.3b. The device performance based on μCP Au nanoparticles has been compared with the devices fabricated with thermally evaporated Au nanoparticles and electrostatic layer-by-layer self-assembled Au nanoparticles. The electrical characteristics of the devices are shown in Figure 9.3c–f. The μCP device possessed the largest memory window among the three devices, due to the largest trapping site density and almost no lateral connection in nanofloating layer. The μCP floating gate memory also showed excellent *P*/*E*

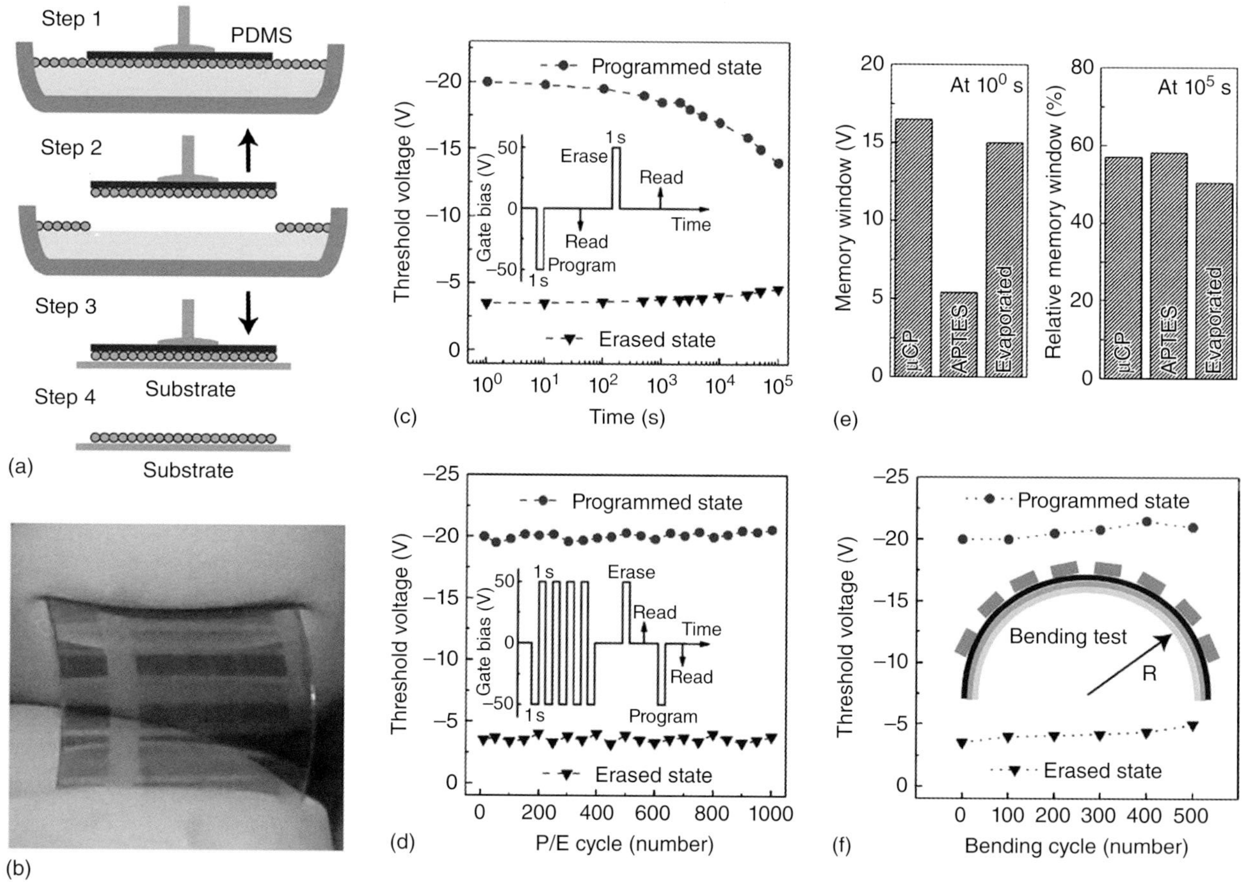

Figure 9.3 (a) Schematic illustration of the nanoparticle printing process. (b) Optical image of the flexible μCP floating gate memory. (c) Threshold voltage of the μCP floating gate memory with respect to the elapsed time. Inset: the pulse sequence for retention test. (d) Threshold voltage of the μCP floating gate memory as a function of the number of P/E cycles. Inset: the test pulse sequence for endurance test. (e) Comparison of the retention properties of different floating gate memories. (f) Flexibility test of the μCP floating gate memory. (Wei *et al*. 2012 [3]. Reproduced with permission of American Chemical Society.)

endurance property and long data retention capability. The μCP approach is a good candidate for fabricating flexible electronics and can scale down the current nanofloating gate memory devices.

9.6 Flexibility of Floating Gate Memory

In flexible electronics, mechanical flexibility is a very important parameter. Therefore, the electrical performances of the floating gate memories need to be carefully investigated and understood at various bending states. Figure 9.4 demonstrates the substrate that is bent in convex (tensile state) and concave (compressive state) direction. When we investigate a device on the surface of a flexible substrate with a bending radius of R, the strain S is given by the equation:

$$S = \frac{(t_L + t_S)(1 + 2\eta + \chi\eta^2)}{2R(1 + \eta)(1 + \chi\eta)}$$

where $\eta = t_L/t_S$, t_L is the thickness of the device layer, t_S is the thickness of the flexible substrate, $\chi = Y_L/Y_S$, Y_L is the Young's modulus of the device layer, and Y_S is the Young's modulus of the flexible substrate [41–43]. S can be simply expressed as $D/2R$ where D is the thickness of the flexible substrate.

Bending experiments can be carried out to investigate the electrical and data storage performance of the flexible floating gate memories on PET at different strains [44]. The PET films were bent along the device channel transport axis, as illustrated in Figure 9.5. Real time characterization of the electrical properties can be carried out during the bending test. The applied compressive and tensile strain

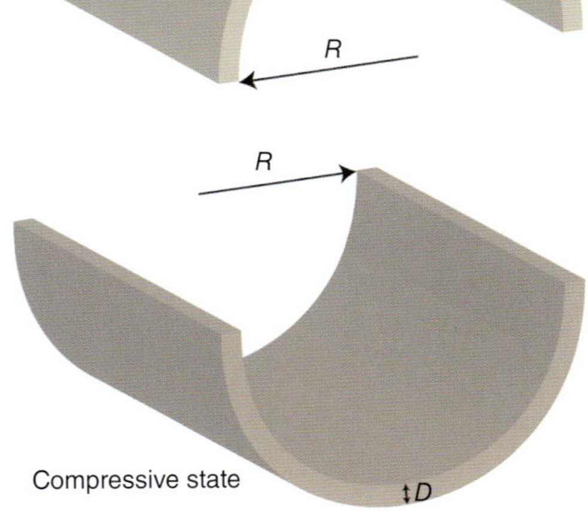

Figure 9.4 Schematic diagram of the flexible substrate at tensile state and compressive state.

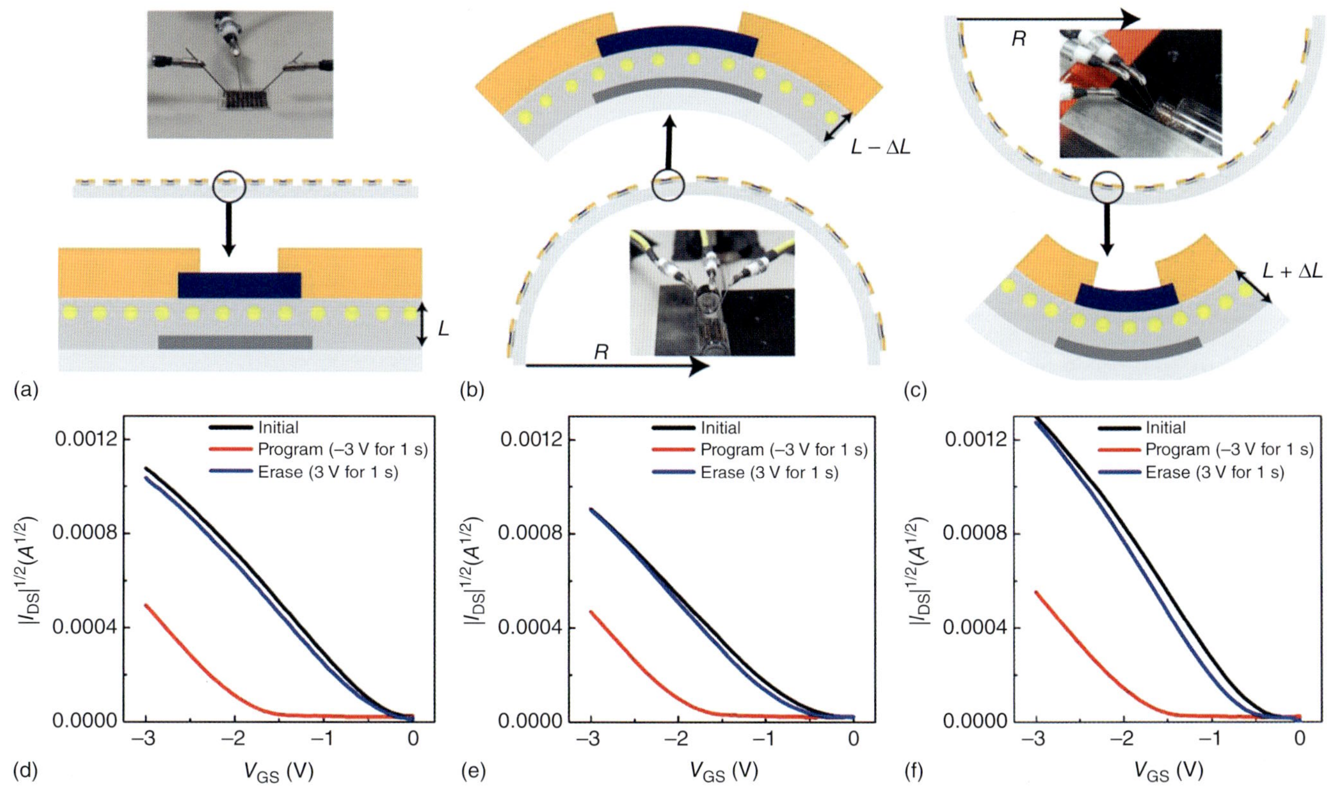

Figure 9.5 (a) Schematic diagram of the flat floating gate memory; (b) schematic diagram of the floating gate memory at negative strain; (c) schematic diagram of the floating gate memory at positive strain; (d) electrical performances of the flat floating gate memory; (e) electrical performances of the floating gate memory at negative strain; (f) electrical performances of the floating gate memory at positive strain. (Zhou *et al*. 2013 [44]. Reproduced with permission of Royal Society of Chemistry.)

on the memory device were ±1.1%. The respective transfer characteristics of the floating gate memory at different states are also shown in Figure 9.5. At compressive strain, the I_{DS} of the nanofloating gate memory increases; in contrast, at tensile strain the I_{DS} decreases.

In the bending test for floating gate memory, the result is reproducible and the change in the current is reversible. Therefore, this phenomenon cannot be related with the time-dependent drift of transistor performance or the degradation of electrical performance. The varied I_{DS} of the floating gate memory can be explained by the transport properties of the semiconductor. When the floating gate memory is at compressive strain, the energy barrier for charge carriers hopping has been reduced since the distance between pentacene molecules get smaller. At the tensile strain, the mobility of the semiconductor decreases for the reason that the spacing get larger. At tensile strain, V_{th} of the floating gate memory shifts to the most negative value after the programming operation. At compressive strain, V_{th} of the floating gate memory shifts to the least negative value. This result can be explained by the lowest mobility of pentacene at negative strain and highest mobility at positive strain. Owing to the Poisson effect, the effective thickness of the tunneling dielectric layer reduces at negative strain and increases at positive strain, which may also lead to the observed electrical performance under different strain [45]. The negatively shifted V_{th} compared with the zero strain can be attributed to the reduced tunneling barrier of the charge carriers at tensile strain. In contrast, the positively shifted V_{th} compared with the zero strain can be attributed to the increased tunneling barrier of the charge carriers at compressive strain. For the electrical performance after erasing operation, at tensile strain, V_{th} of the floating gate memory is easiest to go back to the initial condition, due to the lowest barrier of the tunneling dielectric layer. Meanwhile, at compressive strain, V_{th} is hardest to turn back to the initial condition due to the highest energy barrier of the tunneling dielectric layer.

9.7 Conclusion

With the development of information technology, it becomes clear that memory devices play an important role in portable and wearable electronics. In this chapter, we discuss the materials selection and structure design of the floating gate memory on flexible substrates. The electrical performances of the memory devices under different applied strains are also described. Flexible floating gate memory with novel nanostructure materials should be quite promising for future advanced flexible electronics. With proper materials and structure design, memory devices can be used in stretchable, foldable, and wearable electronic devices of any substrate materials and geometry.

References

1 Bao, Z. and Chen, X. (2016) Flexible and stretchable devices. *Adv. Mater.*, **28**, 4177.

2 Zhou, Y., Han, S.-T., Chen, X., Wang, F., Tang, Y.-B., and Roy, V.A.L. (2014) An upconverted photonic nonvolatile memory. *Nat. Commun.*, **5**, 4720.
3 Wei, Q., Lin, Y., Anderson, E.R., Briseno, A.L., Gido, S.P., and Watkins, J.J. (2012) Additive-driven assembly of block copolymer–nanoparticle hybrid materials for solution processable floating gate memory. *ACS Nano*, **6**, 1188.
4 Han, S.-T., Zhou, Y., Xu, Z.-X., Huang, L.-B., Yang, X.-B., and Roy, V.A.L. (2012) Microcontact printing of ultrahigh density gold nanoparticle monolayer for flexible flash memories. *Adv. Mater.*, **24**, 3556.
5 Lee, J.-S. (2010) Recent progress in gold nanoparticle-based non-volatile memory devices. *Gold Bull.*, **43**, 189.
6 Guo, Y., Yu, G., and Liu, Y. (2010) Functional organic field-effect transistors. *Adv. Mater.*, **22**, 4427.
7 Lee, J.-S., Kim, Y.-M., Kwon, J.-H., Shin, H., Sohn, B.-H., and Lee, J. (2009) Tunable memory characteristics of nanostructured, nonvolatile charge trap memory devices based on a binary mixture of metal nanoparticles as a charge trapping layer. *Adv. Mater.*, **21**, 178.
8 Cottrell, P.E., Troutman, R.R., and Ning, T.H. (1979) Hot-electron emission in n-channel IGFETs. *IEEE J. Solid-State Circuits*, **14**, 442.
9 Eitan, B. and Frohman-Bentchkowsky, D. (1981) Hot-electron injection into the oxide in n-channel MOS devices. *IEEE Trans. Electron Devices*, **28**, 328.
10 Tam, S., Ko, P.-K., Hu, C., and Muller, R.S. (1982) Correlation between substrate and gate currents in MOSFET's. *IEEE Trans. Electron Devices*, **29**, 1740.
11 Liu, Z., Xue, F., Su, Y., Lvov, Y.M., and Varahramyan, K. (2006) Memory effect of a polymer thin-film transistor with self-assembled gold nanoparticles in the gate dielectric. *IEEE Trans. Nanotechnol.*, **5**, 379.
12 Esaki, L. (1974) Long journey into tunnelling. *Proc. IEEE*, **62**, 825.
13 Lenzlinger, M. and Snow, E.H. (1969) Fowler-Nordheim tunneling into thermally grown SiO_2. *J. Appl. Phys.*, **40**, 278.
14 Moll, J. (1964) *Physics of Semiconductors*, McGraw-Hill, New York.
15 Ando, T., Fowler, A.B., and Stern, F. (1982) Electronic properties of two-dimensional systems. *Rev. Mod. Phys.*, **54**, 437.
16 Sune, J., Olivo, P., and Ricco, B. (1992) Quantum-mechanical modeling of accumulation layers in MOS structure. *IEEE Trans. Electron Devices*, **39**, 1732.
17 Lanzoni, M., Sune, J., Olivo, P., and Ricco, B. (1993) Advanced electrical-level modeling of EEPROM cells. *IEEE Trans. Electron Devices*, **40**, 951.
18 Kahng, D. and Sze, S.M. (1967) A floating gate and its application to memory devices. *Bell Syst. Tech. J.*, **46**, 1288.
19 Sekitani, T., Yokota, T., Zschieschang, U., Klauk, H., Bauer, S., Takeuchi, K., Takamiya, M., Sakurai, T., and Someya, T. (2009) Organic nonvolatile memory transistors for flexible sensor arrays. *Science*, **326**, 1516.
20 Han, S.-T., Zhou, Y., Wang, C., He, L., Zhang, W., and Roy, V.A.L. (2013) Layer-by-layer-assembled reduced graphene oxide/gold nanoparticle hybrid double-floating-gate structure for low-voltage flexible flash memory. *Adv. Mater.*, **25**, 872.

21 Leong, W.L., Lee, P.S., Lohani, A., Lam, Y.M., Chen, T., Zhang, S., Dodabalapur, A., and Mhaisalkar, S.G. (2008) Non-volatile organic memory applications enabled by in situ synthesis of gold nanoparticles in a self-assembled block copolymer. *Adv. Mater.*, **20**, 2325.

22 Tang, X., Krzeminski, C., Lecavelier des Etangs-Levallois, A., Chen, Z., Dubois, E., Kasper, E., Karmous, A., Reckinger, N., Flandre, D., Francis, L.A., Colinge, J.-P., and Raskin, J.-P. (2011) Energy-band engineering for improved charge retention in fully self-aligned double floating-gate single-electron memories. *Nano Lett.*, **11**, 4520.

23 Talapin, D.V., Lee, J.-S., Kovalenko, M.V., and Shevchenko, E.V. (2009) Prospects of colloidal nanocrystals for electronic and optoelectronic applications. *Chem. Rev.*, **110**, 389.

24 Wang, S.M., Leung, C.W., and Chan, P.K.L. (2010) Nonvolatile organic transistor-memory devices using various thicknesses of silver nanoparticle layers. *Appl. Phys. Lett.*, **97**, 023511.

25 Baeg, K.-J., Noh, Y.-Y., Sirringhaus, H., and Kim, D.-Y. (2010) Controllable shifts in threshold voltage of top-gate polymer field-effect transistors for applications in organic nano floating gate memory. *Adv. Funct. Mater.*, **20**, 224.

26 Lee, J.-S., Cho, J., Lee, C., Kim, I., Park, J., Kim, Y.-M., Shin, H., Lee, J., and Caruso, F. (2007) Layer-by-layer assembled charge-trap memory devices with adjustable electronic properties. *Nat. Nanotechnol.*, **2**, 790.

27 Kim, S.-J., Park, Y.-S., Lyu, S.-H., and Lee, J.-S. (2010) Nonvolatile nano-floating gate memory devices based on pentacene semiconductors and organic tunneling insulator layers. *Appl. Phys. Lett.*, **96**, 033302.

28 Novembre, C., Guerin, D., Lmimouni, K., Gamrat, C., and Vuillaume, D. (2008) Gold nanoparticle-pentacene memory transistors. *Appl. Phys. Lett.*, **92**, 103314.

29 Leong, W.L., Mathews, N., Mhaisalkar, S.G., Chen, T.P., and Lee, P.S. (2008) Charging dynamics of discrete gold nanoparticle arrays self-assembled within a poly (styrene-b-4-vinylpyridine) diblock copolymer template. *Appl. Phys. Lett.*, **93**, 222908.

30 Di, C.-A., Yu, G., Liu, Y., Guo, Y., Wang, Y., Wu, W., and Zhu, D. (2008) High-performance organic field-effect transistors with low-cost copper electrodes. *Adv. Mater.*, **20**, 1286.

31 Elias, D.C., Gorbachev, R.V., Mayorov, A.S., Morozov, S.V., Zhukov, A.A., Blake, P., Ponomarenko, L.A., Grigorieva, I.V., Novoselov, K.S., Guinea, F., and Geim, A.K. (2011) Dirac cones reshaped by interaction effects in suspended graphene. *Nat. Phys.*, **7**, 701.

32 Balandin, A.A., Ghosh, S., Bao, W., Calizo, I., Teweldebrhan, D., Miao, F., and Lau, C.N. (2008) Superior thermal conductivity of single-layer graphene. *Nano Lett.*, **8**, 902.

33 Novoselov, K.S., Geim, A.K., Morozov, S.V., Jiang, D., Zhang, Y., Dubonos, S.V., Grigorieva, I.V., and Firsov, A.A. (2004) Electric field effect in atomically thin carbon films. *Science*, **306**, 666.

34 Schedin, F., Geim, A.K., Morozov, S.V., Hill, E.W., Blake, P., Katsnelson, M.I., and Novoselov, K.S. (2007) Detection of individual gas molecules adsorbed on graphene. *Nat. Mater.*, **6**, 652.

35 Zhang, Y., Tan, Y.-W., Stormer, H.L., and Kim, P. (2005) Experimental observation of quantum Hall effect and Berry's phase in graphene. *Nature*, **438**, 201.
36 Gómez-Navarro, C., Weitz, R.T., Bittner, A.M., Scolari, M., Mews, A., Burghard, M., and Kern, K. (2007) Electronic transport properties of individual chemically reduced graphene oxide sheets. *Nano Lett.*, **7**, 3499.
37 Hwang, H., Joo, P., Kang, M.S., Ahn, G., Han, J.T., Kim, B.-S., and Cho, J.H. (2012) Highly tunable charge transport in layer-by-layer assembled graphene transistors. *ACS Nano*, **6**, 2432.
38 Jo, K., Lee, T., Choi, H.J., Park, J.H., Lee, D.J., Lee, D.W., and Kim, B.-S. (2011) Stable aqueous dispersion of reduced graphene nanosheets via non-covalent functionalization with conducting polymers and application in transparent electrodes. *Langmuir*, **27**, 2014.
39 Yang, J., Kim, J.-W., and Shin, H.S. (2012) Facile method for rGO field effect transistor: selective adsorption of rGO on SAM-treated gold electrode by electrostatic attraction. *Adv. Mater.*, **24**, 2299.
40 Wang, S., Ang, P.K., Wang, Z., Tang, A.L.L., Thong, J.T.L., and Loh, K.P. (2009) High mobility, printable, and solution-processed graphene electronics. *Nano Lett.*, **10**, 92.
41 Suo, Z., Ma, E.Y., Gleskova, H., and Wagner, S. (1999) Mechanics of rollable and foldable film-on-foil electronics. *Appl. Phys. Lett.*, **74**, 1177.
42 Gleskova, H., Wagner, S., and Suo, Z. (1999) Failure resistance of amorphous silicon transistors under extreme in-plane strain. *Appl. Phys. Lett.*, **75**, 3011.
43 Jedaa, A. and Halik, M. (2009) Toward strain resistant flexible organic thin film transistors. *Appl. Phys. Lett.*, **95**, 103309.
44 Zhou, Y., Han, S.-T., Xu, Z.-X., and Roy, V.A.L. (2013) The strain and thermal induced tunable charging phenomenon in low power flexible memory arrays with a gold nanoparticle monolayer. *Nanoscale*, **5**, 1972.
45 Sekitani, T., Kato, Y., Iba, S., Shinaoka, H., Someya, T., Sakurai, T., and Takagi, S. (2005) Bending experiment on pentacene field-effect transistors on plastic films. *Appl. Phys. Lett.*, **86**, 073511.

10

Flexible and Stretchable Wireless Systems

Aftab M. Hussain and Muhammad M. Hussain

King Abdullah University of Science and Technology (KAUST), Bldg. 3, Level 3, Rm 3274, Thuwai 23955-6900, Makkah Province, Kingdom of Saudi Arabia

10.1 Introduction

Wireless communication has transformed the way we live, work, and play. Over the past few decades, exponential progress in wireless communication systems has brought about a paradigm shift in our interactions with each other and with our surroundings. Wireless systems rely on information communicated by propagating electromagnetic radiation through space. Early breakthroughs by James Clerk Maxwell, Albert Michaelson and Edward Morley helped explain the basic theory of generation and propagation of electromagnetic waves. In the late 1880s, a series of experiments by Heinrich Hertz provided proof of Maxwell's theory and a first glimpse of the propagation and detection of wireless electromagnetic energy. In the 1890s, an Italian electrical engineer named Guglielmo Marconi carried out experiments on wireless signal propagation for communicating information. He developed the first complete wireless system capable of transmitting information over a distance of several kilometers. Later, he moved to England where he worked on much larger systems for transmission over larger distances; the first trans-Atlantic communications were carried out by Marconi in the early 1900s and he received the Nobel Prize in Physics in 1909 for his contributions in wireless communication systems. Thereafter, the early twentieth century saw the rise of reliable wireless communication systems that could communicate information across the Atlantic Ocean. The advent of the world wars saw large amount of funds being directed toward improving radio communication capabilities to obtain a military advantage. Wireless communication systems were particularly attractive to the naval and aviation sectors. With the invention of vacuum tube diodes and amplifiers, the radio became a household device with several radio stations popping up broadcasting everything from entertainment to propaganda.

With the advent of solid-state devices in the 1960s, radios became more compact, mobile, energy efficient, and cost-effective. As a result, radios and early

Flexible and Stretchable Medical Devices, First Edition. Edited by Kuniharu Takei.

television sets based on wireless broadcasting became more popular. Wireless communication eventually entered cellular telephony systems, wireless local area networks (WLAN), and Wi-Fi systems. While there are many examples of wireless technology replacing wired networks, there are some examples of the inverse phenomenon. For example, the early wireless television broadcast systems were replaced by high-quality wired cable networks, but satellite radio stations meant that wireless systems regained dominance in the television segment. Direct device-to-satellite communication has also enabled key technologies, such as global positioning systems (GPS) for navigation, location services, and satellite phones. With the abundance of applications using electromagnetic waves simultaneously, the electromagnetic spectrum has been divided into multiple bands and the spectrum has become a valued "resource" with usage rights being routinely traded among companies. The latest research and development in wireless systems aims at developing wireless power transmission links. In this chapter, we will discuss the basic components of a wireless system and ways of obtaining flexible and stretchable versions of these components.

10.2 The Basics of Wireless Systems

10.2.1 Wireless Systems

Complete wireless systems include the circuit controlling the input signal, the antenna generating electromagnetic radiation, the antenna receiving the electromagnetic radiation, and the circuit processing the output. While this might seem straightforward, understanding the nuances of both transceiving circuits and antennas has demanded more than a hundred years of innovation and design optimization in each field. To understand these nuances, let us take the office Wi-Fi network as an example. Many portable devices connect to a single Wi-Fi node with fixed ranges. These nodes need to be established as an array to cover the entire office space. In theory, the coverage provided by these nodal points is illustrated as a hexagonal region centered at the nodes, with the nodes arranged in a hexagonal lattice. While this may be true for flat and unobstructed terrain (e.g., cellular towers in a field), inside buildings where Wi-Fi routers are placed based on space availability, efficiency is limited by line-of-sight propagation, shadowing, and number of users. (Devices automatically connect to the best Wi-Fi router in terms of signal strength and not physical distance.)

Wireless networks consist of two key components: a circuit for encoding/decoding information and an antenna for transmitting/receiving electromagnetic waves. Circuits have evolved from spark-gap transmitters and vacuum-tube-based diodes to sophisticated silicon complementary metal-oxide semiconductor (CMOS) circuits. These circuits are available in a multitude of configurations, data rates, and frequencies and their use could be optimized by designing application-specific integrated circuits. In most modern communication systems, the circuit is a variation of a superheterodyne radio. The radio frequency signal is received, preamplified within its domain and converted into an intermediate frequency (IF) signal. This IF signal can then be amplified with a high-gain narrow-frequency band array, which is easier to design than a wideband array. The signal is then converted into a baseband signal that can be demodulated or converted into a digital signal using an analog-to-digital converter. With advancements in silicon circuits, the IF signals are now directly converted into digital signals for processing by microprocessors. Hence, functional components, such as mixers, filters, demodulators, and amplifiers, can be implemented using microprocessor software rather than hardware. This configuration, called software-defined radio (SDR), provides more flexibility to the RF designers to change the demodulation, filtration, and amplification parameters dynamically based on the input signal received. In case of transmission, a similar circuit is employed in the reverse order: the baseband signal is modulated, mixed, and amplified in the IF domain and then transmitted using an antenna after further amplification and matching circuits in the radio frequency domain.

Because even basic circuit components, such as resistors, capacitors, inductors, and transistors, behave very differently at high frequencies, they need to be designed accordingly. In fact, even a simple wire can change the impedance offered to a signal with frequency, because of the skin effect and self-inductance. Transistors used in commercial radio frequency circuits can be fabricated using two approaches: field-effect transistors (FETs) or bipolar junction transistors (BJTs). FETs have a capacitive gate, which produces an electrostatic field in the semiconductor channel to modulate the resistance of the channel. Because the current through FETs is dependent on voltage, they are considered to be voltage-controlled devices. Hence, because no current is consumed by the gate terminal to keep the transistor switched on and because of the inherent limit on electrostatic modulation of the channel current (limited subthreshold slope) FETs usually consume less power (i.e., current) and are slower than BJTs. Meanwhile, BJTs have abrupt junctions across which current flows due to an applied potential and the gradient in carrier concentrations. Because the current through BJTs is dependent on the current injected at the base terminal, they are considered to be current-controlled devices. Although both transistors can be incorporated into silicon chips using standard fabrication processes, their monolithic integration with state-of-the-art processor technology nodes is challenging. In any case, because silicon is predominantly used as a substrate for radio frequency circuit fabrication, the flexing and stretching of these circuits depend on the flexing and stretching of the host substrate. In the next sections, we will investigate ways of obtaining flexible and stretchable silicon-based circuits.

10.2.2 Antennas

Antennas are usually passive metallic structures used for radiating or capturing electromagnetic energy of a certain frequency. Antennas range from being a simple wire to comprising complicated fractal patterns. In general, antennas have an input signal pin, which is connected to a transmitter circuit to obtain the signal to be radiated, and grounding pins for reference. Maxwell's equations explain how a simple wire can create electromagnetic waves. Consider a metallic wire

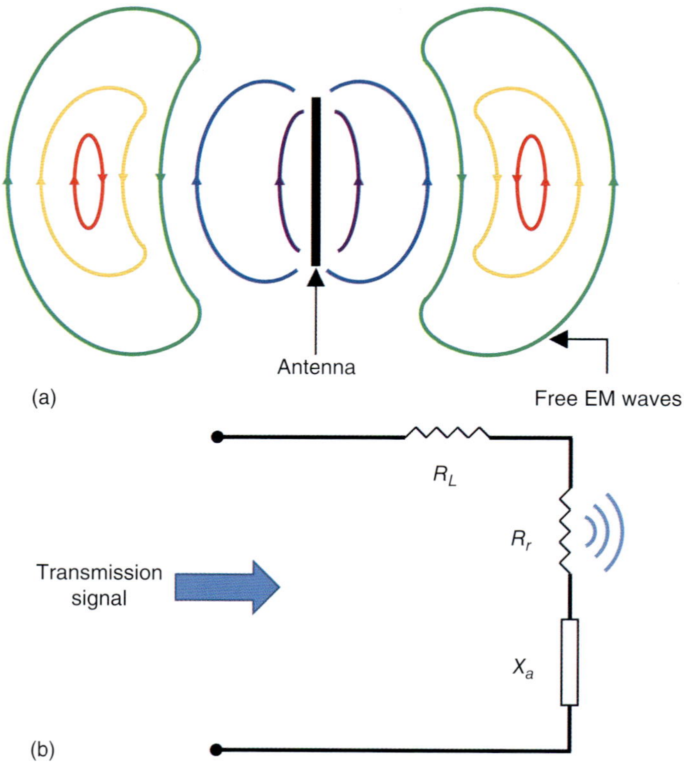

Figure 10.1 (a) Generation of electromagnetic waves in free space from an antenna. (b) The Thevenin-equivalent circuit of an antenna as seen from the side of the transmission signal.

connected to a source of electromotive force (EMF). If the signal is periodically oscillating (AC voltage), the charges in the wire will oscillate at the same frequency. This oscillation leads to an acceleration of electrons, which creates an accelerating electric field. According to Maxwell's equations, an accelerating electric field produces a magnetic field and an accelerating magnetic field produces an electric field. When coupled, these fields travel across free space at the speed of light and are called electromagnetic waves. Quantum mechanics associates chargeless, massless (rest mass = 0) particles called photons with this wavefront. Figure 10.1a illustrates how electromagnetic radiation is produced in this way. Note that an electric field accelerating at a constant or polynomial rate will only produce a transient wavefront while a sinusoidally accelerating field can produce a continuous stream of electromagnetic waves, as long as the source is sustained.

In circuit terms, the antenna and the EMF source can be represented by the Thevenin-equivalent circuit shown in Figure 10.1b. In transmitting mode, the antenna can be represented by the following equation [1]:

$$Z_a = (R_r + R_L) + jX_a,$$

where Z is the total impedance of the antenna, R_r is the radiation resistance of the antenna and is used to represent the power radiated by the antenna, R_L is the loss associated with the conduction and parasitics of the antenna, and X_a is used to describe the imaginary part of the antenna impedance. The antenna will receive maximum power for radiation if it is conjugate-matched to the EMF source. In this case, half the power is transferred to the antenna, where it gets distributed between R_r and R_L. In general, efficient radiation requires that R_r be maximized and R_L be minimized. Because antennas are metallic structures, there are various ways in which they can be made flexible and stretchable. Free-form antennas coupled with free-form radio frequency circuits can produce completely flexible, stretchable wireless systems.

10.2.3 Antenna Parameters

It is essential to quantitatively analyze antennas for their performance in terms of efficiency of radiation and the directions in which they radiate most effectively. This requires the definition of certain performance parameters that can quantitatively predict the performance of an antenna. One of the key performance metrics of an antenna is its radiation pattern. The radiation pattern is the field strength or power density at a given spatial coordinate in the far-field of the antenna. The radiation pattern is generally represented most conveniently in a spherical co-ordinate system with the power density normalized with respect to the maximum power density. The normalized power density is generally reported in decibels (dB), so as to highlight the shape and directionality of side lobes (regions of relatively weak radiation intensity) compared to the main lobes. An antenna with perfectly equal radiation intensity in all directions is called an isotropic radiator. It is an ideal antenna, which cannot be fabricated physically, but is used as a reference for comparing other antennas. Antenna parameters are defined based on the basic concepts of radiation pattern and isotropic antennas:

- Directivity is the ratio the radiation intensity at a point to the radiation intensity of an isotropic antenna at the same point in the far-field. Directivity can be more than 1 if the radiation is more "focused" along a particular direction.
- Gain is the ratio of the radiation intensity at a point to the radiation intensity of an isotropic distribution of input power. Gain of an antenna is, by definition, a dimensionless quantity, but is represented in decibels (dB) as:

  $$G(\text{dB}) = 10\log_{10}[G(\text{dimensionless})].$$

  Gain represents the directivity of the antenna as well as the losses associated with the antenna because gain is calculated with respect to input power. The losses associated with radiation can be represented using an efficiency term, hence, gain and directivity are related as:

  $$G = \eta D,$$

  where, G is the gain, η is the radiation efficiency and D is the directivity. It should be noted that the definition of gain does not include the antenna as seen from the transmission line, hence, reflection losses are not included in the definition. The term η only includes conductor and dielectric losses associated with the antenna.

Because the antenna and the transmission line form a two-port network, the power exchange at the interface can be quantified with the help of the corresponding Scattering parameters (or S-parameters). These parameters are commonly quoted for antennas to quantify reflection losses. In general, for a two-port network, if x represents the input power and y represents the output power, with 1 and 2 representing the port numbers, the output power can be expressed in terms of input power as:

$$\begin{bmatrix} y_1 \\ y_2 \end{bmatrix} = \begin{bmatrix} S_{11} & S_{12} \\ S_{21} & S_{22} \end{bmatrix} \begin{bmatrix} x_1 \\ x_2 \end{bmatrix}.$$

The matrix S is known as the S-parameter matrix and represents the efficiencies of transmission or reflection of power across the network. In case of antenna systems, the parameter S_{11} is commonly reported because it represents the power reflected back to the transmission line as seen in the following linear equation:

$$y_1 = S_{11}x_1 + S_{12}x_2,$$

where y_1 is the power reflected, x_1 is the power input from the transmission line, and x_2 is the power input from the antenna side. In case of a transmitting antenna, x_2 is zero, thus the return loss or reflection loss of the antenna transmission line junction is represented by S_{11}. In general, S_{11} is a dimensionless quantity and is represented in decibels (dB). S_{11} is highly dependent on frequency, thus is routinely reported to define the radiation frequency and bandwidth of an antenna. If S_{11} is 0 dB, all the input power is reflected back to the transmission line, hence no radiation takes place; thus, the radiation frequency is the frequency at which S_{11} is lowest. Also, the bandwidth is defined as the region of frequency where S_{11} is below a certain value (say −10 dB).

10.3 Flexible, Stretchable Circuits

As discussed in the previous section, most radio frequency circuits are made using silicon as a substrate. The transistors may be voltage (FET) or current controlled (BJT) depending on the specific application requirements. In general, FETs consume less power but are slower than BJTs. These factors need to be considered before designing a wireless transceiver circuit. In addition, the behavior of each component is different at different frequencies and a thorough equivalent circuit is advisable for precise modeling of the circuit. FETs are typically preferred for flexible and stretchable wireless systems because power consumption and battery life are key constraints in wearable applications. Circuits made using a silicon substrate and FET transistors can be flexed in many ways. Furthermore, the use of semiconductor channels made from different materials provides the opportunity for innovative fabrication techniques. In this section, an overview of these techniques is presented.

10.3.1 Flexible, Stretchable Silicon Circuits

Single-crystal silicon substrates are generally obtained using the Czochralski process pioneered by Jan Czochralski in 1916. In this process, a single-crystal silicon

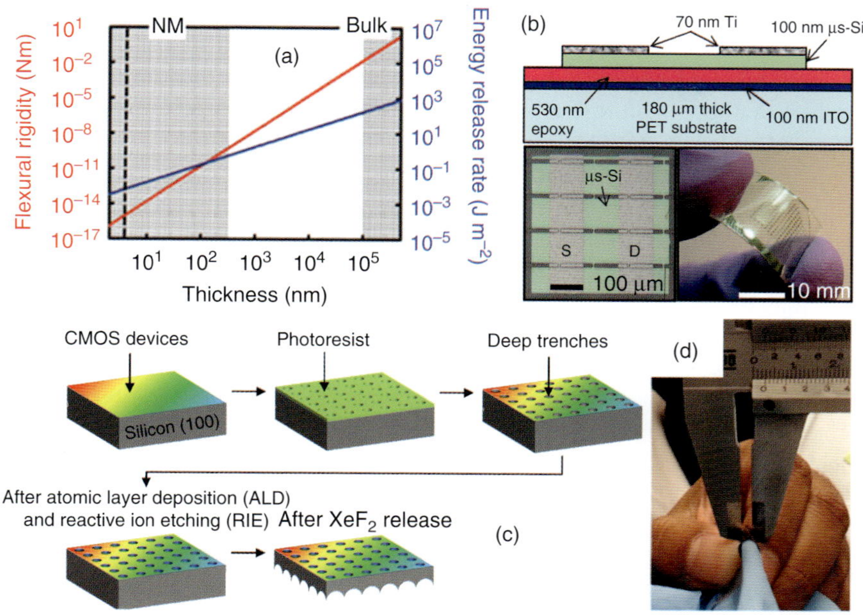

Figure 10.2 (a) The relationship between flexural rigidity of a material with decreasing thickness and energy release rate. (Rogers *et al.* 2011 [2]. Reproduced with permission of Nature Publishing Group.) (b) Structural and optical image of a flexible FET fabricated on silicon nanomembranes using a device last approach. (Menard *et al.* 2005 [3]. Reproduced with permission of AIP Publishing.) (c) Schematic process flow for the "trench-protect-etch-release" (TPER) process. (Hussain and Hussain 2016 [4]. Reproduced with permission of John Wiley & Sons.) (d) Optical image of a flexible FinFET fabricated using the "soft etch back" (SEB) process. (Torres Sevilla 2014 [5]. Reproduced with permission of American Chemical Society.)

seed is used to "pull" a single-crystal ingot from a molten silicon feed. The substrate can be obtained in a number of orientations depending on the orientation of the seed and the direction in which the ingot is cut. Silicon (100) with the (100) plane normal to the substrate surface is by far the most popular silicon substrate in the CMOS industry because of the balance between electron and hole mobilities and low defect densities at the semiconductor–dielectric interface. Silicon wafers are rigid and brittle, thus, the radio frequency circuits made on them are also rigid; however, silicon substrates can be made flexible by reducing their thickness below a certain value (Figure 10.2a) [2, 4]. Using thinned, flexible substrates to make device components conducive for fabrication of flexible radio frequency circuits is a popular approach (Figure 10.2b) [3, 6–14]. The state-of-the-art fabrication processes necessary to produce these thinned silicon wafers requires thousands of individual steps, some of which can be at very high temperatures (>1000 °C). These temperature variations, coupled with inherent stresses in the thin films deposited on the substrates, can cause severe bowing of the prethinned wafer during processing. Hence, for circuits with large transistor counts, standard thickness silicon wafers have to be used first to complete the circuits and be later thinned.

After device fabrication, silicon wafers can be thinned using the trench-protect-etch-release process (TPER) [15–18]. In this process, silicon wafers with prefabricated devices are patterned at predetermined locations and deep trenches in the silicon substrates are made using deep reactive-ion etching (DRIE). The wafers are then subjected to conformal deposition of a protective layer using atomic layer deposition. The protective layer is etched anisotropically using directional reactive ion etching to remove the protective layer from only those faces normal to the surface of the wafer (the top surface and the bottom of the trenches, thus, keeping the walls of the trenches protected). The wafer is then subjected to isotropic etching of silicon using XeF_2 gas. The etching process proceeds at equal speed in all directions, laterally under-cutting the wafer and when the lateral etch holes come together, the top surface of silicon is released. A schematic illustration of this process is shown in Figure 10.2c. Alternatively, silicon wafers may be thinned using the soft etch back (SEB) process [5, 19], which requires that the wafer be flipped post device fabrication and etched using DRIE. Because this process is highly controllable, wafer thickness can be engineered with micrometer precision. Silicon pieces with state-of-the-art FinFETs, flexed using this process are shown in Figure 10.2d. Both of these processes are compatible with state-of-the-art CMOS manufacturing and are meticulously designed to induce no damage to pre-existing devices.

Because in a silicon substrate the silicon atoms are tightly bound in a diamond lattice with no slip planes to absorb any lateral force, the substrate is inherently brittle and does not support stretchability. When single-crystalline silicon is stretched, the silicon atoms move away from each other, slightly lengthening the bonds. Because of the strength of Si—Si bonds, a large applied force causes only a small amount of strain, hence, silicon has a high Young's modulus of 169 GPa [20]. Although the yield strain for silicon is $\sim$1%, and therefore considered to be inherently unstretchable, materials like silicon can be made to stretch and withstand a large amount of deformation strain by micromachining them into specific shapes; for example, lateral spring structures may be periodically introduced into thin films to make them stretchable. The most popular of these spring designs is the "horse-shoe" or "meandering" and "serpentine" structures (Figure 10.3a) [21]. When a lateral force is applied to these structures, they twist out of plane at certain points absorbing the work done in straining as deformation potential. Other spring structures reported in the literature for obtaining stretchable silicon circuits include spiral spring structures (Figure 10.3b) [22], and the leaf arm design (Figure 10.3c) [23]. These structures can be obtained by micromachining silicon substrates after device fabrication to obtain device-first stretchable silicon circuits.

10.3.2 Non-Silicon-Based Channels

While silicon is by far the preferred semiconductor material of choice for circuit manufacturing, several other materials have begun to show promise. One of the most studied alternative channel material for high-frequency electronics is graphene. Graphene is an allotrope of carbon with atomically thin sheets of sp^2-hybridized carbon atoms. Carbon atoms form a two-dimensional (2D)

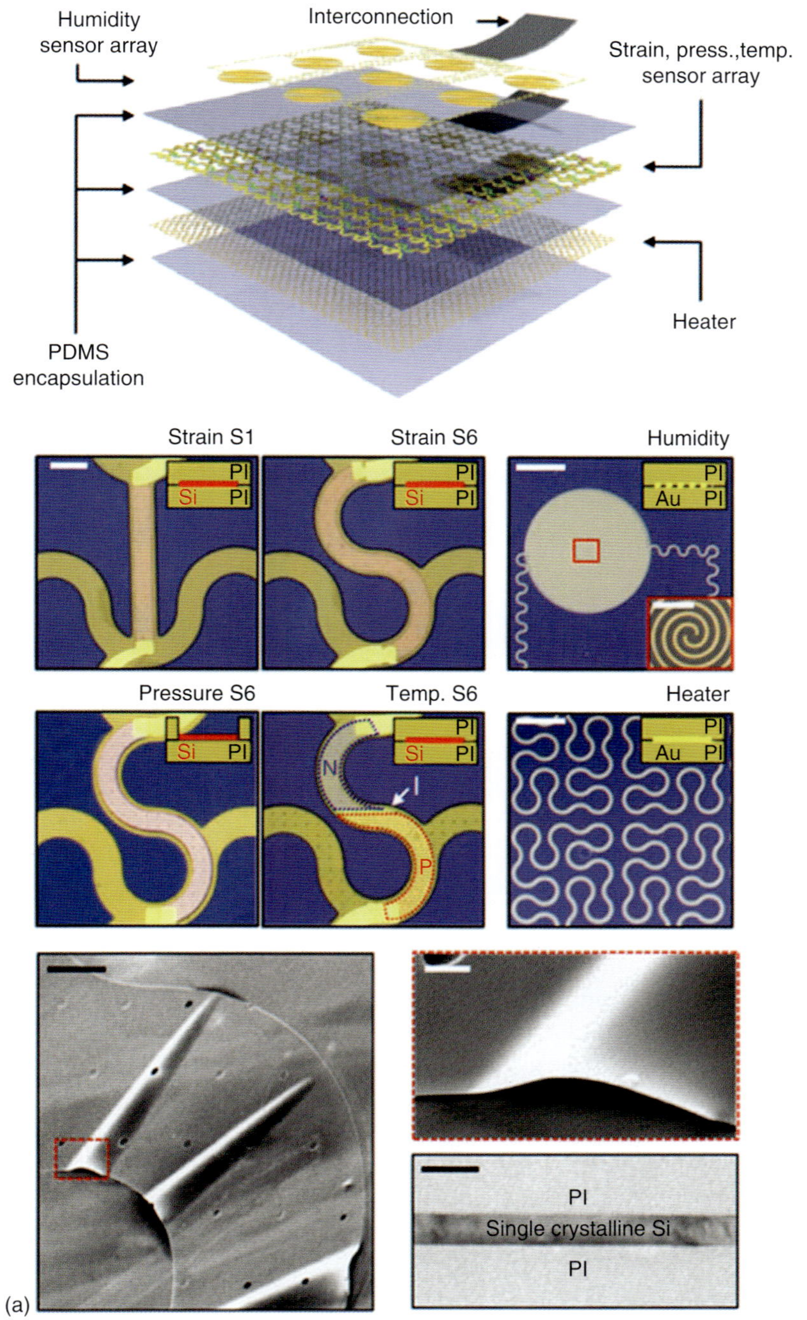

Figure 10.3 (a) Design, optical images, and scanning electron micrograph (SEM) images of stretchable sensors fabricated using lateral spring structures of silicon nanomembranes. (Kim *et al*. 2014 [21]. Reproduced with permission of Nature Publishing Group.) (b) and (c) Optical images of stretchable silicon fabricated using (b) spiral interconnects and (c) the leaf arm design. (Panel (b): Rojas *et al*. 2014 [22]. Reproduced with permission of AIP Publishing. Panel (c): Dinyari *et al*. 2008 [23]. Reproduced with permission of AIP Publishing.)

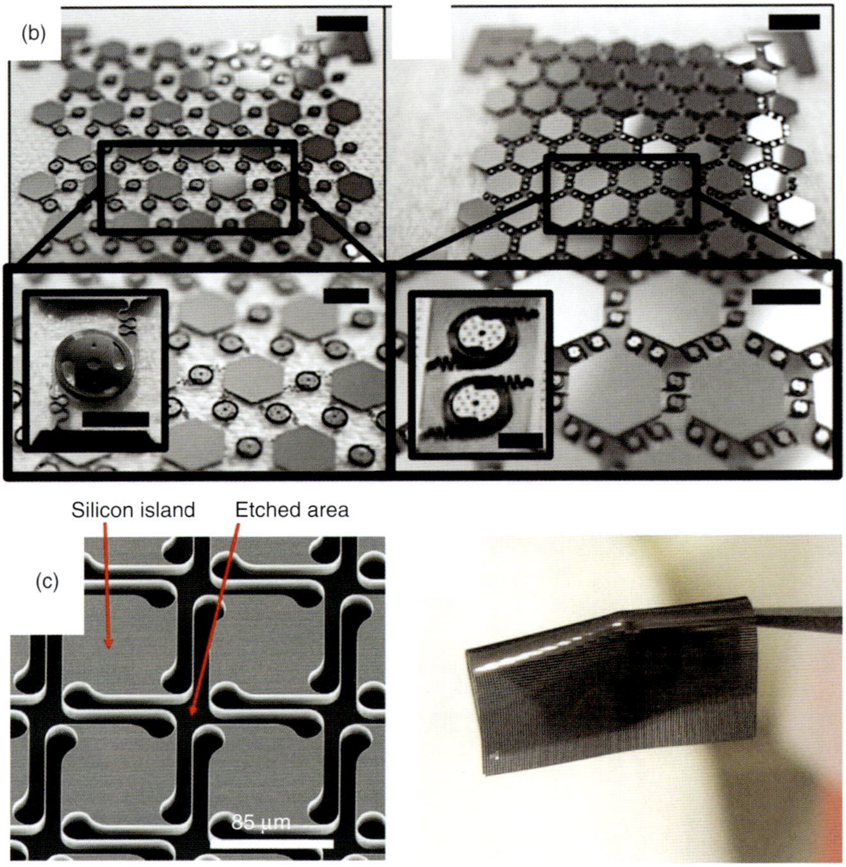

Figure 10.3 (*Continued*)

honeycomb structure with an out-of-plane p_z orbital. When these p_z orbitals hybridize to form a π-band, graphene's peculiar electrical and thermal properties are observed. Graphene has high electron mobility and conductivity, making it an attractive option for transistors with a high switching speed. Hence, several studies have reported the use of graphene to fabricate high-speed radio frequency circuits [24–31]. Carbon nanotube (CNT) is another allotrope of carbon studied widely for radio frequency applications [32–37]. CNTs have a cylindrical structure with walls formed from atomically thin sheets of sp^2-hybridized carbon atoms. Because the bond structure is very similar to that of graphene, CNTs have electronic properties that are similar to those of graphene.

Other materials include 2D atomic crystal structure (2D ACS) materials in the transition metal chalcogenide family (e.g., MoS_2, WS_2, WSe_2) [38–40], oxide-based semiconductors (e.g., ZnO) [41–44], group IV alloys (e.g., SiGe, SiSn, GeSn, etc.) [45–50], and organic and polymeric thin films (e.g., pentacene) [51–53]. Unlike the Czochralski process or the float zone process used for silicon, some of these materials can be used to fabricate thin films at relatively low temperatures, followed by a low thermal budget process of producing a flexible transceiver circuit. Although this enables thin sheets of these materials to be integrated directly onto the flexible substrate, their basic charge transport characteristics are relatively poor compared to silicon. Also, these materials do not have a robust theoretical model for charge transport or charge injection mechanisms, limiting the circuit designer's ability to simulate large-scale circuits using these semiconductors. Furthermore, very few studies have showcased their performance in the radio frequency regime, and subsequently, these materials are yet to be used in commercial radio frequency transceiver circuits.

10.4 Flexible Antennas

Antennas are metallic structures capable of radiating electromagnetic waves at a desired resonant frequency. For antennas to be flexible, they must be made of flexible metallic structures that can conform to nonplanar and asymmetric surfaces. Microstrip patch antennas (MPAs) are low-profile antennas that generally comprise a metallic patch, a microstrip feed line, and a ground plane [54]. They can be fabricated using simple and inexpensive technology, designed according to any surface for conformal attachment, and can be flexible or mechanically rigid and robust based on the specific application. MPAs can be designed using sophisticated photolithography and etching techniques to obtain dimensions up to nanometer precision. This gives designers versatility to design complicated shapes to obtain specific antenna parameters, such as resonant frequency, bandwidth, polarization, and impedance. Further improvements in their design can be brought about by adding switching elements to dynamically varying antenna parameters. One of the major advantages of MPAs is their compatibility with modern CMOS-integrated circuit fabrication, making them the antenna of choice for system-on-package and system-on-chip devices and applications. They are a popular choice in today's technology because they are very robust and reliable over time; however, they have low efficiency and bandwidth (high-quality factor). MPAs were launched by the printed circuit board industry with the aim of using the existing technology and infrastructure to make radiating elements, transmission lines, and integrated circuit interconnects. Early studies reporting MPAs began to emerge in the early 1970s [55], but their low bandwidth precluded them from popularity. During the 1980s, antenna and radio frequency circuit designers began to realize the advantages of using MPAs directly on printed circuit boards. In the past four decades, extensive research has improved their bandwidth, efficiency, and reliability. Accurate modeling techniques afforded by high-speed super-computing clusters have enabled the design of MPAs to be fine-tuned for specific applications.

MPAs are ideal radiating components for fabricating flexible or stretchable wireless systems for devices, such as body-mounted electronics, implanted electronics, and for applications in aviation, military, and satellite technology. They comprise a patterned metallic patch, which connects to the signal using a metal microstrip. If these metallic patches are fabricated on flexible substrates, the resulting patch antenna can be flexible. Several techniques have been reported for fabricating MPAs on various flexible substrates. In this section, some of the key technologies will be discussed.

10.4.1 Micromachined Flexible Antennas

Several methods can be used to micromachine conductive metallic patches onto flexible substrates. These include sputtering, evaporation, electrodeposition, and etching of metallic films on plastic, polymer (e.g., PDMS, polyimide, PEN, PET) or paper substrates. One of the ways of micromachining MPAs is by the use of flexible printed circuit boards (fPCBs). Printed circuit boards, used in the electronics industry for decades, are insulating substrates (often made with glass epoxy) metalized with copper thin films. PCBs are used to mechanically support electronic circuit components and provide electrical conductive paths for interconnects and pads. fPCBs have a thin polyimide base and copper metallization has been introduced for flexible and conformal electronics applications. The thickness of both the insulating base and copper metallization is lower in flexible PCBs to afford overall flexibility. These flexible circuit boards can easily be patterned to fabricate on-board MPAs for any desired set of antenna parameters [56–59]. This method is favorable because the board already supports the desired radio frequency circuit components that are to be connected to the antennas and hence the interconnection between the antenna and the rest of the circuit is very simple.

Flexible MPAs can also be fabricated starting with a silicon substrate base and then releasing a metallic thin film to obtain flexibility [60]. Alternatively, liquid crystal polymers (LCPs) can provide a suitable base for flexible antennas due to their low dielectric constant, low loss tangent and low cost [61, 62]. Flexible MPAs can be made by selectively metalizing a flexible polymer or textile substrate [63–66], or by integrating conductive and nonconductive textiles together [67].

10.4.2 Inkjet-Printed Antennas

Inkjet printers use droplets of ink propelled from a chamber to obtain images on a substrate. Most printers use a piezoelectric drop-on-demand (DOD) technique wherein the ink chamber contains a piezoelectric element that expands upon the application of a voltage and creates a pressure pulse in the fluid to force a droplet out of the nozzle. The process is schematically illustrated in Figure 10.4a. Metallic conductive lines are obtained using specially made conductive inks that use silver or gold nanoparticle dispersions in solvents. The physical properties of these inks, such as viscosity and surface tension, have to be tightly controlled to obtain stable droplet formation using a particular nozzle diameter. The ink is then cured using UV exposure or heating to remove excess solvent and to obtain a continuous conductive layer. The printing process is highly suitable for low-temperature, low-cost and highly scalable manufacturing of a specific patch design on any given flexible substrate. The printed design can be closely controlled and does not require expensive photolithography, laser etching equipment, or a cleanroom environment. Hence, this method is being heavily investigated for its application for flexible antenna fabrication.

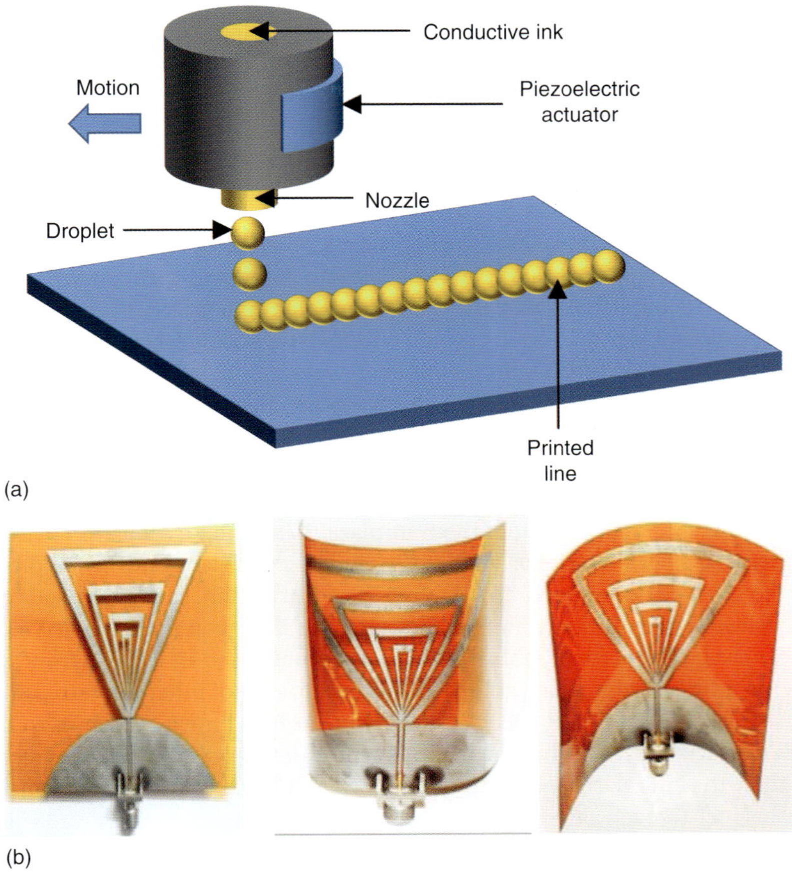

Figure 10.4 (a) Schematic illustration of the inkjet printing process. (b) Optical images of flexible antennas fabricated using inkjet printing on Kapton. (Ahmed *et al.* 2015 [68]. Reprinted with permission from IEEE.)

The versatility afforded by this technique has been used to fabricate antennas on several substrates, including paper [69–71], Kapton (Figure 10.4b) [68], cardboard [72], and textiles [73–75]. These studies report using silver nanoparticle ink with some curing or sintering at 100–120 °C [76]. The inks generally contain 30–60% silver nanoparticles dispersed in an organic solvent with overall viscosity in the centipoise range. While silver-nanoparticle-based inks are the most commonly used, gold-nanoparticle-based inks [77, 78] and CNT-based inks [79] have also been reported. The planar structure obtained using inkjet printing can be folded up to obtain interesting three-dimensional shapes that retain the characteristics of the antennas [80]. However, printed designs have a more limited resolution than do laser-etched or lithography-based designs. Also, porous substrates, such as paper and textiles, absorb the ink droplets, preventing a continuous film of metallic nanoparticles from depositing on the surface. Because this leads to discontinuous and nonconductive lines, a screening layer is typically printed on the textile prior to printing. Also, photo-paper is used instead of regular paper to reduce ink absorption.

10.5 Stretchable Antennas

Skin-mounted electronics must be stretchable because human skin undergoes large amounts of strain (up to 50%) during muscle movement [81]. Hence, it is important to design materials and patterns that can withstand high amounts of strain reversibly. Stretchability can either be an inherent material property, as in the case of polymers and rubbers, or can be obtained through designing and patterning otherwise unstretchable materials, such as metal springs. In the case of polymers, the bulk material is formed from polymer chains that are thousands of monomers long, entangled and connected to each other by crosslinks, weak Van der Waal's interactions, and hydrogen bonds. When a lateral force is applied to the polymer, the polymer chains get displaced by the force because there is no strong chemical interaction to hold them in place. When the force is removed, the polymer snaps back into its original position to maximize its entropy, as dictated by the laws of thermodynamics. For antenna fabrication, there is a need to reversibly stretch metallic thin films while retaining their conductive behavior during stretching. However, metal thin films commonly used in the electronics industry, including copper, silver, gold, and aluminum, are not inherently stretchable. These materials form polycrystalline thin films, which have a regular crystal structure in individual grains, but these grains are randomly oriented with respect to each other. The boundaries of these grains are weakly bonded, hence, the grains slip with respect to each other when a lateral force is applied to the thin film. After a certain strain (usually <10%), the grains separate causing the metallic film to crack and lose conductivity. Thus, metal thin films need to be patterned to obtain stretchability. Hence, stretchability by material and design are the two main approaches taken by the electronics community for fabricating stretchable antennas. In this section, some of the processes and materials associated with these approaches will be discussed.

10.5.1 Material Stretchability

Inherently stretchable materials, such as rubbers, are typically nonconducting and therefore not suitable for radiating electromagnetic waves directly. Instead, one of the key ways of making polymeric materials conductive is to insert conductive particles, nanowires, or flakes into the stretchable polymer matrix. In these polymer composites, conduction of electrons takes place through the continuous conductive paths made by adjoining conductive elements. According to the percolation theory, conductivity strongly depends on the particle volume fraction [82, 83]: when the particle volume fraction is below the percolation limit, the polymer remains insulating because the conductive particles are too sparsely distributed to conduct, but as it surpasses the limit, the polymer becomes conductive as conductive pathways form from one end of the polymer composite to another. After the percolation limit is crossed, further increase in particle volume fraction does not significantly influence conductivity. In general, the percolation limit is affected by several factors including the size and composition of the conductive particles, the chemical composition of the polymer matrix, and the deposition method [84–86].

These conductive polymers can be used to obtain stretchable antennas, as demonstrated using composites of silver nanoparticles with styrene-butadiene-styrene [87], and silver nanowires with PDMS (Figure 10.5a) [88, 91]. In 2015, Li *et al.* demonstrated stretchable antennas using electrically conductive adhesives (composites with silver nanoparticles as conductive particles) [92]. In addition to metallic particles, liquid metals can be embedded in polymer structures to obtain stretchable conductors. Mercury and NaK (sodium potassium alloy) are commonly known metals that are liquid at room temperature; however, due to their toxicity and reactivity, they are not proposed for use in stretchable electronics applications. Recently, a eutectic alloy of gallium and indium (called EGaIn), has been demonstrated to be liquid at room temperature [93]. In 2010, Kubo *et al.* demonstrated a stretchable antenna using EGaIn as the conductive material encapsulated in PDMS and EcoFlex

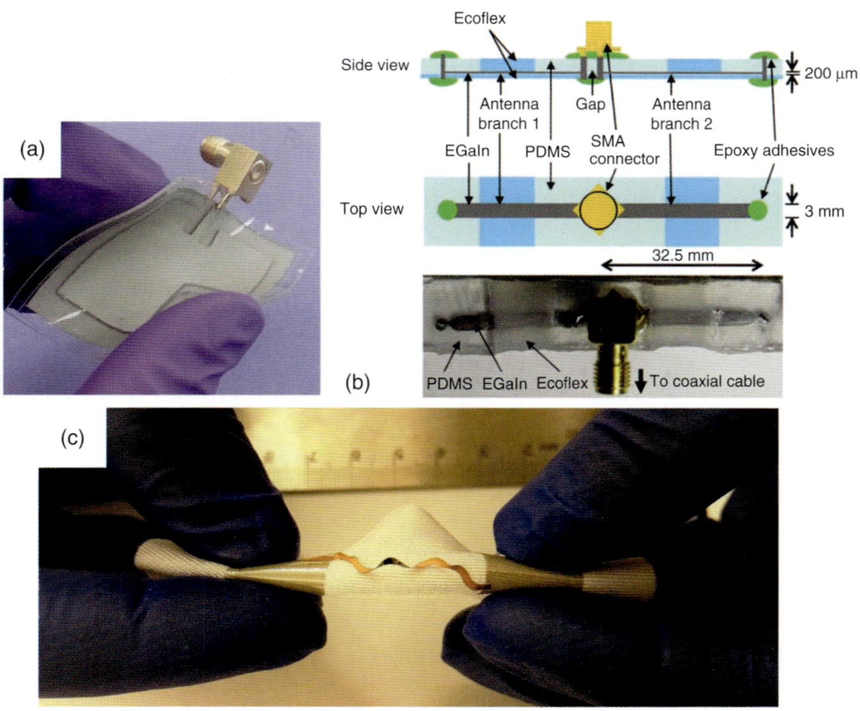

Figure 10.5 (a) Stretchable antenna fabricated using Ag nanowire and PDMS composite. (Song *et al.* 2014 [88]. Reproduced with permission of American Chemical Society.) (b) Design and optical image of a stretchable antenna fabricated using liquid metal EGaIn as the conductive material. (Kubo *et al.* 2010 [89]. Reproduced with permission of John Wiley & Sons.) (c) Optical image of a stretchable metal–polymer bilayer creating an antenna designed for constant frequency communication during straining. (Hussain *et al.* 2015 [90]. Reproduced with permission of John Wiley & Sons.)

substrates (Figure 10.5b) [89]. In addition, a ternary metal alloy formed with gallium, indium, and tin (called Galinstan), which is liquid at room temperature, has been used to fabricate stretchable antennas, mostly utilizing PDMS as the encapsulation polymer [94–97].

10.5.2 Design Stretchability

Although polymer composites and polymer-embedded stretchable antennas can radiate electromagnetic waves continuously during the application of lateral or biaxial strain, the frequency of these radiations invariably shifts due to the deformation of the antenna. Because the resonant frequency of an antenna strongly depends on the length of the antenna, it is expected that straining a stretchable antenna will distort its initial resonant frequency. While this can be useful in certain niche applications, such as for wireless strain sensing, it is highly undesirable for normal communication that involves a fixed frequency transceiver. Indeed, for a stretchable antenna that can communicate at constant frequency irrespective of the strain, the stretchability cannot be obtained using inherent material stretchability. In this section, we will discuss the use of spring structures to obtain stretchable antennas. Lateral spring structures, designed and patterned using micromachining have been demonstrated in the past as stretchable interconnects [98, 99]. When a lateral force is applied to a free-standing lateral spring, the spring elongates and twists out of plane at certain points. The deformation potential associated with this twisting action absorbs the work done in straining, thus, reducing the strain on the metal thin film itself, preventing the metal thin film from physically elongating during the elongation of the lateral spring. However, the spring structure must be free-standing to allow the twisting to take place, otherwise, if the metal thin film is patterned in the form of horseshoe springs on a continuous polymeric substrate, for example, the elongation of the substrate will cause the metal thin film to elongate, negating the potential benefits of the spring design [100].

In 2015, Hussain *et al.* demonstrated a stretchable antenna based on the horseshoe lateral spring structure (Figure 10.5c) [90]. The antenna was fabricated using electrochemically deposited copper as a conductive material and a low-stress polyimide layer as the support. Both the polyimide layer and the copper were patterned in the lateral spring structure and released to obtain a free-standing antenna. Key antenna parameters, such as resonant frequency, gain, bandwidth, and radiation pattern, were shown to remain constant with strain. This process can be used to obtain stretchable antennas with various lateral spring designs and strain-invariant performance parameters. As discussed in Section 2.3, S_{11} is a key antenna parameter that represents the losses associated with the transmission line–antenna junction. The measured S_{11} of the fabricated antenna for the stretched and unstretched case shows virtually no change in the pattern (Figure 10.6a). The antenna is said to "resonate" at a particular frequency if the S_{11} at that frequency is sufficiently low. In the case of the stretchable antenna reported, which was designed to resonate at 2.45 GHz, S_{11} was observed to sharply decline at this frequency for both stretched and unstretched cases. Thus, the resonant frequency has been maintained. Further, the bandwidth was defined

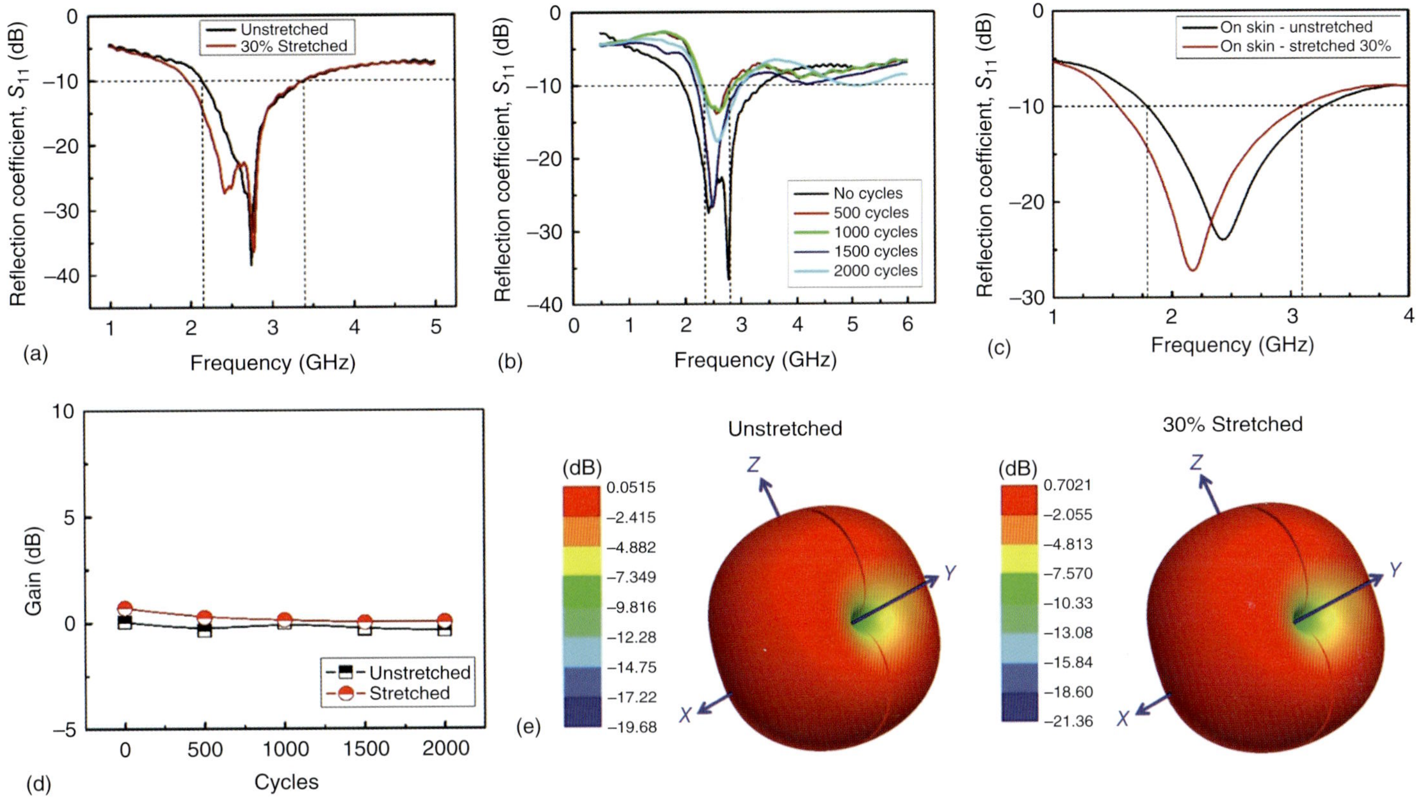

Figure 10.6 (a–c) S_{11} for stretchable antenna measured under various conditions. (d) Variation of gain of the antenna with stretching cycles. (e) Radiation pattern of the stretchable antenna for stretched and unstretched conditions. (Hussain *et al.* 2015 [90]. Reproduced with permission of John Wiley & Sons.)

as the region of frequency where S_{11} is less than 10 dB (shown with a dotted line in Figure 10.6a). This region, and hence the bandwidth, can also be observed to be reasonably invariant with strain. The S_{11} reported for stretching cycles (Figure 10.6b) also shows that the resonant frequency and bandwidth remain invariant. In case of mounting the antenna on a human subject (Figure 10.6c), the resonant frequency shows a slight shift on stretching, which can be attributed to variation in contact impedance due to straining while being worn on the skin. However, because S_{11} of the stretched antenna at the design frequency is still very low (~ -15 dB), the antenna essentially radiates most of the supplied power at the design frequency and can be used for single frequency communication. For the gain of the antenna, the authors report a value of close to 0 dB at maximum point (Figure 10.6d). Because the radiation pattern is that of an omnidirectional antenna (Figure 10.6e), the power is distributed evenly across most of the solid angle around the antenna. Hence, this gain is expected as 0 dB (gain of 1 in dimensionless terms) which means an isotropic antenna with the same input power would radiate with the same intensity in the given direction.

10.6 Future Outlook

The field of flexible and stretchable wireless systems continues to steadily advance. Recent breakthroughs in processing techniques have enabled the circuits and the antennas to be made flexible and stretchable. While these are promising advances, many more challenges need to be resolved before a truly flexible and stretchable wireless communication system can be implemented. Radio frequency circuits and antenna are the key building blocks of any communication system and developing flexible and stretchable versions of these is essential and the right step forward. However, in the near future, it is necessary to use these advances and develop complete wireless systems by interconnecting them. Moreover, for a complete standalone system, we need both a flexible battery and a flexible memory. Although flexible memories have been reported in the literature [101], the field has only just taken off, leaving room for many more advances in memory technology that are needed to reach a flexible, stretchable gigabyte memory. Another key component of the wireless system is the battery, which has become a limiting factor for performance specifications in modern devices. Although silicon processor technology has advanced tremendously paving way for reliable and low power radio frequency transistors to be fabricated, electromagnetic radiation consumes a lot of power itself. Furthermore, the power radiated into free space by wireless communication systems is delivered by battery, placing higher demands on battery lifetime. Several studies have reported flexible and stretchable batteries [98, 102], but their performance is insufficient to be comparable to solid-state batteries. To realize standalone flexible, stretchable wireless systems, continued advancements in flexible, stretchable radio frequency circuits, antennas, memories, and batteries along with advancements in their interconnection methodologies are needed.

References

1 Balanis, C.A. (2005) *Antenna Theory: Analysis and Design*, John Wiley & Sons, Inc.
2 Rogers, J.A., Lagally, M.G., and Nuzzo, R.G. (2011) *Nature*, **477**, 45.
3 Menard, E., Nuzzo, R.G., and Rogers, J.A. (2005) *Appl. Phys. Lett.*, **86**, 093507.
4 Hussain, A.M. and Hussain, M.M. (2016) *Adv. Mater.*, **28**, 4219.
5 Torres Sevilla, G.A., Ghoneim, M.T., Fahad, H., Rojas, J.P., Hussain, A.M., and Hussain, M.M. (2014) *ACS Nano*, **8**, 9850.
6 Yuan, H.-C., Qin, G., Celler, G.K., and Ma, Z. (2009) *Appl. Phys. Lett.*, **95**, 043109.
7 Sun, L., Qin, G., Huang, H., Zhou, H., Behdad, N., Zhou, W., and Ma, Z. (2010) *Appl. Phys. Lett.*, **96**, 013509.
8 Yuan, H.-C. and Ma, Z. (2006) *Appl. Phys. Lett.*, **89**, 212105.
9 Xu, X., Subbaraman, H., Hosseini, A., Lin, C.-Y., Kwong, D., and Chen, R.T. (2012) *Opt. Lett.*, **37**, 1020.
10 Yang, Y., Hwang, Y., Cho, H.A., Song, J.-H., Park, S.-J., Rogers, J.A., and Ko, H.C. (2011) *Small*, **7**, 484.
11 Tilke, A., Rotter, M., Blick, R.H., Lorenz, H., and Kotthaus, J.P. (2000) *Appl. Phys. Lett.*, **77**, 558.
12 Menard, E., Lee, K.J., Khang, D.-Y., Nuzzo, R.G., and Rogers, J.A. (2004) *Appl. Phys. Lett.*, **84**, 5398.
13 Jong-Hyun, A., Hoon-Sik, K., Keon Jae, L., Zhengtao, Z., Menard, E., Nuzzo, R.G., and Rogers, J.A. (2006) *IEEE Electron Device Lett.*, **27**, 460.
14 Zhu, Z.-T., Menard, E., Hurley, K., Nuzzo, R.G., and Rogers, J.A. (2005) *Appl. Phys. Lett.*, **86**, 133507.
15 Rojas, J.P., Torres Sevilla, G.A., Ghoneim, M.T., Inayat, S.B., Ahmed, S.M., Hussain, A.M., and Hussain, M.M. (2014) *ACS Nano*, **8**, 1468.
16 Sevilla, G.A.T., Inayat, S.B., Rojas, J.P., Hussain, A.M., and Hussain, M.M. (2013) *Small*, **9**, 3916.
17 Ghoneim, M.T., Fahad, H.M., Hussain, A.M., Rojas, J.P., Torres Sevilla, G.A., Alfaraj, N., Lizardo, E.B., and Hussain, M.M. (2015) *AIP Adv.*, **5**, 127115.
18 Alfaraj, N., Hussain, A.M., Torres Sevilla, G.A., Ghoneim, M.T., Rojas, J.P., Aljedaani, A.B., and Hussain, M.M. (2015) *Appl. Phys. Lett.*, **107**, 174101.
19 Torres Sevilla, G.A., Almuslem, A.S., Gumus, A., Hussain, A.M., Cruz, M.E., and Hussain, M.M. (2016) *Appl. Phys. Lett.*, **108**, 094102.
20 Hopcroft, M.A., Nix, W.D., and Kenny, T.W. (2010) *J. Microelectromech. Syst.*, **19**, 229.
21 Kim, J., Lee, M., Shim, H.J., Ghaffari, R., Cho, H.R., Son, D., Jung, Y.H., Soh, M., Choi, C., Jung, S., Chu, K., Jeon, D., Lee, S.-T., Kim, J.H., Choi, S.H., Hyeon, T., and Kim, D.-H. (2014) *Nat. Commun.*, **5**, 5747.
22 Rojas, J.P., Arevalo, A., Foulds, I.G., and Hussain, M.M. (2014) *Appl. Phys. Lett.*, **105**, 154101.
23 Dinyari, R., Rim, S.-B., Huang, K., Catrysse, P.B., and Peumans, P. (2008) *Appl. Phys. Lett.*, **92**, 091114.

24 Lin, Y.-M., Valdes-Garcia, A., Han, S.-J., Farmer, D.B., Meric, I., Sun, Y., Wu, Y., Dimitrakopoulos, C., Grill, A., Avouris, P., and Jenkins, K.A. (2011) *Science*, **332**, 1294.

25 Moon, J.S., Curtis, D., Hu, M., Wong, D., McGuire, C., Campbell, P.M., Jernigan, G., Tedesco, J.L., VanMil, B., Myers-Ward, R., Eddy, C., and Gaskill, D.K. (2009) *IEEE Electron Device Lett.*, **30**, 650.

26 Wang, H., Hsu, A., Wu, J., Kong, J., and Palacios, T. (2010) *IEEE Electron Device Lett.*, **31**, 906.

27 Wu, Y., Jenkins, K.A., Valdes-Garcia, A., Farmer, D.B., Zhu, Y., Bol, A.A., Dimitrakopoulos, C., Zhu, W., Xia, F., Avouris, P., and Lin, Y.-M. (2012) *Nano Lett.*, **12**, 3062.

28 Moon, J.S., Curtis, D., Zehnder, D., Kim, S., Gaskill, D.K., Jernigan, G.G., Myers-Ward, R.L., Eddy, C.R., Campbell, P.M., Lee, K.M., and Asbeck, P. (2011) *IEEE Electron Device Lett.*, **32**, 270.

29 Badmaev, A., Che, Y., Li, Z., Wang, C., and Zhou, C. (2012) *ACS Nano*, **6**, 3371.

30 Lin, Y.-M., Dimitrakopoulos, C., Jenkins, K.A., Farmer, D.B., Chiu, H.-Y., Grill, A., and Avouris, P. (2010) *Science*, **327**, 662.

31 Han, S.-J., Jenkins, K.A., Valdes Garcia, A., Franklin, A.D., Bol, A.A., and Haensch, W. (2011) *Nano Lett.*, **11**, 3690.

32 Koswatta, S.O., Valdes-Garcia, A., Steiner, M.B., Lin, Y.M., and Avouris, P. (2011) *IEEE Trans. Microwave Theory Tech.*, **59**, 2739.

33 Rutherglen, C. and Burke, P. (2007) *Nano Lett.*, **7**, 3296.

34 Min, Z., Xiao, H., Chan, P.C.H., Qi, L., and Tang, Z.K. (2006) *IEEE Electron Device Lett.*, **27**, 668.

35 Happy, H., Haddadi, K., Theron, D., Lasri, T., and Dambrine, G. (2014) *IEEE Microwave Mag.*, **15**, 30.

36 Wang, D., Yu, Z., McKernan, S., and Burke, P.J. (2007) *IEEE Trans. Nanotechnol.*, **6**, 400.

37 Akinwande, D., Close, G.F., and Wong, H.S.P. (2006) *IEEE Trans. Nanotechnol.*, **5**, 599.

38 Radisavljevic, B., Whitwick, M.B., and Kis, A. (2011) *ACS Nano*, **5**, 9934.

39 Wang, H., Yu, L., Lee, Y.-H., Shi, Y., Hsu, A., Chin, M.L., Li, L.-J., Dubey, M., Kong, J., and Palacios, T. (2012) *Nano Lett.*, **12**, 4674.

40 Cheng, R., Jiang, S., Chen, Y., Liu, Y., Weiss, N., Cheng, H.-C., Wu, H., Huang, Y., and Duan, X. (2014) *Nat. Commun.*, **5**, 5143.

41 Hanna, A.N., Ghoneim, M.T., Bahabry, R.R., Hussain, A.M., and Hussain, M.M. (2013) *Appl. Phys. Lett.*, **103**, 224101.

42 Hanna, A.N., Ghoneim, M.T., Bahabry, R.R., Hussain, A.M., Fahad, H.M., and Hussain, M.M. (2014) *IEEE Trans. Electron Devices*, **61**, 3223.

43 Hanna, A.N., Hussain, A.M., Ghoneim, M.T., Rojas, J.P., Torres Sevilla, G.A., and Hussain, M.M. (2015) *ECS Trans.*, **67**, 191.

44 Hanna, A.N., Hussain, A.M., Omran, H., Alsharif, S., Salama, K.N., and Hussain, M.M. (2016) *IEEE Electron Device Lett.*, **37**, 193.

45 Hussain, A.M., Fahad, H.M., Singh, N., Sevilla, G.A.T., Schwingenschlögl, U., and Hussain, M.M. (2014) *Phys. Status Solidi RRL*, **8**, 332.

46 Hussain, A.M., Singh, N., Fahad, H., Rader, K., Schwingenschlögl, U., and Hussain, M. (2014) *J. Appl. Phys.*, **116**, 224506.
47 Hussain, A.M., Wehbe, N., and Hussain, M.M. (2015) *Appl. Phys. Lett.*, **107**, 082111.
48 Floyd, B.A., Reynolds, S.K., Pfeiffer, U.R., Zwick, T., Beukema, T., and Gaucher, B. (2005) *IEEE J. Solid-State Circuits*, **40**, 156.
49 Racanelli, M. and Kempf, P. (2005) *IEEE Trans. Electron Devices*, **52**, 1259.
50 Russer, P. (1998) *IEEE Trans. Microwave Theory Tech.*, **46**, 590.
51 Baude, P.F., Ender, D.A., Haase, M.A., Kelley, T.W., Muyres, D.V., and Theiss, S.D. (2003) *Appl. Phys. Lett.*, **82**, 3964.
52 Davis, M.F., Sutono, A., Sang-Woong, Y., Mandal, S., Bushyager, M., Chang-Ho, L., Lim, K., Pinel, S., Maeng, M., Obatoyinbo, A., Chakraborty, S., Laskar, J., Tentzeris, E.M., Nonaka, T., and Tummala, R.R. (2002) *IEEE Trans. Adv. Packag.*, **25**, 136.
53 Schön, J.H. and Kloc, C. (2001) *Appl. Phys. Lett.*, **79**, 4043.
54 Huang, H. (2013) *IEEE Sens. J.*, **13**, 3865.
55 Howell, J. (1975) *IEEE Trans. Antennas Propag.*, **23**, 90.
56 Chia-Ching, L., Gwo-Yun, L., and Kin-Lu, W. (2003) *Electron. Lett*, **39**, 1302.
57 Alrawashdeh, R., Huang, Y., and Cao, P. (2013) *Electron. Lett*, **49**, 1515.
58 Yoon, H.K., Kang, W.S., Yoon, Y.J., and Lee, C.-H. (2007) A CPW-fed flexible monopole antenna for UWB systems. Presented at 2007 IEEE Antennas and Propagation Society International Symposium, June 9–15, 2007.
59 Yoon, H.K., Yoon, Y.J., Kim, H., and Lee, C.H. (2011) *IET Microwaves Antennas Propag.*, **5**, 1463.
60 Lin, C.P., Chang, C.H., Cheng, Y.T., and Jou, C.F. (2011) *IEEE Antennas Wirel. Propag. Lett.*, **10**, 1108.
61 DeJean, G., Bairavasubramanian, R., Thompson, D., Ponchak, G.E., Tentzeris, M.M., and Papapolymerou, J. (2005) *IEEE Antennas Wirel. Propag. Lett.*, **4**, 22.
62 Abbasi, Q.H., Rehman, M.U., Yang, X., Alomainy, A., Qaraqe, K., and Serpedin, E. (2013) *IEEE Antennas Wirel. Propag. Lett.*, **12**, 1606.
63 Trajkovikj, J., Zurcher, J.-F., and Skrivervik, A.K. (2012) Soft and flexible antennas on permittivity adjustable PDMS substrates. Presented at Antennas and Propagation Conference (LAPC), 2012 Loughborough, November, 12–13 2012.
64 Siegel, A.C., Phillips, S.T., Dickey, M.D., Lu, N., Suo, Z., and Whitesides, G.M. (2010) *Adv. Funct. Mater.*, **20**, 28.
65 Hertleer, C., Langenhove, L.V., and Rogier, H. (2008) *Adv. Sci. Technol.*, **60**, 64.
66 Marnat, L. and Shamim, A. (2012) Liquid crystal polymer (LCP) based antenna for flexible system on package (SoP) applications. Presented at Antenna Technology and Applied Electromagnetics (ANTEM), 2012 15th International Symposium on, June 25–28, 2012.
67 Hertleer, C., Tronquo, A., Rogier, H., Vallozzi, L., and Langenhove, L.V. (2007) *IEEE Antennas Wirel. Propag. Lett.*, **6**, 392.
68 Ahmed, S., Tahir, F.A., Shamim, A., and Cheema, H.M. (2015) *IEEE Antennas Wirel. Propag. Lett.*, **14**, 1802.

69 Rida, A., Yang, L., Vyas, R., and Tentzeris, M.M. (2009) *IEEE Antennas Propag. Mag.*, **51**, 13.
70 Mansour, A.M., Shehata, N., Hamza, B.M., and Rizk, M.R.M. (2015) *Int. J. Antennas Propag.*, **2015**, 6.
71 Kim, S., Ren, Y.J., Lee, H., Rida, A., Nikolaou, S., and Tentzeris, M.M. (2012) *IEEE Antennas Wirel. Propag. Lett.*, **11**, 663.
72 Saghlatoon, H., Björninen, T., Sydänheimo, L., Tentzeris, M.M., and Ukkonen, L. (2015) *IEEE Antennas Wirel. Propag. Lett.*, **14**, 325.
73 Whittow, W.G., Chauraya, A., Vardaxoglou, J.C., Li, Y., Torah, R., Yang, K., Beeby, S., and Tudor, J. (2014) *IEEE Antennas Wirel. Propag. Lett.*, **13**, 71.
74 Chauraya, A., Whittow, W.G., Vardaxoglou, J.C., Li, Y., Torah, R., Yang, K., Beeby, S., and Tudor, J. (2013) *IET Microwaves Antennas Propag.*, **7**, 760.
75 Li, Y., Torah, R., Beeby, S., and Tudor, J. (2015) *Electron. Lett*, **51**, 1306.
76 Wunscher, S., Abbel, R., Perelaer, J., and Schubert, U.S. (2014) *J. Mater. Chem. C*, **2**, 10232.
77 Khan, Y., Pavinatto, F.J., Lin, M.C., Liao, A., Swisher, S.L., Mann, K., Subramanian, V., Maharbiz, M.M., and Arias, A.C. (2016) *Adv. Funct. Mater.*, **26**, 1004.
78 Huang, D., Liao, F., Molesa, S., Redinger, D., and Subramanian, V. (2003) *J. Electrochem. Soc.*, **150**, G412.
79 Dragoman, M., Flahaut, E., Dragoman, D., Ahmad, M.A., and Plana, R. (2009) *Nanotechnology*, **20**, 375203.
80 Kimionis, J., Isakov, M., Koh, B.S., Georgiadis, A., and Tentzeris, M.M. (2015) *IEEE Trans. Microwave Theory Tech.*, **63**, 4521.
81 Pawlaczyk, M., Lelonkiewicz, M., and Wieczorowski, M. (2013) *Adv. Dermatol. Allergol.*, **30**, 302.
82 Stauffer, D. and Aharony, A. (1994) *Introduction To Percolation Theory*, Taylor & Francis.
83 Essam, J.W. (1980) *Rep. Prog. Phys.*, **43**, 833.
84 Li, J. and Kim, J.-K. (2007) *Compos. Sci. Technol.*, **67**, 2114.
85 Sandler, J.K.W., Kirk, J.E., Kinloch, I.A., Shaffer, M.S.P., and Windle, A.H. (2003) *Polymer*, **44**, 5893.
86 Yao, S. and Zhu, Y. (2015) *Adv. Mater.*, **27**, 1480.
87 Park, M., Im, J., Shin, M., Min, Y., Park, J., Cho, H., Park, S., Shim, M.-B., Jeon, S., Chung, D.-Y., Bae, J., Park, J., Jeong, U., and Kim, K. (2012) *Nat. Nanotechnol.*, **7**, 803.
88 Song, L., Myers, A.C., Adams, J.J., and Zhu, Y. (2014) *ACS Appl. Mater. Interfaces*, **6**, 4248.
89 Kubo, M., Li, X., Kim, C., Hashimoto, M., Wiley, B.J., Ham, D., and Whitesides, G.M. (2010) *Adv. Mater.*, **22**, 2749.
90 Hussain, A.M., Ghaffar, F.A., Park, S.I., Rogers, J.A., Shamim, A., and Hussain, M.M. (2015) *Adv. Funct. Mater.*, **25**, 6565.
91 Rai, T., Dantes, P., Bahreyni, B., and Kim, W.S. (2013) *IEEE Electron Device Lett.*, **34**, 544.
92 Li, Z., Le, T., Wu, Z., Yao, Y., Li, L., Tentzeris, M., Moon, K.-S., and Wong, C.P. (2015) *Adv. Funct. Mater.*, **25**, 464.

93 Dickey, M.D., Chiechi, R.C., Larsen, R.J., Weiss, E.A., Weitz, D.A., and Whitesides, G.M. (2008) *Adv. Funct. Mater.*, **18**, 1097.

94 Jeong, S., Hjort, K., and Wu, Z. (2014) *Sensors*, **14**, 16311.

95 Cheng, S. and Wu, Z. (2010) *Lab Chip*, **10**, 3227.

96 Mazlouman, S.J., Jiang, X.J., Mahanfar, A.N., Menon, C., and Vaughan, R.G. (2011) *IEEE Trans. Antennas Propag.*, **59**, 4406.

97 Wu, Z., Hjort, K., and Jeong, S.H. (2015) *Proc. IEEE*, **103**, 1211.

98 Xu, S., Zhang, Y., Cho, J., Lee, J., Huang, X., Jia, L., Fan, J.A., Su, Y., Su, J., Zhang, H., Cheng, H., Lu, B., Yu, C., Chuang, C., Kim, T.-i., Song, T., Shigeta, K., Kang, S., Dagdeviren, C., Petrov, I., Braun, P.V., Huang, Y., Paik, U., and Rogers, J.A. (2013) *Nat. Commun.*, **4**, 1543.

99 Hussain, A.M., Lizardo, E.B., Torres Sevilla, G.A., Nassar, J.M., and Hussain, M.M. (2015) *Adv. Healthc. Mater.*, **4**, 665.

100 Arriola, A., Sancho, J.I., Brebels, S., Gonzalez, M., and Raedt, W.D. (2011) *IET Microwaves Antennas Propag.*, **5**, 852.

101 Ghoneim, M. and Hussain, M. (2015) *Electronics*, **4**, 424.

102 Kutbee, A.T., Ghoneim, M.T., Ahmad, S.M., and Hussain, M.M. (2016) *IEEE Trans. Nanotechnol.*, **15**, 402.

11

Conductive Nanosheets for Ultra-Conformable Smart Electronics

Kento Yamagishi[1], *Silvia Taccola*[2], *Shinji Takeoka*[1], *Toshinori Fujie*[3,4], *Virgilio Mattoli*[2], *and Francesco Greco*[1,2]

[1] *Graduate School of Advanced Science and Engineering, Waseda University, TWIns, 2-2 Wakamatsu-cho, Shinjuku, Tokyo 162-8480, Japan*
[2] *Center for Micro-BioRobotics@SSSA, Istituto Italiano di Tecnologia, Viale Rinaldo Piaggio 34, Pontedera, Pisa 56025, Italy*
[3] *Waseda Institute for Advanced Study, Waseda University, 1-6-1 Nishi Waseda, Shinjuku-ku, Tokyo 169-8050, Japan*
[4] *Japan Science and Technology Agency, PRESTO, 4-1-8 Honcho Kawaguchi, Saitama 332-0012, Japan*

11.1 Introduction

Recent studies on flexible electronics have resulted in excellent contributions to a wide variety of applications, especially with regard to personal health monitoring devices, including electronic skins (e-skins) [1–5]; wearable or skin-attachable devices [6–10]; implantable devices [11–13]; and advanced devices with additional unique characteristics such as biocompatibility/biodegradability/bioresorbability [14–16], self-power [17, 18], and self-healing [19, 20]. For all the aforementioned applications, flexible/stretchable/conformable polymer layers have a crucial, significant role in determining the final properties and overall structural characteristics of materials and devices. The significance of layering of thin films increases as the devices become more complex and multifunctional. Although polymeric supporting layers, made of structured metal or other inorganic materials, contribute significantly to mechanical stability, flexibility, stretchability, and conformability, they are often considered as "structural" components of the devices, just acting as supporting layers for the "functional" part.

In an additional approach, namely that of organic electronics and bioelectronics, conducting and semiconducting polymers can play roles of both structural and functional materials. In this regard, poly(3,4-ethylenedioxythiophene) (PEDOT) is probably the most widely used conjugated conductive polymer [21, 22]. Owing to its outstanding electronic, structural, and biocompatible properties, its applications cover a wide range of fields from electronic components to biomedical devices [23, 24]. The availability of this polymer as a readily available aqueous dispersion of PEDOT:PSS (PEDOT doped with poly(styrenesulfonate)) is one of the reasons why PEDOT has become the most successful conductive

Flexible and Stretchable Medical Devices, First Edition. Edited by Kuniharu Takei.

polymer. Partially oxidized PEDOT macromolecules in combination with partially deprotonated PSS as a counter-ion can indeed form a polyion complex made up of core (PEDOT)-shell (PSS) structure [25], thus allowing its stable dispersion in water. A PEDOT:PSS dispersion is produced on an industrial scale and displays versatility in several coating, printing, deposition techniques. Since the early 2000s, the application of PEDOT:PSS has been investigated for its potential as a charge injection layer in organic light emitting diodes (OLEDs) [26, 27], organic field effect transistors (OFETs) [28–31], organic photovoltaics (OPVs) [32, 33], as well as a transparent conductor as an alternative for indium tin oxide (ITO) or other transparent conductive oxides (TCOs) [34].

On the other hand, our groups, since 2007, have developed free-standing polymer ultrathin films (nanosheets) with a thickness of tens to hundreds of nanometers and a huge size-aspect ratio of 10^6 between thickness and width [35–37]. Taking advantage of their large contact area—bilateral structures that allow heterofuctionality by surface modification, and unique physical properties such as physical adhesion, robustness, and flexibility—nanosheets have been used as "nanoadhesive plasters" for biomedical applications such as surgical tools [38–40], cell/tissue engineering [41–45], and drug delivery system [46, 47]. Functional magnetic nanosheets could also be produced by the introduction of superparamagnetic iron oxide nanoparticles (NPs) in a structural polymer matrix [48].

Since 2011, the introduction of electroconductive properties in free-standing nanosheets has been considered suitable for application as ultra-conformable electrodes or electrically responsive membranes. To this aim, we developed PEDOT:PSS based ultrathin and free-standing nanosheets [49–54] (Figure 11.1). The conductive nanosheets can adhere onto various kinds of complex surfaces including human skin, without using any adhesive agents. From the next section, we describe the various methodologies for the preparation of single-layered and multi-layered conductive nanosheets. We also introduce a couple of techniques for patterning of conductive properties in order to define circuits on board of free-standing nanosheets- and to collect free-standing nanosheets

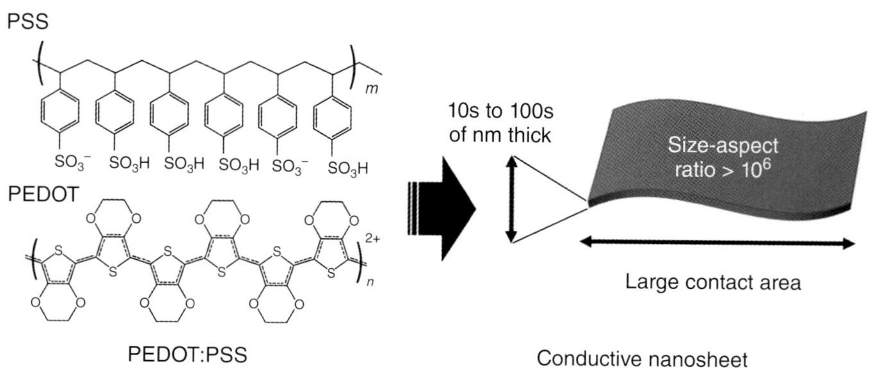

Figure 11.1 General features of a "conductive nanosheet"; a free-standing conductive polymer ultrathin film based on poly(3,4-ethylenedioxythiophene):poly(styrene sulfonate) (PEDOT:PSS).

with a size aspect ratio in excess of 10^6. Electrical, structural, mechanical, and electrochemical characterization of the conductive nanosheets is then presented before to show some applications as ultra-conformable sensors, electroactive actuators, and skin-contact electrodes.

This chapter particularly highlights what kinds of physical, chemical, and electrical properties are exhibited by two-dimensional conductive polymer assemblies, and also describes how such properties can be applied or integrated into smart electronics. The conductive nanosheet technology will open a new avenue toward the development of flexible electronics and devices as the world's thinnest smart electrical interface between biological systems and the external world as in environments, computers, and robots.

11.2 Fabrication of Conductive Nanosheets

11.2.1 Spin-Coating-Processed Conductive Nanosheets

This section starts with the most simple, basic conductive nanosheets; PEDOT:PSS single-layered nanosheets, which were fabricated by spin-coating of a commercially available ready-to-use PEDOT:PSS aqueous dispersion (Clevios™ PH1000, the weight ratio of PEDOT to PSS is 1 : 2.5, Heraeus GmbH) [49]. First, a thin film of PDMS (~800 nm thickness) was formed by spin-coating of a PDMS solution diluted by *n*-hexane (15% in weight) onto silicon substrates. After curing the PDMS (95 °C, 1 h), an air plasma treatment was applied for temporal improvement of the PDMS surface wettability. The PEDOT:PSS solution was filtered (pore size 1.20 μm) and subsequently spin-coated for 60 s over the plasma-treated PDMS thin film. The spin-coating rotation speed was varied between 1000 and 6000 rpm to obtain nanosheets of different thicknesses. The thickness of the nanosheet could be controlled between 30 and 100 nm. Then fabricated nanosheets underwent a thermal treatment (170 °C, 1 h), which made the nanosheets resistant to water and improved their electrical conductivity. The PEDOT:PSS conductive nanosheet was released as a free-standing structure by a water-soluble supporting layer technique [38, 55]. A poly(vinylalcohol) (PVA) supporting layer was formed by casting a PVA aqueous solution (10 wt%) onto the fabricated nanosheets and drying overnight at room temperature. The PEDOT:PSS/PVA bilayered thin film was then peeled off from the substrate and finally released into water to dissolve the PVA layer, resulting in free-standing PEDOT:PSS single-layered conductive nanosheet (Figure 11.2a and b). After recollecting them onto various substrates, the conductive nanosheets showed good conformability against smooth and rough, soft and rigid surfaces (Figure 11.2c–e).

Taking advantage of this technique, we embedded other polymers to fabricate multilayered conductive nanosheets such as PEDOT:PSS/poly(lactic acid) (PLA) bilayered nanosheets; the PLA layer (tens to hundreds of nanometer thickness) acts as a mechanical supporting layer that enhances robustness of the free-standing nanosheet [50]. The PEDOT:PSS/PLA nanosheet was prepared by modifying a fabrication process of single-layered PEDOT:PSS nanosheets. After

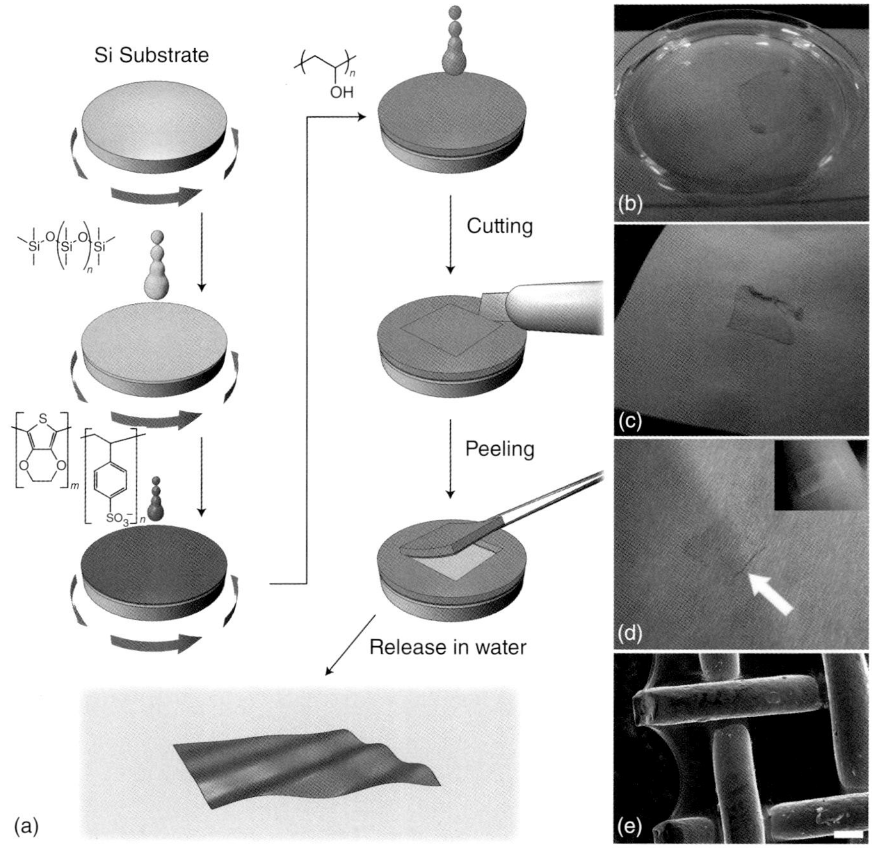

Figure 11.2 (a) Schematic illustration of the spin-coating process for the preparation of a free-standing single-layered conductive nanosheet. (b) A free-standing PEDOT:PSS nanosheet in water. PEDOT:PSS nanosheets collected onto (c) paper, (d) human skin, and (e) steel mesh (scale bar 100 μm). (Greco *et al.* 2011 [49]. Reproduced with permission of Royal Society of Chemistry.)

the thermal treatment of PEDOT:PSS nanosheets, a PLA solution in organic solvent (e.g., chloroform, dichloromethane, or ethyl acetate) was spin-coated and then a PVA-supporting layer was deposited by the same protocol as described in the case of single-layered nanosheets for the detachment of the PEDOT:PSS/PLA nanosheet.

Moreover, patterned conductive nanosheets (Figure 11.3a) were obtained by the addition of a step of localized/patterned over-oxidation of the PEDOT:PSS layer to the above-described procedure [50]. In this case, inkjet printing is useful for patterning the surface of nanosheets because it provides a noncontact, maskless process for a large area. Localized/patterned over-oxidation of the PEDOT:PSS layer was carried out by inkjet printing of a sodium hypochlorite (NaClO) aqueous solution (2 wt%) with 0.13 wt% Triton X-100 by using a Dimatix Materials Printer (Fujifilm Co., Japan). The inkjet printing/patterning was performed just before spin-coating the PLA solution. Indeed, upon exposure

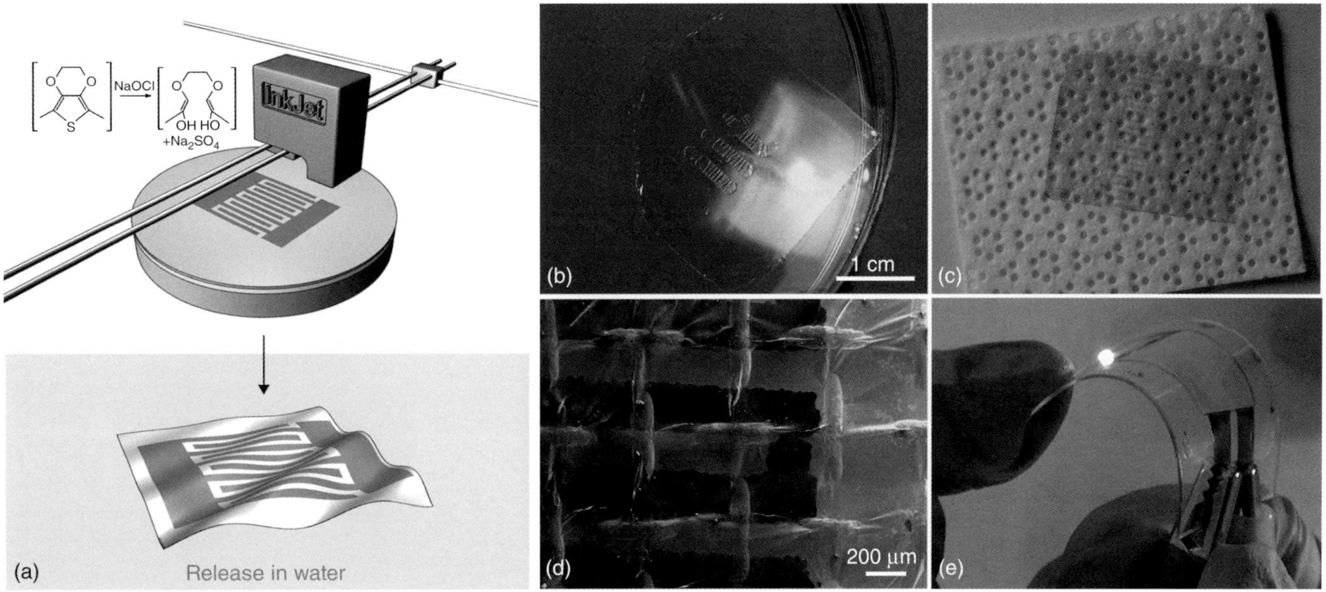

Figure 11.3 (a) Scheme of bilayer PEDOT:PSS/PLA nanosheets subtractive patterning through inkjet printing of a deactivating (overoxidizing) solution of NaClO. (b) Free-standing patterned nanosheet (IIT logo) floating in water. Inkjet patterned nanosheets (interdigitated electrodes pattern with 200 μm gap size) collected onto (c) paper and (d) a steel mesh. (e) Demonstration of functioning of nanosheet as a suspended and bendable conductor membrane: patterned nanosheet (two conducting lines) suspended over a plastic frame and connected to an LED. (Greco *et al*. 2013 [50]. Reproduced with permission of American Chemical Society.)

of PEDOT(:PSS) to NaClO, irreversible deactivation (suppression of electrically conductive properties) is obtained, because of breaking of conjugation in the polythiophene chain; concomitantly, the PEDOT:PSS color is bleached from blue to transparent [56]. In this way, it was possible to fabricate circuits with customizable shape and design onto the surface of free-standing nanosheets. Successful operation was demonstrated as ultra-conformable circuits with the nanosheet on a variety of surfaces (e.g., skin, elastomers, paper, among others) or in a free-standing state, where the printed circuit acted as connectors between a DC voltage supply and an operating light emitting diode (LED) (Figure 11.3b–e).

11.2.2 Roll-to-Roll (R2R) Gravure-Printing-Processed Conductive Nanosheets

It is of crucial importance for real-world applications to extend the processing of the conductive nanosheet technologies to mass-scalable industrial film fabrication techniques. Recently, our groups proposed a methodology for continuous, high-throughput, large-area preparation of PEDOT:PSS single-layered and PEDOT:PSS/Poly(D,L-lactic acid) (PDLLA) bilayered conductive nanosheets based on a Roll-to-Roll (R2R) process [54]. The proposed process employed a gravure-coating system (Tabletop Mini-Labo™ Test Coater, Yasui Seiki Co., Japan, Figure 11.4a).

As regard the single-layer, we obtained free-standing nanosheets by a sacrificial layer technique. Firstly, a cellulose acetate (CA) sacrificial layer was deposited by gravure-printing of a CA solution in acetone onto a poly(ethylene-terephtalate) (PET) film substrate (Lumirror® T60, thickness: 25 μm, Toray Industries, Inc., Japan) and dried under a hot air flow. A PEDOT:PSS dispersion mixed with a nonionic fluorosurfactant, Zonyl® FS-300 (1 vol%) was then deposited over the CA layer. After drying the PEDOT:PSS layer, a thermal treatment (140 °C, 15 min) was carried out on the re-reeled PET film coated with a PEDOT:PSS/CA bilayered film. This R2R technique provided a roll sample with an area of 12 cm × ~20 m (Figure 11.4b) in a typical deposition session. Finally, free-standing PEDOT:PSS single-layered conductive nanosheets were obtained by dissolving the CA sacrificial layer in acetone (Figure 11.4c). The nanosheet thickness could be controlled between 60 and 135 nm by varying the gravure roll rotation speed.

PEDOT:PSS/PDLLA bilayered conductive nanosheets, consisting of a PDLLA mechanical supporting layer and a PEDOT:PSS conducting layer, were also prepared by an R2R process. A PDLLA solution in ethyl acetate was first gravure-printed on a poly(propylene) (PP) film substrate (TORAYFAN® 2500H, thickness: 40 μm, Toray Industries, Inc., Japan). A PEDOT:PSS dispersion mixed with Zonyl® FS-300 (1 vol%) was then gravure-printed over the dried PDLLA layer. Fabricated PEDOT:PSS/PDLLA bilayered nanosheets were detached from the PP substrate by a "tape method" (the schematic procedure is represented in Figure 11.4d) using an adhesive tape frame attached onto the PEDOT:PSS layer, to detach the nanosheets from the plastic substrate (Figure 11.4e). Such suspended membranes could be then transferred onto target surfaces (including skin) with the aid of a reusable wet nylon mesh. The large-size bilayered conductive

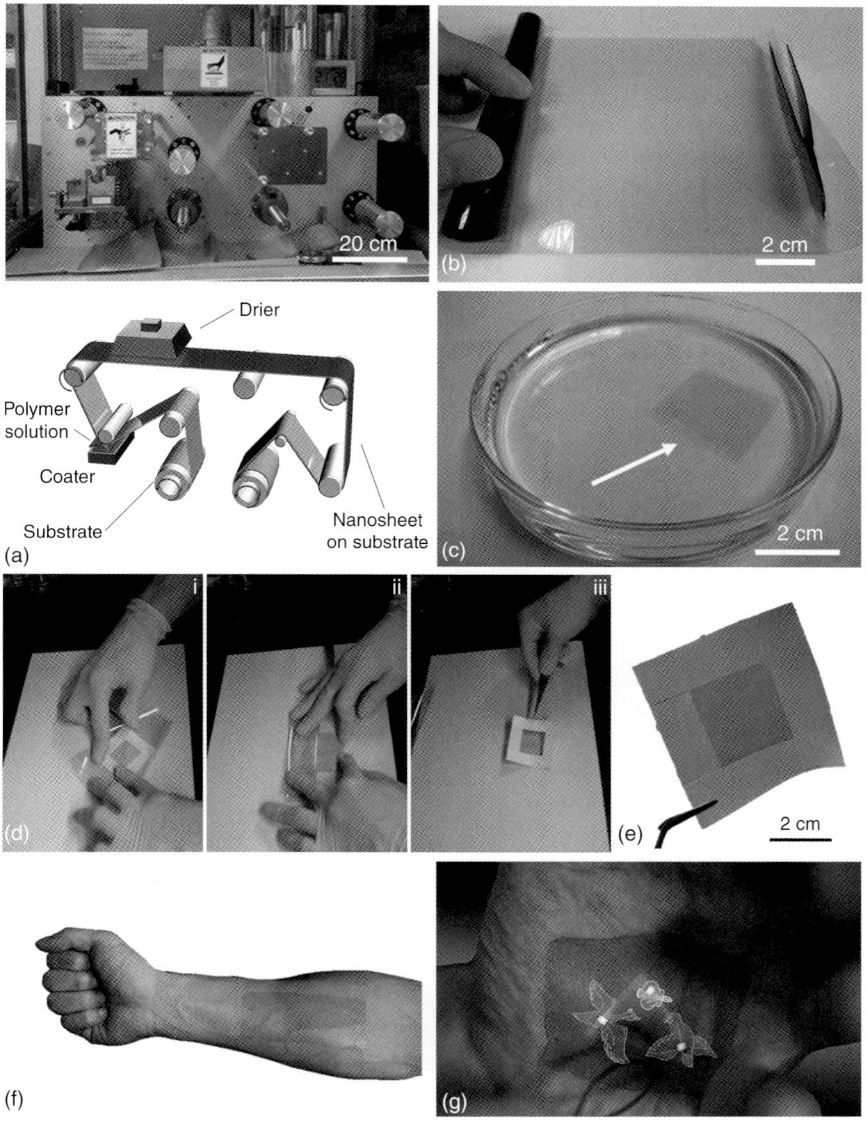

Figure 11.4 (a) Tabletop Mini-Labo™ Test Coater, Yasui Seiki Co., Japan (upper) and schematic illustration of a Roll-to-Roll (R2R) gravure-printing system (bottom). R2R process uses a gravure roll with an engraved texture that allows to print the ink (polymer solution) onto the flexible substrates. (b) R2R processed conductive nanosheets supported on a roll substrate. (c) A free-standing R2R-processed single-layered conductive nanosheet in acetone. (d) Detachment of a PEDOT:PSS/PDLLA bilayered conductive nanosheet from a poly(propylene) (PP) substrate by a "tape method". Four pieces of Scotch® adhesive tape were placed on the nanosheet-printed side of the PP substrate to form a supporting frame for detachment (i). The PP substrate was peeled off from the frame (ii) to obtain a free-standing nanosheet supported by an adhesive tape frame (iii). (e) An R2R conducting nanosheet peeled off from the substrate. (f) Example of a large-area conductive nanosheet transferred onto human skin. (a–f: Zucca *et al*. 2015 [54]. Reproduced with permission of Royal Society of Chemistry.) (g) "Summer Triangle" in Your Hand: an ultra-conformable conductive nanosheet bridging LEDs on the skin. (g: Fujie 2016 [37]. Reproduced with permission of Nature Publishing Group.)

nanosheet transferred onto the skin is shown in Figure 11.4f. The electrical conductive property of the nanosheet was demonstrated by operating LEDs on the skin (Figure 11.4g, the image title: "Summer Triangle" in Your Hand, the cover art for [37]). The thickness of the PEDOT:PSS and the PDLLA layer could be regulated by varying the gravure roll rotation speed and polymer concentration; a total thickness of bilayered nanosheets was between 180 and 300 nm.

Thanks to this R2R technique, we succeeded in scaling up the processing capability of the conductive nanosheets and approached real-world applications. By the combination with other printing methods such as inkjet printing, screen printing, and microcontact printing, fully integrated electronic devices (e.g., electrodes, sensors, and transducers) will be also envisioned on an R2R nanosheet.

11.3 Characterization of Conductive Nanosheets

11.3.1 Electrical Properties of Conductive Nanosheets

Electrical properties of conductive nanosheets are typically investigated by a four-point probe measurement method. Conductivity of the spin-coated single-layered PEDOT:PSS nanosheets measured at different release and recovery steps with different thickness highlighted some peculiar phenomena of these free-standing large-area 2D conductors. The measurements have been performed on the PEDOT:PSS single-layered nanosheets on PDMS (prior to release) and on glass substrates (posterior to release). The measurement was repeated after a thermal treatment at 170 °C for 1 h in order to evaluate the effect of the residual water on the electrical properties. Figure 11.5a shows the obtained values of conductivity of the nanosheets in different situations. Indeed it was possible to appreciate that, while nanosheets having thickness around or over 100 nm show conductivity values that are comparable to bulk PEDOT:PSS samples (i.e., films having thickness of some micrometers or more), a somewhat lower conductivity is observed in thinner nanosheets. This behavior was rationalized by taking into consideration the grain-like structure of PEDOT:PSS in the film (composed of PEDOT-rich cores surrounded by PSS-rich shells, with typical size ~30 nm) and percolative behavior (Figure 11.5b) [49]. From the results shown in Figure 11.5b, we discussed that the fluctuation of conductivity of the PEDOT:PSS nanosheets were strongly associated with the structure of the PEDOT-rich particle assembly in the film. In the range of thickness under 80 nm, the PEDOT-rich cores could not be densely piled up with each other and thus neighboring conductive regions were not well interconnected. Thereby, the increased length of the conducting pathways in the same distance caused the reduction of conductivity. When a percolation threshold was reached, the stacking of the conductive PEDOT-rich particles at larger thickness provided the multiple parallel pathways to form an electrical network thus leading to the improvement of conductivity.

While previous discussions involved the conductive properties of nanosheets made up of PEDOT:PSS (i.e., without any additional functional additive), it is well known that a series of chemical substances called "secondary dopants" have

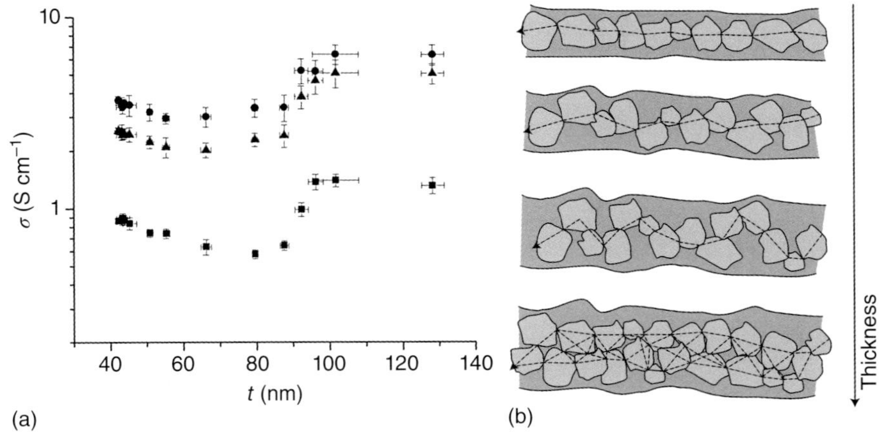

Figure 11.5 (a) The relationship between the thickness t and the conductivity σ of free-standing single-layered conductive nanosheets prepared by a spin-coating process. Nanosheets supported onto PDMS before release, (solid squares); nanosheets after release in water, re-collection on glass (solid circles), and after a subsequent thermal treatment, (solid triangles). (b) Schematic representation of the percolative mechanism in single-layered PEDOT:PSS nanosheet structure composed of PEDOT-rich particles surrounded by the PSS matrix. Length of conducting pathways between neighbor PEDOT particles (dashed line) increases as its thickness comes up to a percolation threshold, thus establishing multiple parallel pathways. (Greco *et al.* 2011 [49]. Reproduced with permission of Royal Society of Chemistry.)

a relevant effect on improving the electrical properties of PEDOT:PSS [21]. The term "secondary dopant" refers to an additive reagent that increases the conductivity of a conjugated polymer that already includes a "primary" dopant by up to 2–3 orders of magnitude. Primary dopant (as PSS in PEDOT:PSS) is indeed introduced as a counter-ion during the synthesis of the material, usually an oxidative chemical polymerization or electrochemical polymerization. In order to enhance the conductivity of the films fabricated by depositing PEDOT:PSS dispersions, several organic solvents such as ethylene glycol (EG) [57–59], dimethyl sulfoxide (DMSO) [60], and N-methyl-2-pyrrolidone (NMP) [61] have been investigated as secondary dopants. Ouyang *et al.* [62] summarized the effect of various secondary dopants on the conductivity of PEDOT:PSS films. There are also some reports about the secondary doping effect of sorbitol [63] and polyethylene glycol (PEG) [64, 65]. The reasons why highly polar moieties enhance the conductivity are thought to be as follows: "(i) a screening effect between positive-charged PEDOT chains and negative-charged PSS; leading to the reduction of the Coulombic interaction between them, (ii) an inductive effect on the orientation of PEDOT by replacing PSS molecules with the high polar moieties, (iii) an enhancement of the dispersibility, and (iv) a formation of the conducting paths by regulating superstructure of PEDOT" [62]. More recently, ionic liquids [66] and electrolyte salts [67] also proved to be efficient secondary dopants to PEDOT:PSS.

The effect of two different secondary dopants was tested on conductive polymer nanosheets: (i) DMSO, a conventional secondary dopant and (ii) butylene

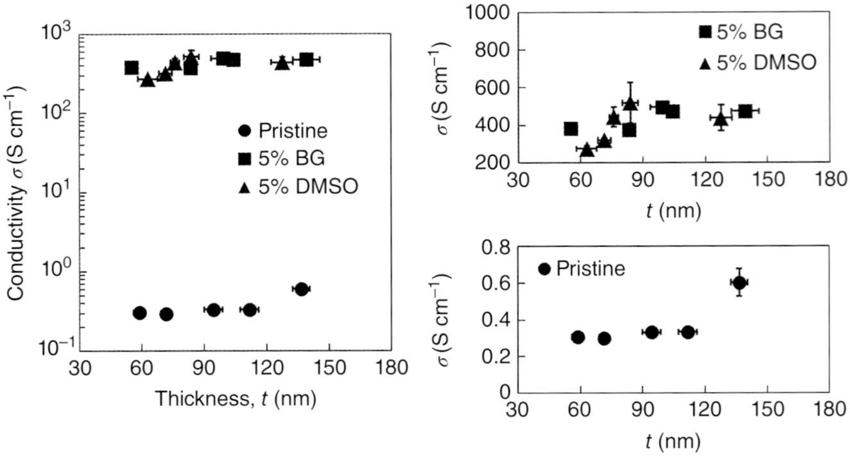

Figure 11.6 Conductivity σ of free-standing single-layered conductive nanosheets prepared by an R2R gravureprinting process as a function of their thickness t; comparison among different formulations of a PEDOT:PSS dispersion: pristine (solid circles), 5% BG-doped (solid squares), and 5% DMSO-doped (black circles). On the right side detailed trends for secondary doped (up) and pristine (bottom) formulations of PEDOT:PSS.

glycol (BG). The latter was especially selected from the view point of skin-contact applications since BG is included in several skin-applied cosmetic products as a dermatologically approved ingredient [68]. Moreover, it was foreseen as a biocompatible alternative to a well-known secondary dopant, EG, because of structural and physico-chemical similarity. DMSO or BG was added as 5 vol% additives to the original PEDOT:PSS aqueous dispersion. Doped nanosheets were prepared by an R2R gravure-printing process to evaluate conductivity and compare it with that of pristine samples. As shown in Figure 11.6, the effect of both DMSO and BG was clearly demonstrated by the higher conductivity that was three orders of magnitude as compared with that of the pristine samples. This secondary doping effect on the electrical properties was totally in agreement with the previous report for PEDOT:PSS films containing similar dopants [63]. The conductivity of the nanosheets slightly increased as the thickness increased, similar to the results observed in spin-coated nanosheets. This fact can be rationalized by the above-described percolation effect observed at small thickness, comparable with the size of PEDOT-rich particles [69].

11.3.2 Structural Properties of Conductive Nanosheets

Structure and surface micro/nanotopography of the spin-coated single-layered conductive nanosheets were investigated before and after being released in water in order to observe the change in their thickness and surface morphology. Interestingly, an average 12% decrease in thickness was observed independently on the original thickness. This effect is ascribable to the loss of excess PSS (e.g., a typical PEDOT:PSS water dispersion Clevios™ PH1000 contains 2.5 times larger weight of PSS than PEDOT) during water-rinsing or releasing process of the nanosheet. Indeed, it is known that the excess PSS causes phase separation from the PEDOT:PSS complex and forms a top PSS-rich layer in the film (10% of total film thickness) [70, 71]; a previous report showed that such excess amount of the PSS outer layer can be removed by a water rinse [69]. According to this report, by considering the Beer–Lambert law behavior of the PEDOT:PSS films, a 1 : 2.5 mass ratio of PEDOT to PSS in the films made from a PEDOT:PSS water dispersion changed into 1 : 1.4 after a water rinse [69]. We also confirmed the PSS removal by the surface morphological change after releasing the PEDOT:PSS free-standing nanosheets in water, as observed by atomic force microscope (AFM) measurements (images are shown in Figure 11.7a). Upon removal of the surface PSS-rich layer, the distinct grain-like structure of PEDOT:PSS emerged clearly, and, at the same time, the surface roughness (R_a) increased from 1.02 to 1.47 nm, when the thickness changed from 78.6 to 70.1 nm [49]. Nevertheless, even after release in water, the surface of free-standing PEDOT:PSS nanosheets was still rather smooth ($R_a < 2$ nm), which feature has beneficial implications in ultraconformability, adhesion, and electrical interface with target surfaces onto which nanosheets are recollected.

The morphological changes associated with the addition of the secondary dopants have also been investigated by several groups. Crispin *et al.* reported that the addition of diethylene glycol (DEG) reduced excess PSS from the surface of the PEDOT:PSS particles by phase separation, leading to the enhancement of conductivity of the films from 0.006 S/cm (pristine) to 10 S/cm (0.3 wt% DEG) [72]. They observed elongated fiber-like islands in AFM images due to the segregation of the excess PSS surrounded by a PEDOT:PSS phase. A more recent study using EG and PEG as a secondary dopant also showed similar AFM phase images [65]. According to these studies, a screening effect, described in the previous section, was produced by the addition of glycol derivatives, thus allowing the formation of the well-separated fiber-like structure probably derived from the phase separation between PEDOT and PSS. Here, we show AFM phase images of BG-doped PEDOT:PSS nanosheets (Figure 11.7b). As described before, BG was selected as a dermatologically approved glycol derivative, envisaging biomedical uses of the conductive nanosheets. While the pristine PEDOT:PSS nanosheet showed a small phase separation consisting of PEDOT:PSS grain-like structure, the nanosheets containing a 5 vol% BG showed a highly-connected fiber-like structure which can be associated with a very different percolative behavior. The results suggested that the enhancement of the conductivity can be related to the structural change of PEDOT:PSS nanosheets at the nanoscale caused by the BG treatment. This drastic effect of BG is probably explained by the same theory that was reported in previous studies.

11.3.3 Mechanical Properties of Conductive Nanosheets

Investigation of mechanical properties in free-standing nanosheets is particularly relevant. Mechanical properties play a key role in the ability of an ultrathin film to maintain its structural and functional integrity as a free-standing or partially supported membrane or to conformably adhere to the target surfaces. Despite the wide usage of PEDOT:PSS in several relevant technological applications, there have not been many studies focusing on the mechanical properties of

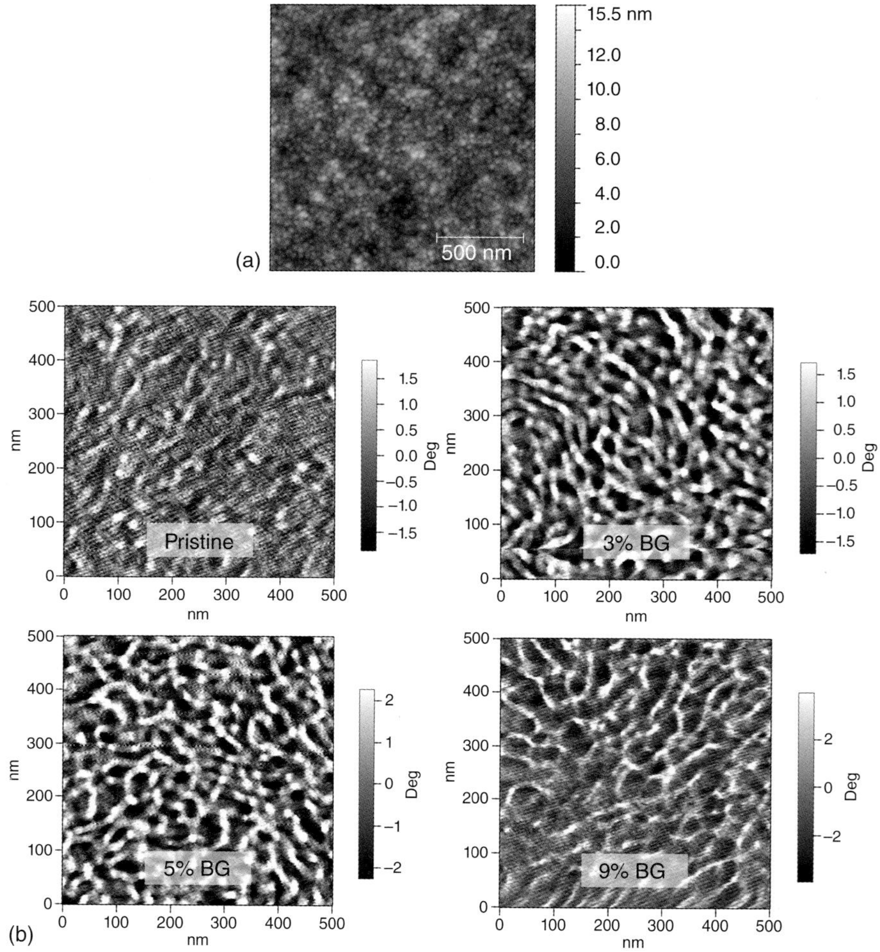

Figure 11.7 (a) AFM topographic images (1.5 μm × 1.5 μm) of single-layered PEDOT:PSS nanosheet (spin-coating-processed) collected on Si after its release in water. Surface topography made up of individual grains is evidenced. (Greco *et al.* 2011 [49]. Reproduced with permission of Royal Society of Chemistry.) (b) AFM phase images (500 nm × 500 nm) of the surface morphology of conductive nanosheets: comparison among different concentrations of a secondary dopant BG; pristine, 3%, 5%, and 9% BG-doped.

PEDOT:PSS thin films. Moreover, most studies did not investigate the properties of ultrathin films, but rather focused on relatively thick films. For instance, Okuzaki *et al.* performed a tensile test for free-standing microfibers (10 μm diameter) or cast films (20 – 30 μm thickness) of PEDOT:PSS, to investigate the Young's modulus and tensile strength [73, 74]. Additionally, Lang *et al.* showed that the mechanical properties of PEDOT:PSS cast films (25 μm thickness) varied depending on the humidity [75]. Thus, no previous studies addressed the mechanical behavior of PEDOT:PSS nanosheets before the report, by our groups, of a methodology for preparation of free-standing PEDOT:PSS nanosheets [49]. In this study, regarding the free-standing single-layered PEDOT:PSS nanosheets, the mechanical properties were characterized by "strain-induced buckling instability for mechanical measurements" (SIEBIMM) [76], a special technique developed to measure the Young's modulus of polymer-based ultrathin films. The SIEBIMM is based on analyzing the buckled surface of polymer thin films. When the thin film is re-collected onto a prestretched elastic substrate (i.e., a PDMS slab), strain relaxation induces buckling of the film, with periodic wrinkles. By measuring the wrinkle wavelength λ on the film surface, the Young's modulus E of the film is calculated using the following formula:

$$E_{\mathrm{n}} = \frac{3(E_{\mathrm{s}}(1 - \nu_{\mathrm{n}}^2))}{(1 - \nu_{\mathrm{s}}^2)} \left(\frac{\lambda}{2\pi t}\right), \tag{11.1}$$

where E is the Young's modulus, ν is the Poisson's ratio, t is the thickness of the nanosheet, and subscripts n and s refer to nanosheet and substrate (PDMS in this case), respectively. As regards PEDOT:PSS nanosheets, evaluation of Young's modulus by SIEBIMM employed $E_{\mathrm{s}} = 1.8\,\mathrm{MPa}$, $\nu_{\mathrm{n}} = 0.33$, and $\nu_{\mathrm{s}} = 0.50$, by following a previous report [77]. The measurements were performed at 50% relative humidity (RH).

The measured buckling wavelength and the Young's modulus of each samples with different thicknesses, calculated by Eq. (1), are displayed in Figure 11.8a and b, respectively. The increment of buckling wavelength depending on the increase of the thickness was observed as expected. The calculated Young's modulus values of the nanosheets (0.81, 1.02, and 1.02 GPa for 37, 58, 77 nm thick samples, respectively) is in good agreement with the values measured with other techniques on 25 μm-thick cast films at 55% humidity condition (0.9 GPa) reported in a previous study [75]. The lower Young's modulus in the thinner samples is probably derived from the structural variation of the films as discussed in Section 11.3.1 using Figure 11.5b, On the other hand, the Young's modulus values of PEDOT:PSS nanosheets were relatively lower compared to those of other polymer ultrathin films with tens to hundreds of nanometers thickness evaluated by SIEBIMM such as polystyrene (*ca.* 3.5 GPa) [76], polyelectrolyte multilayer films (*ca.* 2.7 GPa) [77], and PDLLA (*ca.* 3 GPa) [78]. This can be attributed to the presence of moisture-sensitive hydrophilic PSS.

Adhesion properties of nanosheets made from polyelectrolyte multilayers is strongly associated with their thickness and mechanical properties [38]. Interestingly, we found that the adhesive strength of nanosheets drastically increased as their thickness decreased below 200 nm due to the decrement of their elasticity. This unique characteristic of the nanosheets provides physical adhesion against various substrates including human skin without any adhesive or surface functionalization. The high adhesive strength of the ultrathin and low Young's modulus free-standing PEDOT:PSS nanosheets was demonstrated and quantified by the evaluation using a microscratch tester [79]. The adhesion properties of the nanosheets were evaluated by investigating the critical load required to detach them from an SiO_2 substrate. Such evaluation was carried on R2R-processed single-layered PEDOT:PSS, PDLLA, and PEDOT:PSS/PDLLA bilayered nanosheets with different thicknesses of the PDLLA layer.

As shown in Figure 11.8c–f, we observed that the normalized critical load (i.e., obtained values were divided by the nanosheet thickness) increased depending

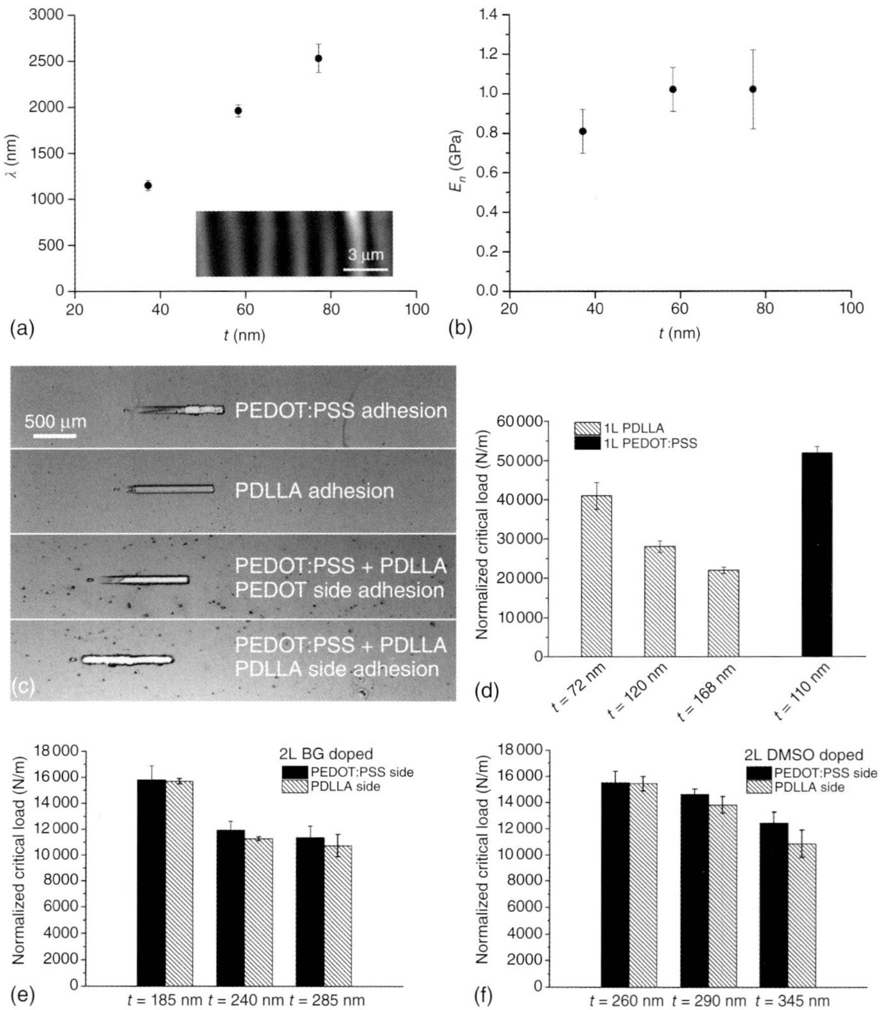

Figure 11.8 Mechanical properties of the single-layered PEDOT:PSS conductive nanosheets with different thicknesses *t* evaluated by the SIEBIMM [76] measurement. The relationship between thickness *t* and (a) the buckling wavelength *λ*, that is, the distance between two consecutive ripple maxima and (b) the Young's modulus En of the nanosheets. Inset shows an example of strain-induced buckling on a 77.1 nm thick conducting nanosheet sample (topographic image obtained by AFM). (a and b: Greco *et al.* 2011 [49]. Reproduced with permission of Royal Society of Chemistry.) Evaluation of adhesive strength of the conductive nanosheets recollected onto SiO_2 substrates using a microscratch tester. (c) Images of representative scratch samples. Normalized critical load for (d) single-layered nanosheets, comparison among various thicknesses of PDLLA layer for PEDOT:PSS; PEDOT:PSS/PDLLA bilayered nanosheets with (e) BG and (f) DMSO as secondary dopants in the PEDOT:PSS dispersion, comparison among nanosheets with different thicknesses of the PDLLA layer for both PDLLA and PEDOT:PSS sides attached to the substrates. (c–f: Zucca *et al.* 2015 [54]. Reproduced with permission of Royal Society of Chemistry.)

on the decrement of the thickness for both single-layered and bi-layered nanosheets. As regards the single-layered PDLLA nanosheets, the critical load decreased from *ca.* 40 000 N/m to *ca.* 22 000 N/m as the thickness increased from 72 to 168 nm (Figure 11.8d). Instead, the single-layered PEDOT:PSS nanosheet with a thickness of 110 nm showed a higher critical load (*ca.* 51 000 N/m) than PDLLA nanosheets (Figure 11.8d). When comparing similar thickness, the adhesive strength of PEDOT:PSS nanosheets (110 nm thick) was around 1.8 times higher than that of PDLLA nanosheets (120 nm thick, critical load: *ca.* 28 000 N/m). In the case of a bilayer, we compared the results between bilateral sides of the nanosheets. Regardless of the secondary dopants (DMSO and BG), higher values of critical loads were found when the PEDOT:PSS side was attached to the substrate rather than the PDLLA side (Figure 11.8e and f). It is suggested that the higher adhesive strength of the PEDOT:PSS side is derived from the surface energy and the mechanical properties, that is, the higher hydrophilicity and the lower elastic (Young's) modulus of the PEDOT:PSS compared to those of PDLLA. Such hetero-surface properties will be an important aspect to transfer the conductive nanosheet to biological tissues with appropriate mechanical properties.

11.3.4 Electrochemical Properties of Conductive Nanosheets

In addition to the conductive properties, PEDOT:PSS has unique electrochemical properties as ionic conductors. Owing to its twofold functionality, this conductive polymer has been used as a transducer at the biotic/abiotic interface; that is, between the wet biological world (e.g., cells, organs, and skin) and dry electronic devices (e.g., electrodes, sensors, actuators, and drug delivery systems). Basically, these applications are based on the "switching" of the redox state of PEDOT:PSS by electrochemical activation. Interestingly, many properties such as transparency (i.e., color), surface energy (i.e., wettability), protein/cell adhesiveness can be fully reversibly regulated by applying a relatively low voltage (0–1 V) to this material. Taking advantage of this unique electrochemical behavior, PEDOT:PSS has been recently applied in the field of smart biointerfaces such as electronic controlled cell detachment [80], ions transport [81], and other organic bioelectronic materials [82, 83].

As a demonstration of electrochemical switching of free-standing conductive nanosheets, cyclic voltammograms (CV) curves were obtained at different scan rates (Figure 11.9a) [50]. In this case, a patterned conductive nanosheet separated into two electrically isolated regions was re-collected on a polytetrafluoroethylene (PTFE) ring-shaped frame equipped with sputtered gold electrodes and wires for contacting each region of the nanosheet. One region acted as a working electrode and the other as a counter electrode in cyclic voltammetry experiments. Typical reduction/oxidation peaks and the color change of the PEDOT:PSS (dark blue for the reduced state in comparison with light blue for the oxidized) were observed due to its electrochromic properties. Alternate reversible switching redox reaction of each region was also observed with the corresponding electrochromic color change.

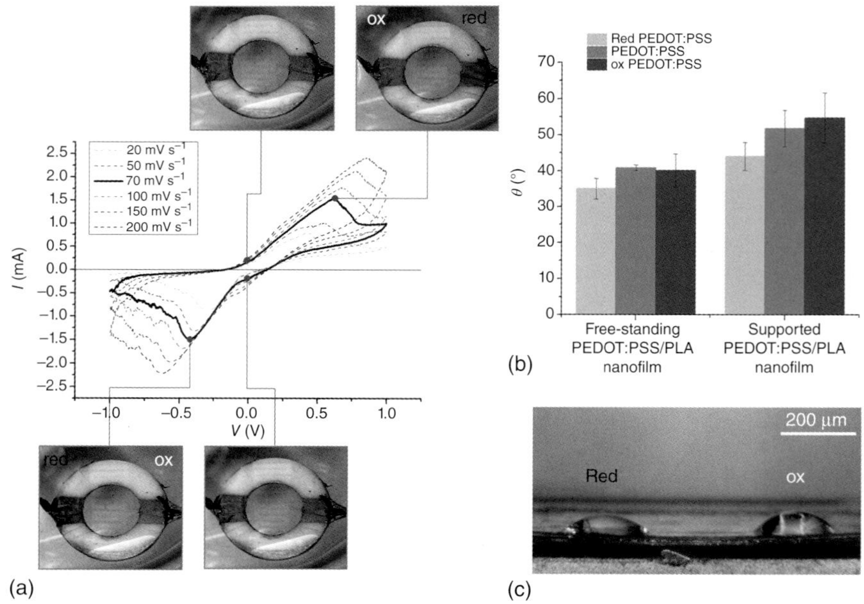

Figure 11.9 (a) Electrochemical properties of conductive nanosheets. The nanosheet, patterned with an interdigitated electrodes design, was suspended onto a Teflon ring that provided electrical contact: left side set as working electrode, right side as counter electrode. Nanosheet was immersed in a 0.1 M NaCl solution in water and Cyclic voltammograms (CV) were recorded at different scan rates. Pictures depict the electrochromic behavior of PEDOT:PSS/PLA patterned nanosheets at each redox state during CV experiment. Electrochemical switching of wettability on conductive nanosheets surface; (b) variation of contact angle θ depending on the redox state of free-standing or supported nanosheets: (c) side-view of a free-standing PEDOT:PSS/PLA patterned nanosheet showing different contact angle for drops placed on the reduced or the oxidized portion of the film. (Greco *et al.* 2013 [50]. Reproduced with permission of American Chemical Society.)

The modulation of the surface energy of the conductive nanosheets depending on different redox states of PEDOT:PSS was tested by comparing the values of a contact angle. For both free-standing and supported (i.e., recollected on bulk polystyrene sheets) nanosheets, higher contact angle θ was observed in the case of the oxidized state than the reduced (Figure 11.9b and c) [50]. The results were in agreement with a previous similar study on PEDOT:tosylate films [84]. The wettability of the electrochemically active surface such as PEDOT:PSS is strongly associated with a change in the binding characteristics between dipolar species (PEDOT main chains) and doping ions (sulfonate ions of PSS). A lower surface energy (i.e., higher contact angle) of the oxidized surface is attributed to a greater anchoring between the PEDOT chains and the sulfonate ions of PSS. In the reduced state, on the contrary, the PSS with sulfonate ions are more easily exposed on the surface to approach the water droplet, resulting in improvement of surface energy/wettability.

Therefore, electrochemical redox switching of the patterned conductive nanosheets was demonstrated by showing the modulation of the surface energy.

This unique electrochemical property of the conductive nanosheets will be used as smart biointerfaces for the electrical regulation of cell adhesion and differentiation.

11.4 Applications of Conductive Nanosheets

11.4.1 Surface Electromyogram (EMG) Recording Using Conductive Nanosheets

The recent development of wearable electronic devices permits to envision an unprecedented series of applications as personal monitoring systems in healthcare and sports. For example, by integrating a variety of wearable (on body) sensors and communication systems onto suitable on body platforms, remote health monitoring systems have been realized. Moreover, given the fact that we are facing super-aging society, the health maintenance management is demanded for the promotion of healthy life expectancy, improving the quality of life of elderly people, reducing the need of hospitalization. In this regard, recently sheet-like skin-attachable electronic devices have been developed in the field of flexible, stretchable, and conformable electronics [6–10]. While a variety of technological strategies and applications have been reported in this research field so far, a common goal of these developments has been to provide a seamless interface with the body (usually skin) so that the device can be unperceivable for the user.

As a first demonstration of skin-contact applications of R2R-processed BG-doped PEDOT:PSS/PDLLA bilayered conducting nanosheets for monitoring human activity and personal healthcare, they were tested as surface electromyogram (sEMG) electrodes. As shown in Figure 11.10a, the conductive nanosheet electrodes adhered to skin were connected to a standard EMG set-up through planar connectors made up of thin Au-sputtered polyimide films (12.5 μm thickness); these unperceivable nanosheet electrodes were successful in recording the electrical muscle activity of a healthy subject. Standard clinical approved pregelled Ag/AgCl electrodes were also used to obtain a meaningful comparison with the nanosheets. A stepwise increase of sEMG signal intensity was recorded depending on the increment of the pressure applied by a hand grasping an analog pressure gauge (Figure 11.10a). After removal of the nanosheets, no signals were recorded. Notably, the conductive nanosheets detected sEMG from a healthy subject with as high a signal-to-noise ratio (SNR) as control pregelled electrodes. This demonstration of the bilayered conductive nanosheets as ultra-conformable skin-contact electrodes for monitoring of human activity will open up the future toward not only healthcare applications but also other attractive fields such as prosthetic limbs and wearable robots.

In order to test the feasibility of the nanosheet technology in this field of application in a real-world scenario, we investigated how the electrical properties of skin-adhered conducting nanosheets are affected in daily life. Firstly, we evaluated the stability of electrical resistance of the nanosheets adhered on flexural parts of the body (the wrist and the finger) against repetitive cycles of flexion. The mechanical stress during exercise is probably a main damage source to the

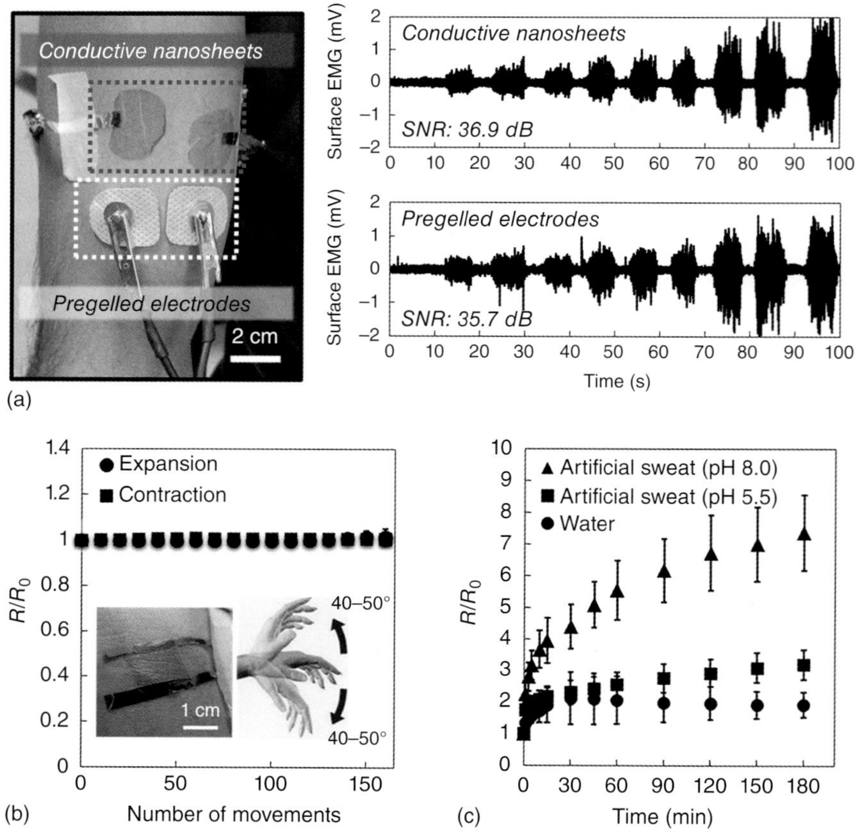

Figure 11.10 (a) Surface EMG recording of muscle activity on the arm; comparison between (BG-doped) PEDOT:PSS/PDLLA bilayered conductive nanosheets and standard pregelled Ag/AgCl electrodes. The signal-to-noise ratio (SNR) of a recorded signal demonstrating similar performances. (b) Stability of the conductive nanosheet against mechanical stress: normalized resistance variation (R/R_0) of the nanosheet during repeated (160 times) exercise for wrist contraction/expansion (the nanosheet placed on wrist, flexion ±40°–50° with respect to the relaxed state). (c) Stability of the conductive nanosheet against sweat: normalized resistance variation (R/R_0) of the nanosheet collected on a silicon-based artificial skin model and submerged in a bath containing water (circles), artificial sweat—pH 5.5 (squares) and pH 8.0 (triangles). (Zucca *et al.* 2015 [54]. Reproduced with permission of Royal Society of Chemistry.)

integrity and the function of the nanosheets. The results in the case of the wrist are summarized in Figure 11.10b. Notably, after 160 cycles of exercise, slight variations in resistance were observed on the wrist (expansion/contraction on a 40°–50°). In the case of finger contraction (flexion 70°), the resistance increment was up to 10% after 160 cycles and 20% after 250 cycles. Such incremental resistance can be derived from the formation of small cracks that interrupt the electric pathways of the conductive nanosheet at its interface with external connectors (Au-sputtered polyimide films). The mechanical mismatch between ultrathin, ultra-conformable nanosheets and relatively stiffer and thicker (~10μm) connectors is detrimental for maintaining the structural integrity of electrodes. Indeed, the integration of stable and compliant connectors or wires for interfacing with external electronic devices still poses technological challenges.

A second source of variation/damage is represented by water and sweat. The electrical stability of the PEDOT:PSS/PDLLA bilayered conductive nanosheets was evaluated by measuring the electrical resistance versus the immersion time in MilliQ water (18 MΩcm) and artificial sweat solutions with two different pH states; physiological skin pH (pH 5.5) and particular conditions such as dry skin, aging, or some pathologies (pH 8.0) [85]. Figure 11.10c shows the normalized resistance variations of the nanosheet when immersed in each liquid for 180 min. Immersion in MilliQ water caused a gradual increase of nanosheet resistance, up to 2.1 times higher than the intact (dry) one (sheet resistance (R_s): 150–200 Ω/□) after 30 min. Then, the resistance became almost constant. In case of acidic artificial sweat solution, a similar profile was observed; however, the nanosheet resistance continued to increase even after 30 min, reaching a value that is 3.2 times higher (R_s: 500–700 Ω/□) than the intact one after 180 min. In case of alkaline sweat, the resistance increase rate was faster than in previous cases. The resistance reached 4.4-fold (R_s: 600–900 Ω/□) at 30 min and 7.4-fold (R_s: 1–1.5 kΩ/□) at 180 min, with respect to the intact value.

These results can be rationalized taking into consideration the hygroscopic and water absorbing properties of PEDOT:PSS nanosheets. A previous research reported that exposure of a PEDOT:PSS film to water resulted in an increment of the resistivity [86]. Moreover, according to a previous study on the effect of pH on the electrical property of PEDOT:PSS films, the increase of pH in a solution in contact with PEDOT:PSS causes the replacement of H^+ of sulfonate groups in PSS with Na^+, and changes the local environment around positively charged PEDOT chains [87]. These results suggested that alkaline components (such as NaOH) in the artificial sweat solution caused the decrease of the carrier density and the carrier mobility. Despite the harsh experimental condition, that is, a worse condition than real human sweating on skin, the conductive nanosheets demonstrated their structural integrity and still retained their electrical properties ($R_s < 2\,k\Omega/\square$ even after 180 min immersion in the alkaline sweat). These results strongly suggest that the BG-doped PEDOT:PSS/PDLLA bilayered conductive nanosheets have a potential to be used in a real-world application in the future.

Finally, envisaging the application in the field of sports science, the stability of the conductive nanosheets adhered on the skin was evaluated by observing the morphological changes before and after exercise in hot and humid environment. After exercise (15 min × 4 games of football) under high temperature (26.5 °C) and humidity (71%), a PEDOT:PSS/PDLLA bilayered nanosheet adhered on the forearm of the subject while the PEDOT:PSS side attached to the skin stayed adhered without formation of cracks. Moreover, no allergic skin reactions such as inflammation and rash were observed after the removal of the nanosheet (by rubbing with a wet towel). Therefore, this demonstration proved not only the mechanical stability and durability against sweating but also a low skin-sensitizing potential of PEDOT:PSS, which strongly indicated that the conductive nanosheets are highly expected to be applied toward real-time monitoring of athletes' health or performance during a training or a match.

11.4.2 Humidity Sensors

As previously mentioned, PEDOT:PSS is a water-absorbing material changing its physical properties, such as volume and electrical resistance, depending upon the RH of the surrounding air [86, 88–90]. Such properties provide the basic ideas and applications of PEDOT:PSS nanosheets in humidity-responsive systems, that is, ultrathin humidity sensors or hydromorphic actuators, both widely investigated by our group [51, 91].

On the other hand, in addition to the fabrication techniques reported above, we developed an original simple technique for obtaining free-standing multifunctional PEDOT:PSS/iron oxide NPs nanosheets [51]. The insertion of iron oxide NPs with *ca.* 10 nm diameter was expected to increase the surface roughness of the nanosheets, providing a larger exposed surface than pristine PEDOT:PSS nanosheets. The fabrication process is simple enough to spin-coat a stable mixture of NPs colloids and the polymer in a suitable solvent, by maintaining the same processes used for unloaded nanosheets [48]. The incorporation of magnetic NPs in a nanosheet largely alters the morphology, evidencing NP clustering phenomenon and the increase of thickness and surface roughness depending on the amount of NPs embedded in the structure [48, 51]. Despite this, PEDOT:PSS/iron oxide NPs nanosheets maintain the peculiar properties of their purely polymeric counterpart, such as manipulability in water, flexibility, conformability, and good conductivity (Figure 11.11a–e) [51].

In this framework, PEDOT:PSS and PEDOT:PSS/iron oxide NPs nanosheets were evaluated as ultrathin humidity sensors in the range between 30% and 70% RH, demonstrating that their resistance linearly increased when exposed to increasing values of RH (Figure 11.11f and g). PEDOT:PSS/iron oxide NPs composites demonstrated better sensitivity than pristine PEDOT:PSS for both suspended membranes and nanosheets collected on solid substrates (glass, polystyrene, or paper stripes with complex surface topography), confirming that the response was independent from the substrate. The observed sensitivity enhanced by the composites is ascribable to the nanostructure of the nanosheets, that is, the insertion of iron oxide NPs largely changed their morphology and surface roughness [51]. The development of such simple and reliable humidity sensors with facile transferability onto various substrates including flexible or stretchable substrates with any given shape and surface texture, can open up the way toward many different applications such as comfort sensors, safety/security purposes, and quality assessment of food and pharmaceutical products.

11.4.3 Microactuators

Free-standing PEDOT:PSS nanosheets are particularly appealing for the development of new all-polymer bilayer electrochemical microactuators because, compared to thick actuators, the use of submicron films improves electrochemical actuation properties such as velocity, stress output, and so on [24]. Since the volume-change-based actuation is ascribable to the diffusion of ions and the solvent through the film upon electrochemical redox reactions, thick films are affected by slow responses and limited performances that restrict the applicability of conductive polymer actuators.

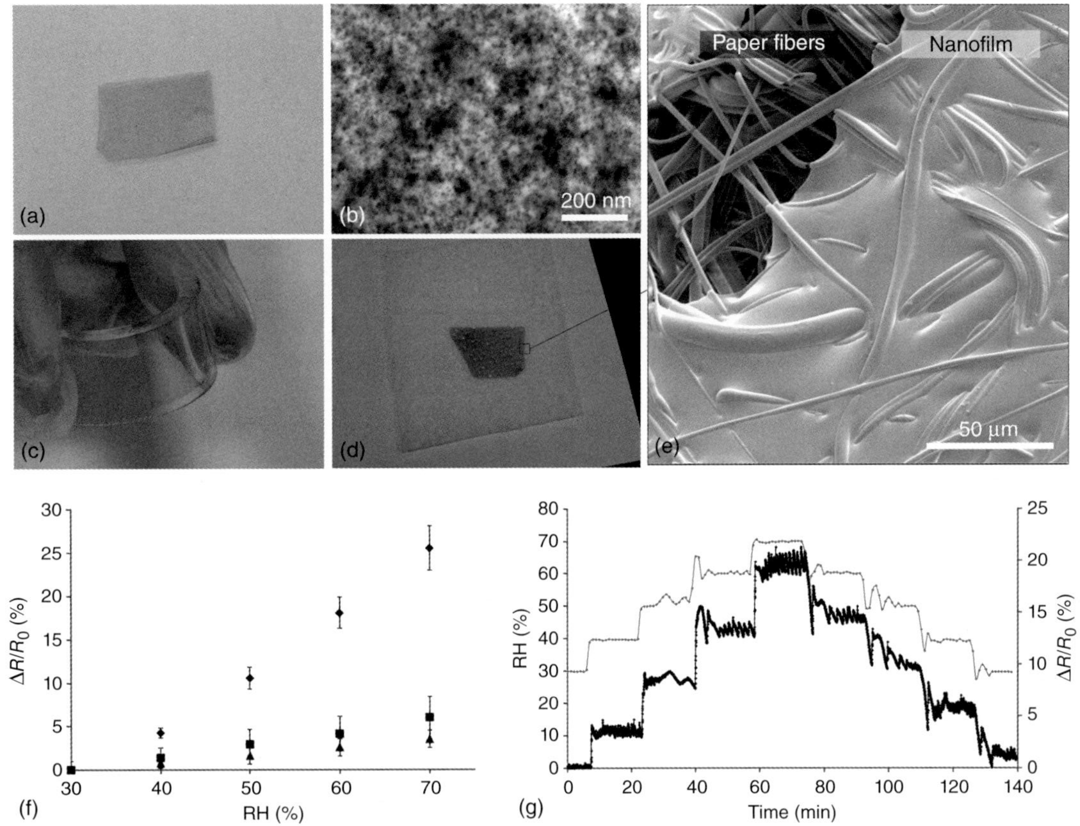

Figure 11.11 Pictures of (a) free-standing PEDOT:PSS/iron oxide NPs nanosheet floating in water after release; (b) STEM images showing NPs dispersion within nanocomposite PEDOT:PSS nanosheet; nanosheet collected onto (c) flexible PDMS and (d) paper. (e) SEM image showing the conformal adhesion of nanosheet re-collected on paper. (f) Resistance response to relative humidity variation in pure PEDOT:PSS and PEDOT:PSS/iron oxide NPs composite nanofilms at different NP concentrations (x): $x = 0$ (▲); 1 (■); 5 (◆) mg mL^{-1}. (g) Resistance variation (black curve, right vertical axis) of a PEDOT:PSS/iron oxide NPs nanosheet (5 mg mL^{-1}) during humidity step-change experiments (gray curve, left vertical axis) in the range of 30–70% RH. (Taccola *et al.* 2013 [51]. Reproduced with permission of American Chemical Society.)

In this framework, we developed free-standing PEDOT:PSS/SU8 bilayer microactuators patterned in the form of microfingers. The fabrication process, which consists of a combination of standard microfabrication procedures such as photolithography and wet etching, is schematically illustrated in Figure 11.12a [92].

The photoresist SU8 was used at the same time for patterning the PEDOT:PSS nanosheets by photolithography and as the passive layer in a bilayer configuration (Figure 11.12b). The choice of SU8, that is widely employed as a structural material in microfabricated devices, is due to a good combination of many different properties such as biocompatibility, good mechanical properties, thermal and chemical stability, and so on. Microfingers movements, both bending and curling, were evidenced during electrochemical oxidation/reduction cycles, demonstrating the reversible actuation capabilities of the PEDOT:PSS microactuators. In particular, a contraction/bending was observed in the oxidized state and an expansion/straightening in the reduced state (Figure 11.12c). This work opens up the possibility to realize micrometer-sized soft actuators, which could be employed for a number of applications in the field of microrobotics as well as in microsurgery and cell handling.

11.4.4 Tattoo Conductive Nanosheets for Skin-Contact Applications

The developments reviewed so far in this chapter have demonstrated the feasibility of realizing conformable electronic devices, electrodes, sensors, actuators based on free-standing conducting polymer nanosheets. Nevertheless, the release, manipulation, and transfer of these ultrathin conductive membranes still impose practical challenges, especially in applications on the human skin or other biological organs/tissues.

Indeed, while the release of nanosheets from a temporary substrate is quite easy—supporting layer dissolution while submerging in water for spin-coated, dry "tape frame" method for R2R nanosheets—having faster and more reliable methods for their recollection/transfer on target surfaces would be beneficial for the development of real-world applications. In the quest for cheap, simple, and mass-scalable technological solutions permitting easy, fast, and reliable transfer of nanosheets onto skin, an idea to use a novel unconventional substrate was conceived, that is, decal transfer paper (temporary tattoo (TT) paper). The TT paper is employed for standard TT stickers for children or fashion: pressing it against the target skin surface and wetting it with a small amount of water allow to release and cause adhesion of the tattoo with a printed drawing. The TT paper is available on the market as paper sheets that can be fed onto inkjet printers. Noteworthy, it consists of three layers: (i) paper, (ii) starch-dextrin coating (water soluble layer) and (iii) ethylcellulose (EC) . Wetting the TT paper with water causes the dissolution of starch-dextrin resulting in the release of a submicrometer thick EC film.

Ultra-conformable conductive tattoo nanosheets with submicrometric thickness were fabricated on top of the TT paper by modifying and optimizing fabrication and patterning processes developed in earlier studies concerning conducting nanosheets. Conductive nanosheets were prepared by inkjet printing of a conductive polymer PEDOT:PSS. To this aim, a highly conductive PEDOT:PSS aqueous dispersion optimized for inkjet printing was employed and

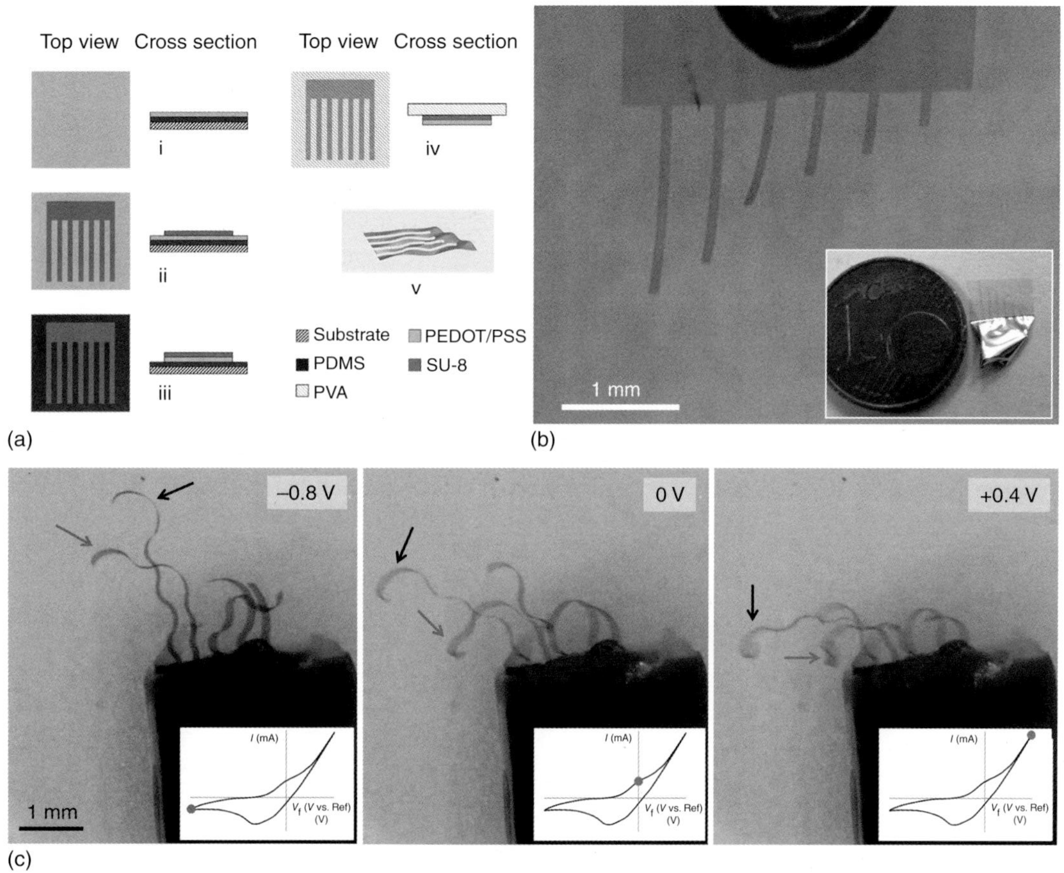

Figure 11.12 (a) Fabrication procedure for PEDOT:PSS/SU8 bilayer microactuators: (i) PEDOT:PSS deposition on PDMS layer; (ii) SU-8 deposition and photolithographic patterning; (iii) wet chemical etching of PEDOT:PSS; (iv) bilayer microactuator peeling off by using temporary PVA support layer; (v) free-standing PEDOT:PSS/SU8 microactuators released in water. (b) Picture of PEDOT:PSS/SU8 microactuator released in water after PVA dissolution (in inset the actuator before water immersion supported by PVA layer). (c) Movements of PEDOT:PSS/SU8 microactuators during cyclic voltammetry at different potentials and oxidation states (from oxidation $V = +0.4$ V to reduction $V = -0.8$ V). (© 2013 IOP Publishing Ltd.)

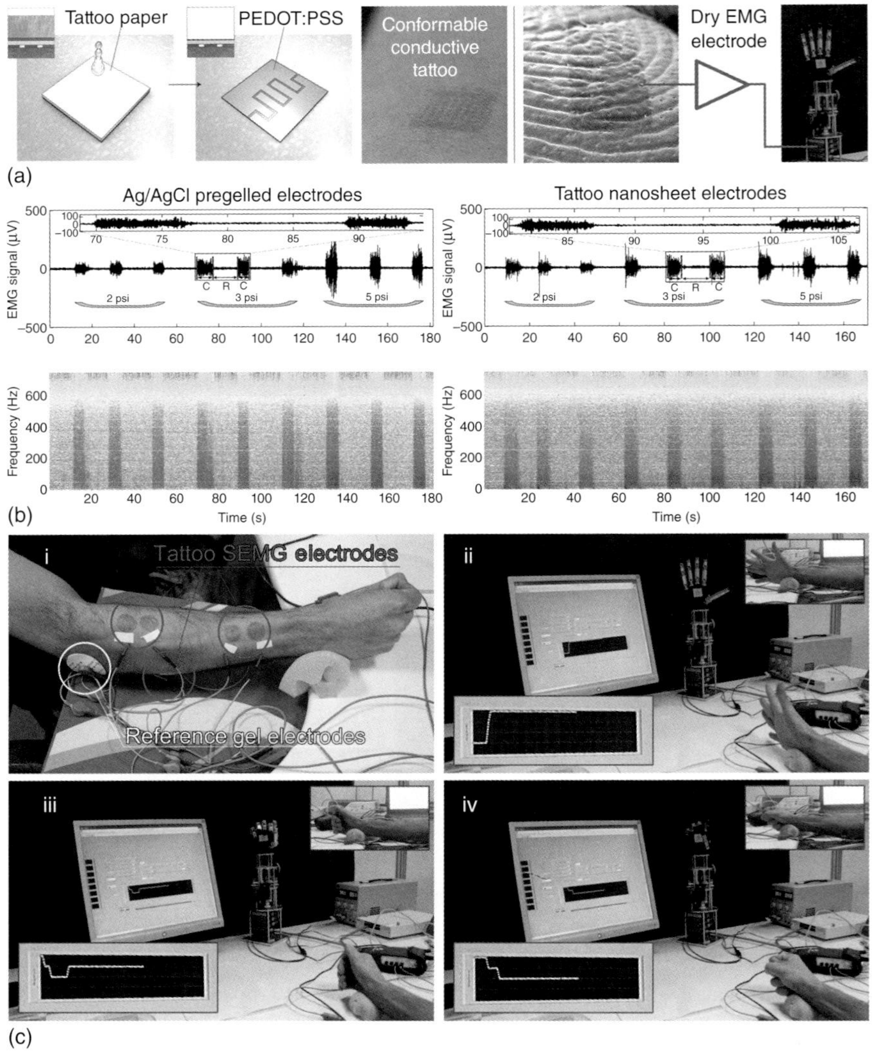

Figure 11.13 (a) Concept of temporary tattoo conductive nanosheet as skin-contact ultra-conformable electrodes. (b) Comparison of recording of electrical activity of muscles performed with EMG dry electrodes based on tattoo nanosheets and standard pregelled Ag/AgCl electrodes. (c) Example of use of EMG dry tattoo electrodes for the control of a prosthetic limb: multiple movements are correctly reproduced by the robotic hand, by using four pairs of tattoo electrodes placed on the forearm of the test subject to pick up muscle activation signals. (Zucca *et al.* 2015 [52]. Reproduced with permission of John Wiley & Sons.)

used in additive and subtractive deposition techniques. Details about fabrication can be found elsewhere [52].

The basic conducting tattoo nanosheet is therefore composed of an EC layer (about 480 nm thickness) and a PEDOT:PSS layer (50–300 nm thickness, depending on application). Several modifications of the process permit to obtain multilayer tattoo nanosheets, comprising, for example, a top electrically insulating layer or multiple layers of PEDOT:PSS. Tattoo conductive nanosheets were fully characterized, assessing their good electrical properties, high conformability onto the skin even when dry, ultralightweight, and good feasibility of transfer. Scanning electron microscopy (SEM) images reported in Figure 11.13a shows conformal adhesion of tattoo nanosheets on the epidermal crests of a skin replica. Thus, tattoo nanosheets are considered to be a very convenient, ultra-conformable, and unperceivable skin-contact human–machine interface for personal physiological monitoring (Figure 11.13b). They were particularly tested for recording the muscle activity as dry electrodes for sEMG, by comparing their performances with standard pregelled Ag/AgCl electrodes in use in clinical applications (Figure 11.13b). Tattoo nanosheet electrodes showed similar results compared with bulky state-of-the-art EMG electrodes, demonstrating their use as unperceivable bioelectrodes to detect the signal in the spectrum of the EMG. Moreover, as one of the fascinating uses of EMG is in the control of prosthetic limbs, we proved the control of multiple movements of a robotic hand prosthesis by EMG recording from four pairs of nanosheet tattoo electrodes on a healthy subject arm (Figure 11.13c) [52].

11.5 Concluding Remarks

To summarize, we have reviewed here our investigations on conductive nanosheets—free-standing ultrathin films based on a conductive polymer PEDOT:PSS—and their applications envisaging the development of ultraconformable electronics. Owing to their ultrathinness, huge size-aspect ratio, and high flexibility, the conductive nanosheets attain conformal and stable physical adhesion onto virtually any target surface, as well as unperceivability on skin, without using any adhesive agents. Firstly, the original concept and technologies for the preparation of single-layered and bilayered conductive nanosheets *via* spin-coating was explained, and R2R gravure-printing process was also introduced taking account of the industrial production of the conductive nanosheets. In addition, selective patterning of PEDOT:PSS using an inkjet printing technique permitted to draw circuits onto free-standing nanosheets, opening the way to advanced applications. Secondly, we have reviewed investigations on the electrical, structural, mechanical, and electrochemical properties of the conductive nanosheets highlighting their unique characteristics including the distinguishing properties of polymer nanosheets, namely, high flexibility and physical adhesion. Notably, functional properties of conductive nanosheets (conductivity, being the crucial one) are fully retained in the nanosheets when released as free-standing, as partially supported suspended membrane or recollected onto target surfaces, thus opening the way to several applications. In fact, we have demonstrated their use in biomedicine and healthcare by testing conductive nanosheets as unperceivable electrodes attached on human skin for recording bioelectric signals such as sEMG. Similar applications as electrical interfaces on skin can be foreseen in the field of personal monitoring for healthcare and sport. In addition to the skin-contact applications, the conductive nanosheets were successfully tested as ultra-conformable sensors in air and electroactive actuators in electrolyte solutions. Therefore, the integration of the electronic/ionic conductive properties into the free-standing polymer nanosheets has made them promising materials for various applications. It is evisaged that conductive nanosheets will contribute to the future progress of nanobioelectronics as an ultra-conformable smart interface between biosystems and electronics/robotics.

Acknowledgments

This work was supported by JSPS Core-to-Core Program from MEXT, Japan (K.Y., S.T., T.F., and F.G.), Unit for Energy and Nanomaterials, Top Global University Program, Waseda University from MEXT, Japan (F.G.), Institute of Advanced Active Aging Research, Waseda University (K.Y., S.T., and T.F.), the Leading Graduate Program in Science and Engineering, Waseda University from MEXT, Japan (K.Y.), JSPS KAKENHI (grant number 15H05355 for T.F.) from MEXT, Japan, Grant-in-Aid for JSPS Fellows (grant number 16J07140 for K.Y.) from MEXT, Japan, the Precursory Research for Embryonic Science and Technology (PRESTO) from the Japan Science and Technology Agency (JST; grant number JPMJPR152A for T.F.), Mizuho Foundation for the Promotion of Sciences (T.F.), and Mitsubishi Materials Research Grant (K.Y. and T.F.). The authors sincerely acknowledge Professor Hiroyasu Iwata and Associate Professor Eiji Iwase at Waseda University, Dr. Alessandra Zucca, Dr. Sudha and Mr. Jonathan Barsotti at the Istituto Italiano di Tecnologia, and Professor Christian Cipriani and Mr. Sergio Tarantino at the Biorobotics Institute, Scuola Superiore Sant'Anna.

References

1 Takei, K., Takahashi, T., Ho, J.C., Ko, H., Gillies, A.G., Leu, P.W., Fearing, R.S., and Javey, A. (2010) Nanowire active-matrix circuitry for low-voltage macroscale artificial skin. *Nat. Mater.*, **9**, 821.
2 Wang, C., Hwang, D., Yu, Z., Takei, K., Park, J., Chen, T., Ma, B., and Javey, A. (2013) User-interactive electronic skin for instantaneous pressure visualization. *Nat. Mater.*, **12**, 1.
3 Someya, T., Sekitani, T., Iba, S., Kato, Y., Kawaguchi, H., and Sakurai, T. (2004) A large-area, flexible pressure sensor matrix with organic field-effect transistors for artificial skin applications. *Proc. Natl. Acad. Sci. U.S.A.*, **101**, 9966.
4 Schwartz, G., Tee, B.C.-K., Mei, J., Appleton, A.L., Kim, D.H., Wang, H., and Bao, Z. (2013) Flexible polymer transistors with high pressure sensitivity for application in electronic skin and health monitoring. *Nat. Commun.*, **4**, 1859.
5 Lipomi, D.J., Vosgueritchian, M., Tee, B.C.-K., Hellstrom, S.L., Lee, J.A., Fox, C.H., and Bao, Z. (2011) Skin-like pressure and strain sensors based on transparent elastic films of carbon nanotubes. *Nat. Nanotechnol.*, **6**, 788.

6 Kim, D.-H., Lu, N., Ma, R., Kim, Y.-S., Kim, R.-H., Wang, S., Wu, J., Won, S.M., Tao, H., Islam, A., Yu, K.J., Kim, T.-I., Chowdhury, R., Ying, M., Xu, L., Li, M., Chung, H.-J., Keum, H., McCormick, M., Liu, P., Zhang, Y.-W., Omenetto, F.G., Huang, Y., Coleman, T., and Rogers, J.A. (2011) Epidermal electronics. *Science*, **333**, 838.

7 Yeo, W.H., Kim, Y.S., Lee, J., Ameen, A., Shi, L., Li, M., Wang, S., Ma, R., Jin, S.H., Kang, Z., Huang, Y., and Rogers, J.A. (2013) Multifunctional epidermal electronics printed directly onto the skin. *Adv. Mater.*, **25**, 2773.

8 Son, D., Lee, J., Qiao, S., Ghaffari, R., Kim, J., Lee, J.E., Song, C., Kim, S.J., Lee, D.J., Jun, S.W., Yang, S., Park, M., Shin, J., Do, K., Lee, M., Kang, K., Hwang, C.S., Lu, N., Hyeon, T., and Kim, D.-H. (2014) Multifunctional wearable devices for diagnosis and therapy of movement disorders. *Nat. Nanotechnol.*, **9**, 397.

9 Stoppa, M. and Chiolerio, A. (2014) Wearable electronics and smart textiles: a critical review. *Sensors*, **14**, 11957.

10 Takamatsu, S., Lonjaret, T., Ismailova, E., Masuda, A., Itoh, T., and Malliaras, G.G. (2016) Wearable keyboard using conducting polymer electrodes on textiles. *Adv. Mater.*, **28**, 4485.

11 Il Park, S., Brenner, D.S., Shin, G., Morgan, C.D., Copits, B.A., Chung, H.U., Pullen, M.Y., Noh, K.N., Davidson, S., Oh, S.J., Yoon, J., Jang, K.-I., Samineni, V.K., Norman, M., Grajales-Reyes, J.G., Vogt, S.K., Sundaram, S.S., Wilson, K.M., Ha, J.S., Xu, R., Pan, T., Kim, T., Huang, Y., Montana, M.C., Golden, J.P., Bruchas, M.R., Gereau, R.W., and Rogers, J.A. (2015) Soft, stretchable, fully implantable miniaturized optoelectronic systems for wireless optogenetics. *Nat. Biotechnol.*, **33**, 1280.

12 Minev, I.R., Musienko, P., Hirsch, A., Barraud, Q., Wenger, N., Moraud, E.M., Gandar, J., Capogrosso, M., Milekovic, T., Asboth, L., Torres, R.F., Vachicouras, N., Liu, Q., Pavlova, N., Duis, S., Larmagnac, A., Vörös, J., Micera, S., Suo, Z., Courtine, G., and Lacour, S.P. (2015) Electronic dura mater for long-term multimodal neural interfaces. *Science*, **347**, 159.

13 Liu, J., Fu, T., Cheng, Z., Hong, G., Zhou, T., Jin, L., Duvvuri, M., Jiang, Z., Kruskal, P., Xie, C., Suo, Z., Fang, Y., and Lieber, C.M. (2015) Syringe-injectable electronics. *Nat. Nanotechnol.*, **10**, 629.

14 Kang, S., Murphy, R.K.J., Hwang, S., Lee, S.M., Daniel, V., Shin, J., Gamble, P., Cheng, H., Yu, S., Liu, Z., Mccall, J.G., Stephen, M., Ying, H., Kim, J., Park, G., Webb, R.C., Lee, C.H., Chung, S., Wie, D.S., Gujar, A.D., Vemulapalli, B., Kim, A.H., Lee, K., Cheng, J., Huang, Y., Lee, S.H., and Paul, V. (2016) Bioresorbable silicon electronic sensors for the brain. *Nature*, **530**, 71.

15 Hwang, S., Huang, X., Seo, J., Song, J., Kim, S., Hage-Ali, S., Chung, H., Tao, H., Omenetto, F.G., Ma, Z., and Rogers, J.A. (2013) Materials for bioresorbable radio frequency electronics. *Adv. Mater.*, **25**, 3526.

16 Kim, D.-H., Viventi, J., Amsden, J.J., Xiao, J., Vigeland, L., Kim, Y.-S., Blanco, J.A., Panilaitis, B., Frechette, E.S., Contreras, D., Kaplan, D.L., Omenetto, F.G., Huang, Y., Hwang, K.-C., Zakin, M.R., Litt, B., and Rogers, J.A. (2010) Dissolvable films of silk fibroin for ultrathin conformal bio-integrated electronics. *Nat. Mater.*, **9**, 511.

17 Yang, Y., Zhang, H., Lin, Z.H., Zhou, Y.S., Jing, Q., Su, Y., Yang, J., Chen, J., Hu, C., and Wang, Z.L. (2013) Human skin based triboelectric nanogenerators for harvesting biomechanical energy and as self-powered active tactile sensor system. *ACS Nano*, **7**, 9213.

18 Fan, F.R., Lin, L., Zhu, G., Wu, W., Zhang, R., and Wang, Z.L. (2012) Transparent triboelectric nanogenerators and self-powered pressure sensors based on micropatterned plastic films. *Nano Lett.*, **12**, 3109.

19 Tee, B.C.-K., Wang, C., Allen, R., and Bao, Z. (2012) An electrically and mechanically self-healing composite with pressure- and flexion-sensitive properties for electronic skin applications. *Nat. Nanotechnol.*, **7**, 825.

20 Benight, S.J., Wang, C., Tok, J.B.H., and Bao, Z. (2013) Stretchable and self-healing polymers and devices for electronic skin. *Prog. Polym. Sci.*, **38**, 1961.

21 Elschner, A., Kirchmeyer, S., Lövenich, W., Merker, U., and Reuter, K. (2011) *PEDOT Principles and Applications of Intrinsically Conductive Polymer*, CRS Press.

22 Kirchmeyer, S. and Reuter, K. (2005) Scientific importance, properties and growing applications of poly(3,4-ethylenedioxythiophene). *J. Mater. Chem.*, **15**, 2077.

23 Guimard, N.K., Gomez, N., and Schmidt, C.E. (2007) Conducting polymers in biomedical engineering. *Prog. Polym. Sci.*, **32**, 876.

24 Smela, B.E. (2003) Conjugated polymer actuators for biomedical applications. *Adv. Mater.*, **15**, 481.

25 Takano, T., Masunaga, H., Fujiwara, A., Okuzaki, H., and Sasaki, T. (2012) PEDOT nanocrystal in highly conductive PEDOT:PSS polymer films. *Macromolecules*, **45**, 3859.

26 Jonda, C.H., Mayer, A.B.R., and Stolz, U. (2000) Surface roughness effects and their influence on the degradation of organic light emitting devices. *J. Mater. Sci.*, **35**, 5645.

27 White, M.S., Kaltenbrunner, M., Głowacki, E.D., Gutnichenko, K., Kettlgruber, G., Graz, I., Aazou, S., Ulbricht, C., Egbe, D.A.M., Miron, M.C., Major, Z., Scharber, M.C., Sekitani, T., Someya, T., Bauer, S., and Sariciftci, N.S. (2013) Ultrathin, highly flexible and stretchable PLEDs. *Nat. Photonics*, **7**, 811.

28 Khodagholy, D., Gurfinkel, M., Stavrinidou, E., Leleux, P., Herve, T., Sanaur, S., and Malliaras, G.G. (2011) High speed and high density organic electrochemical transistor arrays. *Appl. Phys. Lett.*, **99**, 99.

29 Wan, A.M., Inal, S., Williams, T., Wang, K., Leleux, P., Estevez, L., Giannelis, E.P., Fischbach, C., Malliaras, G.G., and Gourdon, D. (2015) 3D conducting polymer platforms for electrical control of protein conformation and cellular functions. *J. Mater. Chem. B*, **3**, 5040.

30 Khodagholy, D., Rivnay, J., Sessolo, M., Gurfinkel, M., Leleux, P., Jimison, L.H., Stavrinidou, E., Herve, T., Sanaur, S., Owens, R.M., and Malliaras, G.G. (2013) High transconductance organic electrochemical transistors. *Nat. Commun.*, **4**, 2133.

31 Khodagholy, D., Doublet, T., Quilichini, P., Gurfinkel, M., Leleux, P., Ghestem, A., Ismailova, E., Hervé, T., Sanaur, S., Bernard, C., and Malliaras, G.G. (2013)

In vivo recordings of brain activity using organic transistors. *Nat. Commun.*, **4**, 1575.
32 Kaltenbrunner, M., White, M.S., Głowacki, E.D., Sekitani, T., Someya, T., Sariciftci, N.S., and Bauer, S. (2012) Ultrathin and lightweight organic solar cells with high flexibility. *Nat. Commun.*, **3**, 770.
33 Becker, E., Parashkov, R., Ginev, G., Schneider, D., Hartmann, S., Brunetti, F., Dobbertin, T., Metzdorf, D., Riedl, T., Johannes, H.H., and Kowalsky, W. (2003) All-organic thin-film transistors patterned by means of selective electropolymerization. *Appl. Phys. Lett.*, **83**, 4044.
34 Paetzold, R., Heuser, K., Henseler, D., Roeger, S., Wittmann, G., and Winnacker, A. (2003) Performance of flexible polymeric light-emitting diodes under bending conditions. *Appl. Phys. Lett.*, **82**, 3342.
35 Fujie, T., Okamura, Y., and Takeoka, S. (2007) Ubiquitous transference of a free-standing polysaccharide nanosheet with the development of a nano-adhesive plaster. *Adv. Mater.*, **19**, 3549.
36 Takeoka, S., Okamura, Y., Fujie, T., and Fukui, Y. (2008) Development of biodegradable nanosheets as nanoadhesive plaster. *Pure Appl. Chem.*, **80**, 2259.
37 Fujie, T. (2016) Development of free-standing polymer nanosheets for advanced medical and health-care applications. *Polym. J.*, **48**, 773.
38 Fujie, T., Matsutani, N., Kinoshita, M., Okamura, Y., Saito, A., and Takeoka, S. (2009) Adhesive, flexible, and robust polysaccharide nanosheets integrated for tissue-defect repair. *Adv. Funct. Mater.*, **19**, 2560.
39 Okamura, B.Y., Kabata, K., Kinoshita, M., Saitoh, D., and Takeoka, S. (2009) Free-standing biodegradable poly (lactic acid) nanosheet for sealing operations in surgery. *Adv. Mater.*, **21**, 4388.
40 Miyazaki, H., Kinoshita, M., Saito, A., Fujie, T., Kabata, K., Hara, E., Ono, S., Takeoka, S., and Saitoh, D. (2012) An ultrathin poly(L-lactic acid) nanosheet as a burn wound dressing for protection against bacterial infection. *Wound Repair Regen.*, **20**, 573.
41 Niwa, D., Fujie, T., Lang, T., Goda, N., and Takeoka, S. (2012) Heterofunctional nanosheet controlling cell adhesion properties by collagen coating. *J. Biomater. Appl.*, **27**, 131.
42 Fujie, T., Mori, Y., Ito, S., Nishizawa, M., Bae, H., Nagai, N., Onami, H., Abe, T., Khademhosseini, A., and Kaji, H. (2014) Micropatterned polymeric nanosheets for local delivery of an engineered epithelial monolayer. *Adv. Mater.*, **26**, 1699.
43 Shi, X., Fujie, T., Saito, A., Takeoka, S., Hou, Y., Shu, Y., Chen, M., Wu, H., and Khademhosseini, A. (2014) Periosteum-mimetic structures made from freestanding microgrooved nanosheets. *Adv. Mater.*, **26**, 3290.
44 Fujie, T., Shi, X., Ostrovidov, S., Liang, X., Nakajima, K., Chen, Y., Wu, H., and Khademhosseini, A. (2015) Spatial coordination of cell orientation directed by nanoribbon sheets. *Biomaterials*, **53**, 86.
45 Ventrelli, L., Fujie, T., Del Turco, S., Basta, G., Mazzolai, B., and Mattoli, V. (2013) Influence of nanoparticle-embedded polymeric surfaces on cellular adhesion, proliferation , and differentiation. *J. Biomed. Mater. Res. Part A*, **102**, 2652.

46 Fujie, T., Saito, A., Kinoshita, M., Miyazaki, H., Ohtsubo, S., Saitoh, D., and Takeoka, S. (2010) Dual therapeutic action of antibiotic-loaded nanosheets for the treatment of gastrointestinal tissue defects. *Biomaterials*, **31**, 6269.

47 Kashiwagi, K., Ito, K., Haniuda, H., Ohtsubo, S., and Takeoka, S. (2013) Development of latanoprost-loaded biodegradable nanosheet as a new drug delivery system for glaucoma. *Invest. Ophthalmol. Visual Sci.*, **54**, 5629.

48 Taccola, S., Desii, A., Pensabene, V., Fujie, T., Saito, A., Takeoka, S., Dario, P., Menciassi, A., and Mattoli, V. (2011) Free-standing poly(L-lactic acid) nanofilms loaded with superparamagnetic nanoparticles. *Langmuir*, **27**, 5589.

49 Greco, F., Zucca, A., Taccola, S., Menciassi, A., Fujie, T., Haniuda, H., Takeoka, S., Dario, P., and Mattoli, V. (2011) Ultra-thin conductive free-standing PEDOT/PSS nanofilms. *Soft Matter*, **7**, 10642.

50 Greco, F., Zucca, A., Taccola, S., Mazzolai, B., and Mattoli, V. (2013) Patterned free-standing conductive nanofilms for ultraconformable circuits and smart interfaces. *ACS Appl. Mater. Interfaces*, **5**, 9461.

51 Taccola, S., Greco, F., Zucca, A., Innocenti, C., De Julián Fernández, C., Campo, G., Sangregorio, C., Mazzolai, B., and Mattoli, V. (2013) Characterization of free-standing PEDOT:PSS/iron oxide nanoparticle composite thin films and application as conformable humidity sensors. *ACS Appl. Mater. Interfaces*, **5**, 6324.

52 Zucca, A., Cipriani, C., Tarantino, S., Ricci, D., Mattoli, V., and Greco, F. (2015) Tattoo conductive polymer nanosheets for skin-contact applications. *Adv. Healthcare Mater.*, **4**, 983.

53 Greco, F., Mattoli, V., Dario, P., Menciassi, A., and Zucca, A. (2013) Process for the preparation of biocompatible, free-standing nanofilms of conductive polymers. International application deposited on 2011, Protocol Number PCT/IB2011/055288. WO2012070016 (Also published as US2012306114). EP2643395 A1.

54 Zucca, A., Yamagishi, K., Fujie, T., Takeoka, S., Mattoli, V., and Greco, F. (2015) Roll to roll processing of ultraconformable conducting polymer nanosheets. *J. Mater. Chem. C*, **3**, 6539.

55 Stroock, A.D., Kane, R.S., Weck, M., Metallo, S.J., and Whitesides, G.M. (2003) Synthesis of free-standing quasi-two-dimensional polymers. *Langmuir*, **19**, 2466.

56 Yoshioka, Y. and Jabbour, G.E. (2007) in *Conjugated Polymers: Processing and Applications* (eds T.A. Skotheim and J.R. Reynolds), CRS Press, Boca Raton, FL, pp. 3-1–3-21 doi: 10.1017/CBO9781107415324.004.

57 Ashizawa, S., Horikawa, R., and Okuzaki, H. (2005) Effects of solvent on carrier transport in poly(3,4-ethylenedioxythiophene)/poly(4-styrenesulfonate). *Synth. Met.*, **153**, 5.

58 Hohnholz, D., Okuzaki, H., and MacDiarmid, A.G. (2005) Plastic electronic devices through line patterning of conducting polymers. *Adv. Funct. Mater.*, **15**, 51.

59 Murakami, T., Mori, Y., and Okuzaki, H. (2011) Effect of ethylene glycol on structure and carrier transport in highly conductive poly(3,4-ethylene dioxythiophene)/poly(4-styrenesulfonate). *Trans. Mater. Res. Soc. Jpn*, **36**, 165.

60 Kim, J.Y., Jung, J.H., Lee, D.E., and Joo, J. (2002) Enhancement of electrical conductivity by a change of solvents. *Synth. Met.*, **126**, 311.
61 Louwet, F., Groenendaal, L., Dhaen, J., Manca, J., Van Luppen, J., Verdonck, E., and Leenders, L. (2003) Synthesis, characterization, properties and applications. *Synth. Met.*, **135–136**, 115.
62 Ouyang, J., Xu, Q., Chu, C.W., Yang, Y., Li, G., and Shinar, J. (2004) On the mechanism of conductivity enhancement in poly(3,4- ethylenedioxythiophene):poly(styrene sulfonate) film through solvent treatment. *Polymer*, **45**, 8443.
63 Jönsson, S.K.M., Birgerson, J., Crispin, X., Greczynski, G., Osikowicz, W., Denier van der Gon, A.W., Salaneck, W.R., and Fahlman, M. (2003) The effects of solvents on the morphology and sheet resistance in poly(3,4-ethylenedioxythiophene)-polystyrenesulfonic acid (PEDOT-PSS) films. *Synth. Met.*, **139**, 1.
64 Wang, T., Qi, Y., Xu, J., Hu, X., and Chen, P. (2005) Effects of poly(ethylene glycol) on electrical conductivity of poly(3,4-ethylenedioxythiophene)-poly (styrenesulfonic acid) film. *Appl. Surf. Sci.*, **250**, 188.
65 Alemu Mengistie, D., Wang, P.-C., and Chu, C.-W. (2013) Effect of molecular weight of additives on the conductivity of PEDOT:PSS and efficiency for ITO-free organic solar cells. *J. Mater. Chem. A*, **1**, 9907.
66 Badre, C., Marquant, L., Alsayed, A.M., and Hough, L.A. (2012) Highly conductive poly(3,4-ethylenedioxythiophene):poly (styrenesulfonate) films using 1-ethyl-3-methylimidazolium tetracyanoborate ionic liquid. *Adv. Funct. Mater.*, **22**, 2723.
67 Onishi, K. and Nakajima, S. (2010) Enhancement of conductivity on PEDOT/salt hybrid films. *IEEJ Trans. Fundam. Mater.*, **130**, 217.
68 Fan, W., Kinnunen, T., Niinimäki, A., and Hannuksela, M. (1991) Skin reactions to glycols used in dermatological and cosmetic vehicles. *Am. J. Contact Dermat.*, **2**, 181.
69 Delongchamp, D.M., Vogt, B.D., Brooks, C.M., Kano, K., Obrzut, J., Richter, C.A., Kirillov, O.A., and Lin, E.K. (2005) Influence of a water rinse on the structure and properties of poly(3,4-ethylene dioxythiophene):poly(styrene sulfonate) films. *Langmuir*, **21**, 11480.
70 Higgins, A.M., Martin, S.J., Jukes, P.C., Geoghegan, M., Jones, A.L., Langridge, S., Cubitt, R., Kirchmeyer, S., Ox, U.K., Laue-langevin, I., Horowitz, J., and Cedex, F.-G. (2003) Interfacial structure in semiconducting polymer devices. *J. Mater. Chem.*, **13**, 2814.
71 Jukes, P.C., Martin, S.J., Higgins, A.M., Geoghegan, M., Jones, R.A.L., Langridge, S., Wehrum, A., and Kirchmeyer, S. (2004) Controlling the surface composition poly (styrene sulfonate) blends by heat treatment. *Adv. Mater.*, **16**, 807.
72 Crispin, X., Marciniak, S., Osikowicz, W., Zotti, G., Danier van der Gon, A.W., Louwet, F., Fahlman, M., Groenendaal, L., De Schryver, F., and Salaneck, W.R. (2003) Conductivity, morphology, interfacial chemistry, and stability of poly(3,4-ethylene dioxythiophene)–poly(styrene sulfonate): a photoelectron spectroscopy study. *J. Polym. Sci., Part B: Polym. Phys.*, **41**, 2561.

73 Okuzaki, H. and Ishihara, M. (2003) Spinning and characterization of conducting microfibers. *Macromol. Rapid Commun.*, **24**, 261.

74 Okuzaki, H., Suzuki, H., and Ito, T. (2009) Electrically driven PEDOT/PSS actuators. *Synth. Met.*, **159**, 2233.

75 Lang, U., Naujoks, N., and Dual, J. (2009) Mechanical characterization of PEDOT:PSS thin films. *Synth. Met.*, **159**, 473.

76 Stafford, C.M., Harrison, C., Beers, K.L., Karim, A., Amis, E.J., VanLandingham, M.R., Kim, H.-C., Volksen, W., Miller, R.D., and Simonyi, E.E. (2004) A buckling-based metrology for measuring the elastic moduli of polymeric thin films. *Nat. Mater.*, **3**, 545.

77 Nolte, A.J., Cohen, R.E., and Rubner, M.F. (2006) A two-plate buckling technique for thin film modulus measurements: Applications to poly electrolyte multilayers. *Macromolecules*, **39**, 4841.

78 Fujie, T., Kawamoto, Y., Haniuda, H., Saito, A., Kabata, K., Honda, Y., Ohmori, E., Asahi, T., and Takeoka, S. (2013) Selective molecular permeability induced by glass transition dynamics of semicrystalline polymer ultrathin films. *Macromolecules*, **46**, 395.

79 Baba, S., Midorikawa, T., and Nakano, T. (1999) Unambiguous detection of the adhesion failure of metal films in the MST by waveform analysis of the friction signal. *Appl. Surf. Sci.*, **144–145**, 344.

80 Persson, K.M., Karlsson, R., Svennersten, K., Löffler, S., Jager, E.W.H., Richter-Dahlfors, A., Konradsson, P., and Berggren, M. (2011) Electronic control of cell detachment using a self-doped conducting polymer. *Adv. Mater.*, **23**, 4403.

81 Nilsson, D., Robinson, N.D., Isaksson, J., All, P.K.J., Berggren, M., and Richter-dahlfors, A. (2007) Electronic control of Ca2+ signalling in neuronal cells using an organic electronic ion pump. *Nat. Mater.*, **6**, 673.

82 Berggren, M. and Richter-Dahlfors, A. (2007) Organic bioelectronics. *Adv. Mater.*, **19**, 3201.

83 Wan, A.M.D., Schur, R.M., Ober, C.K., Fischbach, C., Gourdon, D., and Malliaras, G.G. (2012) Electrical control of protein conformation. *Adv. Mater.*, **24**, 2501.

84 Saltó, C., Saindon, E., Bolin, M., Kanciurzewska, A., Fahlman, M., Jager, E.W.H., Tengvall, P., Arenas, E., and Berggren, M. (2008) Control of neural stem cell adhesion and density by an electronic polymer surface switch. *Langmuir*, **24**, 14133.

85 Herrmann, F. and Mandol, L. (1955) Studies of pH of sweat produced by different forms of stimulation. *J. Invest. Dermatol.*, **24**, 225.

86 Huang, J., Miller, P.F., Wilson, J.S., De Mello, A.J., De Mello, J.C., and Bradley, D.D.C. (2005) Investigation of the effects of doping and post-deposition treatments on the conductivity, morphology, and work function of poly(3,4-ethylenedioxythiophene)/poly(styrene sulfonate) films. *Adv. Funct. Mater.*, **15**, 290.

87 De Kok, M.M., Buechel, M., Vulto, S.I.E., Van De Weyer, P., Meulenkamp, E.A., De Winter, S.H.P.M., Mank, A.J.G., Vorstenbosch, H.J.M., Weijtens, C.H.L., and Van Elsbergen, V. (2004) Modification of PEDOT:PSS as hole injection layer in polymer LEDs. *Phys. Status Solidi A*, **201**, 1342.

88 Kawano, K., Pacios, R., Poplavskyy, D., Nelson, J., Bradley, D.D.C., and Durrant, J.R. (2006) Degradation of organic solar cells due to air exposure. *Sol. Energy Mater. Sol. Cells*, **90**, 3520.

89 Daoud, W.A., Xin, J.H., and Szeto, Y.S. (2005) Polyethylenedioxythiophene coatings for humidity, temperature and strain sensing polyamide fibers. *Sens. Actuators, B*, **109**, 329.

90 Liu, J., Agarwal, M., Varahramyan, K., Berney, E.S. IV, and Hodo, W.D. (2008) Polymer-based microsensor for soil moisture measurement. *Sens. Actuators, B*, **129**, 599.

91 Taccola, S., Greco, F., Sinibaldi, E., Mondini, A., Mazzolai, B., and Mattoli, V. (2015) Toward a new generation of electrically controllable hygromorphic soft actuators. *Adv. Mater.*, **27**, 1668.

92 Taccola, S., Greco, F., Mazzolai, B., Mattoli, V., and Jager, E.W.H. (2013) Thin film free-standing PEDOT: PSS / SU8 bilayer microactuators. *J. Micromech. Microeng.*, **23**, 117004.

12

Flexible Health-Monitoring Devices/Sensors

Minjeong Ha, Seongdong Lim, and Hyunhyub Ko

Ulsan National Institute of Science and Technology (UNIST), School of Energy and Chemical Engineering, 50, UNIST-gil, Eonyang-eup, Ulju-gun, 44919 Ulsan, Republic of Korea

12.1 Introduction

Recently, people are becoming increasingly interested in healthcare because of concerns about their quality of life and longevity. Although the demand for healthcare is increasing significantly because of a rapid growth of aging population, the medical man power, facility, and accessibility are insufficient to allow unrestricted individual health monitoring on a daily basis. This prompts the notion of a personal healthcare system for the real-time monitoring of patients who suffer from chronic diseases, for the training and managing of professional athletes, and for the public who wish to maintain or raise their fitness levels. In addition, the monitoring and recording of periodic data from bio-signals such as heart rate (HR), body temperature, respiratory rate, and secretory pH variations would allow for earlier diagnosis, and thus, for the possible prevention of severe diseases.

Personal health monitoring requires portable, miniaturized, and user-friendly healthcare devices to replace conventional health-monitoring systems, which are usually bulky, expensive, and have to be operated by medical professionals. The development of flexible and wearable devices would enable a reduction in healthcare expenditure and allow professional health monitoring to be implemented more easily both in hospitals and at home. Wearable devices are now commercially available in the form of watches, bands, textiles, and glasses [1–3], which include sensors for detecting activity and vital signs. However, these devices are still underdeveloped in terms of their rigidity due to circuit-board/power-supply/storage requirements, their relatively low sensitivity and reliability due to imperfect skin contact, and their limited functionality for detecting multiple bio-signals [4–6]. More practical health monitoring requires more convenient, conformal, and reliable wearable devices to be developed using mechanically flexible materials modified with micro/nanoscale morphologies [7–10] and consisting of ultrathin and lightweight components for closer contact with the body [11–14]. Such devices would improve comfort, reliability, and

Flexible and Stretchable Medical Devices, First Edition. Edited by Kuniharu Takei.

sensitivity because of the immediate transduction of bio-signals from the body to sensors. This next generation of wearable health-monitoring devices would also enable telemedicine [15], self-diagnosis [16] and home healthcare [17] for all.

In this chapter, we focus on flexible sensors for personal health-monitoring systems that can detect human activity and physiological vital signs. We discuss the recent work on flexible health-monitoring devices based on organic, inorganic, and hybrid materials whose structural modification and sensing mechanism depend on the method of signal transduction. We also discuss noninvasive or minimally invasive design approaches to highly flexible, wearable, and body-attachable healthcare devices for different body sites in terms of enhanced functionalities that can detect and distinguish multiple bio-signals with high sensitivity. Finally, we consider areas of practical application for such flexible healthcare sensors and suggest possible future health-monitoring systems.

12.2 Flexible Sensors for Health Monitoring

Monitoring of human bio-signals is an essential part of any daily healthcare regime. Thus, considerable efforts have been made to develop highly sensitive flexible sensors for tracking physical activities and physiological vital signs. In this section, we classify three types of bio-signals: physical, biochemical, and electrophysiological (Figure 12.1). We also summarize the recent progress in flexible sensor technology and associated sensing techniques in terms of their materials and sensor types, with specific signal transduction methods being matched to individual body sites.

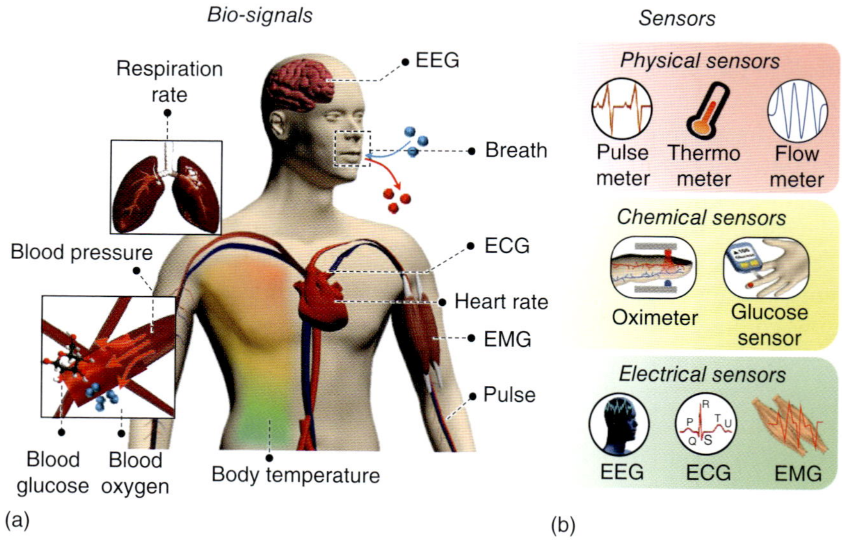

Figure 12.1 *Human bio-signals and types of healthcare sensors.* Representative bio-signals from the human body sites (a) and types of healthcare sensors depending on the detection approaches for physical, biochemical, and electrophysiological vital signs (b).

12.2.1 Detection Approaches for Physical Bio-Signals

The human body has many physical health parameters associated with habitual motion, muscle movement, and changes in body temperature. Here, we consider advanced technologies for pressure, strain, and temperature sensors that incorporate high sensitivity and mechanical flexibility for the detection of human physical bio-signals.

12.2.1.1 Pressure and Strain Sensors for Health Monitoring

In order to detect body movements, various pressure and strain sensors have been developed in flexible, wearable, and patchable forms with structurally modified materials and different signal-transduction mechanisms.

Materials Typical pressure and strain sensors are composed of elastomeric polymers or their hybrid forms by adding active materials to establish both high flexibility and functionality. Polydimethylsiloxane is a commonly used elastomer for the active sensing element and a flexible platform for pressure and strain sensors [18]. It is readily available, easily fabricated, and has excellent properties in terms of mechanical flexibility and stretchability [19, 20], chemical inertness [21, 22], and optical transparency [23]. Other active materials with suitable functionalities are semiconducting [24, 25] or metallic nanostructures [8, 26, 27], carbon materials such as carbon nanotubes (CNTs) [28] and graphene [29], and semiconducting or conducting polymers such as poly(3-hexylthiophene) [30], polyaniline (PANI) [31], poly(3,4-ethylenedioxythiophene) poly(styrenesulfonate) (PEDOT:PSS), and polypyrrole. Metal and semiconducting materials are usually considered mechanically stiff, fragile, and unsuitable for flexible devices despite their outstanding electrical properties. However, effective structural and geometrical modifications of such materials can confer sufficient mechanical flexibility [27] and stretchability [12, 13].

Signal transduction Depending on the stress-induced variation in a material's electrical properties, its signal-transduction mechanism can be classified as one of the following [32].

1) Resistivity
   Resistive transduction is one of the frequent signal-readout methods due to its simple working principle to detect the variations of pressure and strain. The representative mechanism of resistive transduction depends on the changes of intrinsic electrical properties of materials or the structural-deformation-induced resistance change. For example, the typical semiconducting CNTs undergo electrical resistance changes due to a deformed band structure [33]. The electrically conductive CNT composite films exhibit the stress-induced contact resistance differences [34].
2) Capacitance
   Generally, capacitance indicates the stored amount of electric charges between the dielectric materials and corresponding electrodes under an applied voltage [32]. Even though capacitance depends on the several

variables such as dielectric constant of materials, area, and distance of electrodes, the pressure-induced distance change is properly used for capacitive-type of pressure and strain sensors [35].

3) Piezo/tribo-electricity
Piezoelectric and triboelectric effects are widely known for energy harvesting methods, which usually generate a voltage according to the applied pressure and strain. Firstly, the piezoelectric transduction is achievable through the piezoelectric materials that enable to form the separated dipoles and the induced polarization in response to the external force. Thus, the compensating charges build up in the corresponding electrodes [7, 9, 32, 36]. Similarly, the triboelectric transduction sensor perceives the dynamic pressure and motion through the induced polarization from the contact-separation between the two materials with different triboelectric charges [7, 32, 36].

In order to design pressure and strain sensors for health-monitoring devices, it is important to select a material based on its signal-transduction method and to modify its structural dimensions so as to effectively detect the desired bio-signals at specific body sites, for example, joints, cardiac muscle, and lungs. Here, we discuss the recent progress in developing pressure and strain sensors for the detection of the following physical bio-signals: human motion and activity, HR and blood pressure (BP), and respiration rate.

Motion and activity Tracking human motion and activity is often the simplest way to detect health problems. Indicators such as an uneven gait or hand tremors can be critical in diagnosing and preventing chronic diseases. In addition, the real-time monitoring of body motion and daily activities is useful for physical therapy, rehabilitation, and athletic training. Thus, pressure and strain sensors that are fast, directional, and highly sensitive are required. Ultrastretchable and highly sensitive fiber [28, 37] and fiber-based [38–40] fabric strain sensors have been suggested as wearable motion sensors. Cheng *et al.* [37] developed highly sensitive graphene-based resistive fiber sensors (Figure 12.2a) with a gauge factor (GF) of 35 (0.2% strain) and a sensing range of up to 100% strain, that were capable of detecting multiple forms of human motion (Figure 12.2b). Wang *et al.* [40] demonstrated highly sensitive resistive strain sensors based on carbonized silk fabric (Figure 12.2c) with a GF of 37.5 (250–500% strain), a wide sensing range (≤500% strain), and fast response (<70 ms) for monitoring vigorous knee-joint motion (Figure 12.2d). In order to facilitate the precise detection of subtle human motion, Roh *et al.* [23] developed a resistive patchable strain sensor based on CNT composites and conductive elastomers of polyurethane (PU)-PEDOT:PSS (Figure 12.2e) that can detect minuscule facial movements as part of recognizing human emotional expressions (Figure 12.2f). Moving beyond simple planar structures, novel designs of bio-inspired structures have been proposed to enhance the sensitivity and functionality of pressure and strain sensors [8, 9, 41, 42]. Kang *et al.* [8] developed an ultrasensitive crack-based pressure sensor inspired by the spider's sensory system (Figure 12.2g) that can differentiate between high-frequency speech patterns (Figure 12.2h).

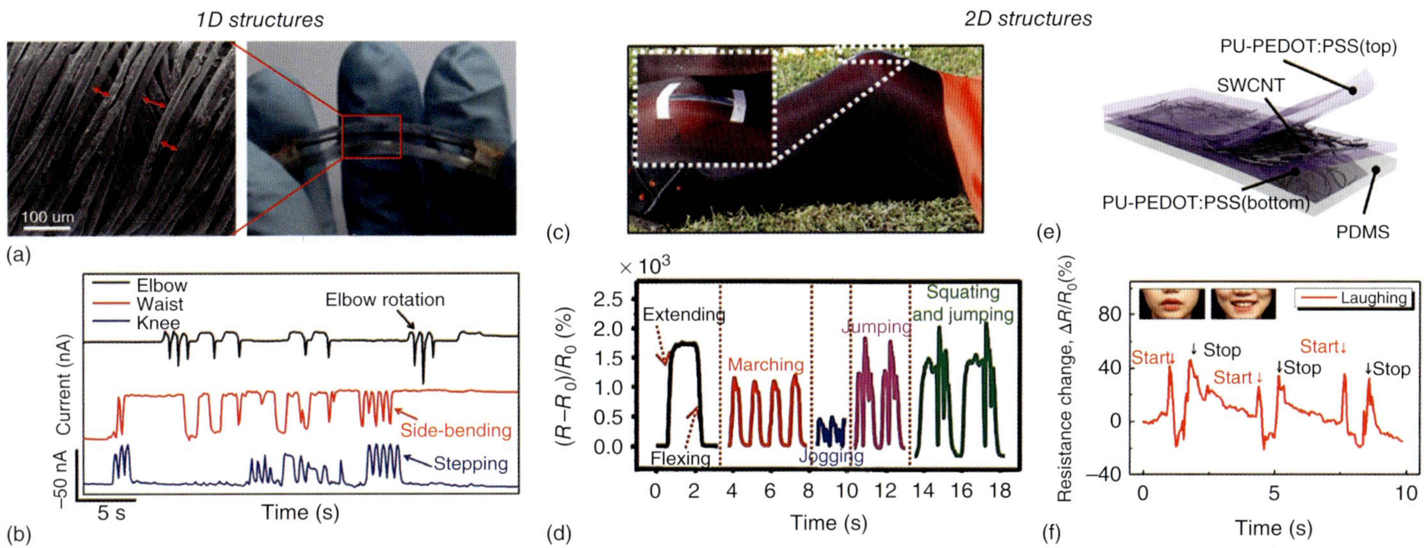

Figure 12.2 *Flexible pressure and strain sensors with structural modification for detecting human motion and activities.* 1D structures: (a) 1D fiber structures based on graphene at 50% strain and (b) response curves of a wearable sensor corresponding to motion. (a,b: Cheng *et al.* 2015 [37]. Reproduced with permission of John Wiley & Sons.) 2D structures: (c) carbonized-silk-fabric-based wearable strain sensors and (d) detection of various human motions, (e) patchable strain sensor consisting of CNTs and conductive elastomers and (f) sensing facial expressions. (c,d: Li *et al.* 2016 [40]. Reproduced with permission of John Wiley & Sons; e,f: Roh *et al.* 2015 [23]. Reproduced with permission of American Chemical Society.) Bioinspired structures: (g) spider's slit organs inspired a crack-based sensor and (h) sound recognition, (i) human-skin inspired electronic skin and (j) stress-direction sensitivity. (g,h: Kang *et al.* 2014 [8]. Reproduced with permission of Nature Publishing Group; i,j: Park *et al.* 2014 [41]. Reproduced with permission of American Chemical Society.)

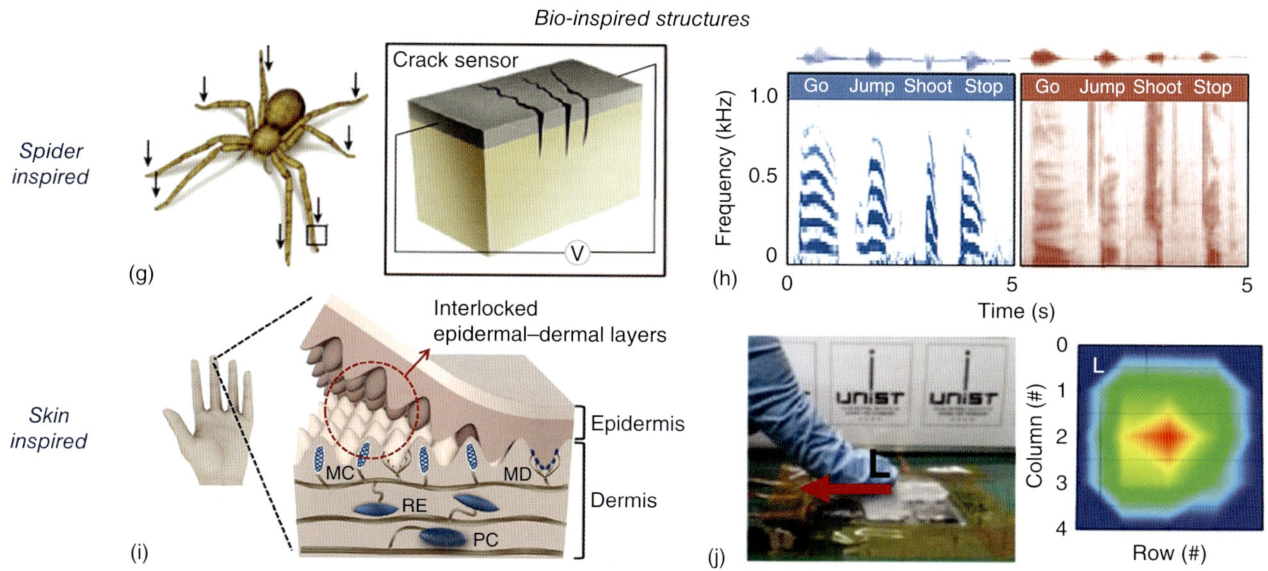

Figure 12.2 (*Continued*)

Park *et al.* [41] developed a directional pressure sensor inspired by the internal interlocking structure of human skin (Figure 12.2i) that can precisely detect external stress depending on the force direction (Figure 12.2j).

Heart rate and blood pressure A cardiovascular condition is assessed through monitoring of the HR and BP. Such vital signs are easily measured in a hospital environment. However, it is more difficult to monitor them on a continuous, long-term basis in order to avoid sudden heart attack, stroke, and death. Therefore, various pressure/strain sensors are used for HR/BP detection in personal and practical use. The periodic HR and vascular BP can be detected at various sites around the chest and blood vessels. Analysis of HR/BP patterns can quantify arterial stiffness for the diagnoses of hypertension and arrhythmia [43, 44]. To detect minuscule HR/BP signals with a noninvasive or minimally invasive approach, a fast and highly sensitive pressure sensor is required. Park *et al.* [42] demonstrated a flexible ferroelectric skin that can accurately detect the radial arterial pulse waveform from the systolic, diastolic, and reflected wave pressures (Figure 12.3a). In addition, they provided a quantitative evaluation of the pulse wave velocity and arterial stiffness from the augmentation index of pulse intensity for application in the diagnosis of cardiovascular diseases. Pang *et al.* [10] suggested a highly sensitive ($\sim 0.58\,\mathrm{kPa}^{-1}$) capacitive microhair sensor that can detect the deep-lying internal jugular venous pulse (JVP) for the diagnosis of arrhythmias and pericardial diseases (Figure 12.3b).

Respiration rate Health abnormalities such as asthma, apnea, and chronic lung diseases are most readily diagnosable via respiration rate [46, 47]. This can be detected by pressure and strain sensors on the body to measure thoracic-cavity expansion/contraction [48], trachea movement [45], or expiratory/inspiratory breathing phases [34]. Hwang *et al.* [45] developed a highly sensitive (GF = 12.26 at 2% strain) resistive patchable strain sensor that can detect inhalation/exhalation via trachea muscle movement (Figure 12.3c). Boland *et al.* [48] proposed resistive strain sensors based on graphene/rubber composites that have high tolerance (GF = 35 for >800% strain) and exceptionally high strain-rate detectability for subtle human breathing motions.

From the above discussion, it is clear that significant efforts have gone into developing high-performance pressure/strain sensors that are fast, highly sensitive, and have superior mechanical properties for the detection of physical bio-signals. However, the challenge remains for differentiating between the bio-signals themselves and simultaneous motion artifacts such as gestures, walking, and speaking.

12.2.1.2 Temperature Sensors for Health Monitoring

Human body temperature varies subtly within a narrow ($\sim 1\,°\mathrm{C}$) range [49], but is nevertheless a crucial indicator of activity level, emotion, and illness. While the normal body temperature of a healthy person is almost constant within 36.5–37.5 °C, a person suffering from hypothermia or fever shows a more irregular temperature variation [50, 51]. Thus, high-resolution and ultrasensitive temperature sensors are required. Furthermore, anatomical body temperatures

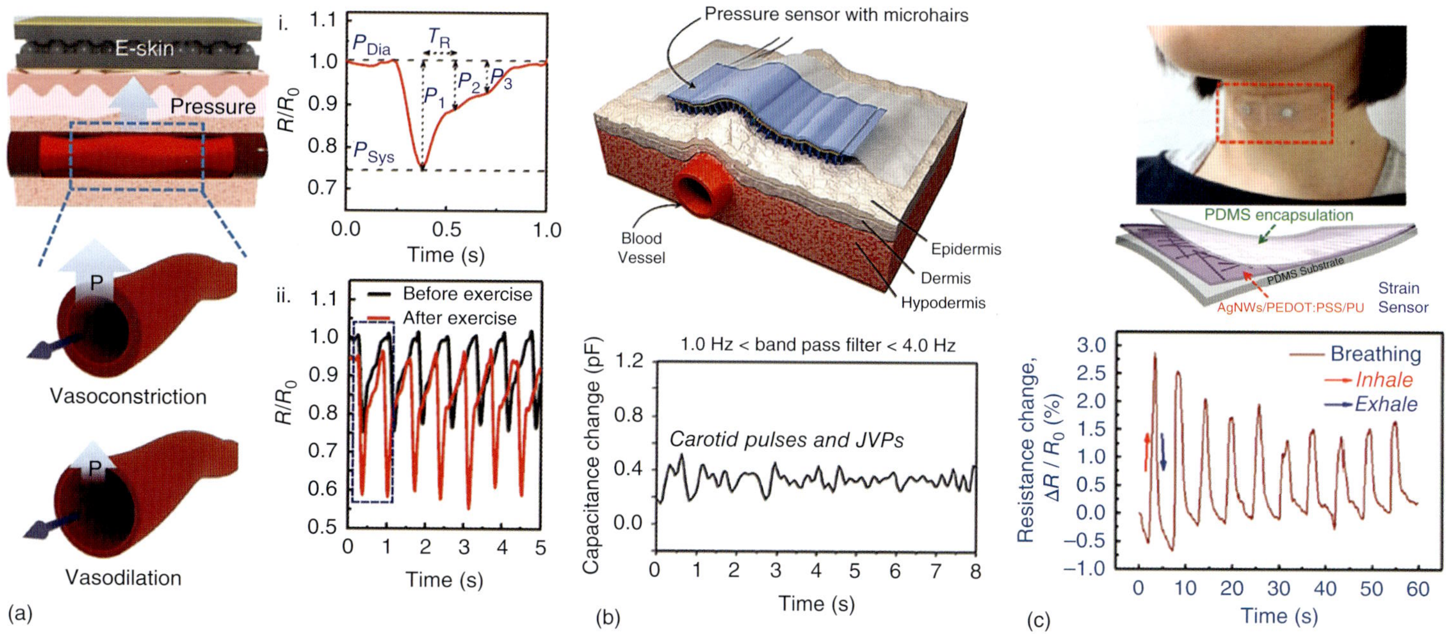

Figure 12.3 *Detection of physical vital signs with pressure and strain sensors.* (a) Schematic illustration for detection of blood pressure with fingertip skin-inspired ferroelectric skins and the detection of artery pulse pressure (i) and variation in pulse waveforms before and after exercise (ii). (Reproduced from Ref. [42]. with permission; Copyright 2015, American Association for the Advancement of Science.) (b) Skin-conformal microhair sensor enables recognition of carotid pulse and jugular venous pulse (JVP). (Pang *et al*. 2015 [10]. Reproduced with permission of John Wiley & Sons.) (c) Monitoring the respiration rate based on patchable strain sensors with perception of muscle movement of trachea and esophagus. (Hwang *et al*. 2015 [45]. Reproduced with permission of American Chemical Society.)

vary internally and externally [52, 53]. For example, the typical temperatures inside the ear and on the wrist are approximately 37 and 32 °C, respectively [54]. Because environmental factors affect the body's exterior more than the internal organs, noninvasive wearable temperature sensors are required to have anatomically specific temperature detection ranges.

Flexible temperature sensors for wearable and body-attachable applications are widely studied in terms of thermistors [55, 56], thermocouples [57], the thermoelectric effect [58], and optical approaches [59]. Thermistors, which detect temperature variations through changes in electrical resistance, come in two types: positive temperature coefficient (PTC) for increased resistance with increasing temperature [56, 60] and negative temperature coefficient (NTC) for decreased resistance with increasing temperature [61, 62]. Yokota *et al.* [56] developed a temperature sensor based on PTC-type polymer composites that has high resolution (<0.1 °C) for 30–50 °C, fast response time (<100 ms), and good repeatability (Figure 12.4a). Trung *et al.* [61] developed a body-attachable temperature sensor (30–80 °C) based on NTC-type reduced graphene oxide (rGO)-PU composites that has a sensitivity of 1.34% per °C and excellent stability after 10 000 stretch cycles (Figure 12.4b). The thermoelectric effect—the conversion of temperature difference into electrical voltage [63, 64]—can be used for both temperature detection and self-powered sensors [58]. Zhang *et al.* [58] developed a highly stable thermoelectric temperature sensor based on PEDOT:PSS-porous PU with a high resolution (<0.1 °C) for 25–75 °C and a negligible environmental-temperature-dependent Seebeck coefficient for 0–100 °C (Figure 12.4c).

A more practical use of temperature sensors is the spatio-temporal imaging of body temperature using commercially well-established infrared (IR) camera technology. However, current IR cameras are typically rigid, bulky, and expensive, and therefore, unsuitable for wearable and body-attachable applications. Therefore, the development of flexible visual temperature sensors based on optical approaches has also been attempted. Gao *et al.* [59] proposed a flexible temperature sensor based on thermochromic liquid crystals with ±50 mK precision in the body-temperature range (32–39 °C). When applied to the human wrist, this produces a spatially high-resolution temperature-distribution image, which can be used to detect occlusions (Figure 12.4d).

12.2.2 Detection Approaches for Biochemical Signals

The human body is composed of various chemical elements, which maintain its compositional balance due to homeostasis and are metabolized biochemically to activate living organs and muscles. Therefore, any imbalance in the chemical composition or unusual internal/external biochemical signals is an indicator of body condition and potential illness. Although there are the same practical and economic motivations for flexible and wearable chemical sensors as for the types already discussed, research on chemical sensors is not as well developed as it is for physical ones.

A personal healthcare sensor that can monitor biochemical signals would greatly assist in disease diagnosis and monitoring. For example, monitoring

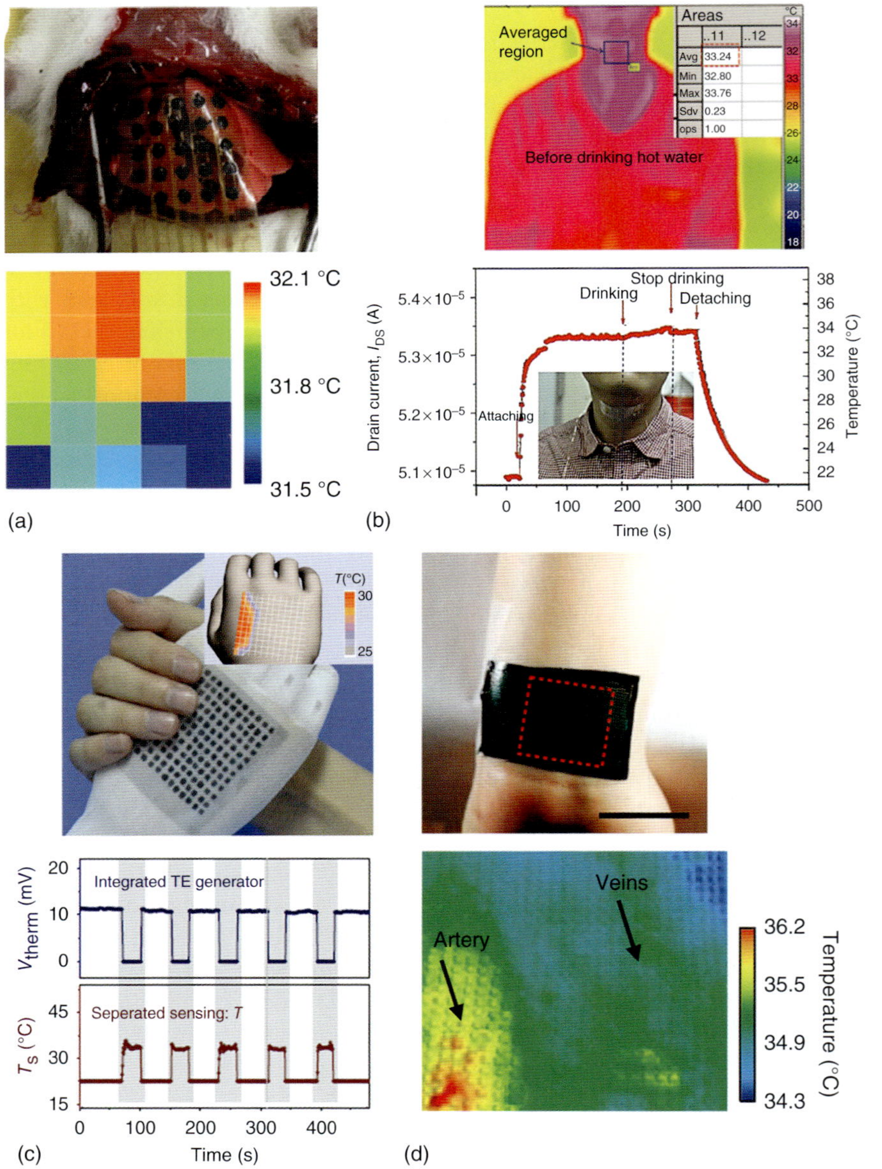

Figure 12.4 *Types of flexible temperature sensors for body temperature distribution*. (a) Temperature mapping of rat lung using flexible and printable thermal sensors. (Reproduced from Ref. [56]. with permission; Copyright 2015, National Academy of Sciences.) (b) Monitoring of temperature change of neck skin during drinking of hot water with body-attachable temperature sensor. (Trung *et al*. 2016 [61]. Reproduced with permission of John Wiley & Sons.) (c) Thermoelectric voltage and temperature responses of organic thermoelectric-material-based arrays to finger-touch cycles. (Reproduced from Ref. [58]. with permission; Copyright 2015, Nature Publishing Group.) (d) Epidermal colorimetric temperature sensors applicable for a reactive hyperemia test on the wrist. (Gao *et al*. 2014 [59]. Reproduced with permission of Nature Publishing Group.)

glucose levels and the volatile organic chemicals (VOCs) [65, 66] in breath, perspiration, and tears can detect diabetes and cancer in relatively early stages. We now introduce the various biochemical signals that are indicative of human diseases and discuss the recently developed flexible chemical sensors for their detection.

12.2.2.1 Flexible pH Sensors

Human bodily fluids are important for processes such as digestion, lubrication, and protection. Given that bodily acidity levels are also critical to the activation of functional fluids, pH levels are carefully controlled at specific anatomical sites. For example, a pH level of 1.0–3.5 persists in the stomach to activate gastric secretion, whereas the heart, liver, brain, and skeletal muscles are pH neutral. Therefore, pH monitoring is important for distinguishing between normal and abnormal health.

Recently, various researchers have considered flexible pH sensors involving the integration of nanomaterials such as PANI [67], graphene [68, 69], and metal oxide [70–72] on flexible substrates. Such sensors mainly use an electrochemical technique (similar to that of commercial pH meters) to measure bodily pH variations. Liu *et al.* [73] reported a flexible transistor based on indium–zinc oxide (IZO) for a highly sensitive (~105 mV/pH), fast (~5 ms), and low-power (15.6–103 pJ/spike for pH 10–4) pH sensor (Figure 12.5a). In their approach, a pH buffer solution on a nanogranular SiO_2 electrolyte film acted as a sensing gate, resulting in changes in the IZO FET source–drain current with the buffer pH level. Note that modulating the biases of the sensing (G1) and control (G2) gates enhances the pH sensitivity. The enhanced sensitivity is related to the amplified capacitive coupling factors between the two gates in the IZO-based transistor. The high sensitivity and low power consumption of this miniaturized pH sensor facilitates an implantable sensory system, leading to potential wearable applications.

Bandodkar *et al.* [67] suggested a tattoo-based epidermal pH monitoring platform using PANI as an ion-selective electrode (Figure 12.5b). PANI is a widely used conducting polymer that has an advantageous pH-sensitive electrical conductivity based on a reversible transition of emeraldine salt and base. The tattoo sensor maintained an acceptably constant potential difference and responded nearly instantaneously to pH 3–7 variations. Furthermore, it showed a well-maintained pH response even after the degree of mechanical deformation (180° bending and 10% stretching) associated with skin surface during exercise.

In terms of practical applications of flexible pH sensors, such as monitoring of wound healing and real-time measurement of perspiration, there have been various efforts to develop a visual flexible pH meter whose color changes with pH. Tamayol *et al.* [74] created an epidermal colorimetric pH sensor based on biocompatible hydrogel microfibers loaded with pH-responsive beads (Figure 12.5c). This sensor showed a distinct color change from dark red (basic pH 8.2) to yellow (acidic, pH 6.2) corresponding to the pH variation in human skin (pH 4–9). In addition, a biocompatible hydrogel-based flexible pH sensor would be suitable for skin-attachable applications because of its high porosity and oxygen permeability.

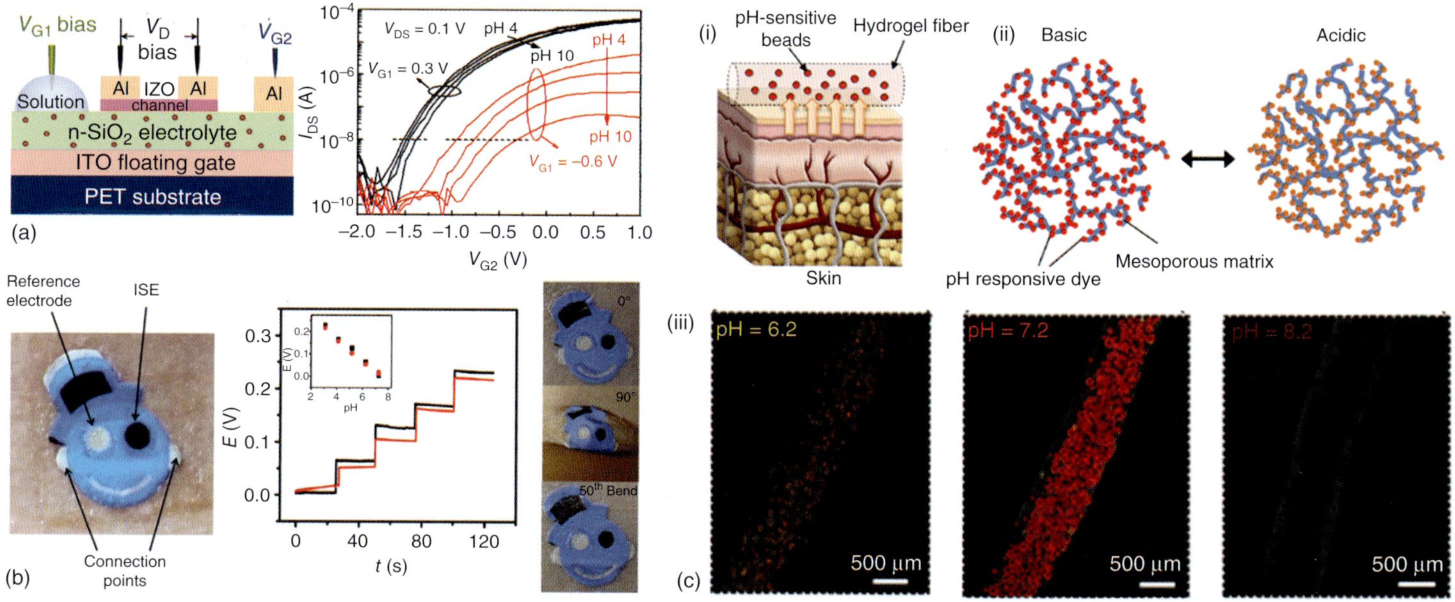

Figure 12.5 *Flexible pH sensors and detection of biochemical signals*. (a) Schematic illustration of pH-sensitive IZO-based neuromorphic transistor measured in dual-gate synergic modulation mode and pH-dependent transfer curves of the device measured by sweeping control gate voltage (G2) at $V_{DS} = 0.1$ V with different fixed sensing gate voltages (G1). (Reproduced from Ref. [73]. with permission; Copyright 2015, Nature Publishing Group.) (b) Photograph of the tattoo-based pH sensor on the skin and pH-responsive behaviors of the sensor over pH range of 3–7 before (black) and after (red) 50 cycles of repeated bending. (Bandodkar *et al*. 2013 [67]. Reproduced with permission of Royal Society of Chemistry.) (c) Schematic illustration of pH-responsive hydrogel microfibers on the skin (i) and expected color change mechanism of mesoporous polyester beads with pH-sensitive dyes in different pH solutions (ii). (iii) Visualized color difference of fabricated wound dressings sprayed with different pH solutions. (Tamayol *et al*. 2016 [74]. Reproduced with permission of John Wiley & Sons.)

12.2.2.2 Flexible Blood Sugar Sensors

Diabetes is a serious disease globally that threatens the health of hundreds of millions of people. Its main symptom is an inveterately raised blood sugar (glucose) level that can induce severe complications such as nervous disorders, coronary artery disease, stroke, and peripheral vascular diseases. Therefore, the self-monitoring of blood sugar is essential for adequate management of the disease. Currently, this is generally done with portable finger-prick blood testers. Although these provide accurate glucose data, it is an inconvenient, painful, and invasive method that is unsuitable for continuous monitoring. Therefore, various researchers have tried to create a highly sensitive, convenient, real-time sensor in flexible form.

One noninvasive approach is to detect glucose levels from perspiration or tears. However, as these secretions have much lower glucose levels than that of blood, this type of noninvasive platform requires greater sensitivity. Recently, Bandodkar *et al.* [75] demonstrated a flexible tattoo-based glucose sensor for epidermal diagnosis (Figure 12.6a). Interstitial skin fluid (including glucose) was first extracted by reverse iontophoresis using a mild current. Glucose levels were then electrochemically analyzed using the current generated by an enzymatic glucose reaction. In this way, they successfully monitored glucose levels before/after eating with an on-body version of the sensor. Rim *et al.* [70] developed a conformal biosensing platform with ultrathin (~3.5 nm) indium oxide (In_2O_3)-based FETs on a thin polyimide substrate (Figure 12.6b). They created a highly sensitive glucose sensor by chemical modification with functional groups (glucose oxidase with a glutaraldehyde linker) on the surface of an In_2O_3 channel. In principle, D-glucose is oxidized by an enzymatic reaction with glucose oxidase, resulting in a pH variation followed by proton production. Such highly sensitive and adhesive conformal glucose sensors can be used for skin-attachable applications or a lens-type sensor for glucose sensing from tears [76, 77].

12.2.2.3 Flexible Pulse Oximeters

Oxygen is an essential component for health, being directly related to metabolism. The cells and tissues that make up the skin, muscles, bones, and other organs in the human body age and die without sufficient oxygen, resulting in various disorders. Nowadays, many people suffer from oxygen deficiency due to external factors such as environmental pollution, stress, lack of exercise, and smoking. Therefore, the analysis of blood oxygen concentration is important for disease prevention.

Recently, portable, noninvasive, and flexible oximeters have been developed for the personal monitoring of oxygen concentration. Optical approaches are generally used to measure how much hemoglobin is oxygenated in the blood. Because oxy- and deoxy-hemoglobin have different absorption properties at red/green wavelengths (Figure 12.7a,b) [78, 79], oximeters typically comprise light-emitting diodes (LEDs) and photodetectors (PDs). There have been some trials to integrate flexible polymer-based LEDs and PDs in oximeters for reasons of flexibility, large-area scalability, and low-cost fabrication [78, 80, 81]. Lochner *et al.* [78] proposed a pulse oximeter that combines red/green organic light-emitting diodes (OLEDs) and an organic photodetector (OPD). The idea was for red/green

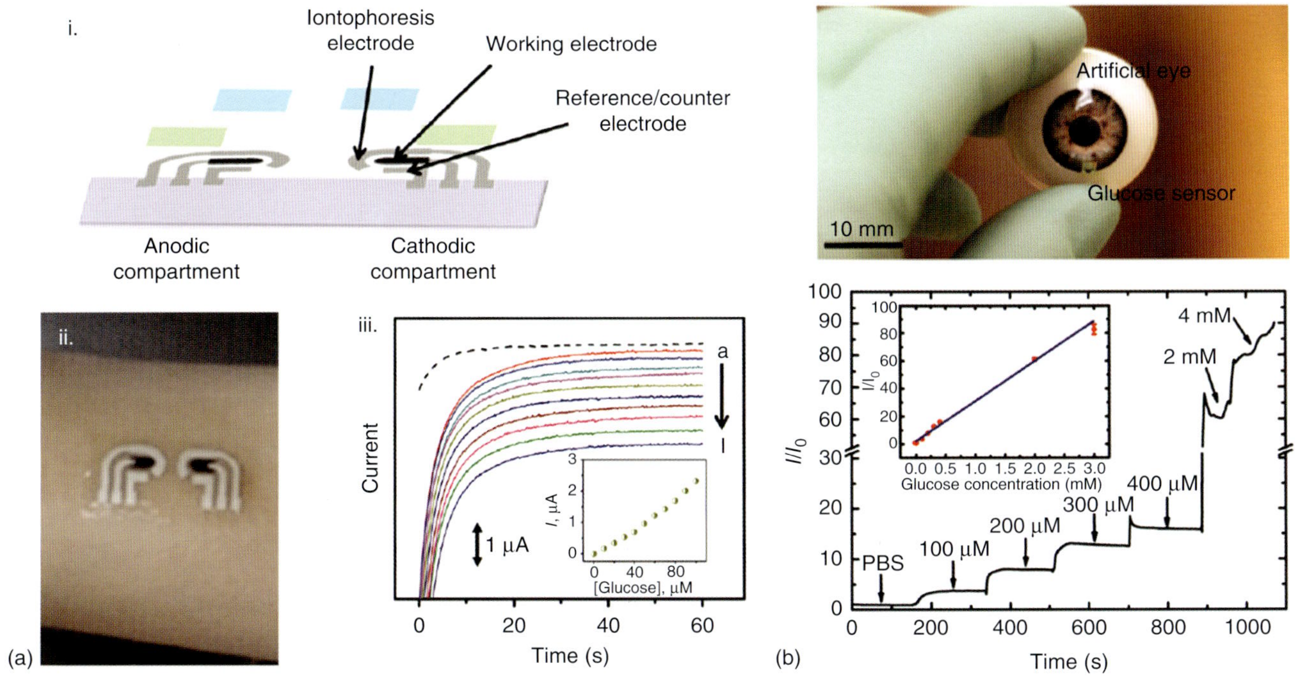

Figure 12.6 *Flexible glucose sensors and detection of blood sugar level.* (a) Schematic illustration of the tattoo-based glucose sensors (i) and photograph of the sensor attached to human skin (ii). (iii) Chronoamperometric response of the sensor with increase of glucose levels from 0 to 100 μM. (Reproduced from Ref. [75]. with permission; Copyright 2014, American Chemical Society.) (b) Photograph of conformally contacted In_2O_3 FET-based glucose sensor on an artificial eye for conceptual suggestion of glucose sensing in tears and representative current changes in the device depending on the glucose levels. (Rim *et al.* 2015 [70]. Reproduced with permission of American Chemical Society.)

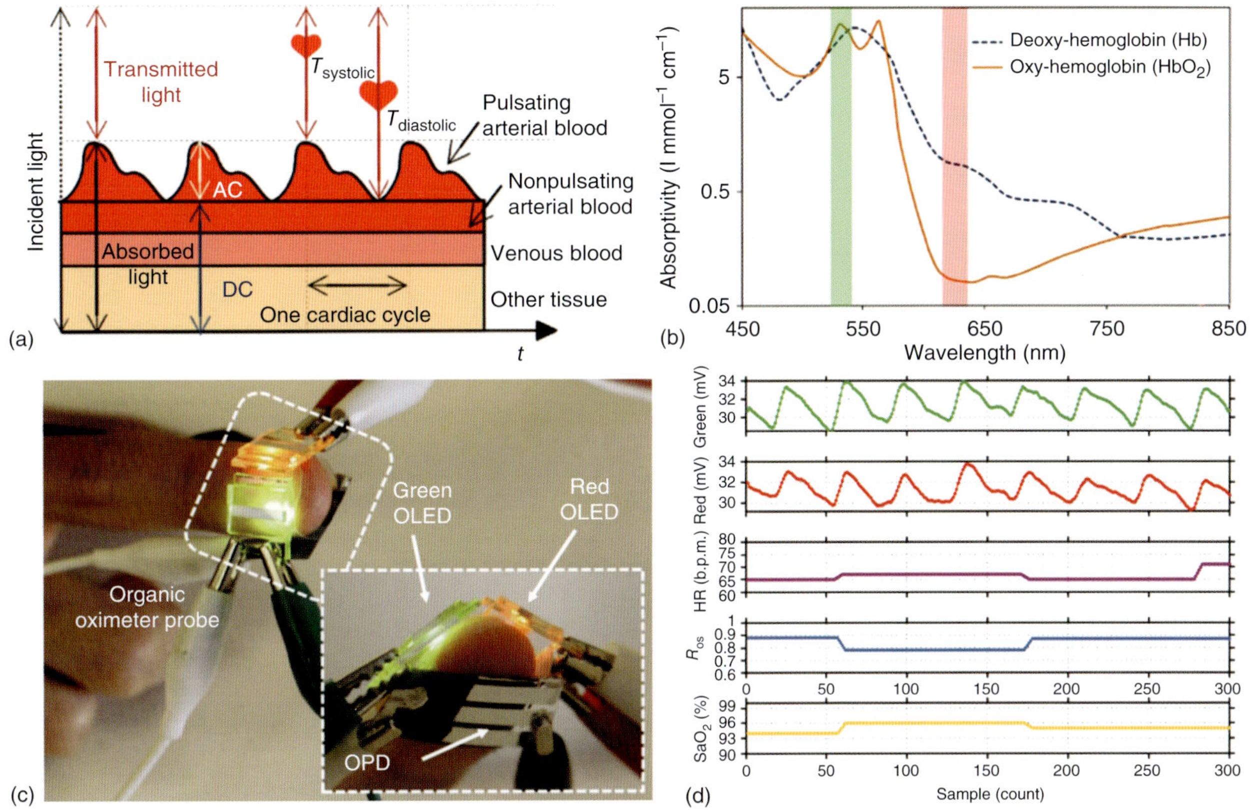

Figure 12.7 *Flexible blood oximeters and detection of oxygenation in human body*. (a) Schematic illustration of a model for penetrated light path from oximeter through skin and blood vessel. (b) The absorptivity of deoxygenated and oxygenated hemoglobin in arterial blood. (c) Photograph of integrated OLED and OPD on subject's finger to monitor the level of blood oxygen concentration. (d) The measured pulsating photoplethysmogram (PPG) signal by all-organic pulse oximetry system. The heart rate and saturation level of blood oxygen were converted from the PPG signal. (Lochner *et al*. 2014 [78]. Reproduced with permission of Nature Publishing Group.)

OLEDs to reflect light on the surface of a fingertip and for the OPD to collect it to calculate the amount of oxy-hemoglobin (Figure 12.7c). The pulsating photoplethysmogram (PPG) signal was measured by using red/green OLEDs and OPD, which could be possible to detect one's HR and the saturation level of arterial blood oxygen (Figure 12.7d). This all-organic oximeter was $\leq$2% accurate compared with a commercial inorganic oxygen sensing system. Lately, Yokota *et al.* [80] developed an ultraflexible and conformable optoelectronic skin for oxygen monitoring. This skin was prepared by integrating polymer light-emitting diodes (PLEDs) and OPDs onto a few-microns-thick highly flexible parylene substrate. Once the OPD detected the reflected light from the finger, the distinguishable optical signals (oxy/deoxy-hemoglobin) could be measured with 99% and 90% oxygenated blood, respectively. Furthermore, they achieved high repeatability and air stability by capping the device with a passivation layer.

12.2.2.4 Other Flexible Chemical Sensors to Detect Volatile Organic Compounds

The analysis of VOCs from urine, skin, blood, and exhaled breath has attracted much attention as another simple and noninvasive approach for early diagnosis of serious diseases such as cancer and diabetes. In particular, exhaled breath includes various VOCs that are useful for monitoring health. Halitosis sufferers and diabetic patients exhibit much higher concentrations of hydrogen sulfide and acetone in their breath than do healthy people [82, 83]. Therefore, various flexible gas sensors have been suggested for real-time monitoring of VOCs in wearable and patchable platforms.

There are two important parameters to assess the performance of gas sensors for breath analysis. First, such sensors should be sensitive to below part-per-million (ppm) levels because the VOC concentration in human breath ranges from ppm to part-per-trillion (ppt). Therefore, many research groups have studied highly sensitive gas sensors based on functionalized nanomaterials that provide large surface areas by control of their variable structures and morphologies, allowing the material properties to be easily tuned by surface functionalization. Xing *et al.* [84] presented a highly sensitive gas sensor based on hybrid In_2O_3/Au nanorods that can detect 0.1 ppm of acetone and 0.05 ppm of ethanol. The reduced amount of acetone or ethanol gas induced the transfer of electrons from the reactive oxygen ions at the surface to the In_2O_3/Au nanorods. Thus, the resistance of In_2O_3-/Au-based gas sensor decreased with the thinning of depletion layer, which enabled the detection of gas molecules. The one-dimensional (1D) nanorods enabled high gas accessibility owing to their large surface area, resulting in high gas sensitivity (Figure 12.8a). In addition, they confirmed significant differences in the acetone/ethanol levels between healthy and atypical individuals who were either intoxicated or suffered from diabetes. Similarly, Kim *et al.* [85] reported a two-dimensional (2D) MoS_2-based chemiresistive gas sensor that was highly susceptible to VOCs including ethanol, propionaldehyde (propanal), acetone, toluene, and hexane (Figure 12.8b). In addition to its excellent sensing performance, they proposed tunable sensing by surface functionalization of MoS_2 treated with thiolated ligand conjugation. The ligand differentiated the electrical responses of the gas sensor according to

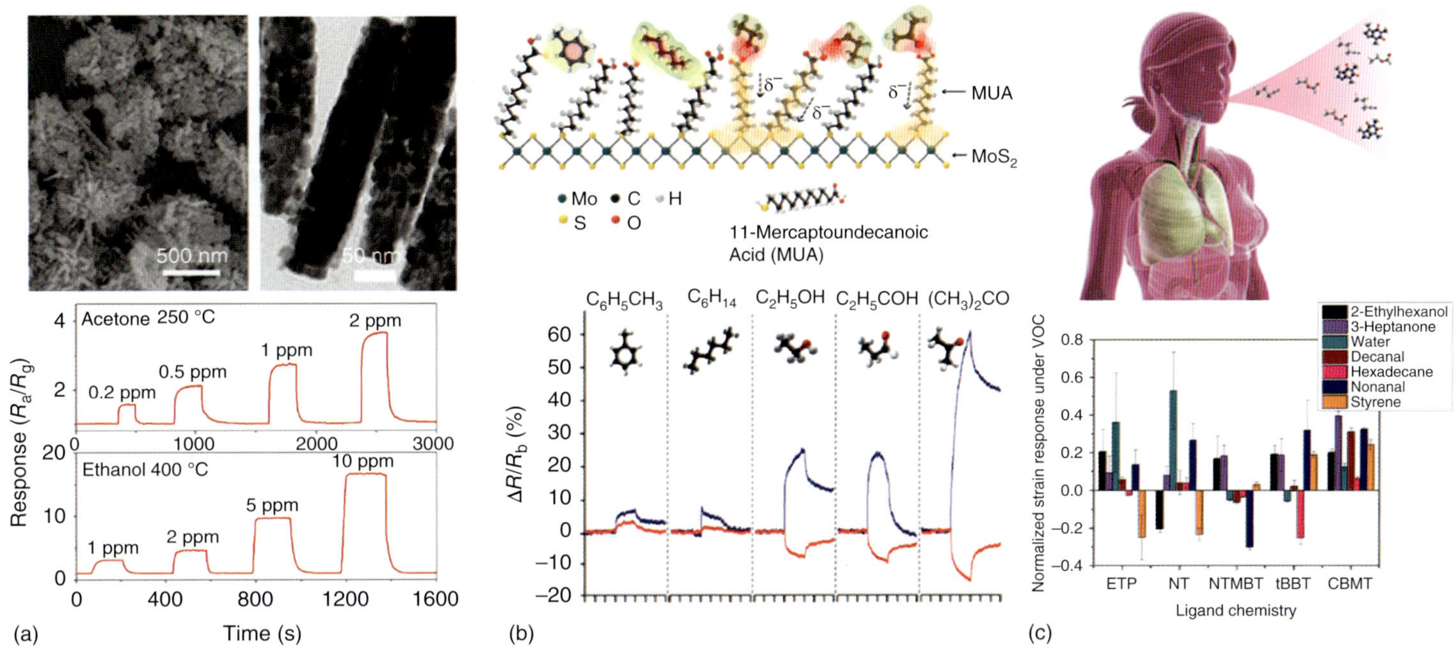

Figure 12.8 *Flexible biochemical sensors and detection of various VOCs.* (a) Scanning electron microscope (SEM) and transmission electron microscope (TEM) images of In_2O_3/Au nanorods with large surface area and dynamic responses of In_2O_3/Au nanorod-based gas sensors under exposure of acetone and ethanol, respectively. (Reproduced from Ref. [84]. with permission; Copyright 2015, Nature Publishing Group.) (b) A schematic illustration of mercaptoundecanoic acid (MUA)-conjugated MoS_2 with target VOC molecules and sensing behaviors of primitive and MUA-conjugated MoS_2-based gas sensors for toluene, hexane, propionaldehyde (propanal), and acetone. (Kim *et al*. 2014 [85]. Reproduced with permission of American Chemical Society.) (c) Schematic illustration of VOC mixture from exhaled breath and bending responses of Au-nanoparticle-based gas sensors functionalized by five thiolated ligands under exposure of 2-ethylhexanol, 3-heptanone, water, decanal, hexadecane, nonanal, and styrene. (Kahn et al. 2015 [86]. Reproduced with permission of American Chemical Society.)

the type of VOC. For example, oxygen-functionalized VOCs such as ethanol, propanal, and acetone showed different responsive behaviors to those of organic compounds of toluene and hexane.

The second important requirement of gas sensors is a high selectivity for each VOC because these generally exhibit in a mixed state. Although there have been various attempts to enhance the selectivity of gas sensors for targeted VOCs [87], it is difficult to achieve a perfectly selective sensor that can distinguish between several hundred VOCs. Instead, Kahn *et al.* [86] suggested multiple arrays of chemiresistive gas sensors based on surface-modified Au nanoparticles (AuNPs) on a flexible substrate. In essence, the surface of the AuNPs was functionalized with five thiol ligands, resulting in a selective gas sensor with different responsive behaviors according to the different types of VOC (Figure 12.8c). Even though each individual gas sensor was not sufficiently selective, the gas-sensing arrays with various responsive features provided more reliable results for breath diagnosis through their complementary analyses. Therefore, they successfully discriminated between an ovarian cancer group and a control group via breath analysis.

12.2.3 Detection Approaches for Electrophysiological Signals

In addition to the physical and chemical bio-signals that have already been discussed, electrophysiological signals from the human body also contain useful information about various organs, for example, electrocardiograms (ECGs) [88–91], electroencephalography (EEG) [92, 93], electromyography (EMG) [94, 95], and electrooculography (EOG) [96]. When muscles contract for some functional purpose, electrical depolarization signals are transmitted to the skin. Thus, a wearable and skin-attachable electrode system enables the detection of the electrical potential changes from the skin, and thus, the possible early diagnosis of disorders. Because of its noninvasive and simple process, electrophysiological examination is frequently used even in hospitals.

Above all, ECG is a widely used technique for assessing the cardiovascular system. An ECG signal comprising specific peak points (P, Q, R, S, and T) of different peak intensities, regular intervals, shape, and periodicity provides crucial data about heart condition. Similarly, EEG signals are analyzed to monitor and record brain activity. Xu *et al.* [88] fabricated a flexible and stretchable microfluidic device by integrating sensors, a circuit, and a wireless system onto an elastomeric substrate. By mounting such devices on the sternum and forehead, ECG and EEG signals, respectively, were clearly measured. For a long-term monitoring of ECG, Takamatsu *et al.* [89] developed a smart textile patterned with PEDOT:PSS electrodes, which had a low impedance contact with the human skin (Figure 12.9a). The biocompatible textile ECG sensors recorded and monitored accurate ECG signals over 3 days. Further to single-point detection, Viventi *et al.* [92] successfully mapped neural activity by using flexible and high-resolution multiplexed electrode arrays (Figure 12.9b). They implanted flexible electrode arrays on the cortical surfaces of cats and visualized real-time brain activity *in vivo*, including sleep spindles and electrographic seizures.

In addition, considerable attention has been given to the analysis of EMG and impedance because of the growing interest in fitness. In particular, EMG signals

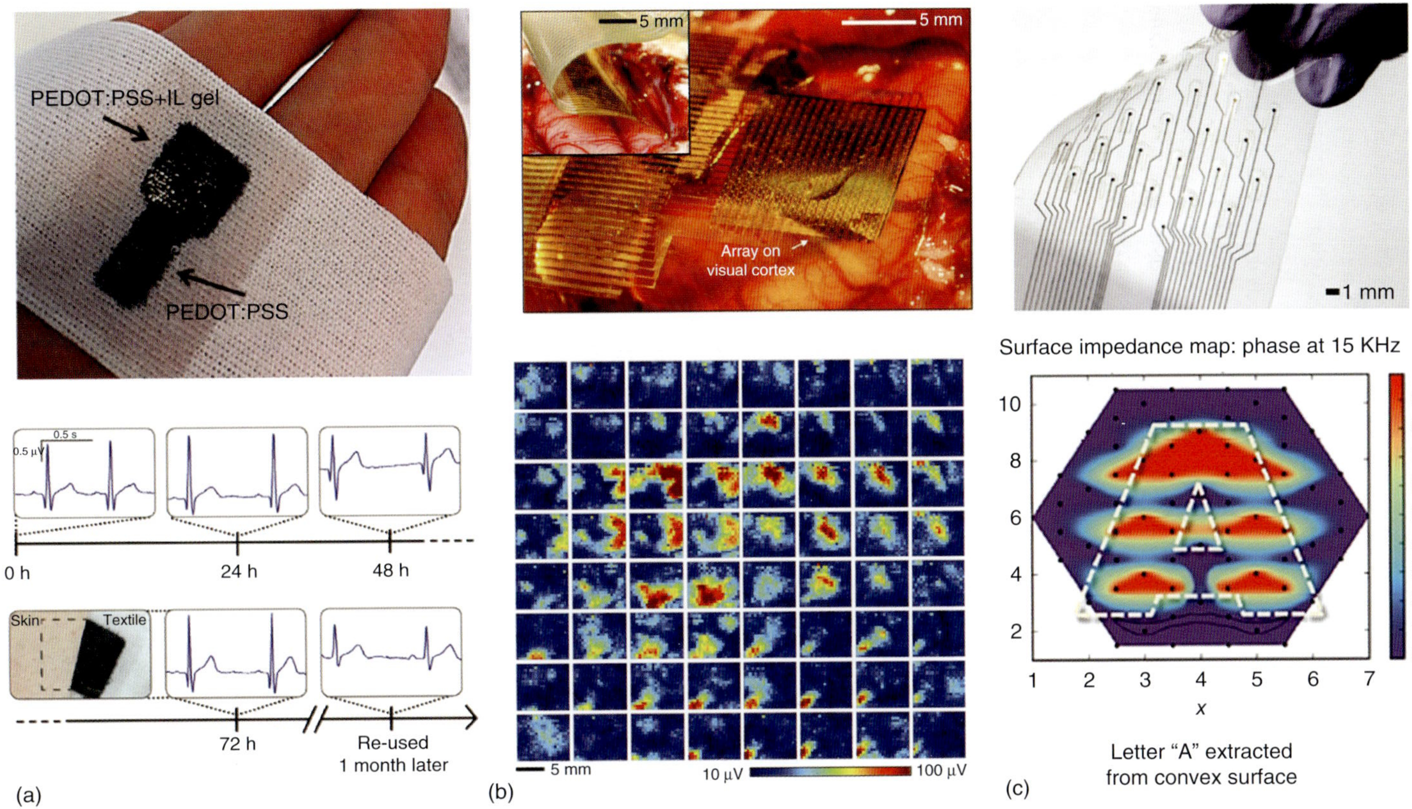

Figure 12.9 *Flexible electrophysiological sensors and detection of electrophysiological signals.* (a) Photograph of patterned PEDOT:PSS electrode on knitted textile for long-term monitoring of ECG and acquired ECG signals over 3 days. (Reproduced from Ref. [89]. with permission; Copyright 2015, Nature Publishing Group.) (b) Photograph of flexible and high-resolution multiplexed electrode arrays on the visual cortex and obtained EEG map images. (Viventi *et al*. 2011 [92]. Reproduced with permission of Nature Publishing Group.) (c) Printed flexible electrode arrays on a PEN substrate after laser cutting process and impedance map image on a 5-mm convex surface. (Khan *et al*. 2016 [97]. Reproduced with permission of John Wiley & Sons.)

represent the movement of skeletal muscles and human gestures, and thus, have huge potential in applications for rehabilitation, human–machine interfaces, and robotics. As a result, various global companies have developed wearable fitness devices. InBody Co., Ltd., is a representative company in the commercial field of body composition analysis based on bioelectrical impedance. Their analysis technique provides quantitative information about the wearer's hydration, proteins, minerals, and body fat. Khan *et al.* [97] recently reported a flexible bioelectronic interface based on inkjet-printed Au electrode arrays (Figure 12.9c). The proposed devices were specially designed with flexure cuts that enabled clear mapping of electrical impedance on 2D surfaces regardless of the mechanical bending state.

12.3 Multifunctional Flexible Sensors for Multiple Bio-Signals

Until now, we have discussed various forms of physical, biochemical, and electrophysiological bio-signals from the human body and their specific detection approaches with mono-, bi-, or tri-functionalities. In general, the human body shows not single but multiple bio-signals, even in a specific area of the body. For example, a runner experiences an increased pulse and temperature and a rapid reduction in glucose levels simultaneously in almost every part of her/his body. Therefore, future personal healthcare sensors should exist in a single system that can detect multiple bio-signals. Some leading research groups have demonstrated advanced wearable healthcare sensors with multifunctional sensing abilities [98–104]. From a technical viewpoint, multifunctional sensing devices require sophisticated techniques to integrate diverse sensors and to design multiple sensing modes in a single system. The state-of-the-art technology in multifunctional flexible sensors has the advantages of high accessibility and usability for consumers, as well as allowing more reliable self-diagnoses of diseases via complementary analysis of multiple bio-signals.

Choi *et al.* [98] suggested a skin-attachable multifunctional medical sensor (Figure 12.10a) that can monitor almost every type of vital sign, such as physical muscle movements, pulse, temperature, and respiration, as well as electrophysiological behavior from an ECG sensor (Figure 12.10b). In particular, a smart patch with ultralow modulus (~108 kPa) was inspired by a cephalopod's suction cups, resulting in a significant improvement in skin adhesion for practical applications. This multifunctional patch was also combined with a commercial smart band that provided wireless transmission of recorded vital signs to mediate the remote control of a drug injection.

In addition, Gao *et al.* [99] developed multiplexed perspiration sensor arrays by integrating electrochemical sensors for the likes of glucose, lactate, sodium, and potassium with resistive temperature sensors on a flexible printed circuit board (FPCB) (Figure 12.10c). The five electrochemical and temperature sensors integrated on the FPCB had sufficient sensitivities to detect human perspiration signals ($\leq$200 μM of glucose, $\leq$30 μM of lactate, 10–160 mM of Na^+, 1–32 mM

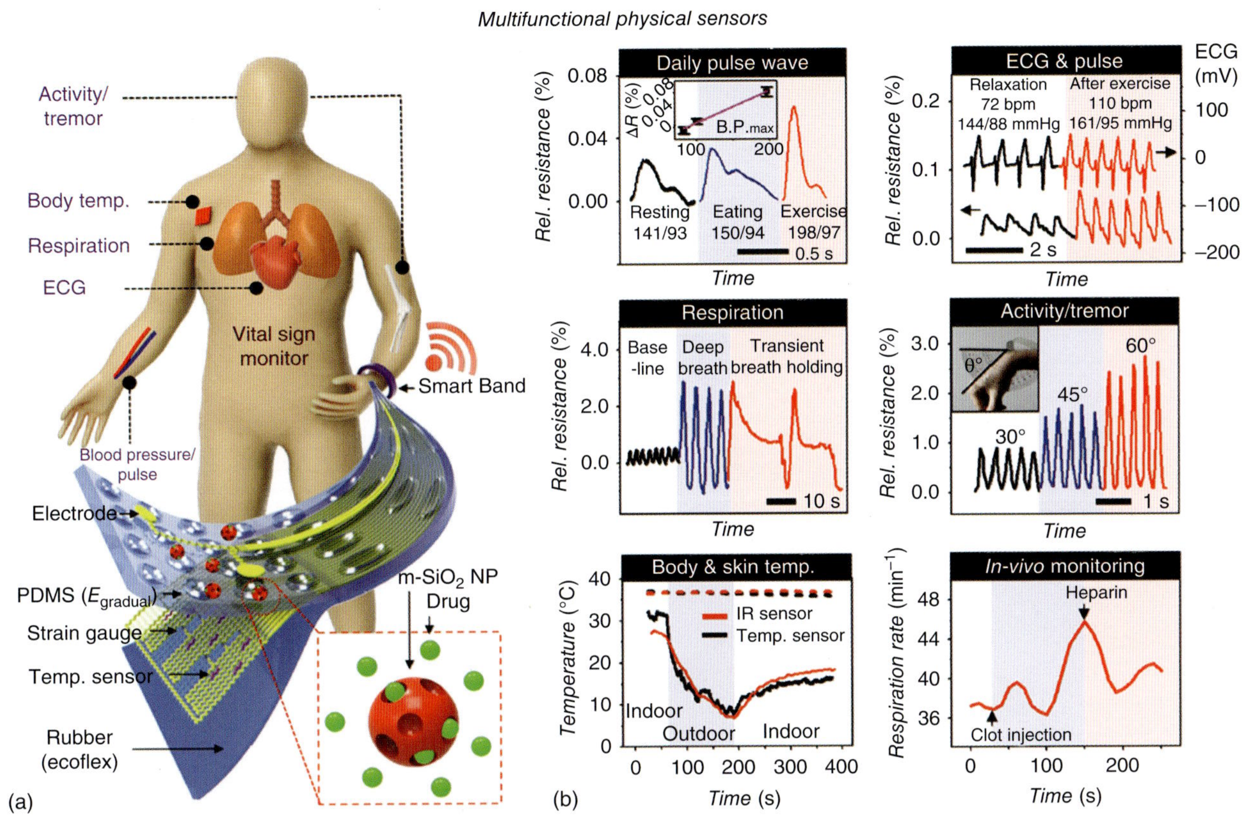

Figure 12.10 *Multifunctional sensors for detection of multiple bio-signals.* (a) Schematic illustration of bioinspired dry-adhesive-based multifunctional electronic patch for monitoring vital signs, wireless signal transmission, and drug delivery. (b) Detection of acute medical conditions with multifunctional patch. (a,b: Choi *et al*. 2016 [98]. Reproduced with permission of John Wiley & Sons.) (c) Photograph and schematic illustration of flexible integrated sensing arrays for perspiration analysis. (d) Selective detection of four types of chemicals (glucose, lactate, sodium, and potassium) and temperature. (e) Real-time perspiration monitoring during cycling using smart wristband. (c–e: Gao *et al*. 2016 [99]. Reproduced with permission of Nature Publishing Group.)

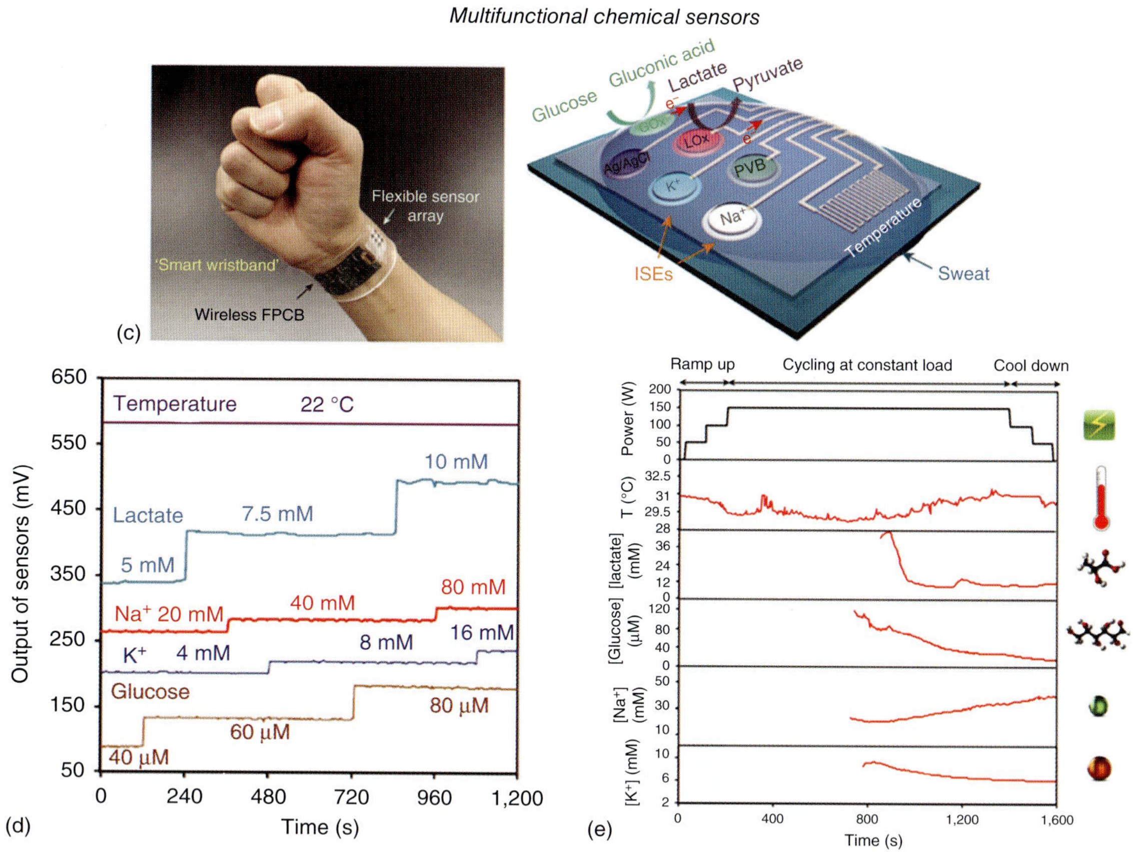

Figure 12.10 (*Continued*)

of K^+, and temperatures of 20–40 °C with high selectivity (Figure 12.10d). Moreover, they fabricated smart wrist- and head-bands for real-time monitoring and perspiration analysis. These multifunctional smart bands successfully monitored on-body real-time perspiration during cycling (Figure 12.10e) and running by using wireless communication with mobile devices.

12.4 Practical Applications of Flexible Health-Monitoring Devices

Ready-fabricated flexible healthcare sensors can be used in several application fields to improve both wellness and usability. Body-wearable/attachable health-monitoring devices have already been developed [105] and have been studied actively with human–machine interface systems to create more interactive healthcare devices [106–108]. Sports/fitness coaching, rehabilitation and prosthetics, wound therapy, and medical diagnosis are the various application fields that introduce promising and practical uses of flexible health-monitoring devices .

12.4.1 Sports and Fitness

Body-wearable and skin-attachable sensors in accessories, textile or epidermal electronics can be used for athletic training or the general improvement of fitness [109, 110]. The accessory-type of motion sensors, such as the smart band, ring, watch, textiles, and glasses, has already been commercialized in this application field [111]. In terms of research, more effective and comfortable forms of pressure and strain sensors combined with textiles enable the monitoring of daily activities during stretching, walking, running, sprinting, and cooling down (Figure 12.11a) [38]. Self-powered textiles integrated with super-capacitors can even supply power to operate the sensors without the need for an external power source. Thus, human interactive and independent healthcare sensors for fitness applications would be beneficial to the public as well as for professional athletes. In addition, Figure 12.11b shows tattoo biosensors that have electrochemical lactate sensors, which were developed with the aim of assessing the physical performance for an athlete [110]. The epidermal lactate sensors with noninvasive manner provide useful information about the dynamics of sweat lactate production during physical activity/exercise, thereby having considerable prospect for sports and healthcare application.

12.4.2 Prosthetics and Rehabilitation

The development of tactile/motion sensors has shown progess in areas such as touch screens, robotics, prosthetics, and medical rehabilitation. In particular, many of the current bulky and uncomfortable fitted prosthetic devices can be replaced with smaller wearable ones. A tactile-sensitive prosthesis resembling human skin can be used to create artificial limbs that move freely and appropriately under the control of the human nervous system via tactile sensors.

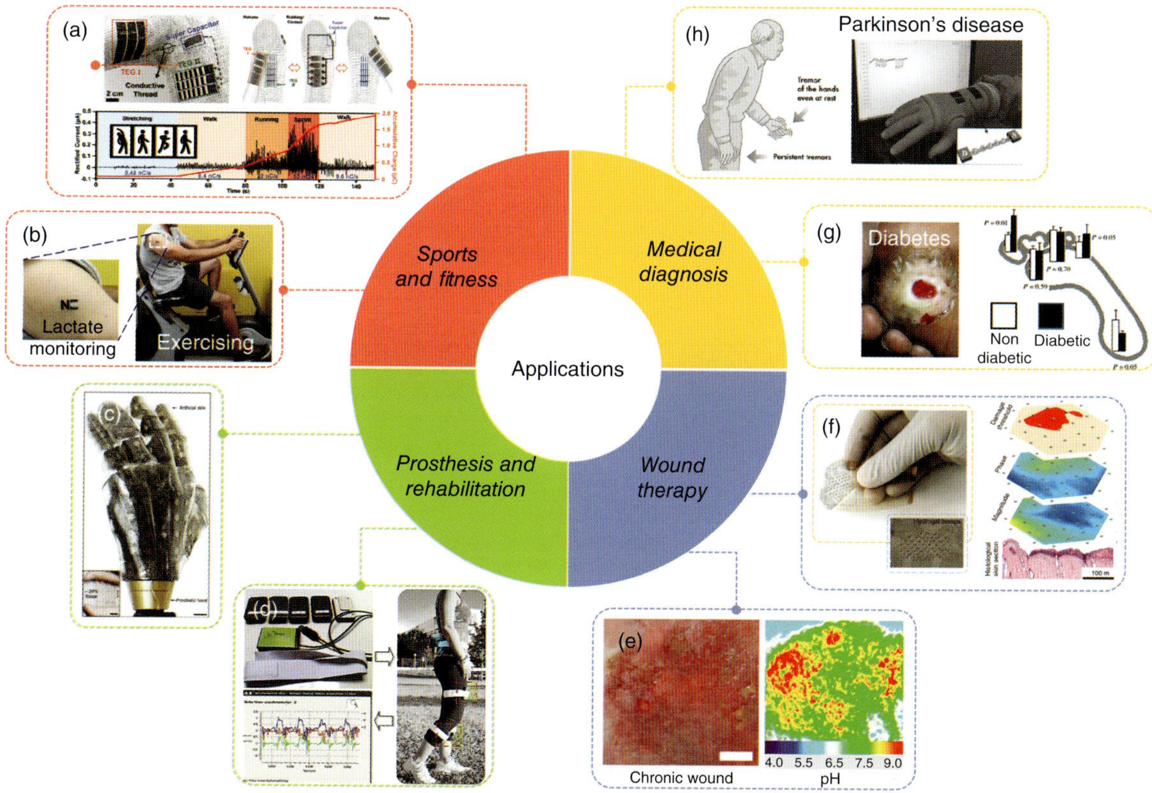

Figure 12.11 *Practical applications of health-monitoring devices.* (a) Fabric-based wearable activity monitors for fitness applications. (Jung *et al*. 2014 [38]. Reproduced with permission of John Wiley & Sons.) (b) Electrochemical tattoo biosensors for noninvasive lactate sensing during exercise. (Jia *et al*. 2013 [110]. Reproduced with permission of American Chemical Society.) (c) Skin prosthesis mimicking the role of human sensory receptors. (Kim *et al*. 2014 [103]. Reproduced with permission of Nature Publishing Group.) (d) Wearable multi-sensor system for physical rehabilitation of patients. (Reproduced from Ref. [112] with permission; Copyright 2013, Multidisciplinary Digital Publishing Institute.) (e) Photograph and 2D luminescence image of pH level of chronic wound. (Reproduced from Ref. [113] with permission; Copyright 2011, National Academy of Sciences.) (f) Bandage-type impedance sensor for early diagnosis of pressure ulcers. (Swisher *et al*. 2015 [114]. Reproduced with permission of Nature Publishing Group.) (g) Potential application of diagnosis and treatment for diabetic patients by monitoring the pressure location of their foot. (Cavanagh *et al*. 2005 [115]. Reproduced with permission of Elsevier; Pataky *et al*. 2005 [116]. Reproduced with permission of John Wiley & Sons.) (h) Early diagnosis of Parkinson's disease showing symptoms of shaking wrists and uneven gait

Figure 12.11c shows a skin prosthesis composed of ultrathin silicon nanoribbon sensors for strain, pressure, temperature, and humidity, representing the multifunctional sensing properties of human skin [103]. This skin prosthesis allows the wearer to feel various external stimuli by stimulating the corresponding peripheral nervous system through a low-impedance multi-electrode array. The field of rehabilitation is generally concerned with long-term care under the supervision of physical therapists; hence, portable and wearable healthcare devices are required [112, 118, 119]. Even though a physical therapist can professionally assess and evaluate a patient's posture, accurate decisions often require more than a visual assessment. In addition, it is often difficult or even impossible for a patient to attend continuous and long-term hospital/clinic-based monitoring. Therefore, as shown in Figure 12.11d, for the rehabilitation of patients suffering from a severe injury, one approach is to have a wearable multisensor system integrated with accelerometers and wireless communications to provide real-time monitoring and analysis of the bodily movements with an objective feedback [112].

12.4.3 Wound Therapy

There are many external factors that affect a wound healing process, including pressure, temperature, pH, moisture, and oxygen concentration. For example, the tracking of skin pH levels enables the healing status of a wound to be estimated. The wounded area has a more alkaline pH level to protect it from infection, whereas the normal state of skin is slightly acidic (pH 4–6). Therefore, the pH level around the wound changes from alkaline to acidic during the healing process. Oxygen also plays an important role in wound healing, such as NADPH oxidases and oxidative phosphorylation [120].

Therefore, noninvasive and body-attachable pH sensors or oximeters can be utilized to confirm the status of a wound in order to prevent chronic illness. Schreml *et al.* [121, 122] suggested 2D luminescence imaging of pH level and wound oxygenation as tools to monitor wound healing status (Figure 12.11e). Their approach of luminescence-based optical imaging enabled noninvasive and bio-compatible detection of pH level and oxygenation on the wounded area. Furthermore, Kassal *et al.* [113] developed a bandage-type electrochemical sensor to detect uric acid. This smart bandage was enabled with wireless communication to transmit the uric acid level of a wound to the patient's mobile devices, thus allowing for personal wound care. In addition to monitoring the status of a wound, Swisher *et al.* [114] developed a smart bandage based on an impedance sensor that enabled early diagnosis of pressure ulcers (Figure 12.11f).

12.4.4 Telemedicine and Self-Diagnosis of Disease

Reliable and highly sensitive healthcare sensors can be used in telemedicine and the self-diagnosis of diseases for early detection and increased convenience [15, 123]. In particular, sufferers of chronic diseases such as asthma, cancer, Parkinson's disease (PD), and diabetes would benefit from the continuous monitoring of their disease progression by personal healthcare devices in order to prevent severe complications [17]. For example, patients who suffer from diabetes are usually also affected by foot ulcers caused by acute mechanical and thermal trauma due to the repetitive concentration of mechanical stress in their feet (Figure 12.11g) [115, 116]. In addition, the increasingly common neurodegenerative PD can be detected at an early stage by monitoring shaking hands or an uneven gait. As shown in Figure 12.11h, highly sensitive fiber-based strain sensors can recognize the muscle movement driven by the shaking of the human wrist, which is a common symptom of PD [117].

12.5 Conclusions and Future Perspective

In this chapter, we investigated the recent progress in flexible healthcare sensors for human bio-signals such as motion and activity; the physical vital signs of HR, BP, respiration rate, and body temperature changes; biochemical signals for monitoring bodily pH variations, blood sugar level, and other chemicals indicating health conditions; and electrophysiological signals from the various organs. For the development of comfortable and user-friendly health-monitoring devices, miniaturized, body-wearable, and skin-attachable sensors were suggested with novel structural and geometrical modification of the constituent materials and device-fabrication techniques. In addition, the high performance of multifunctional sensors was demonstrated through the detection of multiple bio-signals for various practical applications.

Despite rapid and significant progress in flexible healthcare sensors, there are still certain challenges and limitations to using them in real life. First, the precise detection of desired signals is problematic due to the difficulty of differentiating them from other physiological signs, motion artifacts, and numerous variables in the surrounding environment. Therefore, highly selective and reliable sensors that are capable of removing signal cross-talk must be established for future healthcare devices. In addition, the realization of totally flexible and skin-mountable healthcare devices is limited by indispensable electronic components such as electrodes, circuit boards, energy storage, and communication modules that are usually rigid, take up space, and degrade flexibility and stretchability. Thus, the integration of flexible sensors and energy storage devices with innovative designs for stretchable interconnections and circuit systems need to be developed for realistic applications. Better connection and packaging technologies for sensors, power supplies, data acquisition units, and user-interactive communication systems will facilitate remote management, continuous long-term recording, and real-time monitoring for future health-monitoring devices.

References

1 Sapargaliyev, D. (2015) Learning with wearable technologies: a case of google glass, in *Mobile Learning Voyage - From Small Ripples to Massive Open Waters*, vol. **560** (eds T.H. Brown and H.J. Van Der Merwe), Springer, Gewerbestrasse, pp. 343–350.

2 Akana, J., Andre, B.K., Aoyagi, S., Ashcroft, A.M., Bataillou, J., Coster, D.J., De Iuliis, D., Hankey, M.E., Hoenig, J., and Howarth, R.P. (2015) Wearable device. US Patents 29, 499,088, filed Aug. 11, 2014 and issued Aug. 25, 2015.
3 Jakus, A.E., Secor, E.B., Rutz, A.L., Jordan, S.W., Hersam, M.C., and Shah, R.N. (2015) Three-dimensional printing of high-content graphene scaffolds for electronic and biomedical applications. *ACS Nano*, **9** (4), 4636–4648.
4 Takei, K. (2015) *Wearable Electronics Sensors*, Springer, Gewerbestrasse.
5 Takei, K., Honda, W., Harada, S., Arie, T., and Akita, S. (2015) Toward flexible and wearable human-interactive health-monitoring devices. *Adv. Healthcare Mater.*, **4** (4), 487–500.
6 Rodgers, M.M., Pai, V.M., and Conroy, R.S. (2015) Recent advances in wearable sensors for health monitoring. *IEEE Sens. J.*, **15** (6), 3119–3126.
7 Park, J., Lee, Y., Ha, M., Cho, S., and Ko, H. (2016) Micro/nanostructured surfaces for self-powered and multifunctional electronic skins. *J. Mater. Chem. B*, **4** (18), 2999–3018.
8 Kang, D., Pikhitsa, P.V., Choi, Y.W., Lee, C., Shin, S.S., Piao, L.F., Park, B., Suh, K.Y., Kim, T.I., and Choi, M. (2014) Ultrasensitive mechanical crack-based sensor inspired by the spider sensory system. *Nature*, **516** (7530), 222–226.
9 Ha, M., Lim, S., Park, J., Um, D.S., Lee, Y., and Ko, H. (2015) Bioinspired interlocked and hierarchical design of ZnO nanowire arrays for static and dynamic pressure-sensitive electronic skins. *Adv. Funct. Mater.*, **25** (19), 2841–2849.
10 Pang, C., Koo, J.H., Nguyen, A., Caves, J.M., Kim, M.G., Chortos, A., Kim, K., Wang, P.J., Tok, J.B.H., and Bao, Z.A. (2015) Highly skin-conformal microhairy sensor for pulse signal amplification. *Adv. Mater.*, **27** (4), 634–640.
11 Kim, D.H., Lu, N.S., Ma, R., Kim, Y.S., Kim, R.H., Wang, S.D., Wu, J., Won, S.M., Tao, H., Islam, A., Yu, K.J., Kim, T.I., Chowdhury, R., Ying, M., Xu, L.Z., Li, M., Chung, H.J., Keum, H., McCormick, M., Liu, P., Zhang, Y.W., Omenetto, F.G., Huang, Y.G., Coleman, T., and Rogers, J.A. (2011) Epidermal electronics. *Science*, **333** (6044), 838–843.
12 Kim, D.-H., Song, J., Choi, W.M., Kim, H.-S., Kim, R.-H., Liu, Z., Huang, Y.Y., Hwang, K.-C., Zhang, Y.-W., and Rogers, J.A. (2008) Materials and noncoplanar mesh designs for integrated circuits with linear elastic responses to extreme mechanical deformations. *Proc. Natl. Acad. Sci. U.S.A.*, **105** (48), 18675–18680.
13 Kaltenbrunner, M., Sekitani, T., Reeder, J., Yokota, T., Kuribara, K., Tokuhara, T., Drack, M., Schwoediauer, R., Graz, I., Bauer-Gogonea, S., Bauer, S., and Someya, T. (2013) An ultra-lightweight design for imperceptible plastic electronics. *Nature*, **499** (7459), 458–463.
14 Fukuda, K., Takeda, Y., Yoshimura, Y., Shiwaku, R., Lam Truc, T., Sekine, T., Mizukami, M., Kumaki, D., and Tokito, S. (2014) Fully-printed high-performance organic thin-film transistors and circuitry on one-micron-thick polymer films. *Nat. Commun.*, **5**. doi: 10.1038/ncomms5147

15 Hung, K., Zhang, Y., and Tai, B. (2004) Wearable medical devices for tele-home healthcare. 26th Annual International Conference of the IEEE Engineering in Medicine and Biology Society, San Francisco, CA, Sep 1–4, 2004.

16 Son, D., Lee, J., Qiao, S., Ghaffari, R., Kim, J., Lee, J.E., Song, C., Kim, S.J., Lee, D.J., Jun, S.W., Yang, S., Park, M., Shin, J., Do, K., Lee, M., Kang, K., Hwang, C.S., Lu, N., Hyeon, T., and Kim, D.-H. (2014) Multifunctional wearable devices for diagnosis and therapy of movement disorders. *Nat. Nanotechnol.*, **9** (5), 397–404.

17 Korhonen, I., Parkka, J., and Van Gils, M. (2003) Health monitoring in the home of the future. *IEEE Eng. Med. Biol. Mag.*, **22** (3), 66–73.

18 Schwartz, G., Tee, B.C.K., Mei, J., Appleton, A.L., Kim, D.H., Wang, H., and Bao, Z. (2013) Flexible polymer transistors with high pressure sensitivity for application in electronic skin and health monitoring. *Nat. Commun.*, **4**, 1859.

19 Lotters, J.C., Olthuis, W., Veltink, P.H., and Bergveld, P. (1997) The mechanical properties of the rubber elastic polymer polydimethylsiloxane for sensor applications. *J. Micromech. Microeng.*, **7** (3), 145–147.

20 Schmid, H. and Michel, B. (2000) Siloxane polymers for high-resolution, high-accuracy soft lithography. *Macromolecules*, **33** (8), 3042–3049.

21 Belanger, M.C. and Marois, Y. (2001) Hemocompatibility, biocompatibility, inflammatory and *in vivo* studies of primary reference materials low-density polyethylene and polydimethylsiloxane: a review. *J. Biomed. Mater. Res.*, **58** (5), 467–477.

22 Mata, A., Fleischman, A.J., and Roy, S. (2005) Characterization of polydimethylsiloxane (PDMS) properties for biomedical micro/nanosystems. *Biomed. Microdevices*, **7** (4), 281–293.

23 Roh, E., Hwang, B.-U., Kim, D., Kim, B.-Y., and Lee, N.-E. (2015) Stretchable, transparent, ultrasensitive, and patchable strain sensor for human–machine interfaces comprising a nanohybrid of carbon nanotubes and conductive elastomers. *ACS Nano*, **9** (6), 6252–6261.

24 Takei, K., Takahashi, T., Ho, J.C., Ko, H., Gillies, A.G., Leu, P.W., Fearing, R.S., and Javey, A. (2010) Nanowire active-matrix circuitry for low-voltage macroscale artificial skin. *Nat. Mater.*, **9** (10), 821–826.

25 Wu, W., Wen, X., and Wang, Z.L. (2013) Taxel-addressable matrix of vertical-nanowire piezotronic transistors for active and adaptive tactile imaging. *Science*, **340** (6135), 952–957.

26 Lanzara, G., Salowitz, N., Guo, Z., and Chang, F.-K. (2010) A spider-web-like highly expandable sensor network for multifunctional materials. *Adv. Mater.*, **22** (41), 4643–4648.

27 Gong, S., Schwalb, W., Wang, Y., Chen, Y., Tang, Y., Si, J., Shirinzadeh, B., and Cheng, W. (2014) A wearable and highly sensitive pressure sensor with ultrathin gold nanowires. *Nat. Commun.*, **5**. doi: 10.1038/ncomms4132

28 Steven, E., Saleh, W.R., Lebedev, V., Acquah, S.F.A., Laukhin, V., Alamo, R.G., and Brooks, J.S. (2013) Carbon nanotubes on a spider silk scaffold. *Nat. Commun.*, **4**. doi: 10.1038/ncomms3435

29 Jeong, Y.R., Park, H., Jin, S.W., Hong, S.Y., Lee, S.S., and Ha, J.S. (2015) Highly stretchable and sensitive strain sensors using fragmentized graphene foam. *Adv. Funct. Mater.*, **25** (27), 4228–4236.

30 Han, X., Chen, X., Tang, X., Chen, Y.L., Liu, J.H., and Shen, Q.D. (2016) Flexible polymer transducers for dynamic recognizing physiological signals. *Adv. Funct. Mater.*, **26** (21), 3640–3648.
31 Park, H., Jeong, Y.R., Yun, J., Hong, S.Y., Jin, S., Lee, S.-J., Zi, G., and Ha, J.S. (2015) Stretchable array of highly sensitive pressure sensors consisting of polyaniline nanofibers and Au-coated polydimethylsiloxane micropillars. *ACS Nano*, **9** (10), 9974–9985.
32 Hammock, M.L., Chortos, A., Tee, B.C.K., Tok, J.B.H., and Bao, Z. (2013) 25th anniversary article: the evolution of electronic skin (E-Skin): a brief history, design considerations, and recent progress. *Adv. Mater.*, **25** (42), 5997–6037.
33 Tombler, T.W., Zhou, C.W., Alexseyev, L., Kong, J., Dai, H.J., Lei, L., Jayanthi, C.S., Tang, M.J., and Wu, S.Y. (2000) Reversible electromechanical characteristics of carbon nanotubes under local-probe manipulation. *Nature*, **405** (6788), 769–772.
34 Park, J., Lee, Y., Hong, J., Ha, M., Jung, Y.-D., Lim, H., Kim, S.Y., and Ko, H. (2014) Giant tunneling piezoresistance of composite elastomers with interlocked microdome arrays for ultrasensitive and multimodal electronic skins. *ACS Nano*, **8** (5), 4689–4697.
35 Lipomi, D.J., Vosgueritchian, M., Tee, B.C.K., Hellstrom, S.L., Lee, J.A., Fox, C.H., and Bao, Z. (2011) Skin-like pressure and strain sensors based on transparent elastic films of carbon nanotubes. *Nat. Nanotechnol.*, **6** (12), 788–792.
36 Fan, F.R., Tang, W., and Wang, Z.L. (2016) Flexible nanogenerators for energy harvesting and self-powered electronics. *Adv. Mater.*, **28** (22), 4283–4305.
37 Cheng, Y., Wang, R., Sun, J., and Gao, L. (2015) A stretchable and highly sensitive graphene-based fiber for sensing tensile strain, bending, and torsion. *Adv. Mater.*, **27** (45), 7365–7371.
38 Jung, S., Lee, J., Hyeon, T., Lee, M., and Kim, D.-H. (2014) Fabric-based integrated energy devices for wearable activity monitors. *Adv. Mater.*, **26** (36), 6329–6334.
39 Wang, Y., Wang, L., Yang, T., Li, X., Zang, X., Zhu, M., Wang, K., Wu, D., and Zhu, H. (2014) Wearable and highly sensitive graphene strain sensors for human motion monitoring. *Adv. Funct. Mater.*, **24** (29), 4666–4670.
40 Wang, C., Li, X., Gao, E., Jian, M., Xia, K., Wang, Q., Xu, Z., Ren, T., and Zhang, Y. (2016) Carbonized silk fabric for ultrastretchable, highly sensitive, and wearable strain sensors. *Adv. Mater.* doi: 10.1002/adma.201601572
41 Park, J., Lee, Y., Hong, J., Lee, Y., Ha, M., Jung, Y., Lim, H., Kim, S.Y., and Ko, H. (2014) Tactile-direction-sensitive and stretchable electronic skins based on human-skin-inspired interlocked microstructures. *ACS Nano*, **8** (12), 12020–12029.
42 Park, J., Kim, M., Lee, Y., Lee, H.S., and Ko, H. (2015) Fingertip skin–inspired microstructured ferroelectric skins discriminate static/dynamic pressure and temperature stimuli. *Sci. Adv.*, **1** (9), e1500661.
43 Cohn, J.N., Finkelstein, S., McVeigh, G., Morgan, D., LeMay, L., Robinson, J., and Mock, J. (1995) Noninvasive pulse wave analysis for the early detection of vascular disease. *Hypertens.*, **26** (3), 503–508.

44 White, W.B., Wolfson, L., Guttman, C., Moscufo, N., Wakefield, D., Kaplan, R., and Pearlson, G. (2011) Average daily blood pressure, not office blood pressure, determines the progression of cerebrovascular disease and functional decline in older persons. *J. Am. Coll. Cardiol.*, **57** (14), E490.
45 Hwang, B.-U., Lee, J.-H., Tran Quang, T., Roh, E., Kim, D.-I., Kim, S.-W., and Lee, N.-E. (2015) Transparent stretchable self-powered patchable sensor platform with ultrasensitive recognition of human activities. *ACS Nano*, **9** (9), 8801–8810.
46 Larsson, L.-G., Lindberg, A., Franklin, K., and Lundbäck, B. (2001) Symptoms related to obstructive sleep apnoea are common in subjects with asthma, chronic bronchitis and rhinitis in a general population. *Respir. Med.*, **95** (5), 423–429.
47 O'Donnell, D.E., Revill, S.M., and Webb, K.A. (2001) Dynamic hyperinflation and exercise intolerance in chronic obstructive pulmonary disease. *Am. J. Respir. Crit. Care Med.*, **164** (5), 770–777.
48 Boland, C.S., Khan, U., Backes, C., O'Neill, A., McCauley, J., Duane, S., Shanker, R., Liu, Y., Jurewicz, I., Dalton, A.B., and Coleman, J.N. (2014) Sensitive, high-strain, high-rate bodily motion sensors based on graphene-rubber composites. *ACS Nano*, **8** (9), 8819–8830.
49 Hutchison, J.S., Ward, R.E., Lacroix, J., Hebert, P.C., Barnes, M.A., Bohn, D.J., Dirks, P.B., Doucette, S., Fergusson, D., and Gottesman, R. (2008) Hypothermia therapy after traumatic brain injury in children. *N. Engl. J. Med.*, **358** (23), 2447–2456.
50 Bota, D.P., Ferreira, F.L., Mélot, C., and Vincent, J.L. (2004) Body temperature alterations in the critically ill. *Intensive Care Med.*, **30** (5), 811–816.
51 Kelly, G. (2006) Body temperature variability (Part 1): a review of the history of body temperature and its variability due to site selection, biological rhythms, fitness, and aging. *Altern. Med. Rev.*, **11** (4), 278–293.
52 Lenhardt, R. and Sessler, D.I. (2006) Estimation of mean body temperature from mean skin and core temperature. *Anesthesiology*, **105** (6), 1117–1121.
53 Savage, M.V. and Brengelmann, G.L. (1996) Control of skin blood flow in the neutral zone of human body temperature regulation. *J. Appl. Physiol.*, **80** (4), 1249–1257.
54 Olesen, B.W. (1982) Thermal comfort. *Tech. Rev.*, **2**, 3–37.
55 Harada, S., Kanao, K., Yamamoto, Y., Arie, T., Akita, S., and Takei, K. (2014) Fully printed flexible fingerprint-like three-axis tactile and slip force and temperature sensors for artificial skin. *ACS Nano*, **8** (12), 12851–12857.
56 Yokota, T., Inoue, Y., Terakawa, Y., Reeder, J., Kaltenbrunner, M., Ware, T., Yang, K., Mabuchi, K., Murakawa, T., Sekino, M., Voit, W., Sekitani, T., and Someya, T. (2015) Ultraflexible, large-area, physiological temperature sensors for multipoint measurements. *Proc. Natl. Acad. Sci. U.S.A.*, **112** (47), 14533–14538.
57 Imran, M. and Bhattacharyya, A. (2006) Effect of thin film thicknesses and materials on the response of RTDs and microthermocouples. *IEEE Sens. J.*, **6** (6), 1459–1467.

58 Zhang, F., Zang, Y., Huang, D., Di, C.-A., and Zhu, D. (2015) Flexible and self-powered temperature-pressure dual-parameter sensors using microstructure-frame-supported organic thermoelectric materials. *Nat. Commun.*, **6**, 8356.

59 Gao, L., Zhang, Y., Malyarchuk, V., Jia, L., Jang, K.-I., Webb, R.C., Fu, H., Shi, Y., Zhou, G., Shi, L., Shah, D., Huang, X., Xu, B., Yu, C., Huang, Y., and Rogers, J.A. (2014) Epidermal photonic devices for quantitative imaging of temperature and thermal transport characteristics of the skin. *Nat. Commun.*, **5**, 4938.

60 Shih, W.-P., Tsao, L.-C., Lee, C.-W., Cheng, M.-Y., Chang, C., Yang, Y.-J., and Fan, K.-C. (2010) Flexible temperature sensor array based on a graphite-polydimethylsiloxane composite. *Sensors*, **10** (4), 3597–3610.

61 Trung, T.Q., Ramasundaram, S., Hwang, B.U., and Lee, N.E. (2016) An all-elastomeric transparent and stretchable temperature sensor for body-attachable wearable electronics. *Adv. Mater.*, **28** (3), 502–509.

62 Trung, T.Q., Ramasundaram, S., Hong, S.W., and Lee, N.E. (2014) Flexible and transparent nanocomposite of reduced graphene oxide and P(VDF-TrFE) copolymer for high thermal responsivity in a field-effect transistor. *Adv. Funct. Mater.*, **24** (22), 3438–3445.

63 Kraemer, D., Poudel, B., Feng, H.-P., Caylor, J.C., Yu, B., Yan, X., Ma, Y., Wang, X., Wang, D., Muto, A., McEnaney, K., Chiesa, M., Ren, Z., and Chen, G. (2011) High-performance flat-panel solar thermoelectric generators with high thermal concentration. *Nat. Mater.*, **10** (7), 532–538.

64 Kim, S.J., We, J.H., and Cho, B.J. (2014) A wearable thermoelectric generator fabricated on a glass fabric. *Energy Environ. Sci.*, **7** (6), 1959–1965.

65 Haick, H., Broza, Y.Y., Mochalski, P., Ruzsanyi, V., and Amann, A. (2014) Assessment, origin, and implementation of breath volatile cancer markers. *Chem. Soc. Rev.*, **43** (5), 1423–1449.

66 Amann, A., Mochalski, P., Ruzsanyi, V., Broza, Y.Y., and Haick, H. (2014) Assessment of the exhalation kinetics of volatile cancer biomarkers based on their physicochemical properties. *J. Breath Res.*, **8** (1), 016003.

67 Bandodkar, A.J., Hung, V.W., Jia, W., Valdes-Ramirez, G., Windmiller, J.R., Martinez, A.G., Ramirez, J., Chan, G., Kerman, K., and Wang, J. (2013) Tattoo-based potentiometric ion-selective sensors for epidermal pH monitoring. *Analyst*, **138** (1), 123–128.

68 Mailly-Giacchetti, B., Hsu, A., Wang, H., Vinciguerra, V., Pappalardo, F., Occhipinti, L., Guidetti, E., Coffa, S., Kong, J., and Palacios, T.S. (2013) pH sensing properties of graphene solution-gated field-effect transistors. *J. Appl. Phys.*, **114** (8), 084505.

69 Yan, L., Chang, Y.N., Yin, W., Liu, X., Xiao, D., Xing, G., Zhao, L., Gu, Z., and Zhao, Y. (2014) Biocompatible and flexible graphene oxide/upconversion nanoparticle hybrid film for optical pH sensing. *Phys. Chem. Chem. Phys.*, **16** (4), 1576–1582.

70 Rim, Y.S., Bae, S.H., Chen, H., Yang, J.L., Kim, J., Andrews, A.M., Weiss, P.S., Yang, Y., and Tseng, H.R. (2015) Printable ultrathin metal oxide semiconductor-based conformal biosensors. *ACS Nano*, **9** (12), 12174–12181.

71 Santos, L., Neto, J.P., Crespo, A., Nunes, D., Costa, N., Fonseca, I.M., Barquinha, P., Pereira, L., Silva, J., Martins, R., and Fortunato, E. (2014) WO_3 nanoparticle-based conformable pH sensor. *ACS Appl. Mater. Interfaces*, **6** (15), 12226–12234.

72 Maiolo, L., Mirabella, S., Maita, F., Alberti, A., Minotti, A., Strano, V., Pecora, A., Shacham-Diamand, Y., and Fortunato, G. (2014) Flexible pH sensors based on polysilicon thin film transistors and ZnO nanowalls. *Appl. Phys. Lett.*, **105** (9), 093501.

73 Liu, N., Zhu, L.Q., Feng, P., Wan, C.J., Liu, Y.H., Shi, Y., and Wan, Q. (2015) Flexible sensory platform based on oxide-based neuromorphic transistors. *Sci. Rep.*, **5**, 18082.

74 Tamayol, A., Akbari, M., Zilberman, Y., Comotto, M., Lesha, E., Serex, L., Bagherifard, S., Chen, Y., Fu, G., Ameri, S.K., Ruan, W., Miller, E.L., Dokmeci, M.R., Sonkusale, S., and Khademhosseini, A. (2016) Flexible pH-sensing hydrogel fibers for epidermal applications. *Adv. Healthcare Mater.*, **5** (6), 711–719.

75 Bandodkar, A.J., Jia, W., Yardimci, C., Wang, X., Ramirez, J., and Wang, J. (2015) Tattoo-based noninvasive glucose monitoring: a proof-of-concept study. *Anal. Chem.*, **87** (1), 394–398.

76 Chu, M.X., Miyajima, K., Takahashi, D., Arakawa, T., Sano, K., Sawada, S., Kudo, H., Iwasaki, Y., Akiyoshi, K., Mochizuki, M., and Mitsubayashi, K. (2011) Soft contact lens biosensor for *in situ* monitoring of tear glucose as non-invasive blood sugar assessment. *Talanta*, **83** (3), 960–965.

77 Iguchi, S., Kudo, H., Saito, T., Ogawa, M., Saito, H., Otsuka, K., Funakubo, A., and Mitsubayashi, K. (2007) A flexible and wearable biosensor for tear glucose measurement. *Biomed. Microdevices*, **9** (4), 603–609.

78 Lochner, C.M., Khan, Y., Pierre, A., and Arias, A.C. (2014) All-organic optoelectronic sensor for pulse oximetry. *Nat. Commun.*, **5**, 5745.

79 Zijlstra, W.G., Buursma, A., and Meeuwsen-van der Roest, W.P. (1991) Absorption spectra of human fetal and adult oxyhemoglobin, de-oxyhemoglobin, carboxyhemoglobin, and methemoglobin. *Clin. Chem.*, **37** (9), 1633–1638.

80 Yokota, T., Zalar, P., Kaltenbrunner, M., Jinno, H., Matsuhisa, N., Kitanosako, H., Tachibana, Y., Yukita, W., Koizumi, M., and Someya, T. (2016) Ultraflexible organic photonic skin. *Sci. Adv.*, **2**, e1501856.

81 Bansal, A.K., Hou, S., Kulyk, O., Bowman, E.M., and Samuel, I.D. (2015) Wearable organic optoelectronic sensors for medicine. *Adv. Mater.*, **27** (46), 7638–7644.

82 Tangerman, A. and Winkel, E. (2010) Extra-oral halitosis: an overview. *J. Breath Res.*, **4** (1), 017003.

83 Minh, T.D., Oliver, S.R., Ngo, J., Flores, R., Midyett, J., Meinardi, S., Carlson, M.K., Rowland, F.S., Blake, D.R., and Galassetti, P.R. (2011) Non-invasive measurement of plasma glucose from exhaled breath in healthy and type 1 diabetic subjects. *Am. J. Physiol. Endocrinol. Metabol.*, **300** (6), E1166–E1175.

84 Xing, R., Xu, L., Song, J., Zhou, C., Li, Q., Liu, D., and Song, H.W. (2015) Preparation and gas sensing properties of In_2O_3/Au nanorods for

detection of volatile organic compounds in exhaled breath. *Sci. Rep.*, **5**. doi: 10.1038/srep10717
85 Kim, J.-S., Yoo, H.-W., Choi, H.O., and Jung, H.-T. (2014) Tunable volatile organic compounds sensor by using thiolated ligand conjugation on MoS_2. *Nano Lett.*, **14** (10), 5941–5947.
86 Kahn, N., Lavie, O., Paz, M., Segev, Y., and Haick, H. (2015) Dynamic nanoparticle-based flexible sensors: diagnosis of ovarian carcinoma from exhaled breath. *Nano Lett.*, **15** (10), 7023–7028.
87 Vishinkin, R. and Haick, H. (2015) Nanoscale sensor technologies for disease detection via volatolomics. *Small*, **11** (46), 6142–6164.
88 Xu, S., Zhang, Y., Jia, L., Mathewson, K.E., Jang, K.I., Kim, J., Fu, H., Huang, X., Chava, P., Wang, R., Bhole, S., Wang, L., Na, Y.J., Guan, Y., Flavin, M., Han, Z., Huang, Y., and Rogers, J.A. (2014) Soft microfluidic assemblies of sensors, circuits, and radios for the skin. *Science*, **344** (6179), 70–74.
89 Takamatsu, S., Lonjaret, T., Crisp, D., Badier, J.M., Malliaras, G.G., and Ismailova, E. (2015) Direct patterning of organic conductors on knitted textiles for long-term electrocardiography. *Sci. Rep.*, **5**. doi: 10.1038/srep15003
90 Jung, H.C., Moon, J.H., Baek, D.H., Lee, J.H., Choi, Y.Y., Hong, J.S., and Lee, S.H. (2012) CNT/PDMS composite flexible dry electrodes for long-term ECG monitoring. *IEEE Trans. Biomed. Eng.*, **59** (5), 1472–1479.
91 Yu, Y., Zhang, J., and Liu, J. (2013) Biomedical implementation of liquid metal ink as drawable ECG electrode and skin circuit. *PLoS ONE*, **8** (3), e58771.
92 Viventi, J., Kim, D.-H., Vigeland, L., Frechette, E.S., Blanco, J.A., Kim, Y.-S., Avrin, A.E., Tiruvadi, V.R., Hwang, S.-W., and Vanleer, A.C. (2011) Flexible, foldable, actively multiplexed, high-density electrode array for mapping brain activity *in vivo*. *Nat. Neurosci.*, **14** (12), 1599–1605.
93 Debener, S., Emkes, R., De Vos, M., and Bleichner, M. (2015) Unobtrusive ambulatory EEG using a smartphone and flexible printed electrodes around the ear. *Sci. Rep.*, **5**. doi: 10.1038/srep16743
94 Metallo, C., White, R.D., and Trimmer, B.A. (2011) Flexible parylene-based microelectrode arrays for high resolution EMG recordings in freely moving small animals. *J. Neurosci. Methods*, **195** (2), 176–184.
95 Scalisi, R.G., Paleari, M., Favetto, A., Stoppa, M., Ariano, P., Pandolfi, P., and Chiolerio, A. (2015) Inkjet printed flexible electrodes for surface electromyography. *Org. Electron.*, **18**, 89–94.
96 Paul, G.M., Cao, F., Torah, R., Yang, K., Beeby, S., and Tudor, J. (2014) A smart textile based facial EMG and EOG computer interface. *IEEE Sens. J.*, **14** (2), 393–400.
97 Khan, Y., Pavinatto, F.J., Lin, M.C., Liao, A., Swisher, S.L., Mann, K., Subramanian, V., Maharbiz, M.M., and Arias, A.C. (2016) Inkjet-printed flexible gold electrode arrays for bioelectronic interfaces. *Adv. Funct. Mater.*, **26** (7), 1004–1013.
98 Choi, M.K., Park, O.K., Choi, C., Qiao, S., Ghaffari, R., Kim, J., Lee, D.J., Kim, M., Hyun, W., Kim, S.J., Hwang, H.J., Kwon, S.H., Hyeon, T., Lu, N., and Kim, D.H. (2016) Cephalopod-inspired miniaturized suction cups for smart medical skin. *Adv. Healthcare Mater.*, **5** (1), 80–87.

99 Gao, W., Emaminejad, S., Nyein, H.Y., Challa, S., Chen, K., Peck, A., Fahad, H.M., Ota, H., Shiraki, H., Kiriya, D., Lien, D.H., Brooks, G.A., Davis, R.W., and Javey, A. (2016) Fully integrated wearable sensor arrays for multiplexed *in situ* perspiration analysis. *Nature*, **529** (7587), 509–514.

100 Nassar, J.M., Cordero, M.D., Kutbee, A.T., Karimi, M.A., Sevilla, G.A.T., Hussain, A.M., Shamim, A., and Hussain, M.M. (2016) Paper skin multisensory platform for simultaneous environmental monitoring. *Adv. Mater. Technol.*, **1** (1), 1600004.

101 Choi, M.K., Park, I., Kim, D.C., Joh, E., Park, O.K., Kim, J., Kim, M., Choi, C., Yang, J., Cho, K.W., Hwang, J.-H., Nam, J.-M., Hyeon, T., Kim, J.H., and Kim, D.-H. (2015) Thermally controlled, patterned graphene transfer printing for transparent and wearable electronic/optoelectronic system. *Adv. Funct. Mater.*, **25** (46), 7109–7118.

102 Honda, W., Harada, S., Arie, T., Akita, S., and Takei, K. (2014) Wearable, human-interactive, health-monitoring, wireless devices fabricated by macroscale printing techniques. *Adv. Funct. Mater.*, **24** (22), 3299–3304.

103 Kim, J., Lee, M., Shim, H.J., Ghaffari, R., Cho, H.R., Son, D., Jung, Y.H., Soh, M., Choi, C., Jung, S., Chu, K., Jeon, D., Lee, S.T., Kim, J.H., Choi, S.H., Hyeon, T., and Kim, D.H. (2014) Stretchable silicon nanoribbon electronics for skin prosthesis. *Nat. Commun.*, **5**, 5747.

104 Harada, S., Honda, W., Arie, T., Akita, S., and Takei, K. (2014) Fully printed, highly sensitive multifunctional artificial electronic whisker arrays integrated with strain and temperature sensors. *ACS Nano*, **8** (4), 3921–3927.

105 Stoppa, M. and Chiolerio, A. (2014) Wearable electronics and smart textiles: a critical review. *Sensors*, **14** (7), 11957–11992.

106 Jeong, J.-W., Yeo, W.-H., Akhtar, A., Norton, J.J.S., Kwack, Y.-J., Li, S., Jung, S.-Y., Su, Y., Lee, W., Xia, J., Cheng, H., Huang, Y., Choi, W.-S., Bretl, T., and Rogers, J.A. (2013) Materials and optimized designs for human–machine interfaces via epidermal electronics. *Adv. Mater.*, **25** (47), 6839–6846.

107 Norton, J.J.S., Lee, D.S., Lee, J.W., Lee, W., Kwon, O., Won, P., Jung, S.-Y., Cheng, H., Jeong, J.-W., Akce, A., Umunna, S., Na, I., Kwon, Y.H., Wang, X.-Q., Liu, Z., Paik, U., Huang, Y., Bretl, T., Yeo, W.-H., and Rogers, J.A. (2015) Soft, curved electrode systems capable of integration on the auricle as a persistent brain–computer interface. *Proc. Natl. Acad. Sci. U.S.A.*, **112** (13), 3920–3925.

108 Lim, S., Son, D., Kim, J., Lee, Y.B., Song, J.-K., Choi, S., Lee, D.J., Kim, J.H., Lee, M., Hyeon, T., and Kim, D.-H. (2015) Transparent and stretchable interactive human machine interface based on patterned graphene heterostructures. *Adv. Funct. Mater.*, **25** (3), 375–383.

109 Bächlin, M. and Tröster, G. (2012) Swimming performance and technique evaluation with wearable acceleration sensors. Pervasive Mob. *Comput.*, **8** (1), 68–81.

110 Jia, W.Z., Bandodkar, A.J., Valdes-Ramirez, G., Windmiller, J.R., Yang, Z.J., Ramirez, J., Chan, G., and Wang, J. (2013) Electrochemical tattoo biosensors for real-time noninvasive lactate monitoring in human perspiration. *Anal. Chem.*, **85** (14), 6553–6560.

111 Bruno, T. (2015) *Wearable Technology: Smart Watches to Google Glass for Libraries*, vol. **1**, Rowman & Littlefield, Lanham, MD.

112 Gonzalez-Villanueva, L., Cagnoni, S., and Ascari, L. (2013) Design of a wearable sensing system for human motion monitoring in physical rehabilitation. *Sensors*, **13** (6), 7735–7755.

113 Kassal, P., Kim, J., Kumar, R., de Araujo, W.R., Steinberg, I.M., Steinberg, M.D., and Wang, J. (2015) Smart bandage with wireless connectivity for uric acid biosensing as an indicator of wound status. *Electrochem. Commun.*, **56**, 6–10.

114 Swisher, S.L., Lin, M.C., Liao, A., Leeflang, E.J., Khan, Y., Pavinatto, F.J., Mann, K., Naujokas, A., Young, D., Roy, S., Harrison, M.R., Arias, A.C., Subramanian, V., and Maharbiz, M.M. (2015) Impedance sensing device enables early detection of pressure ulcers *in vivo*. *Nat. Commun.*, **6**, 6575.

115 Cavanagh, P.R., Lipsky, B.A., Bradbury, A.W., and Botek, G. (2005) Treatment for diabetic foot ulcers. *Lancet*, **366** (9498), 1725–1735.

116 Pataky, Z., Assal, J.P., Conne, P., Vuagnat, H., and Golay, A. (2005) Plantar pressure distribution in Type 2 diabetic patients without peripheral neuropathy and peripheral vascular disease. *Diabet. Med.*, **22** (6), 762–767.

117 Guan, L., Nilghaz, A., Su, B., Jiang, L., Cheng, W., and Shen, W. (2016) Stretchable-fiber-confined wetting conductive liquids as wearable human health monitors. *Adv. Funct. Mater.*, **26**, 4511–4517.

118 Motoi, K., Higashi, Y., Kuwae, Y., Yuji, T., Tanaka, S., and Yamakoshi, K. (2006) Development of a wearable device capable of monitoring human activity for use in rehabilitation and certification of eligibility for long-term care. 27th Annual International Conference of the IEEE Engineering in Medicine and Biology Society, Shanghai, China, September 1–4, 2005.

119 Hsueh, Y.H., Yin, C., and Chen, Y.H. (2015) Hardware system for real-time EMG signal acquisition and separation processing during electrical stimulation. *J. Med. Syst.*, **39** (9), 88.

120 Schreml, S., Szeimies, R., Prantl, L., Karrer, S., Landthaler, M., and Babilas, P. (2010) Oxygen in acute and chronic wound healing. *Br. J. Dermatol.*, **163** (2), 257–268.

121 Schreml, S., Meier, R.J., Wolfbeis, O.S., Landthaler, M., Szeimies, R.M., and Babilas, P. (2011) 2D luminescence imaging of pH *in vivo*. *Proc. Natl. Acad. Sci. U.S.A.*, **108** (6), 2432–2437.

122 Schreml, S., Meier, R.J., Wolfbeis, O.S., Maisch, T., Szeimies, R.M., Landthaler, M., Regensburger, J., Santarelli, F., Klimant, I., and Babilas, P. (2011) 2D luminescence imaging of physiological wound oxygenation. *Exp. Dermatol.*, **20** (7), 550–554.

123 Pitsillides, A., Pitsillides, B., Samaras, G., Dikaiakos, M., Christodoulou, E., Andreou, P., and Georgiadis, D. (2006) DITIS: a collaborative virtual medical team for home healthcare of cancer patients, in *M-Health* (eds R.S.H. Istepanian, S. Laxminarayan, and C.S. Pattichis), Springer, Gewerbestrasse, pp. 247–266.

13

Stretchable Health Monitoring Devices/Sensors

Xian Huang

Department of Biomedical Engineering, School of Precision Instrument and Optoelectronic Engineering, Tianjin University, China

13.1 Introduction

Stretchable devices made of elastic materials or structures can be deformed in response to stress without interfering with their normal functions. The devices are typically based on thin laminar that adapts to the mechanics of its host and offers a range of unique properties such as conformal coating, spontaneous adhesion, and adaptive deformation. Stretchable electronic devices have been demonstrated in soft robotics [1–4], consumer electronics [5–7], and biomimic electronics [8–10] with more prominent applications lying in the field of health monitoring, which requires direct interaction with soft and curvilinear human bodies. Stretchable devices can adapt to the mechanics of human bodies and offer maximized compliance to skin and organs, leading to improved comfort and reduced restriction to the daily activities of wearers. Additional features of stretchable devices that outweigh traditional devices based on rigid substrates and packages include intimate contact to the test subjects, fixed measurement positions, and coverage of large curved surface. This chapter introduces important aspects (e.g., materials, structures, formats, and applications) of stretchable health monitoring devices, followed by a brief discussion on the future trends in stretchable health monitoring devices.

13.2 Materials for Stretchable Health Monitoring Devices

Stretchable health monitoring devices are composed of materials that are either intrinsically stretchable as raw materials such as elastomers, liquid metals, and conductive polymers, or are not stretchable in their bulky formats but designed into special structures that comply with stress. These materials are combined to yield stretchable devices that can be used in health monitoring. Additional requirements for these materials include biocompatibility that allows them to be integrated with human bodies safely and capability to be mass fabricated using techniques such as CMOS and surface micromachining.

Flexible and Stretchable Medical Devices, First Edition. Edited by Kuniharu Takei.

13.2.1 Physically Soft and Stretchable Materials

Elastomers are the fundamental materials in stretchable devices, and are mostly used as substrates, binders, adhesion layers, and structural materials. Elastomers are referred to as belonging to a wide range of viscoelastic polymers, which are weak in intermolecular forces and available in different compositions with varied stretchability. Elastomers are low in Young's modulus (from 1 to 150 MPa) [11, 12] and high in failure strain (from 30% to 1000%) [13, 14] (Figure 13.1a), making them ideal materials to construct stretchable devices with minimized constrain to human skin and maximized compliance to human motion.

Liquid metals are intrinsically elastic, and are used as alternatives to conventional metals. Popular liquid metals include eutectic gallium-indium (eGaIn) and gallium-indium-tin (Galinstan), which are low in toxicity and resistivity ($\sim 2.9 \times 10^{-7}\,\Omega\,\text{m}$) [23]. Their melting points are 15.5 °C [24] (wt. 75% Ga and wt. 25% In) and −19 °C [25] (wt. 68.5% Ga, 21.5% In, and 10.0% Sn), respectively, resulting in their liquid states at room temperature. These liquid metals can be injected into microfluidic channels due to their low viscosity ($\sim 2 \times 10^{-3}$ Pa s), forming functional components such as pressure sensor [26–28], strain sensors [29, 30], antennas [31, 32], soft wires [33], and keyboard [34]. Devices made of liquid metals can withstand deformation of the microchannels at very high strain (up to 800%) [35] (Figure 13.1b).

Conductive polymers can be realized using polymers mixed with conductive fillers [15] (Figure 13.1c) or using intrinsically conducting polymers (ICPs)[16] (Figure 13.1d). The first case results in composites with fillers (e.g., metal nanoparticles, metal nanowires, graphite, carbon nanotubes, and graphene) that are tightly packed to their percolation threshold in polymers. Intrinsically conducting polymers are achieved by conjugation of polymer backbone, forming high-energy orbitals with loosely bonded electronics to corresponding atoms. ICPs are represented by synthetic poly(acetylene) (PA), poly(pyrrole) (PPy), poly(thiophene) (PT), poly(aniline) (PANI), and poly-(3,4-ethylenedioxythiophene) (PEDOT). Conductive polymers are subject to the influence of strain, which may lead to increased resistivity with strain. Conductivity of more than $10\,\text{S cm}^{-1}$ under a strain of more than 100% has been achieved using single-wall carbon nanotube (SWNT) bundles as fillers in a fluorinated copolymer [36]. Improved conductivity can be achieved using composited fillers containing silver flakes and multi-wall carbonnanotubes (MWCTs), leading to conductivity of $5710\,\text{S cm}^{-1}$ at 0% strain and $20\,\text{S cm}^{-1}$ at 140% strain [37]. Large conductivity ($\sigma \approx 2200\,\text{S cm}^{-1}$) even under large strain (100% strain) has been demonstrated by Park *et al.* [14] using electrospun poly (styrene-*block*-butadiene-*block*-styrene) (SBS) rubber fibers that contain percolated silver nanoparticles.

13.2.2 Unique Stretchable Structures

Materials such as solid metals, semiconductors, and fibers are not stretchable as raw materials. However, unique designing of these materials yields stretchable structures that work together with intrinsically stretchable materials to construct stretchable devices.

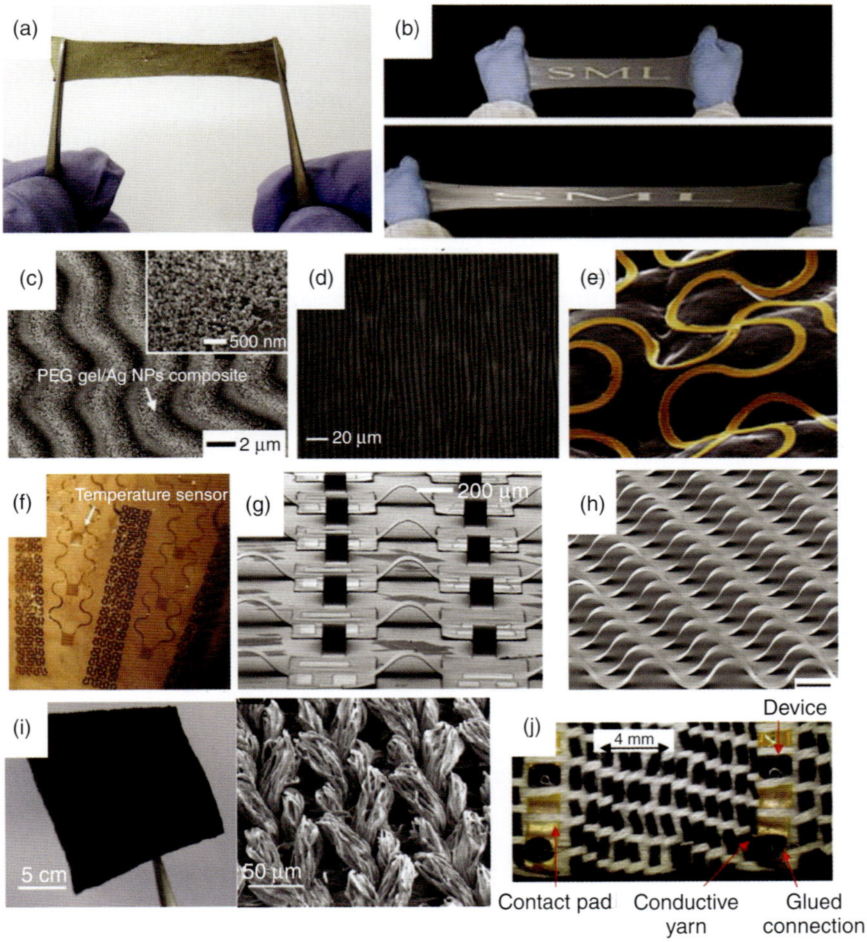

Figure 13.1 Representative materials and structures used in stretchable electronic devices for health monitoring. (a) A highly stretchable elastomer membrane, (Park 2012 [14]. Reproduced with permission of Nature Publishing Group.). (b) A liquid metal pattern in an elastomer membrane, (Bartlett 2016 [13]. Reproduced with permission of John Wiley & Sons.). (c) A electrode made of a silver-filled conductive polymer, (Hyun 2011 [15]. Reproduced with permission of John Wiley & Sons.). (d) A conductive PEDOT:PSS membrane, (Vosgueritchian 2012 [16]. Reproduced with permission of John Wiley & Sons.). (e) A serpentine electrode conformably covered on skin replica, (Yeo 2013 [17]. Reproduced with permission of John Wiley & Sons.) (f) A cardiac sock with fractal interconnects between electrodes. (Xu 2015 [18]. Reproduced with permission of John Wiley & Sons.) (g) A prestrained interconnect that works as bridges to connect functional components on the island together. (Reprinted with permission from Ref. [19] Copyright 2008 National Academy of Sciences.) (h) Aprestrainedsilicon nanoribbon whose strain is released to form bulking structures. (Sun 2006 [20]. Reproduced with permission of Nature Publishing Group.) (i) A conductive fabric made by dipping the fabric into SWNT ink. (Hu *et al.* 2010 [21]. With permission from the American Chemical Society.) (j) Woven fibers that contain electrodes and metal wires (Cherenack 2010 [22]. Reproduced with permission of John Wiley & Sons.)

Solid metals become flexible when they appear as thin films. Stretchability can be achieved when making specially designed metal traces with metallic thin films, which adopt planar or out-of-plane formats of self-similar serpentine [17] (Figure 13.1e), fractal [18] (Figure 13.1f), helical [38] (Figure 13.2B), and prestrained bulking [19] (Figure 13.1g) structures. The elongation of the metal traces is constrained by the fracture strain of the metals (~1%) [41], and can reach more than 100% with optimized design.

Semiconductor materials such as silicon [42], GaAs [43], ZnO [44], InP [45], and GaN [46] can be used to make functional active components such as diodes, transistors, and light-emitting diodes. All these semiconductor materials are rigid in their bulky forms, but their bending stiffness and bending-induced strains at given radii of curvature can be exceptionally small due to cubic and linear scaling of these quantities with thickness. These semiconductor materials are in forms such as nanomembranes [47], nanoribbons [20] (Figure 13.1h), and nanowires [48] with thickness in a scale of hundreds of nanometers, and are functionalized following CMOS fabrication processes.

Woven fabric can be constructed with fibers interlaced together, offering the fabric unique properties such as elasticity, stiffness, and chemical resistance. Conductive threads can be achieved by doping the treads with conductive inks made of conductive particles [21] (Figure 13.1i) or bundling metal wires together with the treads [22, 49] (Figure 13.1j). Woven fabric can be used as sensory elements for strain [50, 51], pressure [52, 53], respiratory [54], and heart rate monitoring [55]. In addition, stretchable skin sensors can be attached to woven fabric to achieve high tensile strain and vapor permeability, while allowing high resistance to surface scratch and humidity [56].

13.3 Health Monitoring Applications of Stretchable Devices

Materials mentioned can be used to construct stretchable health monitoring devices exhibited typically as skin sensors [10, 17, 39, 56–64] (Figure 13.2A), implantable devices [38, 65–72] (Figure 13.2B), and wearable devices without direct coupling to human bodies [40, 73–77] (Figure 13.2C). These devices have demonstrated broad applications in health monitoring with major use in biophysical signal monitoring, biomolecule analysis, brain and neural probes, cardiovascular monitoring, rehabilitation, and daily health tracking.

13.3.1 Skin Sensors

Stretchable devices for health monitoring are predominately realized by skin-mounted devices that are in direct contact with skin and measure diverse skin properties. One innovative type of skin sensors is based on soft and ultrathin materials, whose mechanics are similar as the epidermis of the skin, and, thus, are termed as epidermal electronics [57]. Epidermal electronic devices can be spontaneously attached to skin, and conformably adapt to skin morphology. Epidermal devices have been demonstrated as constituting a conceptual system

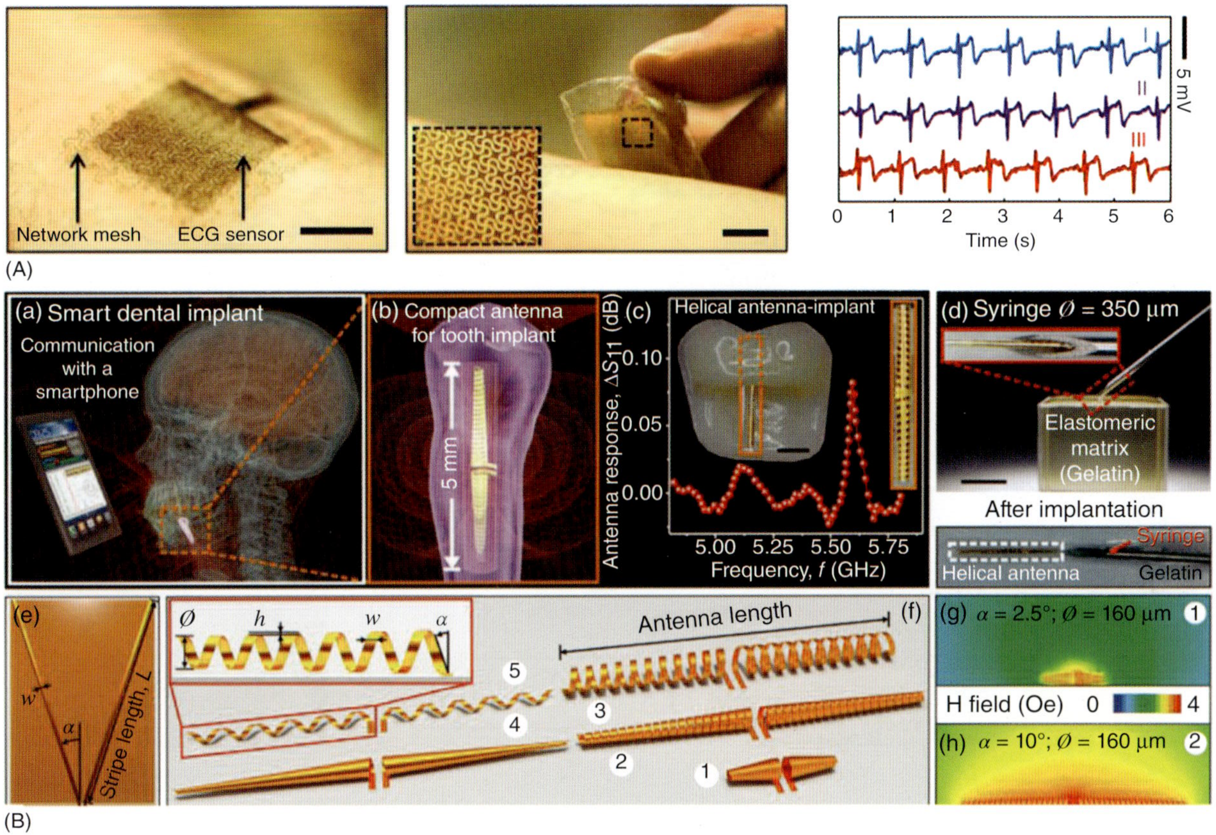

Figure 13.2 Various formats of stretchable health monitoring devices. (A) An epidermal electronic sensor that monitorsbiopotential of the skin. (Jang 2015 [39]. Reproduced with permission of John Wiley & Sons.) (B) A compact helical antenna for smart implant applications. (Karnaushenko *et al.* 2015 [38], http://www.nature.com/am/journal/v7/n6/full/am201553a.html. Used under CC BY 4.0 https://creativecommons.org/licenses/by/4.0/.) (C) A strain sensor based on carbon nanotubes that can be integrated onto various fabrics for human-motion detection. (Yamada 2011 [40]. Reproduced with permission of Nature Publishing Group.)

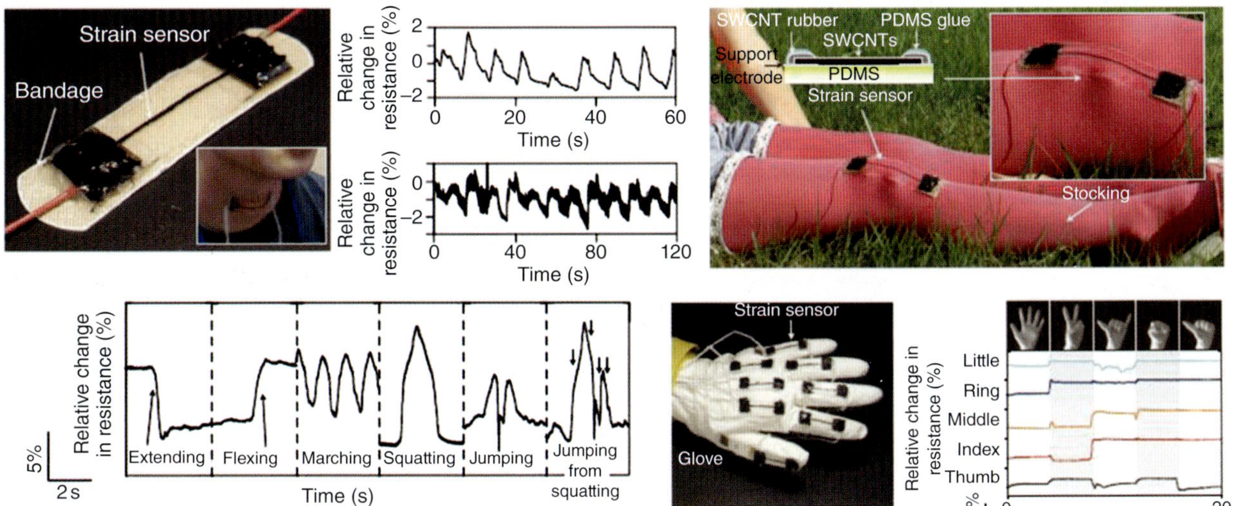

(C)

Figure 13.2 (*Continued*)

that contains multiple sensing components [57] and individual devices as brain–computer interfaces [78, 79], hydration sensors [61–63], temperature sensors [17, 64, 80], and data loggers [81]. Other formats of the skin sensors can be realized by thicker, and thus, less stretchable structures, and use fixtures such as bandages [82, 83] and body straps [84, 85] to realize intimate skin contact. With assistance from silicone adhesive and stretchable fabric, rugged and breathable forms of stretchable electronics can be realized to achieve epidermal or transcutaneous monitoring [56]. Primary use of skin sensors involves biophysical signal sensing and biomolecule analyzing.

13.3.1.1 Skin Biophysical Signal Monitoring

Biopotential Sensing Biopotential sensors measure electrical potential generated across tissues, organs, and cells. Signals such as electrocardiography (ECG) (Figure 13.2A), electromyogram (EMG), and electroencephalography (EEG) [10, 56, 58–60] can be measured to indicate different health conditions such as coronary artery disease [86], pediatric muscle disease [87], muscle fatigue [88], mental states [89], and sleep disorder [90, 91]. These sensors are predominately based on skin-contacted metallic electrodes or meshes made of gold and copper (Figure 13.3a), resulting in highly conformal surface coverage on skin and high signal-to-noise ratio without using any coupling media. A potential issue in the use of metallic electrodes involves skin irritation due to contact allergy to gold [78, 79] and copper [92], leading to alternative methods that use capacitive electrodes, which are separated from skin with a polymeric insulation layer [59]. The sensing mechanism relies on displacement currents induced in electrodes. The resulting signals are captured as voltages measured using an amplification circuit with high input impedance. Other electrode formats include conductive polymer electrodes made of carbon nanotubes [93] or poly(3,4-ethylenedioxythiophene): poly(styrenesulfonate) (PEDOT:PSS) [94], which offer reasonable conductivity and high stretchability.

Hydration Sensing Skin hydration monitoring is an important technique in dermatology to analyze various diseases such as dermatitis [95], psoriasis [96], and pruritus [97]. Hydration measurement is also used for assessing the effectiveness of antiaging and moisturization treatments and other medical therapies. Skin hydration is typically determined by impedance measurement approaches. Huang *et al.* have realized several types of skin impedance sensors that measure skin impedance across two electrodes using alternative electrical current with frequencies from 10 to 100 kHz. The resulting attenuation and phase shift of the electrical current, represented by the impedance of the skin, can be used to assess skin hydration levels, which determine the dielectric properties and conductivities of the skin. Devices capable of conducting differential monitoring [61], regional mapping [62] (Figure 13.3b), and wireless sensing [63] (Figure 13.3c) have been developed based on impedance detection. In addition, hydration can also be assessed by skin thermal conductivity [64], which can be determined through time response of the skin to constant thermal energy input (Figure 13.4a).

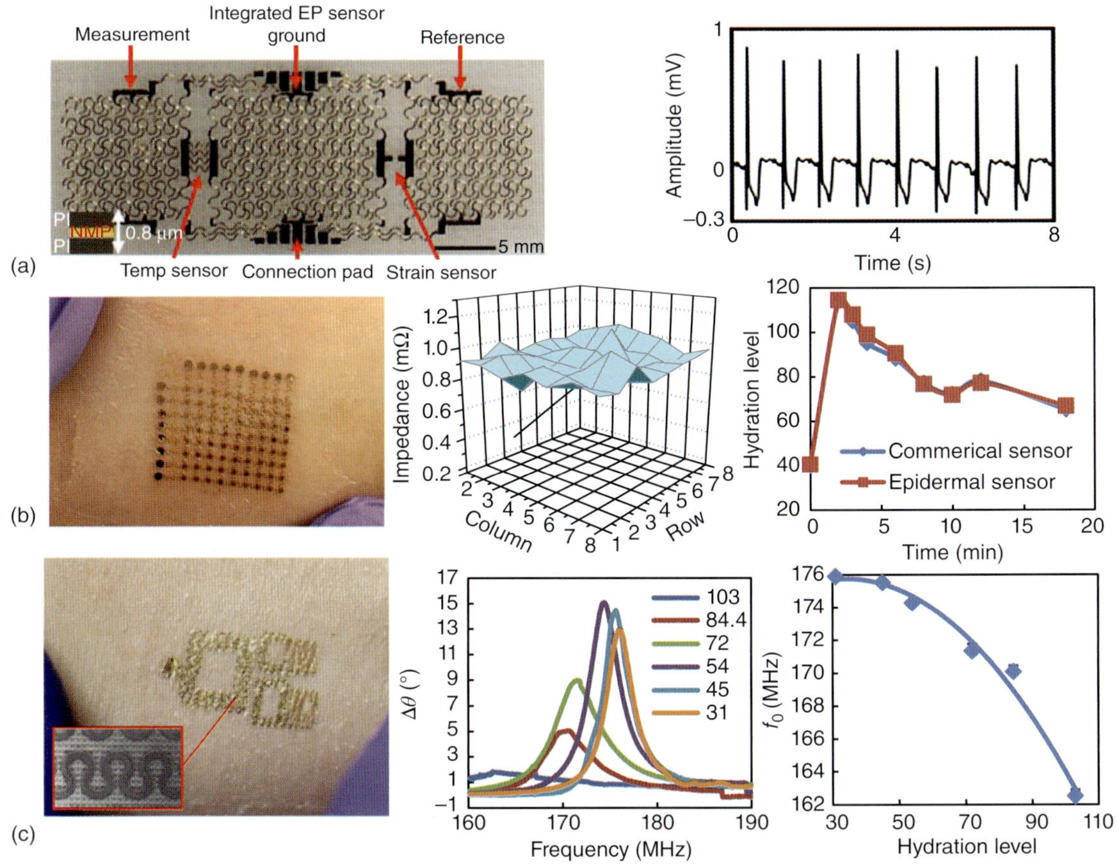

Figure 13.3 Epidermal sensors that can monitor (a) biopotential of skin using metallic meshes (Yeo 2013 [17]. Reproduced with permission of John Wiley & Sons) and hydration levels within skin using impedance measurement approaches based on (b) regional mapping (Huang *et al*. 2013 [62]. With permission from IEEE.) and (c) passive wireless detection (Huang *et al*. 2014 [63]. Reproduced with permission of John Wiley & Sons.)

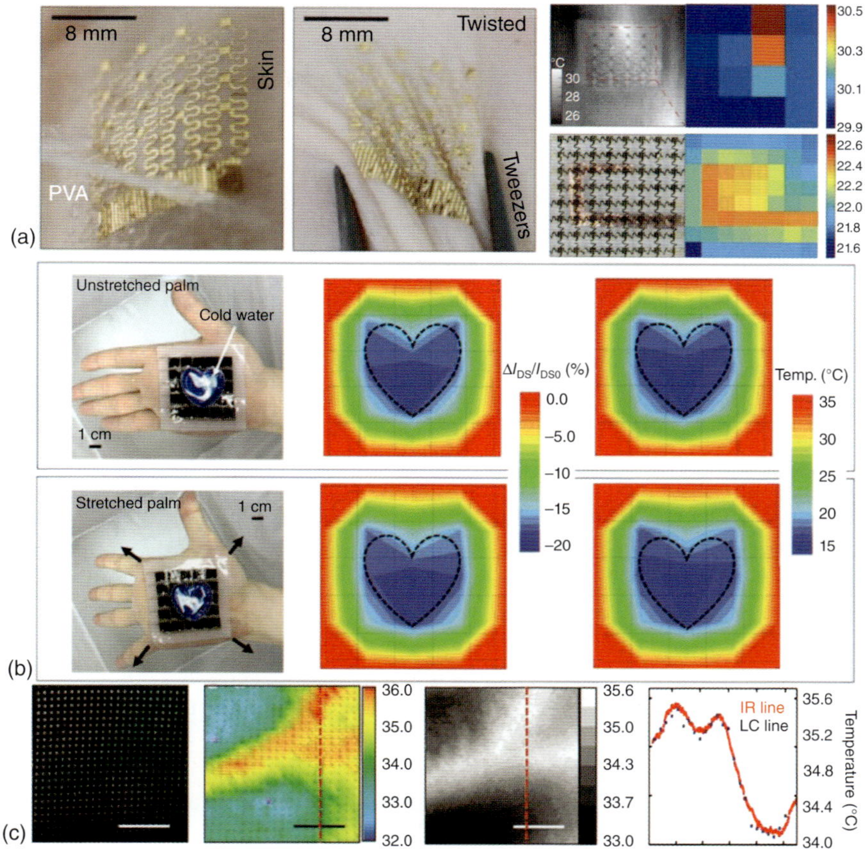

Figure 13.4 Epidermal sensors that can monitor skin temperature using (a) metallic sensors (Webb 2013 [64]. Reproduced with permission of Nature Publishing Group.), (b) organic field-effect transistors (Hong 2016 [98]. Reproduced with permission of John Wiley & Sons.), and (c) thermochromics liquid crystal arrays (Gao 2014 [99]. Reproduced with permission of Nature Publishing Group.)

Temperature Sensing Skin temperature sensors can measure body temperature and skin thermal conductivity as well as effects of blood flow on thermal transport, and can be realized by resistive meander electrodes made of Pt [17] and Au [64] (Figure 13.4a). Skin temperature mapping can be realized by the above-mentioned resistive electrodes integrated with switching diodes or transistors to select individual electrodes. Temperature sensors based on silicon nanomembranes have also been developed [100]. The devices typically contain prestrained lightly or heavily doped silicon nanomembranes, which are released to achieve out-of-plane bulking structures with more than 30% stretchability. Novel approaches to monitor skin temperature also include measuring source/drain current variation of field-effect transistors [98, 101–103] (Figure 13.4b), which undergo temperature-induced property changes in gate dielectrics. Besides electronic devices, skin temperature mapping can also be realized by powerless colorimetric approaches, for example, Gao *et al.* combined high-density thermochromics liquid crystal arrays with metallic antennas that can locally heat the skin by harvesting electromagnetic waves [99] (Figure 13.4c). The resulting device achieves noninvasive spatial mapping of skin temperature with ±50 mK precision and submillimeter spatial resolution.

Other Skin Sensing Applications Stretchable skin sensors also have other health monitoring applications, including oximetry [56, 104, 105], wound healing monitoring [106, 107], pressure sensing [108, 109], and strain sensing [110, 111]. Transdermal pulse oximetry [104] uses LED to emit green or red light, and photo detectors to receive the transmitted light on close proximity to the LED (Figure 13.5a). A ratio between the intensities of transmitted light and emitted LED light (calibrated by applied voltage) can be used to indicate the peripheral capillary oxygen saturation. Skin sensors have also been realized for wound healing. Hattori *et al.* developed an epidermal sensor that can monitor time-dynamic skin temperature and thermal conductivity [106] that are related to the inflammation phase during a wound healing process. Lin *et al.* developed a hydrogel-based smart wound dressing that can sense temperature at various skin locations and deliver different drugs to these locations [107] (Figure 13.5b). Pressure sensors can be used to measure blood pulses. Gong *et al.* demonstrated a pressure sensor based on gold nanowires that are impregnated into tissue paper sandwiched between a black PDMS and a patterned PDMS sheet with interdigitated electrode arrays [108]. The device offers a pressure sensitivity of 1.14 kPa^{-1} and responds to pressure changes within 0.05 s at a frequency up to 5.5 Hz.

13.3.1.2 Biomolecule Analysis

Stretchable skin sensors have been used to monitor biomolecule levels in sweat [112–120] based on ion-selective electrodes, ion-selective field-effect transistors, electrochemical electrodes, and colorimetry. Biomolecules such as sodium [112–115], potassium [113, 115], ammonium [116, 120], glucose [117, 119], and lactate [115, 121] can be measured as indicators for dietary conditions, liver malfunctions, cystic fibrosis, and diabetes. Huang *et al.* introduced materials and design for ultrathin, stretchable passive wireless sensors, which are attached on porous sponge-like substrates for epidermal analysis of biomolecules in sweat. The porous substrates allow sweat collection through capillary forces, without the need for complex microfluidic handling systems. Colorimetric measurement is achieved in the same system by introducing indicator compounds into the substrates for sensing specific components (OH^-, H^+, Cu^+, and Fe^{2+}) in the sweat [118] (Figure 13.6a). In addition to introducing specific ions, Jia *et al.* developed a real-time lactate sensing method for perspiration monitoring during exercise using a flexible printed tattoo-like electrochemical biosensor. The sensor exhibits chemical selectivity toward lactate with linearity up to 20 mM and demonstrates high resiliency against mechanical deformation and friction [122] (Figure 13.6b). Gao *et al.* present a highly integrated sensor array for *in situ* perspiration analysis. The sensor array can simultaneously and selectively measure sweat metabolites (such as glucose and lactate) and electrolytes (such as sodium and potassium ions) as well as skin temperature for sensor calibration [115] (Figure 13.6c).

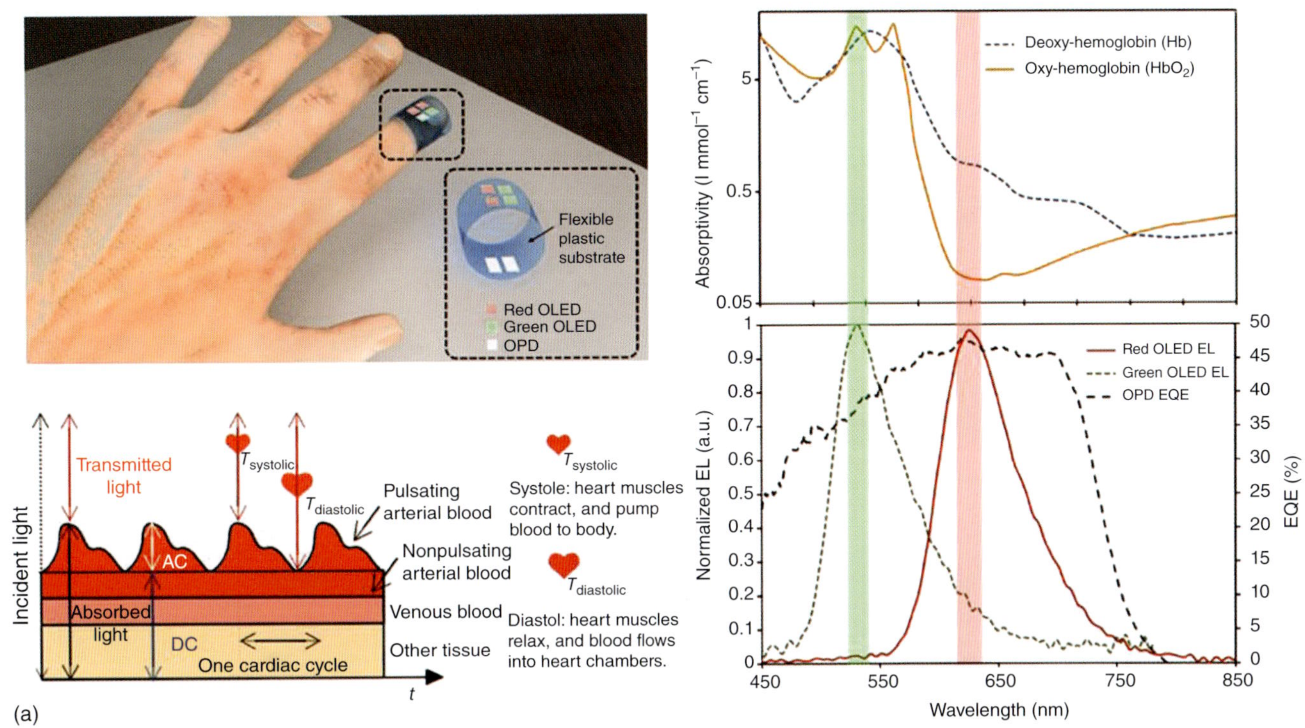

Figure 13.5 Epidermal sensors that can (a) conduct transdermal oximetry measurement using LEDs and photodetectors (Lochner 2014 [104]. Reproduced with permission of Nature Publishing Group.) and (b) assist wound healing (Lin 2016 [107]. Reproduced with permission of John Wiley & Sons.)

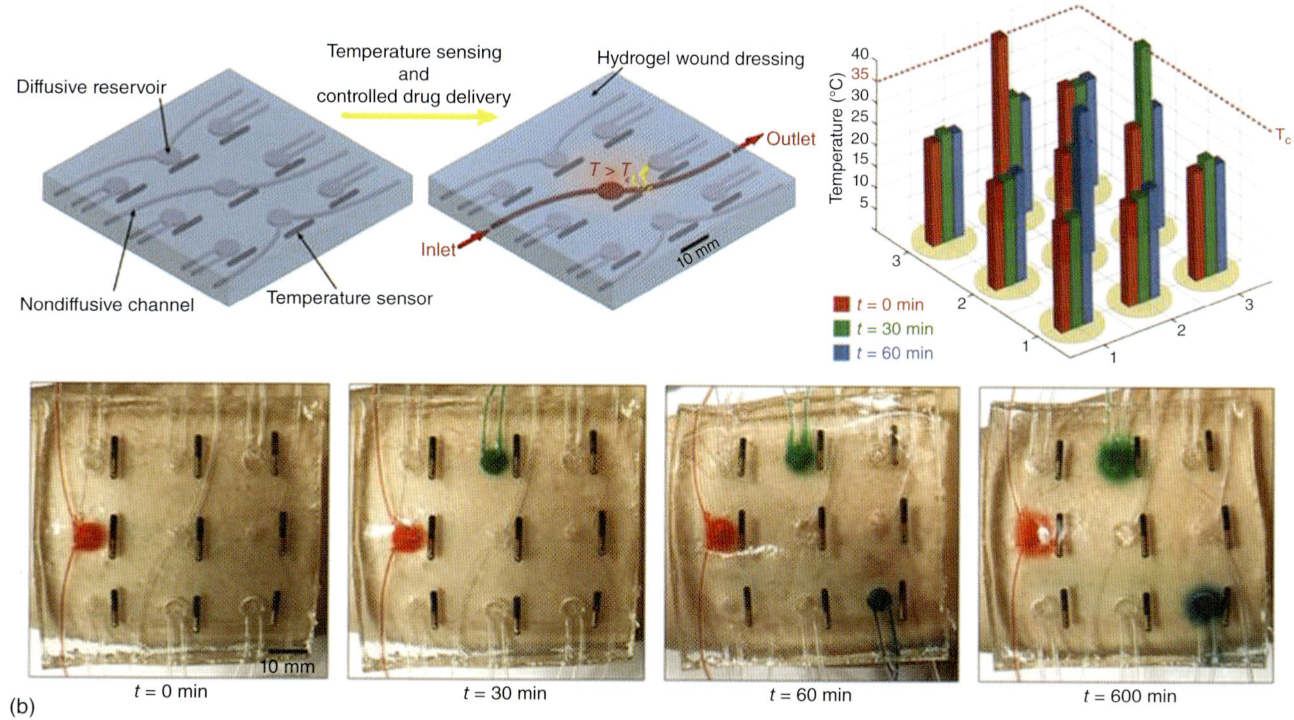

Figure 13.5 (*Continued*)

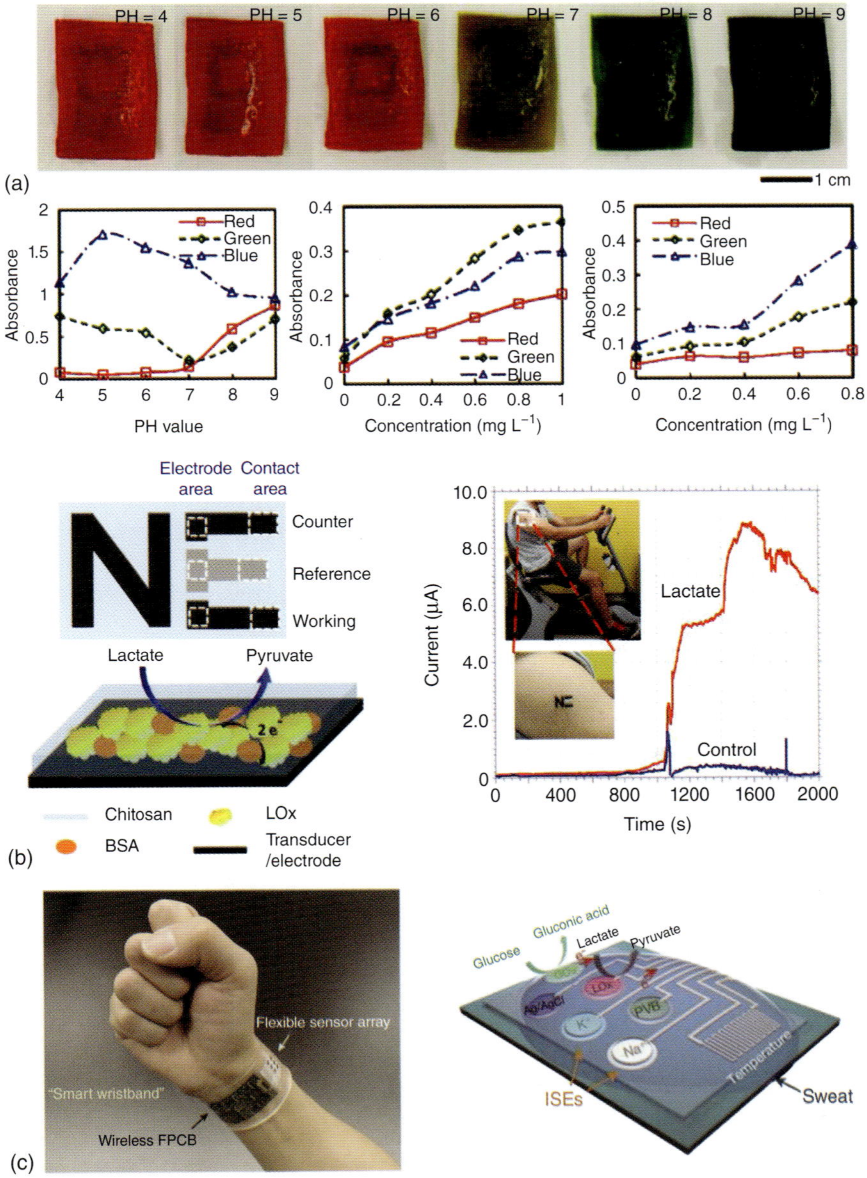

Figure 13.6 Skin sensors that can monitor biomolecules in sweat based on (a) colorimetry approach (Huang 2014 [118]. Reproduced with permission of John Wiley & Sons.) or (b) electrochemical methods (Jia 2013 [122]. Reproduced with permission of American Chemical Society.) (c) A more integrated system that can analyze multiple compositions in sweat simultaneously. (Gao 2016 [115]. Reproduced with permission of Nature Publishing Group..)

13.3.2 Implantable Devices

Stretchable devices can also be implanted into human bodies to conduct measurement internally. The soft and curvilinear formats of the devices match the mechanics and surface morphology of human organs, forming intimate contact with the surface of the organs. These devices can be delivered to tested sites through methods such as using catheters [71], surgery [72, 123], and injection [124, 125]. Implantable devices have very high requirements to the biocompatibility of the devices to minimize potential foreign body reaction. Researchers have developed implantable stretchable devices that can be used continuously within human bodies for over 6 months [126] with major applications in brain and neural probes and cardiovascular monitoring.

13.3.2.1 Brain and Neural Probes

Pioneer works in stretchable electronic devices for brain and neural signal recording typically use metallic electrodes with limited stretchability encapsulated in elastomer membranes [65–69]. These devices in their current format can withstand 5-10% biaxial strain. Guo *et al.* developed a stretchable multielectrode array using a new poly(pyrrole)/polyolborate composite film for electrodes and leads (Figure 13.7a). The resulting polymeric multielectrode array can be stretched up

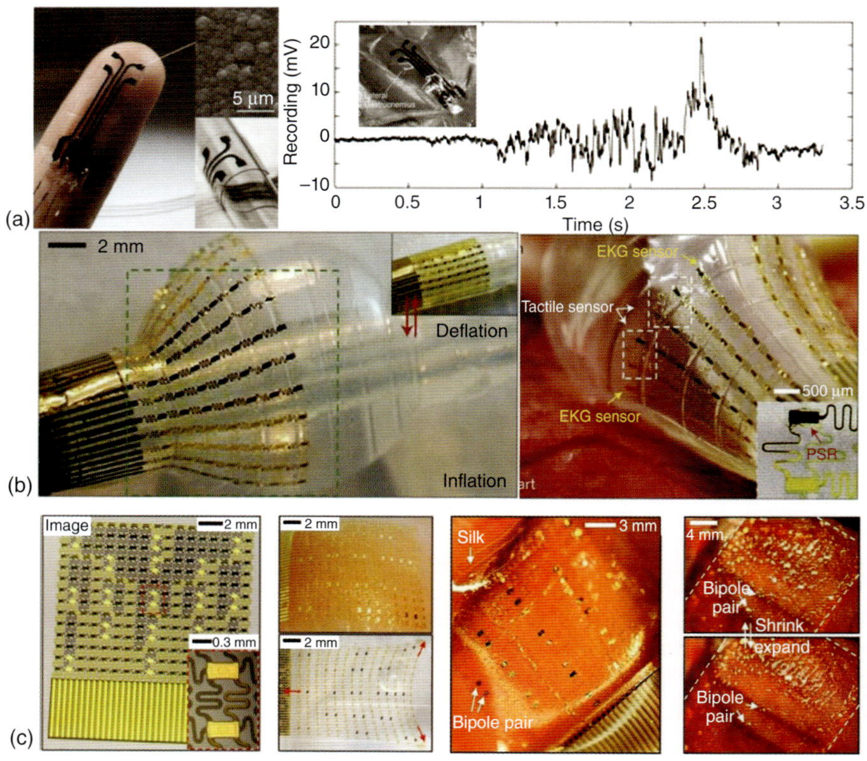

Figure 13.7 Stretchable electronic devices that are used as (a) a neural probe (Guo 2014 [70]. Reproduced with permission of John Wiley & Sons.), (b) a balloon catheter (Kim *et al.* 2011 [71]. Reproduced with permission of Nature Publishing Group.), and (c) cardiovascular mapping webs (Kim *et al.* 2012 [72]. With permission from the National Academy of Sciences.)

to ~23% uniaxial tensile strain with minimal losses in electrical conductivity [70]. Minev *et al.* designed a soft neural interface that can tolerate a strain of 45%. The device mimics the shape and mechanics of the dura mater, and contains stretchable gold interconnects and soft electrodes coated with a platinum–silicone composite. In addition, a microfluidic channel is also integrated within the device. The electrodes and interconnects transfer electrophysiological signals, while the microfluidic channel delivers drugs locally [127].

13.3.2.2 Cardiovascular Monitoring

Stretchable devices are in high demand for monitoring biophysiological signals of heart and blood vessels, which undergo significant deformation during the process of blood circulation. Kim *et al.* developed multifunctional balloon catheters (Figure 13.7b) with capabilities in cardiac electrophysiological mapping and ablation therapy using ultrathin flexible materials such as silicon and metal films [71]. Similar technology can also be used to develop electronic sensing webs [72] (Figure 13.7c) or socks [123] that can wrap around the heart to conduct electrogram mapping for heart beats to determine arrhythmias. Stable and biocompatible conducting polymers such as PEDOT:PSS or graphite–PDMS composites can be used to create bendable, noncytotoxic, and biostable sensor arrays containing up to 60 microelectrodes. Each electrode in the arrays has a thickness below 500 μm, and can reliably capture action potentials (APs) and local field potentials (LFPs) from heart muscle [94].

13.3.3 Body Wearable Devices

Besides skin sensors and implantable sensors, sensors integrated with fabrics or other body wearable gadgets are also performing major roles in stretchable health monitoring devices. These sensors have no direct contact with skin, and, thus, are mostly used to measure human motion with strain [128–130], pressure [131–133], heart rate [134], and respiratory [135] detection. Applications of such kinds of body wearable devices include rehabilitation and daily health tracking in a way that can be worn on bodies in formats such as wristbands [73, 74], glove [75, 133], socks [40], and clothes [129, 130].

13.3.3.1 Rehabilitation

Stretchable devices can assist the rehabilitation processes of the patients. Prominent applications involve hand rehabilitation [136], prosthetics [76], and artificial muscle [137]. The devices are typically in the formats of gloves [75, 138], strips [76, 138] (Figure 13.8a), and wrist-worn meshes [77]. Ryu *et al.* developed highly elastic strain sensing strips that can be used for motion detection during the rehabilitation processes [138]. The strips are based on carbon nanotube bundles that are obtained from dry spinning vertically aligned carbon nanotubes (CNTs) to prestrained (100%) silicone substrates (Figure 13.8a). The CNTs that adhere to the substrates through van der Waals forces are densely packed on the substrates, allowing electrical conduction through tunnel effects with a tolerance of up to 960% strain. Gerratt *et al.* demonstrated a stretchable strip integrated with resistive sensors to monitor finger articulation and capacitive tactile pressure sensors that record pressure distribution along the length of fingers [76]. Attaching the strip to a glove enables precise grasp analysis, which is a critical step

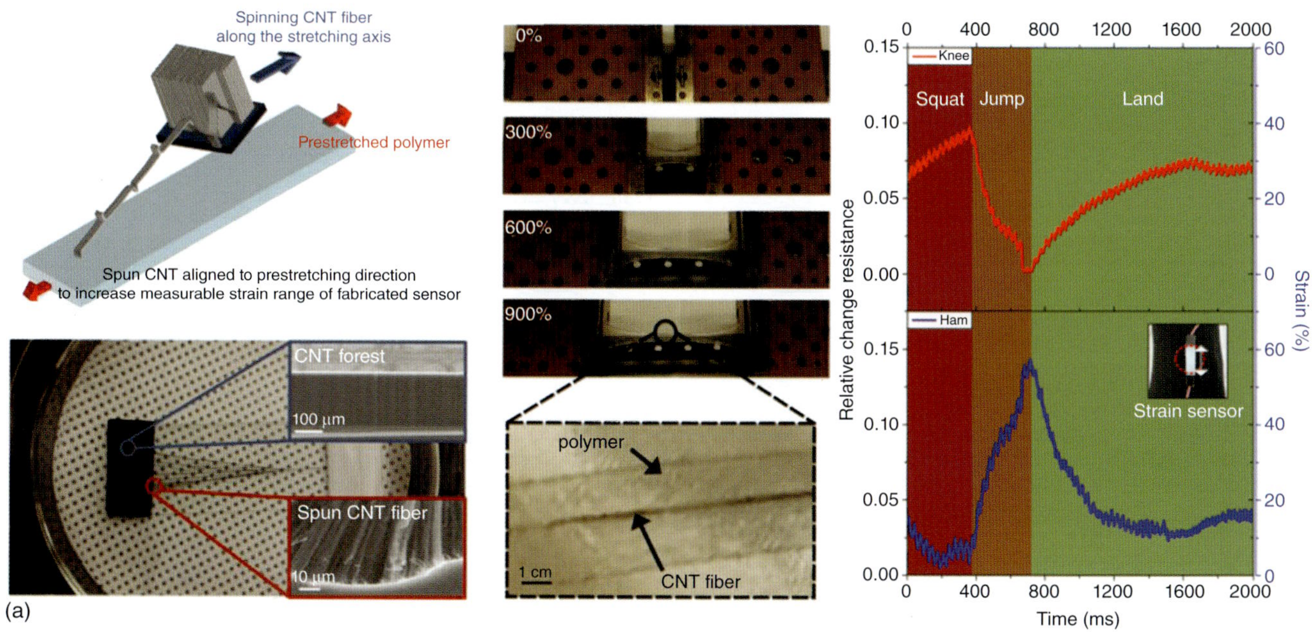

Figure 13.8 Examples of body wearable devices for rehabilitation and health tracking. (a) A carbon nanotube based strain sensor that can be stretched by over 900%. (Ryu *et al*. 2015 [138]. Reproduced with permission of American Chemical Society.) (b) A body motion sensor based on graphene–rubber composites. (Boland *et al*. 2014 [139]. With permission from the American Chemical Society.) (c) Knitted strain sensor textiles of highly conductive all-polymeric fibers (Seyedin *et al*. 2015 [140]. Reproduced with permission of American Chemical Society.)

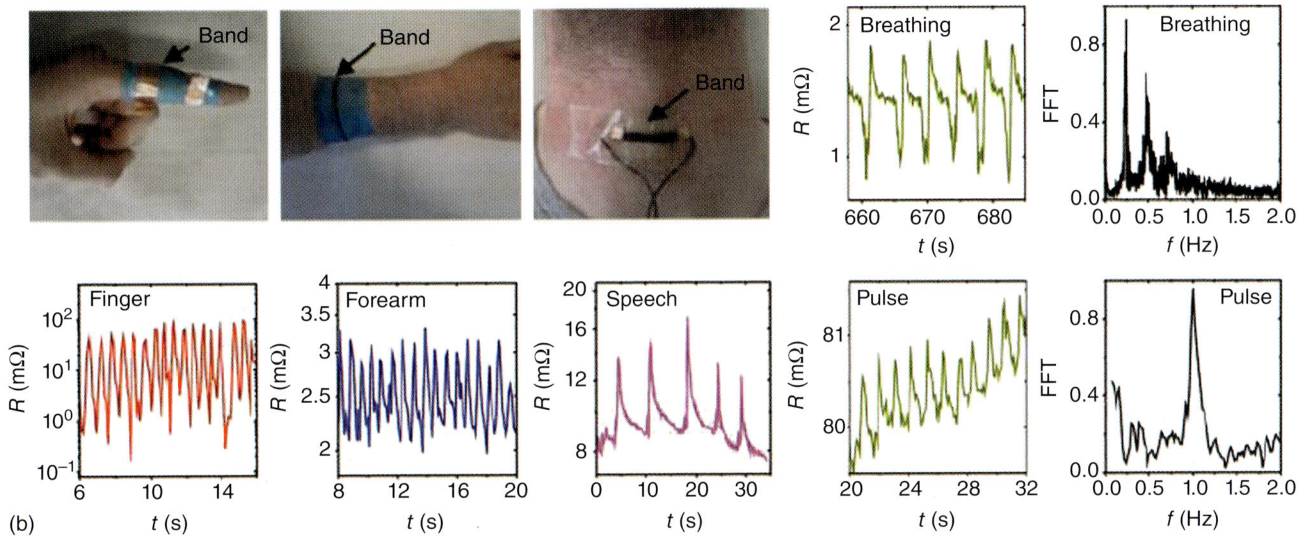

Figure 13.8 (*Continued*)

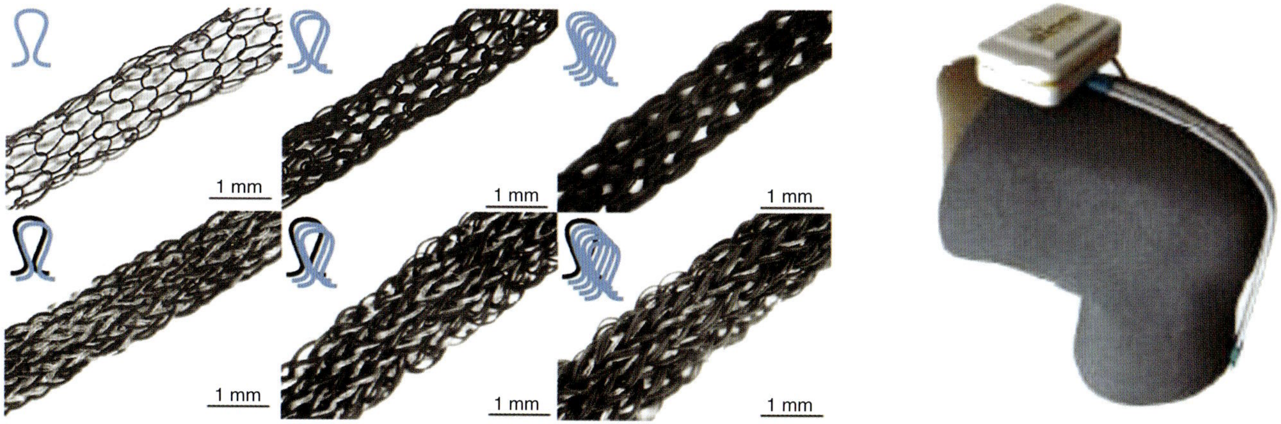

(c)

Figure 13.8 (*Continued*)

in hand prosthesis. Choi *et al.* developed a soft, thin, and stretchable heater for long-term, continuous articular thermotherapy using a nanocomposite of silver nanowires and a thermoplastic elastomer [77]. The nanocomposite is patterned to form serpentinemesh structures capable of conformal lamination on curvilinear joints and of conducting effective heat transfer during wrist motion.

13.3.3.2 Daily Health Tracking

Stretchable devices can appear as garments or accessories worn on bodies to monitor physiological signals to indicate risks or events such as cardiovascular disease, accidental falling, chronic heart failure, diabetes, and sleep disorders. Kim *et al.* demonstrated an electric textile containing planar-fashionable circuit boards (P-FCB), which are made of screen-printed conductive inks onto textile. Passive components such as resistors, capacitors, and inductors can also be printed using the same approach. Potentially, fully integrated circuits with commercial components and printed elements can be achieved to realize garment-based physiological signal sensing [141]. Motion tracking can be realized by strain sensors that assess muscle deformation during the exercise and daily activities [40, 142], and can be achieved through conductive and stretchable polymers using carbon nanotubes as fillers to improve the gauge factor (0.86) as well as the stretchability (280%) of the sensors. Boland *et al.* presented an improved strain gauge that can achieve 800% stretchability using graphene as fillers diffused into natural rubbers, resulting in a gauge factor at ~50 (Figure 13.8b) [139]. The strain gauge is able to detect arm bending, vocal cord vibration, and breathing. Electrically conductive and highly stretchable fibers based on PU/PEDOT:PSS have also been demonstrated (Figure 13.8c), and can be used to knit various textile structures. The knitted textile sensors can distinguish strain up to 160%, and can be integrated with wireless transmitters to realize knee sleeves for personal training and rehabilitation [140].

13.4 Future of Stretchable Electronic Devices

Stretchable electronic devices are targeting many challenges in health monitoring. The future trend of stretchable health monitoring devices lies in solving several critical issues that are causing constrains to the prevalence of such devices. Representative issues include power supplies of stretchable electronic devices, methods of data transmission, device complexity, and lack of system-level solutions. Currently, most of the devices mentioned focus on sensing functions of the stretchable electronic devices. However, power supplies, signal conditioning, data communication, and data storage still largely rely on bulky instruments or integrated circuits based on rigid substrates. Some researches tackle the power issues with stretchable batteries [143, 144], piezoelectric generators [145, 146], and solar cells [6, 147], showing promising future in replacing current bulky power sources with components that mechanically and geometrically match stretchable electronic devices. Work on improving the power density of the above-mentioned methods is also underway, and may eventually lead to construct devices that can stay with human bodies during the entire measurement periods. The complexity of the devices can be further improved by integrating multisensing components as well as commercialoff-the-shelf components that assist signal conditioning and data communication [10], allowing comprehensive assessment of multiple biophysiological signals and improvingthe accuracy of multidegree datain diagnosis and treatment.

References

1 Lu, N. and Kim, D.-H. (2013) *Soft Rob.*, **1**, 53.
2 Majidi, C. (2013) *Soft Rob.*, **1**, 5.
3 Cho, K.-J., Koh, J.-S., Kim, S., Chu, W.-S., Hong, Y., and Ahn, S.-H. (2009) *Int. J. Precis. Eng. Manuf.*, **10**, 171.
4 Suo, Z. (2012) *MRS Bull.*, **37**, 218.
5 Briseno, A.L., Mannsfeld, S.C.B., Ling, M.M., Liu, S., Tseng, R.J., Reese, C., Roberts, M.E., Yang, Y., Wudl, F., and Bao, Z. (2006) *Nature*, **444**, 913.
6 Lipomi, D.J., Tee, B.C.K., Vosgueritchian, M., and Bao, Z. (2011) *Adv. Mater.*, **23**, 1771.
7 Yan, C., Wang, J., Wang, X., Kang, W., Cui, M., Foo, C.Y., and Lee, P.S. (2014) *Adv. Mater.*, **26**, 943.
8 Guo, J., Liu, J., Yang, B., Zhan, G., Kang, X., Tian, H., Tang, L., Chen, X., and Yang, C. (2015) *IEEE Electron Device Lett.*, **36**, 576.
9 Song, Y.M., Xie, Y., Malyarchuk, V., Xiao, J., Jung, I., Choi, K.-J., Liu, Z., Park, H., Lu, C., and Kim, R.-H. (2013) *Nature*, **497**, 95.
10 Xu, S., Zhang, Y., Jia, L., Mathewson, K.E., Jang, K.-I., Kim, J., Fu, H., Huang, X., Chava, P., and Wang, R. (2014) *Science*, **344**, 70.
11 Li, T., Huang, Z., Suo, Z., Lacour, S.P., and Wagner, S. (2004) *Appl. Phys. Lett.*, **85**, 3435.
12 Wagner, S. and Bauer, S. (2012) *MRS Bull.*, **37**, 207.
13 Bartlett, M.D., Fassler, A., Kazem, N., Markvicka, E.J., Mandal, P., and Majidi, C. (2016) *Adv. Mater.*, **28**, 3726.
14 Park, M., Im, J., Shin, M., Min, Y., Park, J., Cho, H., Park, S., Shim, M.-B., Jeon, S., Chung, D.-Y., Bae, J., Park, J., Jeong, U., and Kim, K. (2012) *Nat. Nano*, **7**, 803.
15 Hyun, D.C., Park, M., Park, C., Kim, B., Xia, Y., Hur, J.H., Kim, J.M., Park, J.J., and Jeong, U. (2011) *Adv. Mater.*, **23**, 2946.
16 Vosgueritchian, M., Lipomi, D.J., and Bao, Z. (2012) *Adv. Funct. Mater.*, **22**, 421.
17 Yeo, W.-H., Kim, Y.-S., Lee, J., Ameen, A., Shi, L., Li, M., Wang, S., Ma, R., Jin, S.H., Kang, Z., Huang, Y., and Rogers, J.A. (2013) *Adv. Mater.*, **25**, 2773.
18 Xu, L., Gutbrod, S.R., Ma, Y., Petrossians, A., Liu, Y., Webb, R.C., Fan, J.A., Yang, Z., Xu, R., Whalen, J.J., Weiland, J.D., Huang, Y., Efimov, I.R., and Rogers, J.A. (2015) *Adv. Mater.*, **27**, 1731.
19 Kim, D.-H., Song, J., Choi, W.M., Kim, H.-S., Kim, R.-H., Liu, Z., Huang, Y.Y., Hwang, K.-C., Zhang, Y.-w., and Rogers, J.A. (2008) *Proc. Natl. Acad. Sci. U.S.A.*, **105**, 18675.

20 Sun, Y., Choi, W.M., Jiang, H., Huang, Y.Y., and Rogers, J.A. (2006) *Nat. Nanotechnol.*, **1**, 201.
21 Hu, L., Pasta, M., Mantia, F.L., Cui, L., Jeong, S., Deshazer, H.D., Choi, J.W., Han, S.M., and Cui, Y. (2010) *Nano Lett.*, **10**, 708.
22 Cherenack, K., Zysset, C., Kinkeldei, T., Münzenrieder, N., and Tröster, G. (2010) *Adv. Mater.*, **22**, 5178.
23 Kramer, R.K., Boley, J.W., Stone, H.A., Weaver, J.C., and Wood, R.J. (2014) *Langmuir*, **30**, 533.
24 Dickey, M.D., Chiechi, R.C., Larsen, R.J., Weiss, E.A., Weitz, D.A., and Whitesides, G.M. (2008) *Adv. Funct. Mater.*, **18**, 1097.
25 Liu, T., Sen, P., and Kim, C.J. (2012) *J. Microelectromech. Syst.*, **21**, 443.
26 Park, Y.-L., Majidi, C., Kramer, R., Bérard, P., and Wood, R.J. (2010) *J. Micromech. Microeng.*, **20**, 125029.
27 Khan, M.R., Hayes, G.J., Zhang, S., Dickey, M.D., and Lazzi, G. (2012) *IEEE Microwave Wireless Compon. Lett.*, **22**, 577.
28 Park, Y.-L., Chen, B.-R., and Wood, R.J. (2011) Soft artificial skin with multi-modal sensing capability using embedded liquid conductors. Presented at2011 IEEE Sensors Proceedings.
29 Brown, T.D., Sigal, L., Njus, G.O., Njus, N.M., Singerman, R.J., and Brand, R.A. (1986) *J. Biomech.*, **19**, 165.
30 Cheng, S. and Wu, Z. (2011) *Adv. Funct. Mater.*, **21**, 2282.
31 Cheng, S., Rydberg, A., Hjort, K., and Wu, Z. (2009) *Appl. Phys. Lett.*, **94**, 144103.
32 Mazlouman, S.J., Jiang, X.J., Mahanfar, A.N., Menon, C., and Vaughan, R.G. (2011) *IEEE Trans. Antennas Propag.*, **59**, 4406.
33 Kim, H.-J., Son, C., and Ziaie, B. (2008) *Appl. Phys. Lett.*, **92**, 011904.
34 Kramer, R.K., Majidi, C., and Wood, R.J. (2011) Wearable tactile keypad with stretchable artificial skin. Presented at 2011 IEEE International Conference onRobotics and Automation (ICRA).
35 Zhu, S., So, J.-H., Mays, R., Desai, S., Barnes, W.R., Pourdeyhimi, B., and Dickey, M.D. (2013) *Adv. Funct. Mater.*, **23**, 2308.
36 Sekitani, T., Nakajima, H., Maeda, H., Fukushima, T., Aida, T., Hata, K., and Someya, T. (2009) *Nat. Mater.*, **8**, 494.
37 Chun, K.-Y., Oh, Y., Rho, J., Ahn, J.-H., Kim, Y.-J., Choi, H.R., and Baik, S. (2010) *Nat. Nano*, **5**, 853.
38 Karnaushenko, D.D., Karnaushenko, D., Makarov, D., and Schmidt, O.G. (2015) *NPG Asia Mater.*, **7**, e188.
39 Jang, K.-I., Chung, H.U., Xu, S., Lee, C.H., Luan, H., Jeong, J., Cheng, H., Kim, G.-T., Han, S.Y., Lee, J.W., Kim, J., Cho, M., Miao, F., Yang, Y., Jung, H.N., Flavin, M., Liu, H., Kong, G.W., Yu, K.J., Rhee, S.I., Chung, J., Kim, B., Kwak, J.W., Yun, M.H., Kim, J.Y., Song, Y.M., Paik, U., Zhang, Y., Huang, Y., and Rogers, J.A. (2015) *Nat. Commun.*, **6**, 6566.
40 Yamada, T., Hayamizu, Y., Yamamoto, Y., Yomogida, Y., Izadi-Najafabadi, A., Futaba, D.N., and Hata, K. (2011) *Nat. Nano*, **6**, 296.
41 Kim, D.H., Wang, S., Keum, H., Ghaffari, R., Kim, Y.S., Tao, H., Panilaitis, B., Li, M., Kang, Z., and Omenetto, F. (2012) *Small*, **8**, 3263.
42 Khang, D.-Y., Jiang, H., Huang, Y., and Rogers, J.A. (2006) *Science*, **311**, 208.

43 Sun, Y., Kumar, V., Adesida, I., and Rogers, J.A. (2006) *Adv. Mater.*, **18**, 2857.

44 Park, K., Lee, D.K., Kim, B.S., Jeon, H., Lee, N.E., Whang, D., Lee, H.J., Kim, Y.J., and Ahn, J.H. (2010) *Adv. Funct. Mater.*, **20**, 3577.

45 Wallentin, J., Anttu, N., Asoli, D., Huffman, M., Åberg, I., Magnusson, M.H., Siefer, G., Fuss-Kailuweit, P., Dimroth, F., Witzigmann, B., Xu, H.Q., Samuelson, L., Deppert, K., and Borgström, M.T. (2013) *Science*, **339**, 1057.

46 Hwang, S.-W., Tao, H., Kim, D.-H., Cheng, H., Song, J.-K., Rill, E., Brenckle, M.A., Panilaitis, B., Won, S.M., Kim, Y.-S., Song, Y.M., Yu, K.J., Ameen, A., Li, R., Su, Y., Yang, M., Kaplan, D.L., Zakin, M.R., Slepian, M.J., Huang, Y., Omenetto, F.G., and Rogers, J.A. (2012) *Science*, **337**, 1640.

47 Kim, D.-H. and Rogers, J.A. (2008) *Adv. Mater.*, **20**, 4887.

48 Dasgupta, N.P., Sun, J., Liu, C., Brittman, S., Andrews, S.C., Lim, J., Gao, H., Yan, R., and Yang, P. (2014) *Adv. Mater.*, **26**, 2137.

49 Ouyang, Y. and Chappell, W.J. (2008) *IEEE Trans. Antennas Propag.*, **56**, 381.

50 Cochrane, C., Koncar, V., Lewandowski, M., and Dufour, C. (2007) *Sensors*, **7**, 473.

51 Mattmann, C., Clemens, F., and Tröster, G. (2008) *Sensors*, **8**, 3719.

52 Rothmaier, M., Luong, M., and Clemens, F. (2008) *Sensors*, **8**, 4318.

53 Takamatsu, S., Kobayashi, T., Shibayama, N., Miyake, K., and Itoh, T. (2012) *Sens. Actuators, A*, **184**, 57.

54 Jeong, J.W., Jang, Y.W., Lee, I., Shin, S., and Kim, S. (2009) in *World Congress on Medical Physics and Biomedical Engineering, September 7–12, 2009, Munich, Germany: Vol. 25/5 Information and Communication in Medicine, Telemedicine and e-Health* (eds O. Dössel and W.C. Schlegel), Springer-Verlag, Berlin, Heidelberg, p. 282.

55 Choi, S. and Jiang, Z. (2006) *Sens. Actuators, A*, **128**, 317.

56 Jang, K.-I., Han, S.Y., Xu, S., Mathewson, K.E., Zhang, Y., Jeong, J.-W., Kim, G.-T., Webb, R.C., Lee, J.W., Dawidczyk, T.J., Kim, R.H., Song, Y.M., Yeo, W.-H., Kim, S., Cheng, H., Rhee, S.I., Chung, J., Kim, B., Chung, H.U., Lee, D., Yang, Y., Cho, M., Gaspar, J.G., Carbonari, R., Fabiani, M., Gratton, G., Huang, Y., and Rogers, J.A. (2014) *Nat. Commun.*, **5**, 4779.

57 Kim, D.-H., Lu, N., Ma, R., Kim, Y.-S., Kim, R.-H., Wang, S., Wu, J., Won, S.M., Tao, H., Islam, A., Yu, K.J., Kim, T.-i., Chowdhury, R., Ying, M., Xu, L., Li, M., Chung, H.-J., Keum, H., McCormick, M., Liu, P., Zhang, Y.-W., Omenetto, F.G., Huang, Y., Coleman, T., and Rogers, J.A. (2011) *Science*, **333**, 838.

58 Yang, S., Chen, Y.C., Nicolini, L., Pasupathy, P., Sacks, J., Su, B., Yang, R., Sanchez, D., Chang, Y.F., and Wang, P. (2015) *Adv. Mater.*, **27**, 6423.

59 Jeong, J.W., Kim, M.K., Cheng, H., Yeo, W.H., Huang, X., Liu, Y., Zhang, Y., Huang, Y., and Rogers, J.A. (2014) *Adv. Healthc. Mater.*, **3**, 642.

60 Jeong, J.W., Yeo, W.H., Akhtar, A., Norton, J.J., Kwack, Y.J., Li, S., Jung, S.Y., Su, Y., Lee, W., and Xia, J. (2013) *Adv. Mater.*, **25**, 6839.

61 Huang, X., Yeo, W.-H., Liu, Y., and Rogers, J.A. (2012) *Biointerphases*, **7**, 52.

62 Huang, X., Cheng, H., Chen, K., Zhang, Y., Zhang, Y., Liu, Y., Zhu, C., Ouyang, S.C., Kong, G.W., Yu, C., Huang, Y., and Rogers, J.A. (2013) *IEEE Trans. Biomed. Eng.*, **60**, 2848.

63 Huang, X., Liu, Y., Cheng, H., Shin, W.-J., Fan, J.A., Liu, Z., Lu, C.-J., Kong, G.-W., Chen, K., Patnaik, D., Lee, S.-H., Hage-Ali, S., Huang, Y., and Rogers, J.A. (2014) *Adv. Funct. Mater.*, **24**, 3846.

64 Webb, R.C., Bonifas, A.P., Behnaz, A., Zhang, Y., Yu, K.J., Cheng, H., Shi, M., Bian, Z., Liu, Z., Kim, Y.-S., Yeo, W.-H., Park, J.S., Song, J., Li, Y., Huang, Y., Gorbach, A.M., and Rogers, J.A. (2013) *Nat. Mater.*, **12**, 938.

65 Lacour, S.P., Benmerah, S., Tarte, E., FitzGerald, J., Serra, J., McMahon, S., Fawcett, J., Graudejus, O., Yu, Z., and Morrison, B. (2010) *Med. Biol. Eng. Comput.*, **48**, 945.

66 Graudejus, O., Morrison, B., Goletiani, C., Yu, Z., and Wagner, S. (2012) *Adv. Funct. Mater.*, **22**, 640.

67 Guo, L., Guvanasen, G.S., Liu, X., Tuthill, C., Nichols, T.R., and DeWeerth, S.P. (2013) *IEEE Trans. Biomed. Circuits Syst.*, **7**, 1.

68 Graudejus, O., Yu, Z., Jones, J., Morrison, B., and Wagner, S. (2009) *J. Electrochem. Soc.*, **156**, P85.

69 Lacour, S.P., Tsay, C., Wagner, S., Zhe, Y., and Morrison, B. (2005) Stretchable micro-electrode arrays for dynamic neuronal recording of *in vitro* mechanically injured brain. Presented at IEEE Sensors, *2005*, October 30, 2005–November 3, 2005.

70 Guo, L., Ma, M., Zhang, N., Langer, R., and Anderson, D.G. (2014) *Adv. Mater.*, **26**, 1427.

71 Kim, D.-H., Lu, N., Ghaffari, R., Kim, Y.-S., Lee, S.P., Xu, L., Wu, J., Kim, R.-H., Song, J., Liu, Z., Viventi, J., de Graff, B., Elolampi, B., Mansour, M., Slepian, M.J., Hwang, S., Moss, J.D., Won, S.-M., Huang, Y., Litt, B., and Rogers, J.A. (2011) *Nat. Mater.*, **10**, 316.

72 Kim, D.-H., Ghaffari, R., Lu, N., Wang, S., Lee, S.P., Keum, H., D'Angelo, R., Klinker, L., Su, Y., Lu, C., Kim, Y.-S., Ameen, A., Li, Y., Zhang, Y., de Graff, B., Hsu, Y.-Y., Liu, Z., Ruskin, J., Xu, L., Lu, C., Omenetto, F.G., Huang, Y., Mansour, M., Slepian, M.J., and Rogers, J.A. (2012) *Proc. Natl. Acad. Sci. U.S.A.*, **109**, 19910.

73 Zheng, Y.L., Yan, B.P., Zhang, Y.T., and Poon, C.C.Y. (2014) *IEEE Trans. Biomed. Eng.*, **61**, 2179.

74 Jung, S., Hong, S., Kim, J., Lee, S., Hyeon, T., Lee, M., and Kim, D.-H. (2015) *Sci. Rep.*, **5**, 17081.

75 Kim, J., Lee, M., Shim, H.J., Ghaffari, R., Cho, H.R., Son, D., Jung, Y.H., Soh, M., Choi, C., Jung, S., Chu, K., Jeon, D., Lee, S.-T., Kim, J.H., Choi, S.H., Hyeon, T., and Kim, D.-H. (2014) *Nat. Commun.*, **5**, 5747.

76 Gerratt, A.P., Michaud, H.O., and Lacour, S.P. (2015) *Adv. Funct. Mater.*, **25**, 2287.

77 Choi, S., Park, J., Hyun, W., Kim, J., Kim, J., Lee, Y.B., Song, C., Hwang, H.J., Kim, J.H., Hyeon, T., and Kim, D.-H. (2015) *ACS Nano*, **9**, 6626.

78 Lee, A.Y., Eun, H.C., Kim, H.O., Moon, K.C., Lee, C.H., Kim, G.J., Kim, S.C., and Ham, J.H. (2001) *Contact Dermat.*, **45**, 214.

79 Möller, H. (2010) *Contact Dermat.*, **62**, 193.

80 Chen, Y., Lu, B., Chen, Y., and Feng, X. (2015) *Sci. Rep.*, **5**, 11505.

81 Kim, J., Banks, A., Cheng, H., Xie, Z., Xu, S., Jang, K.I., Lee, J.W., Liu, Z., Gutruf, P., and Huang, X. (2015) *Small*, **11**, 906.

82 Mostafalu, P., Lenk, W., Dokmeci, M.R., Ziaie, B., Khademhosseini, A., and Sonkusale, S.R. (2015) *IEEE Trans. Biomed. Circuits Syst.*, **9**, 670.
83 Kwak, M.K., Jeong, H.E., and Suh, K.Y. (2011) *Adv. Mater.*, **23**, 3949.
84 Joseph, W.M., Yang, W., Russel, T., Neil, G., Gordon, P., Stephen, B., and John, T. (2015) *Smart Mater. Struct.*, **24**, 125028.
85 Zheng, J., Ha, C., and Zhang, Z. (2017) *Med. Biol. Eng. Comput.*, **55**, 283.
86 Das, M.K., Saha, C., El Masry, H., Peng, J., Dandamudi, G., Mahenthiran, J., McHenry, P., and Zipes, D.P. (2007) *Heart Rhythm*, **4**, 1385.
87 Barry, D.T., Gordon, K.E., and Hinton, G.G. (1990) *Muscle Nerve*, **13**, 286.
88 Cifrek, M., Medved, V., Tonković, S., and Ostojić, S. (2009) *Clin. Biomech.*, **24**, 327.
89 Natarajan, K., Acharya, R., Alias, F., Tiboleng, T., and Puthusserypady, S.K. (2004) *BioMed. Eng. OnLine*, **3**, 7.
90 Kupfer, D.J., Foster, F.G., Coble, P., McPartland, R.J., and Ulrich, R.F. (1978) *Am. J. Psychiatry*, **135**, 69.
91 Gillin, J.C., Duncan, W., Pettigrew, K.D., Frankel, B.L., and Snyder, F. (1979) *Arch. Gen. Psychiatry*, **36**, 85.
92 Hostynek, J.J. and Maibach, H.I. (2004) *Dermatol. Ther.*, **17**, 328.
93 Jung, H.C., Moon, J.H., Baek, D.H., Lee, J.H., Choi, Y.Y., Hong, J.S., and Lee, S.H. (2012) *IEEE Trans. Biomed. Eng.*, **59**, 1472.
94 Blau, A., Murr, A., Wolff, S., Sernagor, E., Medini, P., Iurilli, G., Ziegler, C., and Benfenati, F. (2011) *Biomaterials*, **32**, 1778.
95 Sator, P.-G., Schmidt, J.B., and Hönigsmann, H. (2003) *J. Am. Acad. Dermatol.*, **48**, 352.
96 Kim, S., Huh, C., Seo, K., Suh, D., and Youn, J. (2002) *Clin. Exp. Dermatol.*, **27**, 147.
97 Morton, C., Lafferty, M., Hau, C., Henderson, I., Jones, M., and Lowe, J. (1996) *Nephrol. Dial. Transplant.*, **11**, 2031.
98 Hong, S.Y., Lee, Y.H., Park, H., Jin, S.W., Jeong, Y.R., Yun, J., You, I., Zi, G., and Ha, J.S. (2016) *Adv. Mater.*, **28**, 930.
99 Gao, L., Zhang, Y., Malyarchuk, V., Jia, L., Jang, K.-I., Chad Webb, R., Fu, H., Shi, Y., Zhou, G., Shi, L., Shah, D., Huang, X., Xu, B., Yu, C., Huang, Y., and Rogers, J.A. (2014) *Nat. Commun.*, **5**, 4938.
100 Yu, C., Wang, Z., Yu, H., and Jiang, H. (2009) *Appl. Phys. Lett.*, **95**, 141912.
101 Tien, N.T., Jeon, S., Kim, D.-I., Trung, T.Q., Jang, M., Hwang, B.-U., Byun, K.-E., Bae, J., Lee, E., Tok, J.B.H., Bao, Z., Lee, N.-E., and Park, J.-J. (2014) *Adv. Mater.*, **26**, 796.
102 Trung, T.Q., Ramasundaram, S., Hwang, B.-U., and Lee, N.-E. (2016) *Adv. Mater.*, **28**, 502.
103 Someya, T., Kato, Y., Sekitani, T., Iba, S., Noguchi, Y., Murase, Y., Kawaguchi, H., and Sakurai, T. (2005) *Proc. Natl. Acad. Sci. U.S.A.*, **102**, 12321.
104 Lochner, C.M., Khan, Y., Pierre, A., and Arias, A.C. (2014) *Nat. Commun.*, **5**, 5745.
105 Yokota, T., Zalar, P., Kaltenbrunner, M., Jinno, H., Matsuhisa, N., Kitanosako, H., Tachibana, Y., Yukita, W., Koizumi, M., and Someya, T. (2016) *Sci. Adv.*, **2**, e1501856.

106 Hattori, Y., Falgout, L., Lee, W., Jung, S.-Y., Poon, E., Lee, J.W., Na, I., Geisler, A., Sadhwani, D., Zhang, Y., Su, Y., Wang, X., Liu, Z., Xia, J., Cheng, H., Webb, R.C., Bonifas, A.P., Won, P., Jeong, J.-W., Jang, K.-I., Song, Y.M., Nardone, B., Nodzenski, M., Fan, J.A., Huang, Y., West, D.P., Paller, A.S., Alam, M., Yeo, W.-H., and Rogers, J.A. (2014) *Adv. Healthc. Mater.*, **3**, 1597.

107 Lin, S., Yuk, H., Zhang, T., Parada, G.A., Koo, H., Yu, C., and Zhao, X. (2016) *Adv. Mater.*, **28**, 4497.

108 Gong, S., Schwalb, W., Wang, Y., Chen, Y., Tang, Y., Si, J., Shirinzadeh, B., and Cheng, W. (2014) *Nat. Commun.*, **5**, 3132.

109 Vandeparre, H., Watson, D., and Lacour, S.P. (2013) *Appl. Phys. Lett.*, **103**, 204103.

110 Majidi, C., Kramer, R., and Wood, R.J. (2011) *Smart Mater. Struct.*, **20**, 105017.

111 Morteza, A., Yong Jin, Y., and Inkyu, P. (2015) *Nanotechnology*, **26**, 375501.

112 Parrilla, M., Ferré, J., Guinovart, T., and Andrade, F.J. (2016) *Electroanalysis*, **28**, 1267.

113 Parrilla, M., Cánovas, R., Jeerapan, I., Andrade, F.J., and Wang, J. (2016) *Adv. Healthc. Mater.*, **5**, 996.

114 Cazalé, A., Sant, W., Ginot, F., Launay, J.C., Savourey, G., Revol-Cavalier, F., Lagarde, J.M., Heinry, D., Launay, J., and Temple-Boyer, P. (2016) *Sens. Actuators, B*, **225**, 1.

115 Gao, W., Emaminejad, S., Nyein, H.Y.Y., Challa, S., Chen, K., Peck, A., Fahad, H.M., Ota, H., Shiraki, H., Kiriya, D., Lien, D.-H., Brooks, G.A., Davis, R.W., and Javey, A. (2016) *Nature*, **529**, 509.

116 Guinovart, T., Bandodkar, A.J., Windmiller, J.R., Andrade, F.J., and Wang, J. (2013) *Analyst*, **138**, 7031.

117 Kudo, H., Sawada, T., Kazawa, E., Yoshida, H., Iwasaki, Y., and Mitsubayashi, K. (2006) *Biosens. Bioelectron.*, **22**, 558.

118 Huang, X., Liu, Y., Chen, K., Shin, W.-J., Lu, C.-J., Kong, G.-W., Patnaik, D., Lee, S.-H., Cortes, J.F., and Rogers, J.A. (2014) *Small*, **10**, 3083.

119 Lee, H., Choi, T.K., Lee, Y.B., Cho, H.R., Ghaffari, R., Wang, L., Choi, H.J., Chung, T.D., Lu, N., Hyeon, T., Choi, S.H., and Kim, D.-H. (2016) *Nat Nano*, **11**, 566.

120 Bandodkar, A.J., Jeerapan, I., You, J.-M., Nuñez-Flores, R., and Wang, J. (2016) *Nano Lett.*, **16**, 721.

121 Labroo, P. and Cui, Y. (2013) *Biosens. Bioelectron.*, **41**, 852.

122 Jia, W., Bandodkar, A.J., Valdés-Ramírez, G., Windmiller, J.R., Yang, Z., Ramírez, J., Chan, G., and Wang, J. (2013) *Anal. Chem.*, **85**, 6553.

123 Xu, L., Gutbrod, S.R., Bonifas, A.P., Su, Y., Sulkin, M.S., Lu, N., Chung, H.-J., Jang, K.-I., Liu, Z., Ying, M., Lu, C., Webb, R.C., Kim, J.-S., Laughner, J.I., Cheng, H., Liu, Y., Ameen, A., Jeong, J.-W., Kim, G.-T., Huang, H., Efimov, I.R., and Rogers, J.A. (2014) *Nat. Commun.*, **5**, 3329.

124 Koh, A., Gutbrod, S.R., Meyers, J.D., Lu, C., Webb, R.C., Shin, G., Li, Y., Kang, S.-K., Huang, Y., Efimov, I.R., and Rogers, J.A. (2016) *Adv. Healthc. Mater.*, **5**, 373.

125 Kim, T.-i., McCall, J.G., Jung, Y.H., Huang, X., Siuda, E.R., Li, Y., Song, J., Song, Y.M., Pao, H.A., and Kim, R.-H. (2013) *Science*, **340**, 211.

126 Park, S.I., Brenner, D.S., Shin, G., Morgan, C.D., Copits, B.A., Chung, H.U., Pullen, M.Y., Noh, K.N., Davidson, S., Oh, S.J., Yoon, J., Jang, K.-I., Samineni, V.K., Norman, M., Grajales-Reyes, J.G., Vogt, S.K., Sundaram, S.S., Wilson, K.M., Ha, J.S., Xu, R., Pan, T., Kim, T.-i., Huang, Y., Montana, M.C., Golden, J.P., Bruchas, M.R., Gereau, R.W. IV,, and Rogers, J.A. (2015) *Nat. Biotechnol.*, **33**, 1280.

127 Minev, I.R., Musienko, P., Hirsch, A., Barraud, Q., Wenger, N., Moraud, E.M., Gandar, J., Capogrosso, M., Milekovic, T., Asboth, L., Torres, R.F., Vachicouras, N., Liu, Q., Pavlova, N., Duis, S., Larmagnac, A., Vörös, J., Micera, S., Suo, Z., Courtine, G., and Lacour, S.P. (2015) *Science*, **347**, 159.

128 Pang, C., Lee, G.-Y., Kim, T.-i., Kim, S.M., Kim, H.N., Ahn, S.-H., and Suh, K.-Y. (2012) *Nat. Mater.*, **11**, 795.

129 Lee, J., Kim, S., Lee, J., Yang, D., Park, B.C., Ryu, S., and Park, I. (2014) *Nanoscale*, **6**, 11932.

130 Du, D., Li, P., and Ouyang, J. (2016) *J. Mater. Chem. C*, **4**, 3224.

131 Sergio, M., Manaresi, N., Tartagni, M., Guerrieri, R., and Canegallo, R. (2002) A textile based capacitive pressure sensor. Presented at Proceedings of IEEE Sensors, 2002.

132 Ge, J., Sun, L., Zhang, F.R., Zhang, Y., Shi, L.A., Zhao, H.Y., Zhu, H.W., Jiang, H.L., and Yu, S.H. (2016) *Adv. Mater.*, **28**, 783.

133 Lee, J., Kwon, H., Seo, J., Shin, S., Koo, J.H., Pang, C., Son, S., Kim, J.H., Jang, Y.H., Kim, D.E., and Lee, T. (2015) *Adv. Mater.*, **27**, 2433.

134 Paradiso, R. and Caldani, L. (2010) *Res. J. Text. Apparel*, **14**, 9.

135 Narbonneau, F., Jeanne, M., Kinet, D., Witt, J., Krebber, K., Paquet, B., Depre, A., and Logier, R. (2009) OFSETH: smart medical textile for continuous monitoring of respiratory motions under magnetic resonance imaging. Presented at 2009 Annual International Conference of the IEEE Engineering in Medicine and Biology Society.

136 Ko, J., Bhullar, S., Cho, Y., Lee, P.C., and Jun, M.B.-G. (2015) *Smart Mater. Struct.*, **24**, 075027.

137 Stoyanov, H., Kollosche, M., Risse, S., Waché, R., and Kofod, G. (2013) *Adv. Mater.*, **25**, 578.

138 Ryu, S., Lee, P., Chou, J.B., Xu, R., Zhao, R., Hart, A.J., and Kim, S.-G. (2015) *ACS Nano*, **9**, 5929.

139 Boland, C.S., Khan, U., Backes, C., O'Neill, A., McCauley, J., Duane, S., Shanker, R., Liu, Y., Jurewicz, I., Dalton, A.B., and Coleman, J.N. (2014) *ACS Nano*, **8**, 8819.

140 Seyedin, S., Razal, J.M., Innis, P.C., Jeiranikhameneh, A., Beirne, S., and Wallace, G.G. (2015) *ACS Appl. Mater. Interfaces*, **7**, 21150.

141 Kim, Y., Kim, H., and Yoo, H.-J. (2010) *IEEE Trans. Adv. Packag.*, **33**, 196.

142 Cai, L., Song, L., Luan, P., Zhang, Q., Zhang, N., Gao, Q., Zhao, D., Zhang, X., Tu, M., Yang, F., Zhou, W., Fan, Q., Luo, J., Zhou, W., Ajayan, P.M., and Xie, S. (2013) *Sci. Rep.*, **3**, 3048.

143 Xu, S., Zhang, Y., Cho, J., Lee, J., Huang, X., Jia, L., Fan, J.A., Su, Y., Su, J., Zhang, H., Cheng, H., Lu, B., Yu, C., Chuang, C., Kim, T.-I., Song, T.,

Shigeta, K., Kang, S., Dagdeviren, C., Petrov, I., Braun, P.V., Huang, Y., Paik, U., and Rogers, J.A. (2013) *Nat. Commun.*, **4**, 1543.
144 Gaikwad, A.M., Zamarayeva, A.M., Rousseau, J., Chu, H., Derin, I., and Steingart, D.A. (2012) *Adv. Mater.*, **24**, 5071.
145 Lee, J.-H., Lee, K.Y., Gupta, M.K., Kim, T.Y., Lee, D.-Y., Oh, J., Ryu, C., Yoo, W.J., Kang, C.-Y., Yoon, S.-J., Yoo, J.-B., and Kim, S.-W. (2014) *Adv. Mater.*, **26**, 765.
146 Duan, Y., Huang, Y., Yin, Z., Bu, N., and Dong, W. (2014) *Nanoscale*, **6**, 3289.
147 Li, G., Zhu, R., and Yang, Y. (2012) *Nat. Photonics*, **6**, 153.

14

Flexible/Stretchable Devices for Medical Applications

GwanJin Ko, JeongWoong Shin, and Suk-Won Hwang

Korea University, KU R&D Center, Rm.412B, 145 Anam-ro, Seongbuk-gu, Seoul 02841, South Korea

14.1 Introduction

Soft, stretchable electronic systems possess the capability to extend or enlarge beyond the usual or proper limits from a mechanical standpoint, and such excellent characteristics or behavior provide strong means to fulfill various unmet needs that are unable to be addressed by established, existing electronic devices. Recent researches have been focused on requirements that were initially realized by the various accomplishments of materials, devices, and design layouts as well as by the underlying mechanics of flexible, stretchable electronics [1–22], and the resulting advanced developments highlight the need for expanded research scope for potential uses in biomedical systems. Demonstrated examples for biomedicine range from medical implants such as those for monitoring/stimulating/controlling of electrical biopotentials for cardiac [23–28] and neural [29–36] activities, to electronic skin or epidermal electronics [37–46] for personal healthcare system and prosthetic limbs [33, 35] or robotics [46], to power generation [47–53], biomimetic systems [54, 55], and bioresorbable electronics [56–58]. There are two different approaches toward such scientific achievements. The first is to develop new materials, that is, intrinsically soft organic-based components combined with a stretchable rubber resulting in a composite of elastomeric conductor for electrodes, contacts, and interconnects [4, 8, 10, 18, 20, 21]. The second is to devise optimized geometrical configurations of rigid, brittle, inorganic-based materials for interconnects and active constituents, which enable new operational modes for facilitating substantial amounts of mechanical deformations and enhancing conformal contact ability via exploration of curvilinear system layouts to integrate with the human body and/or complex surface/shapes of structures [1, 6, 7, 12, 14, 22]. The fundamental idea is to utilize ultrathin, flexible film or ribbon of materials whose flexural rigidity (bending strain) is inversely proportional to thickness [59–61], thereby making it possible to deform over critical fracture strains.

In this chapter, we summarize the recent advances in the area of flexible, stretchable electronic/optoelectronic devices for widespread applications in

Flexible and Stretchable Medical Devices, First Edition. Edited by Kuniharu Takei.

clinical medicine, for instance for (i) recording/regulating electrical/mechanical/thermal activities associated with heart functions [23–28], (ii) recording/regulating power supply systems and/or pacemakers with the cardiac movements [23, 27], (iii) monitoring electrophysiological information and genetically controlled neuromodulations for brain surgery or related issues [29–36], (iv) electrical/physical interfaces for prosthetics and robotics [33, 35, 46], and (v) real-time, multi-modal monitors of physiological status/conditions [38, 44, 45]. In the beginning, we introduce a brief, comprehensive overview of the materials, their synthesis and composites, manufacturing scheme, and underlying mechanics. Integration of electronic devices, sensors, and systems with biological cells, tissues, and organs supports practical feasibilities of such bioelectronics for prevention, diagnosis, and treatment, as well as for healthcare and wellness. The last section provides conclusions, future directions and an outlook.

14.2 Materials, Synthesis and Composites for Flexible/Stretchable Systems

Figure 14.1a illustrates the approaches for creating ultrathin flexible/stretchable forms of active semiconducting materials and/or devices, applicable to almost any type of electronic system [47]. The top frame highlights the formation of a single crystal silicon microribbon with the thickness of a few microns from a bare (p-type) Si (111) wafer, via a well-known procedure of anisotropic undercut etching with potassium hydroxide (KOH) or tetramethylammonium hydroxide (TMAH)—in case of need to selectively remove a silicon from a silicon oxide such as a silicon on insulator (SOI) wafer. Here, patterning/etching defines the dimension of narrow strips of silicon whose direction of the length requires to be perpendicular to the preferential etching direction of Si <110>, and the thickness of those strips can be determined by the timescale of dry etching. Depositions of appropriate protection layers, for example, silicon oxide, silicon nitride, metal elements, over the top surface as well as sidewalls provide etch masks for the following wet etch in the strong alkaline solvent. The anisotropic removal along the guided direction generates a releasable form of an array of silicon microbars with rigid fixations of support, that is, anchors, at both ends of long axes. The tethered structure of these microcells can be selectively released by physical breaks of the anchors using a polydimethylsiloxane (PDMS) stamp with moderate pressure, and assembled or registered through the transfer printing method onto any kind of desired, foreign materials/substrates, resulting in a complete electronic device. Similar procedure can be applied to a compound semiconductor of gallium nitride (GaN) grown on a silicon wafer, and to an SOI wafer but different plane index with a handle Si (111) wafer, according to a previously reported article [19, 62–64]. This cost-effective, large-scale strategy allows high-temperature process during the course of manufacturing, leading to high-performance flexible, stretchable electronic systems. Another representation of producing an ultrathin sheet of active elements appears in the bottom frame of Figure 14.1a [17]. A variety of growth conditions can control thickness, doping profile, composition, and other properties of layers, and a dry etching with patterned masks provides diverse geometrical options. Employing a sharp contrast of the etching rate in a particular solvent suggests a route to obtain individual pieces/layers of GaAs with predesigned dimensions/layouts from vertically stacked, heterogeneous multi-layers of GaAs and AlAs, by selective removal of AlAs in hydrofluoric acid (HF). Such an analogous process is widely used to extract ultrathin, monocrystalline

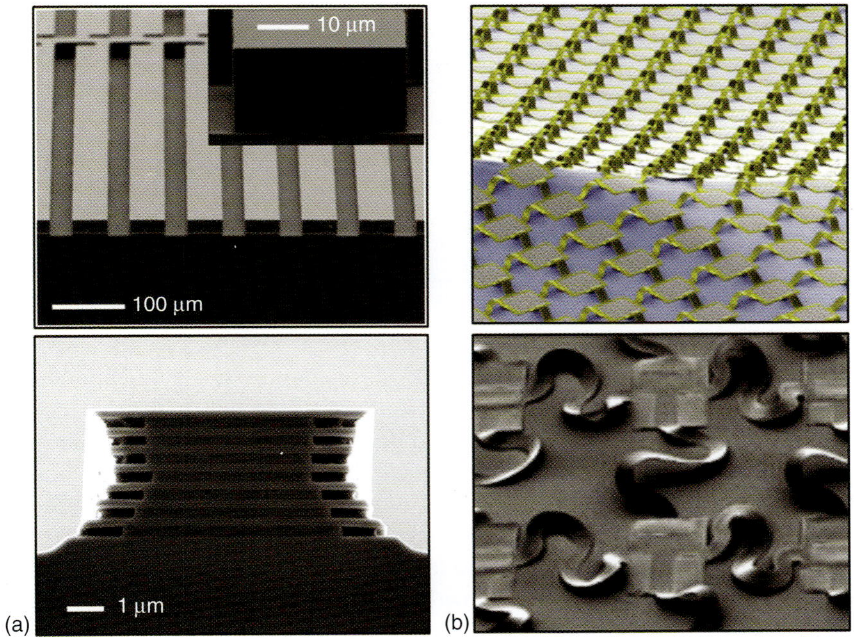

Figure 14.1 Materials, synthesis and composites for flexible/stretchable systems. (a) Top: Tilted scanning electron microscope (SEM) image of an array of ultrathin silicon solar microcells tethered to a mother wafer, right after defining individual cells and undercut etching with potassium hydroxide (KOH). The inset represents a magnified SEM image of a representative microscale solar cell (thickness, ~20 μm). Bottom: Cross-sectional SEM view of multiple stacks of GaAs/AlAs formed by metal organic chemical vapor deposition (MOCVD) during selective etching of the AlAs via hydrofluoric acid (HF). (b) Top: A colorized image of an array of electronic circuits with a pop-up bridge structure to enhance stretchability, conformal interfaces of the system to unusual shapes such as the surface of a golf ball. Bottom: SEM image of an advanced design layout to achieve extreme stretchable capability of an array of silicon CMOS inverters using noncoplanar, serpentine bridges over a large area. Each cell strongly bonds to the PDMS, while serpentine traces are not restricted to the substrate for being stretchable to external forces. (c) Top: A magnified SEM image showing the structure of a representative conductive elastomer, including uniformly distributed single wall carbon nanotubes (SWCTs) in a rubber through multistage manufacturing procedures. Bottom: An optical image of Ag flakes-based elastic ink with high conductivity and stretchability for printed electronics. The electrical and mechanical properties of this elastic conductive ink is determined by its composite materials. (d) Top: Photographs of pliable, patterned SWCTs-based conductors on a PDMS slab for organic electronic devices, with dispersed SWCTs in paste (left) and patterned SWCTS by screen printing (right) in the inset. Bottom: Image of net-shaped conductors enabling excellent contact ability to three-dimensional random configurations, for potentially electronic artificial skin.

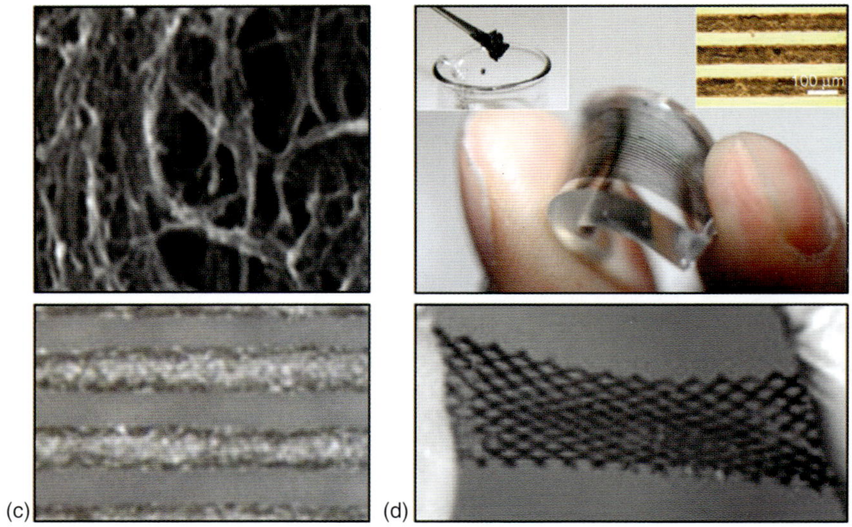

Figure 14.1 (*Continued*)

silicon nanomembranes (Si NMs) from an SOI wafer, by selective elimination of a buried oxide (SiO_2) in HF [5, 11]. In some cases, especially for the case of using a thin sacrificial layer, it is useful to define tiny holes at proper periodic intervals to prevent the membranes from sagging down to the lower membrane, causing to impede propagation of etching solutions, that is, it stops the etching procedure. Deterministic transfer methods described or usage of engineered elastomeric stamp elsewhere [65–67] efficiently conveys each layer of GaAs to any substrates of interest to integrate with other components.

Modifications of mechanical layouts and structural configurations in conventional inorganic-based electronics offer the possibility to transform materials with rigid and fragile nature to become flexible, stretchable, and foldable. An initial step toward accomplishing a soft, stretchable circuit produced a one-dimensional semiconducting material with micron-sized, wavy geometries that enables reversible stretching in a longitudinal direction without significant reduction of the electrical/mechanical/optical properties, although limited to a singular electrical component [5–7]. Developments of wavy and buckled profiles of single crystal silicon nanomembranes (Si NMs) on an elastomeric rubber provide high-performance, stretchable and foldable integrated circuits such as an array of complementary metal-oxide-semiconductor (CMOS), ring oscillator, and differential amplifiers [11, 12]. Analytical mechanics model defines a neutral mechanical plane (NMP) that indicates the geometrical location through the thickness of the device layers, and where strains are zero [11, 12, 14, 15]. Therefore, typical inorganic electronic materials that have high mechanical moduli and low fracture strains can be placed near an NMP to substantially minimize or avoid the degradation of physical/electrical properties during extreme mechanical deformations. More advanced schemes are an extension of such wavy configurations to three dimensions with interconnecting configurations to achieve sophisticated levels of fully functional integrated systems. Figure 14.1b illustrates such examples of noncoplanar pop-up bridges (top) and serpentine traces of interconnects (bottom) [12, 14]. The pop-up structure induced by a prestrain of a receiving elastomer, with a combination of NMP layout that device layers experienced nearly zero strain, could accommodate all of the strains associated with deformations, leading to electronic properties that are independent on externally applied strains. Theoretical analysis by finite element modeling (FEM) reveals that this critical aspect of a design strategy contributes almost no strain to device islands, but generates mechanical loads around interconnects/bridges and/or inactive regions in corresponding electronic systems. Additional deformability can also be obtained via serpentine shape of interconnects/bridges or fractal design strategy [22, 41, 68], enabling to create a geometry that allows the circuit to be folded or stretched in a large scale, and to realize conformal contacts to a variety of complex shapes.

Although structure engineering, in a way that device configuration can accommodate various mechanical deformations with brittle and rigid materials by nature, is a breakthrough for soft electronic systems there might be an approach to ascertain a material that intrinsically contains low flexural rigidity to achieve flexible and stretchable systems relatively independent of externally applied strains [8, 10, 18, 20, 21]. Dramatic reduction in physical dimensions of materials (e.g., nanowires, nanotubes, flakes), combined with an elastic rubber realized such desired mechanical properties, with unprecedented electrical characteristics via optimized synthesis of materials for electrodes/contacts, interconnects, and channel media. Figure 14.1c illustrates examples of such nanomaterials as a SWNT paste (top) from a high purity and aspect ratio of a SWNT [8, 69, 70], and Ag ink (bottom) from commercial Ag flakes, respectively [21]. These conductive paste and ink can be printed on an elastomeric polymer through conventional printing methods (e.g., stencil printing, screen printing, etc.) with desired patterns after chemical surface treatments to improve compatibility of mixture components (Figure 14.1d, top). The mechanical durability can be enhanced by encapsulation of the top surface with an elastomer, which could avoid or minimize delamination of those conductive materials during excessive deformations [8]. A mesh-typed conductive elastomer, instead of a slab of elastic conductor, suggests a way to increase conformal contact to curvilinear shapes, that is, efficiently wrap arbitrary surfaces/shapes of structure (Figure 14.1d, bottom).

14.3 Electronic/Optoelectronic Devices, Sensors and Systems

Advanced electronic components with high performance in unusual shapes and configurations offer new research opportunities in the realm of biomedical implants, wearable devices, and other electronic gadgets, and might be useful in some cases that cannot be realized by conventional, existing electronic systems. Figure 14.2 represents a variety of comprehensive sets of such flexible, stretchable electronic circuits/systems that are capable of accommodating severe

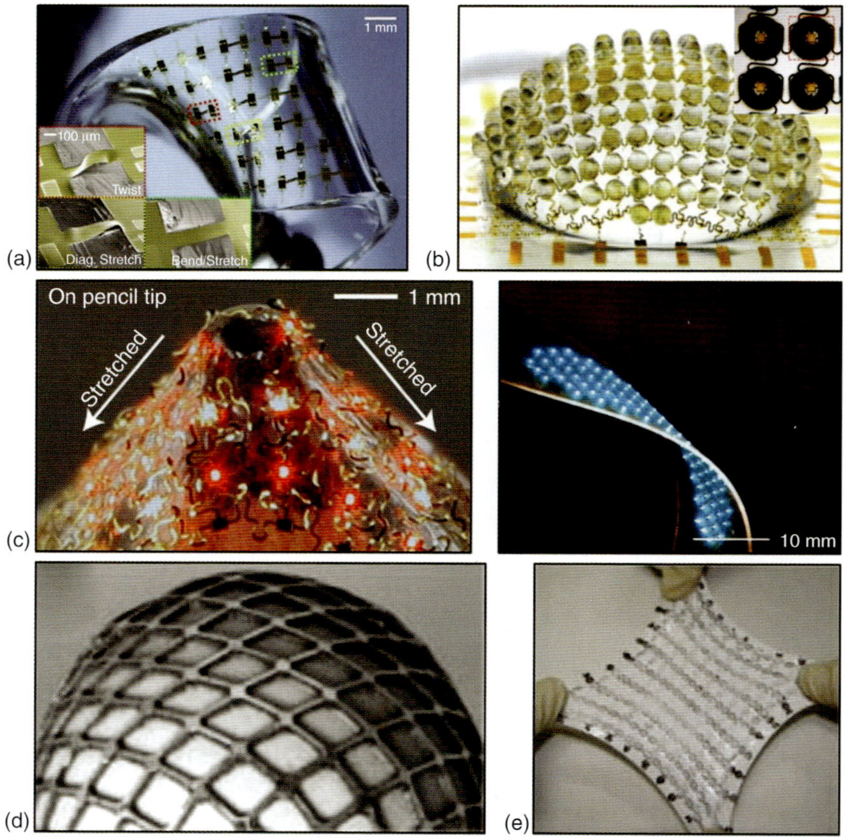

Figure 14.2 Electronic/optoelectronic devices, sensors and systems. (a) An array of stretchable Si CMOS integrated circuits on a PDMS rubber with pop-up bridges as interconnects in a noncoplanar configuration. Chosen materials and design layouts enable to accommodate external mechanical stimulations such as twisting, bending, diagonal stretching, and so on. (b) Description of an artificial digital camera inspired from compound eyes. Combination of silicon photodiodes and blocking diodes in an active matrix array offers elastic hemispherical microlenses system. The inset represents a magnified view of 2 × 2 array of the device connected with serpentine traces for enhanced extension. (c) Photographs of mechanically deformed GaAs- (left) and GaN-based (right) micro-LEDs array. Stretching in a sharp pencil tip and twisting of micro-LEDs exhibit no functional degradation due to the selection of materials and structure configurations. (d) An image of flexible, wearable conductive nets incorporated with organic transistors in the configuration of active matrix addressing on an egg, potentially for pressure, thermal sensors, and artificial electronic skin. (e) Demonstration of stretching tests in uniaxial/biaxial direction of stretchable organic integrated circuits configured in matrix addressing, consisting of organic transistors and SWCTs contacts and interconnects. (f) Photographs of flexible, stretchable large-area organic LED display that is capable of conforming to curvilinear surfaces and/or structures. Deformed states (e.g., folding) do not limit device functionality as shown in the inset.

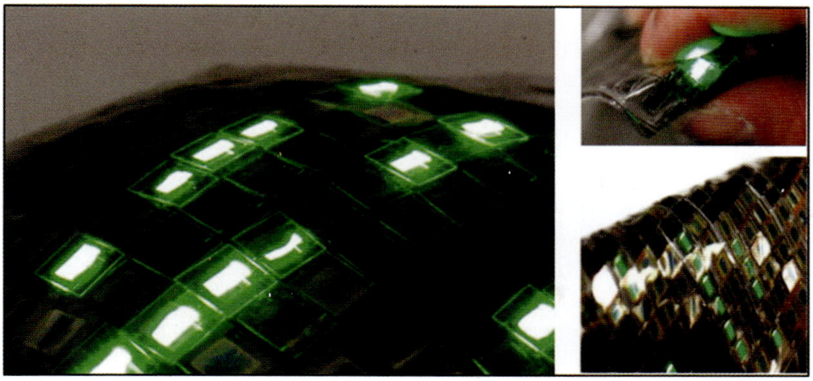
(f)

Figure 14.2 (*Continued*)

mechanical strains such as twisting, bending, stretching, and folding, without any functional degradations in a general operation mode [4, 8, 10, 12, 19, 55, 71]. Examples of inorganic-materials-based electronic and optoelectronic circuits and systems contain monocrystalline silicon nanomembranes (Si NMs)-based CMOS inverters (Figure 14.2a) [12] and an array of photodiodes with blocking diodes for digital cameras (Figure 14.2b) [55], heterogeneous compound semiconductors-based light-emitting diodes (LEDs) (Figure 14.2c; left, GaAs; right, GaN) [19, 71], and are not limited to these components, but include solar cells [17, 47, 48], mechanical/physical/electrochemical sensors/actuators [3, 4, 16, 21, 24, 27, 28, 31, 39, 40], and so on. These electronic devices, sensors, and systems were fabricated by typical semiconductor procedures (e.g., deposition, photolithography, etching, and diffusion) on a rigid, temporary substrate coated with polymeric substances, and after completion of device fabrication, removal of an underlying sacrificial layer, that is, a polymer layer, by immersion in an organic solvent enables to release the device out of a carrier substrate. In this case, a series of manufacturing procedures are limited to a ceiling temperature of 250–300 °C due to polymers as a sacrificial and protective layer, which can be avoided by a fully formed scheme via preferential, anisotropic solution etching with a silicon [47, 63] or SOI wafer [62, 64]. Subsequent procedures of elaborate, rapid transfer printing to prestrained deformable substrates form flexible, stretchable electronic products. As a result, these soft, curvilinear devices exhibit mechanically superior deformability over conventional, bulky devices, and such photography-included processes also afford functional qualities of a variety of components to reach the level required by commercial industry products. More elasticity can be realized by utilizing inorganic materials with fractal-based architectures such as Peano, Hilbert, Moore curves, and Greek cross [22, 41, 68], and these strategies create more opportunities in biomedical electronic systems for organs or tissues with complex, random surfaces.

Materials and phenomena associated to diverse organic electronic devices such as sensors, thin film transistors, LEDs, solar cells, and others have been also studied toward designing large-area, cost-effective flexible, and stretchable electronics. Figure 14.2d represents an organic pressure sensor with a mesh-typed structure designed to improve physical contact ability to a target interface, which will result in the increase of electrical signal quality for electronic artificial skin or biointegrated systems [4] as exceptional enhancements of recorded biopotentials reported elsewhere [29, 38]. Typical fabrication approaches such as evaporations of metal electrodes and a semiconductor layer, and spin coating of an insulator and encapsulation layer on a pliable substrate, form a planar structure with an active matrix of organic field-effect transistors, followed by elimination of inactive electronic regions creating a grid-like structure. A conductive elastomer-based pressure sensor is mechanically shaped as a web-like architecture, and subsequent attachment on the top of the array of organic transistors completes the mesh-type pressure sensor system. The sensor contains sensing areas where both horizontal/vertical lines cross each other, that is, intersection and electrical interconnects (i.e., bit line, word line). Evaluations on mechanical properties emphasized that electrical/mechanical failures in response to external deformations did not occur at intersections but by electrical wires, which can be minimized or prevented through physical dimensions of electrical wires and/or by optimized geometry of removed empty spaces.

A synthesis of carbon nanotubes-based materials with several compatible substances has provided exceptional mechanical/electrical properties, and their uniform distribution in elastomeric polymers offer soft electrical conductors for flexible, stretchable electronic systems [10, 69, 70]. Figure 14.2e illustrates a biaxially stretchable, rubber-like active-matrix transistors, based on composites of organic polymers and carbon nanotubes [10]. Here, super-growth SWNTs with excellent properties [69, 70] are processed through several mechanical/physical/chemical steps to generate superb electrical/mechanical characteristics of an SWNT film as well as SWNT paste. Blending such fabricated SWNT film with a silicone elastomer (PDMS) forms an elastomeric conductor that can serve as interconnects of bit lines and word lines. A highly conductive, adhesive SWNT paste is designed to be utilized for strengthening mechanically vulnerable regions where the gradient of mechanical modulus abruptly changes, that is, between rigid device islands and soft interconnects. An array of actively addressable organic transistors combined with those materials (an elastic conductor and SWNT paste) reveals negligible changes in electrical and mechanical characteristics under uniaxial and biaxial stretching up to 70–80% as well as under repeated applied strains. Similar materials, but with exceptional conductivity and improved viscosity, were able to be coated/patterned on an elastomer for a stretchable, printable elastic conductor, and such a novel strategy was demonstrated as stretchable, bendable, foldable organic LED panels (Figure 14.2f) whose individual pixel can actively be addressed through driving components of a selector and driver transistor, and a capacitor.

14.4 Multifunctional Electronic Sensors and Power Scavenging Circuit for the Heart

Developments of novel materials/structure designs for stretchable electronics have resulted in a three-dimensional web-like electronic sock that could monitor electrophysiological activities and/or vital signs in the heart via a package of various sensors as shown in Figure 14.3a [27]. Multifunctional elements (Figure 14.3a, bottom) enable to detect diverse markers of cardiac conditions, for example, fluctuation of electrical potentials, continuous and real-time alterations in pH value during control of blood supply, temperature variations in cardiac ablation, mechanical deformations (i.e., strain) in response to physical activities of the heart, and recording/mapping cardiac action potentials from optical stimulations. A commercially available 3D printer generates an artificial shape of the heart model after capturing the precise configuration of a heart via an optical scanning approach. Pouring/curing an elastic silicone rubber creates a three-dimensional geometry and a thin membrane sheath as the replica of a rabbit heart, followed by mounting multifunctional electronic components described earlier connected with meander traces in a stretchable format on the top of the model. The engineered heart sock is closely fit to or slightly smaller than the actual organ, which is designed for each electronic constituent to achieve great physical contact with the cardiac surfaces during expanding/contracting the heart. Evaluation of the theoretical study supports the fact that the appropriate pressure of the electronic sock onto the heart provides a stable physical/electrical interface between the entire system and the epicardiac surface. Demonstrations of a number of different functional elements with an isolated perfused rabbit heart show a continuous, spatio-temporal view of electrical activities. Simultaneous recordings with combined use of Si-based piezoresistive strain monitors with electrocardiogram (ECG) electrodes provide correlated responses between mechanical cardiac movements and electrical action potentials (Figure 14.3b); for example, fractional changes in resistance of a Si piezoresistor (blue) well match to the sinus rhythm (top, green), ventricular pacing (middle, green) during normal electrical activity within the heart, while an irregular heart rhythm due to erratic electrical impulses, for example, ventricular fibrillation, induced significant malfunction of pumping chambers (bottom). In addition to investigating electrical and mechanical properties, thermal and chemical characteristics can be demonstrated as temperature mapping and variations during ablation tests, and spatio-temporal pH sensing in response to changes in the blood supply such as in ischemia and reperfusion.

An obstacle or difficulty to be overcome in electronic medical implants as well as in wearable devices would be limited lifetime due to a finite capacity of power sources operating devices/circuits. An ultrathin, flexible piezoelectric circuit shown in Figure 14.3c enables to harvest mechanical energy from constant natural motion of the beating/pulsating heart and lungs, and generate it into electrically stored energy [23]. The energy harvester contains an array of thin ribbons of lead zirconate titanate (PZT)-based active components integrated with a commercial rectifier and microbattery onto a plastic substrate, and each of those peripheral components converts alternating current obtained from PZT ribbons into direct current to charge a microbattery, capable of generating and storing electrical energy. Figure 14.3d exhibits extracted electrical potentials from three different locations of the right ventricle (RV, top), left ventricle (LV, middle), and free wall (bottom) of both animal models of bovine (left, green) and ovine (right, blue) over the cyclic occurrence of expansion and

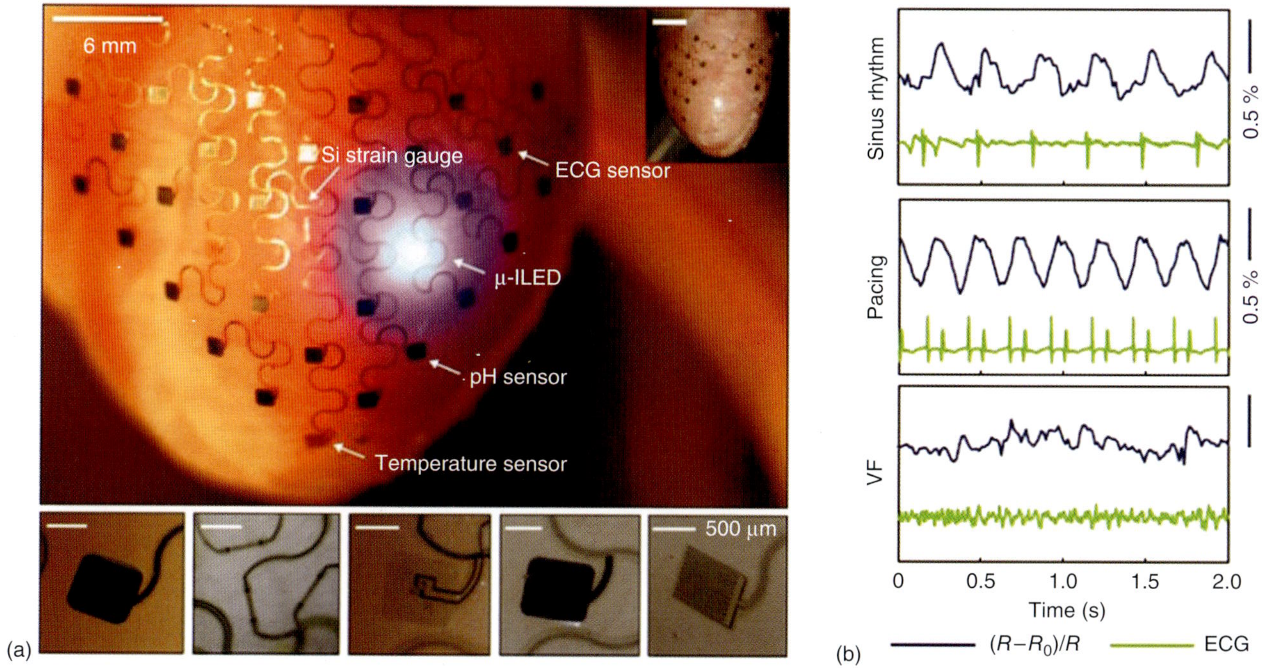

Figure 14.3 Multifunctional electronic sensors and power scavenging circuit for the heart. (a) Optical images of three-dimensional multifunctional integumentary membranes (3D-MIMs) supplying interfaces for physiological mapping and stimulation through wrapping up the entire epicardial surface of the heart, with the view of covering both sides (anterior and posterior) of the heart in the inset. The device includes diverse functional components such as ECG sensor, Si strain gauge, micro-LED (μ-LED), pH sensor, temperature sensor (from left to right). (b) Comparison of measured fractional resistance from a Si strain sensor with recorded signals from ECG sensor during dynamic cardiac movements, for example, sinus rhythm (top), ventricular pacing (middle), and ventricular fibrillation (bottom). (c) Image of *in vivo* attachment of PZT-based mechanical energy harvesters on the right ventricle (RV), left ventricle (LV), and free wall of a bovine heart (left). The whole system consists of a rechargeable microbattery, a rectifier, and PZT MEHs on a flexible substrate (top right), and a magnified view of PZT MEHs connected to anisotropic conductive film (ACF) in a flexible format (bottom right). (d) Measurements of voltage output as a function of time for MEHs by varying the heart rate of bovine (green) and ovine (blue). Voltage characteristics were captured from different locations, RV (top), LV (middle), and free wall (bottom) during expansion and relaxation.

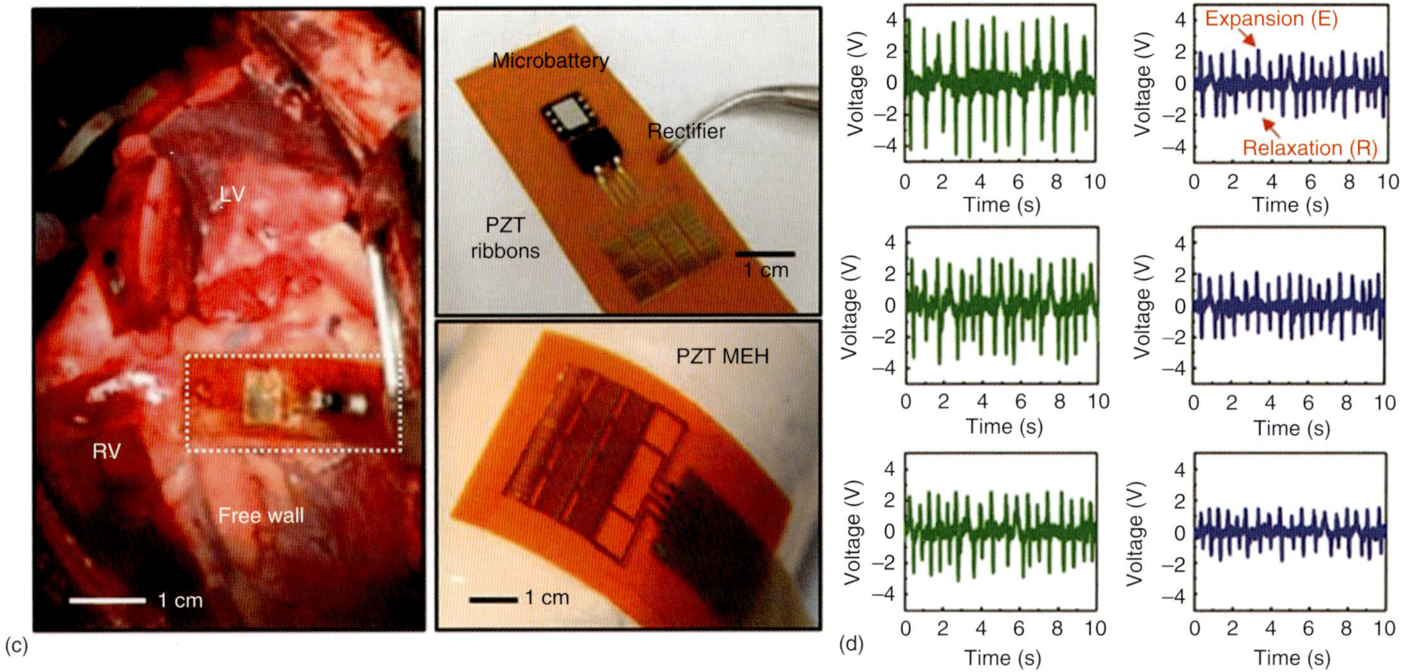

Figure 14.3 *(Continued)*

relaxation of the heart. Each potential spike corresponds to the frequency of dynamic heat beats. The measured output voltages show slightly different peaks of potential depending on the implanted sites since respective regions of the organ have particular motions in direction, shape, dissimilar muscle structures, and thickness of outer surfaces [72, 73]. A few additional factors play a role in measured open-circuit voltages, such as the attached angle of a mechanical energy harvester, the frequency of heart beat as well as the size, mass, and contractile power of the heart. The direction of the device is particularly important due to anisotropic properties of a piezoelectric harvester, and this feature of orientation dependency reveals that the devices placed at the angle of 0° and 45° with regard to the apex of the heart generate higher peak voltages than those placed at 90° due to the specific range of mechanical movements of the muscular tissue of the heart [74, 75]. Additionally, suturing the device with the heart avoids unexpected displacements of this whole system, that is, it assists to fix the location of the harvester, but the fixation does not restrain any functional and mechanical movements of the natural motion of the heart, even though superior mechanical flexibility cannot afford to give rise to any type of delamination during the entire cycle of the motion. As mentioned earlier, implantation of an ultrathin, flexible piezoelectric system onto several organs with different animal models demonstrated the viability of this technology to produce sufficient power for possible use of medical implants such as cardiac pacemakers, cardiac defibrillators, and deep brain stimulators.

14.5 Electrophysiology and Optogenetics for the Brain

The physical/mechanical properties of the brain require consideration of materials selection, device layout, and other factors to implant electronic systems onto the brain surface or into deep brain tissue for fundamental researches of the nervous system. Since conventional tools are less capable of covering large areas of the brain (penetration probe type) or delivering high spatial resolution of electrodes (surface probe type), recent research-introduced approaches have aimed at achieving microelectrode array with high spatial resolution as well as large area coverage. Figure 14.4a shows an array of ultrathin, flexible, and high-density neural electrodes on the surface of the visual cortex in an animal model (top), with insertion of the device into the narrow fissures of the cerebral hemispheres (inset) [30]. Extreme mechanical flexibility of the system allows the folded configuration to measure the electrical potentials from both sides of the hemispheres at the same time (left, before insertion; right, after insertion). Such a neural recording system consists of a flexible array of single-crystal silicon-based field-effect transistors with a few stacks of metal interconnections and interlayer dielectric (ILD) and encapsulation layers, and the thickness of the whole layers can be adjusted to less than ~30 μm to reduce mechanical stiffness. This reduction, therefore, enables the flexible circuit on a plastic substrate to hold the induced strain well below the fracture strain of each electronic component/material during intensive mechanical deformations such as folding, bending, and twisting. The correlation of change in thickness and configuration

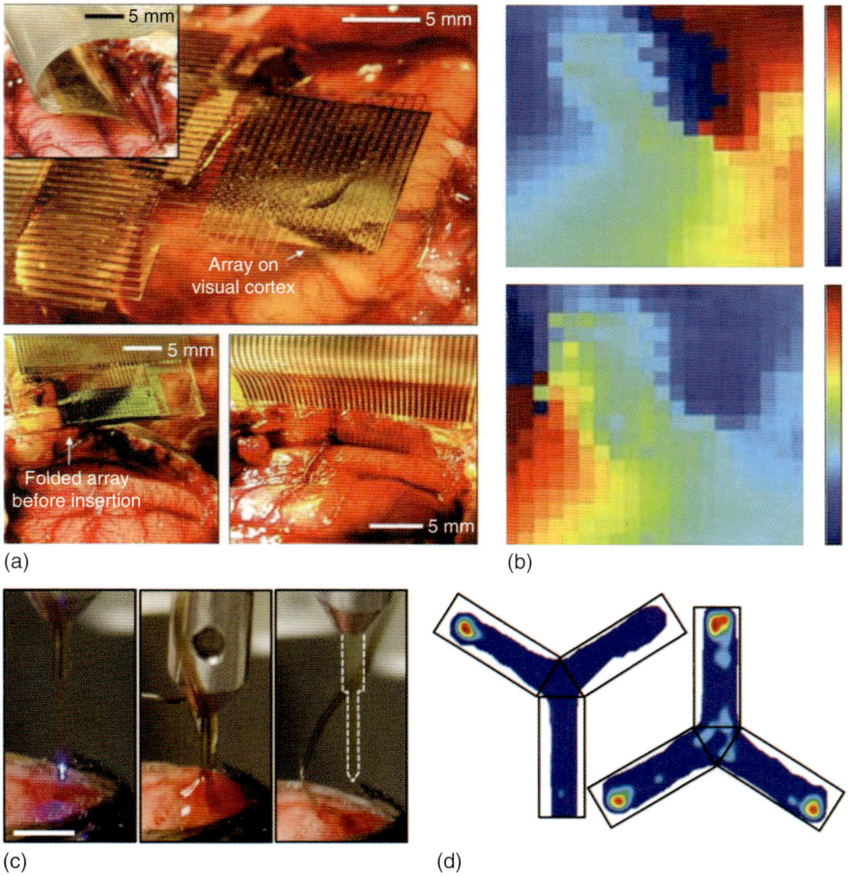

Figure 14.4 Electrophysiology and optogenetics for the brain. (a) *In vivo* animal (feline model) experiments of a flexible, high-density active neural circuit implanted on the visual cortex of the brain, and insertion of the electrode into the interhemispheric fissure (inset). Images of active multiplexing array before (bottom left)/after (bottom right) insertion into the interhemispheric fissure. (b) Recordings of both spiral waveforms, counterclockwise (top) to clockwise (bottom), from active neural electrodes during electrographic seizure, that is, induced seizure via local remedy of the drug (picrotoxin). (c) Images of sequence in a procedure of injection and retraction of microneedle that allows multifunctional, flexible cellular-scale micro-LEDs system to be implanted desirable locations. Attached silk fibroin films on the backside of the micro-LEDs system gradually dissolved during this procedure, leaving the optogenetic system in the targeted area. (d) Experimental results of colorized data map in the Y-shaped maze for the preference of animal behaviors in different conditions. Red colors indicate preferred locations for longer time period than other colors do.

with fracture strain have been well evaluated in previous articles [59–61]. The flexible and foldable neural implant can be utilized to continuously record spatial properties of sudden disorders in the brain such as blows, strokes, and seizure. As a representative example, the system implanted on the visual cortex detected electrical potentials of electrocorticogram (ECoG) over certain time duration after induced seizures using picorotoxin in a cat model. The observed waves during seizures include diverse spatial patterns such as right angle wave, plane wave left to right or vice versa, counter-clockwise spiral (Figure 14.4b, top), and clockwise spiral (Figure 14.4b, bottom).

Besides electrical stimulation and recording, integration of optical devices with electronic components could open up new capabilities in optoelectronic system for unmet applications in the fields of biology and medicine. Figure 14.4c represents sequential insertion stages (left, before injection; middle, after injection; right, retrieval of the microneedle) of an injectable optoelectronic system supported onto a penetrating polymeric microneedle [32]. Individual electronic components in this multifunctional cellular-scale system involve a platinum (Pt)-based electrode for electrical stimulation, recording, and a temperature sensing, and a silicon-based photodetector for detection of changes in light intensity, and all of the components are integrated onto a rigid microneedle with a water-soluble silk fibroin glue that allows a microneedle to release after injection, leaving flexible, thin electronic elements in the brain. From a biological perspective, the functional operations of these diverse components are characterized as having electrical, optical, and thermal properties such as those necessary for power consumption, heat sink, variation of light intensity, and recording action potentials. Integration of such components with wireless modules for radiofrequency (RF) power scavenger such as RF antenna, an impedance-matching inductor, schottky diodes, and capacitors emphasizes the capability of wireless control as demonstrated in various tasks, interactions, and behaviors. As an example of implementation in optogenetic control experiments, Figure 14.4d represents the results of time duration at places in a Y-shape apparatus for animal models. The experimental procedure began to count the number of active nose pokes followed by self-stimulation that indicates active or inactive. Animals with self-stimulation expressing channelrhodopsin-2 (ChR2) provided longer duration at the preferred place (Figure 14.4d, left), while animal models with the same stimulation expressing enhanced yellow fluorescent protein (eYFP) did not show such place preference due to nongeneration of neuronal firing for behavior control (Figure 14.4d, right). These described activities are well correlated to the statistical plots for the number of active nose pokes in the case of active and inactive devices for both groups of ChR2 and eYFP. More sophisticated systems with the current configuration can provide diverse approaches with regard to the central nervous system such as in drug delivery with optical manipulation [34], and mechanically soft, stretchable miniaturized circuit including light and power sources could eliminate physical constraints in a freely moving animal model [36].

14.6 Communication and Regulation for the Nervous System

Figure 14.5a illustrates a skin-inspired artificial mechanoreceptor system that enables to convert mechanical pressure alterations arising in human skins to opto-electrical signals for stimulating somatosensory neurons, to ultimately control or communicate with prosthetic limbs [33]. The basic underlying principle

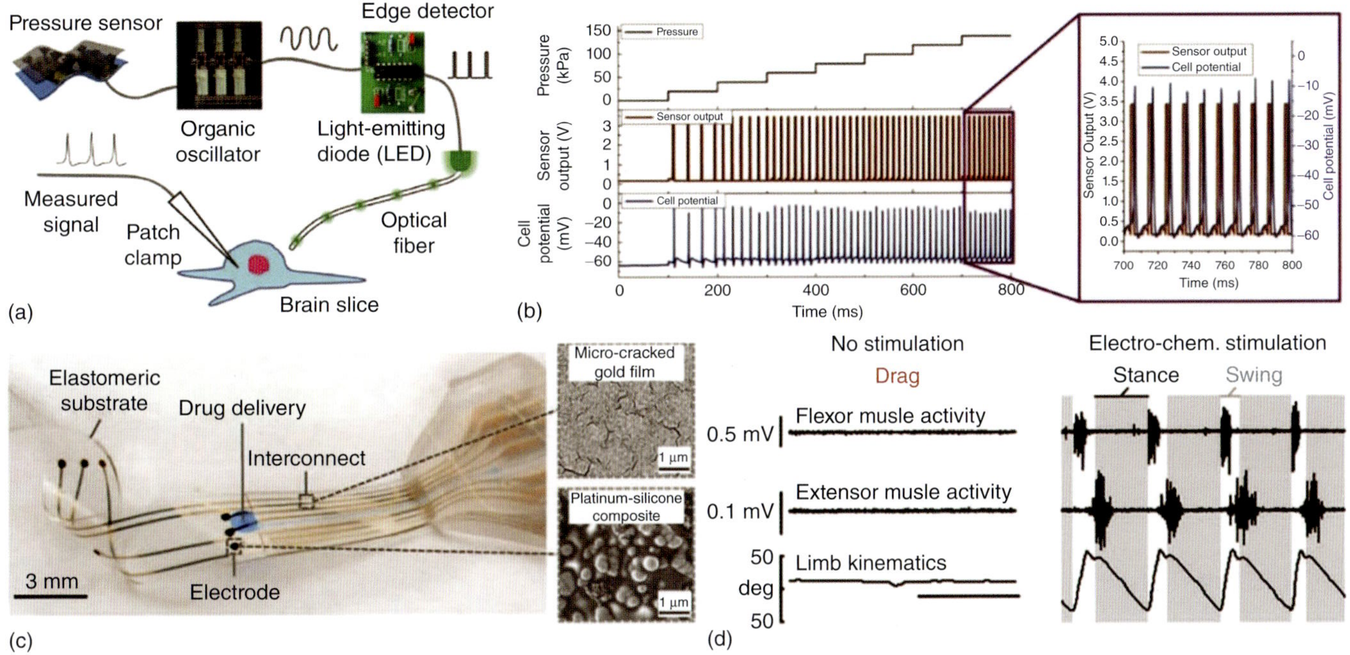

Figure 14.5 Communication and regulation for the nervous system. (a) Illustration of a skin-inspired mechanoreceptor system through pressure-induced somatosensory cortex stimulation circuit for an optoelectronic system, incorporating with a wearable pressure sensor, organic oscillator, light-emitting diode, and optical fiber. (b) Measured correlation data of applied pressure to the digital tactile (DiTact) system, sensor output from the LED, and cell potential from the patch clamp. Sensor output signals are closely related to the recorded action potentials from neurons in the magnified view of data (right). (c) Optical images of soft tissue-like electronic dura mater (e-dura) capable of electrical stimulations as well as drug delivery for injuries related to the nervous system. Materials constituting the system include microcracked gold film for interconnects (top right), composite of platinum nano- and microparticles for electrodes/contacts (bottom right), and a silicone rubber for the substrate. (d) Comparison of response to the electrochemical stimulations from implanted e-dura, with severely injured spinal cord in a rat. Measurement recording signals from walking tests represent obvious recovery capability with (left)/without (right) electrochemical stimulation, from flexor/extensor muscle and hindlimb movements.

and system configuration is that mechanical forces applied to a pressure sensor introduce electrical signals that convert to light pulsations by organic oscillator and edge detector, navigating through an optical fiber. The delivered light pulses at particular frequency range induce action potentials as firing light-responsive neurons in a brain slice, and the resulting evoked potentials were achieved by a commercial patch clamp demonstrating the feasibility as an optogenetic tool. This procedure emulates a complex system of nerve cells (sensory receptors), that is, somatosensory system, responding to variation at the external or internal state of the body via sending/receiving signals to/from the brain. The correlation between pressure and frequency was supported by conforming experiments, such as voltage versus frequency and impedance, which experimental values are consistent with numerical analysis. Figure 14.5b presents simultaneous changes in measurement in correlated numerical values and an evaluation of their relationship. Time-dependent stepwise increase of externally applied pressure causes the frequency of the output potential to gradually increase as a function of time, and the transmitting voltage at periodic interval plays a role of stimulating neurons in an acute slice of somatosensory cortex leading to narrow spiking activity of the cell potential. The magnified view (inset on the right) of measured output voltages and cell potentials indicates that both properties are well correlated with each other.

Elastic modulus of elements in medical implants is one of the key parameters since the magnitude of interfacial strains between soft biological tissues and stiff electronic elements often have probability of contributing to aggravate inflammation or other side effects at implantation sites, particularly for a long-term, continuous monitoring system. Figure 14.5c suggests a model of medically useful implantations to minimize the above-mentioned issues by adjustment of shape and elasticity inspired from dura mater—the tough fibrous layer covering the brain and spinal cord and lining the interior surface of the skull [35]. The electronic dura (E-dura) consists of gold electrodes coated with a composite of platinum and elastomer for electrical stimulation as well as for monitoring physiological states and microfluidic channels for delivery of drugs at topical and specific sites, and interconnects onto a thin sheet of elastomer. Magnified images of microstructure of a microcracked gold layer and a composite of platinum-elastomer in the inset. This type of soft engineered neuroprosthesis enables to testify multiple functions and advantages over nonelastic implants via several experiments for brain-related injuries. Such tests including the motion of a body, biological reconstruction, inflammatory responses and mechanical models show superior properties of the soft implant compared to those of stiff ones. Comparative characteristics were achieved by using three different models: no implants, soft materials-based implants, and hard materials-based implants, implanted beneath the dura mater (subdural) of lower back region (lumbosacral region of the spine) in a rat. During 6 weeks implantation, the assessment of the resulting behaviors based on the capability of the movements showed that the animal model with stiff implant exhibited abnormal locomotion including improper steps on the ladder, while the animal with soft implant did not show any unusual gaits as similar to the control model. The study to investigate biocompatibility revealed inflammatory response with stiff implant, indicating significant increase in the density of microglia and astrocytes. Exploration and scope for development of the soft electronic dura system can be extended to stimulation, recording, and drug delivery associated with the brain and spinal cord. For example, an e-dura system integrated with a light source can provide spatio-resolved information on ECoG through activating particular neurons at local sites, and a similar device implanted near the spinal cord measured electrospinogram via electrical stimulation of the motor cortex. Advanced multifunctional system also offers a strategy that is useful for disabling injury such as paralyzed legs. Evaluation of comparison results as shown in Figure 14.5d represents that electro-chemical stimulations using stimulating electrodes and drug delivery circuit delivered dramatic changes in measured potentials through several activities, indicating that mechanically soft implant is a desired approach for the restoration of the central nervous system-related malfunctions.

14.7 Skin-Like Electronics/Optoelectronics

Figure 14.6a shows an array of mechanically flexible and integrated sensors for multiplexed perspiration analysis via measurements of sweat metabolites (e.g., glucose, lactate) and electrolytes (e.g., sodium, potassium ions) in a simultaneous and selective manner, as well as the skin temperature as a calibration factor of the sensors [44]. This smart wristband system involves two main parts: (i) multifunctional, wearable electrochemical sensors and (ii) a commercially available silicon-based components on a pliable printed circuit board. A skin-like wearable electrochemical sensor was formed by deposition, pattering, and etching of electrodes (Au for working electrodes, Ag/AgCl for reference and counter electrodes) with selected materials on a plastic substrate of polyethylene terephthalate (PET), incorporated with appropriate surface treatments of enhancement of responses to ions and analytes of interest (e.g., Na+, Ka+, glucose, lactate). A flexible integrated circuit board was installed with diverse commercial modules, such as a filter, amplifier, inverter, microcontroller and bluetooth transceiver to exploit signal processing/transduction as well as wireless data transmission, as a real-time monitoring of physiological conditions of human subjects. Characterizations of various concentrations, temperatures, and other conditions with sensing materials verify the performance of individual sensor components for long-term continuous monitoring of physical/chemical states. Practical experiments in Figure 14.6b were performed to evaluate the operation capability of a smart wearable system mounted on the head (i.e., "smart headband") during outdoor group running. In this case, the mounted smart headbands were applied to two different groups: one that ran with water intake (top), the other without water intake (bottom). Real-time measurements of concentration level of electrolytes, Na^+ and K^+, in the perspiration of test subjects provide gradual increase of ionic concentration of sodium at the time scale of 5000 s, but not obvious changes in the case of potassium ions. The result is that dehydration is quite relevant with increments of both sodium and potassium ions, which is consistent with a previous study [76].

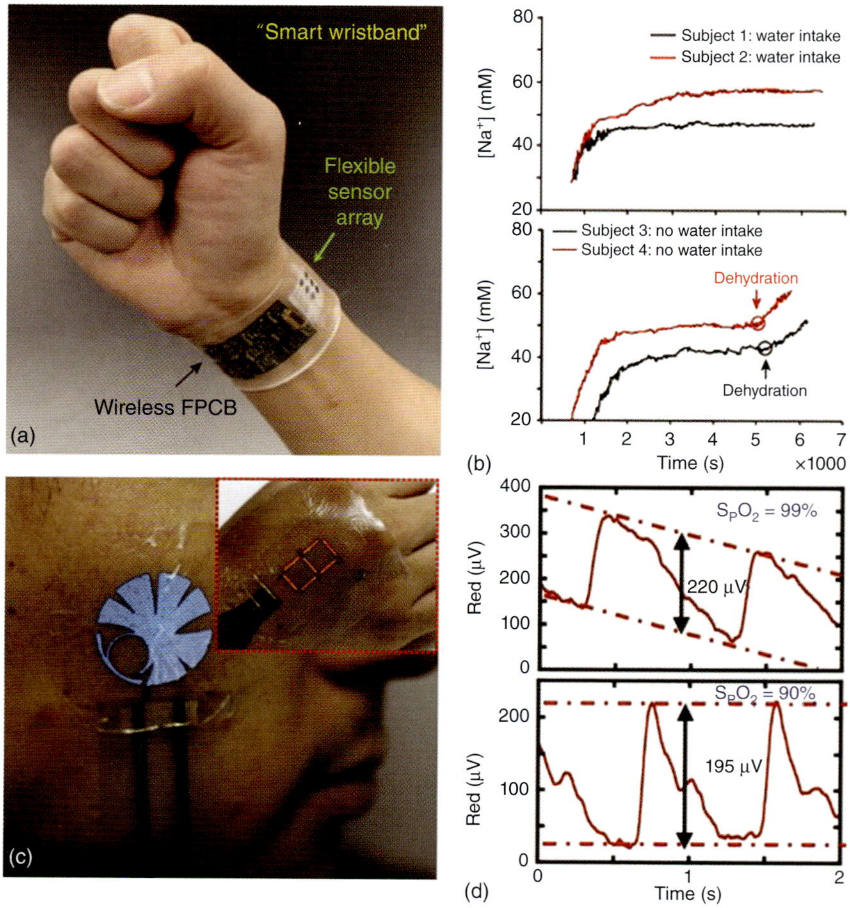

Figure 14.6 Skin-like electronics/optoelectronics. (a) Demonstration of a smart wearable wristband for a real-time, wireless integrated healthcare monitoring system. The wristband consists of an array of multifunctional sensors to measure various analytes (glucose, lactate, sodium, potassium) in perspiration and skin temperature, and commercial electronic components-based flexible printed circuit board. (b) Comparison of real-time plots of sodium concentrations for tracing hydration/dehydration levels from flexible sensor arrays during group outdoor running, in the case of water intake and no water intake. (c) Illustrations of ultrathin, flexible polymer light-emitting diodes (PLEDs) laminated onto human skin with conformal contacts, capable of displaying user's health conditions and other information received from integrated sensors. Representative examples of device functionality exhibit a blue logo and red number (inset) with external power connections. (d) Electrical characterizations of different oxygen concentrations in blood through organic photodetectors (OPDs). Light emissions from green and red PLEDs reflected from blood, which depends on the concentration of oxygen in blood (top, 99%: bottom, 90%). (e) Schematic description of a soft, stretchable electronic robot that is capable of displaying color differences in response to changes of pressure. This soft robot includes an actuator system (pneumatic chambers with strain limited layer) for a locomotion that leads to changes of capacitances to display the robot's status or surrounding conditions. (f) A series of optical images to describe soft robot's locomotion with independent color segments. As underlying pneumatic chambers are in inflation/deflation states, top layers including electroluminescent layer become stretched/expanded leading to increase of illuminance of the system.

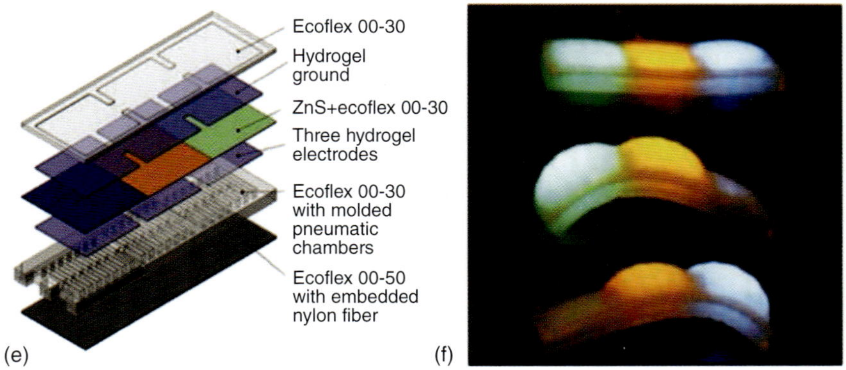

Figure 14.6 (*Continued*)

Figure 14.6c represents images of ultrathin optoelectronic skin sensors that are able to attach easily to the human body (the cheek; the hand in the inset) with their superior mechanical properties [45]. Representative examples of analog/digital displays consist of several independent segments that are capable of indicating various information on different combinations of color and intensity. The entire thickness of this system is in a range of a few microns, enabling to mount on almost any type of surface and shape without any mechanical/electrical impairs. Demonstration platforms include a conjugated polymer-based polymer light-emitting diodes (PLEDs) with three different colors of red, green, and blue, and semiconducting polymers-based organic photodetectors (OPDs) on an extremely thin parylene substrate (thickness, ~1 μm), and integration of those elements formed a pulse oximetry via emission and detection of the lights. A number of characteristics of fabricated circuits were evaluated under ambient conditions and mechanical deformations, providing long duration, reliability, and less variation in stable function. A blood-oxygen monitor was realized by placing a reflective pulse oximetry at a fingertip, and it was observed that absorption of two different wavelengths of light emitted from PLEDs (i.e., red and green) was different between oxygenated and deoxygenated hemoglobin, allowing photodetectors to respond to different intensities of reflected lights. Irradiation of the red and green light alternately turns on and off in regular sequence, thereby the amount of both reflected lights is separately detected by photodetectors. The measured oscillating amplitudes of a red light in time domain (Figure 14.6d) exhibit that electrical potentials proportionally decreased with reduction (99–90%) of peripheral oxygen saturation (S_pO_2), verifying detection capability of blood occupied or unoccupied with oxygen. Similar behavior was observed by using green LEDs, supporting that PLEDs-based pulse oximetry approach is useful for recording the level of oxygen saturation in clinical use.

Beyond current wearable electronics, soft robots incorporated with intelligent features are able to do many things that existing systems cannot. The skins inspired from nature, such as various marine mollusks of the class of cephalopods (e.g., octopus, squid, cuttlefish) have fascinating properties containing highly flexible/stretchable and color-variation components for self-preservation, that is, camouflage systems. Figure 14.6e illustrates a schematic description of materials, design layout of a locomotive, electroluminescent soft robot [46]. The structure consists of (i) a hyperelastic light-emitting capacitor (HLEC) that is capable of changing illuminance and capacitance in response to mechanical deformations during locomotive actions. ZnS-embeded dielectric elastomer serves as an emitting layer, sandwiched by top and bottom electrodes with ionic hydrogels made of aqueous lithium chloride (LiCl) for conductor and polyacrylamide (PAM) for elastomeric matrix. These materials are well known for high conductivity and ionic strength, and for transparency and toughness [77]; (ii) a connection of fluidic chambers for actuation and composite-materials-embedded extension-limited layer [46]. Pneumatic chambers are inflated and deflated by external fluidic stimuli, which is restricted by the strain-limiting layer, inducing outward bending moments for undulating movements. This reaction mechanism was exploited to form mobile ability of a soft robot with colorized segments as a series of sequential images as illustrated in Figure 14.6f. Evaluations of electro-mechanical properties were performed to clarify the correlation between mechanical deformations and electrical capacitances. Since pressure changes from actuation and/or touch induces associated deformations in dielectric elastomer layers, alternations in dimensions (shared area between conductive and dielectric layers, and thickness of a dielectric layer) lead to changes in capacitance. The resulting properties could be applied for sensitive artificial skin system for displaying personal physiology conditions and communicating with prosthetics by converting mechanical movements into electrical signals.

14.8 Transient, Bioresorbable Systems

A class of silicon electronics that is water soluble and biocompatible, opens up completely new opportunities for semiconductor devices with regard to a new kind of implantable medical device designed to accelerate wound healing and prevent infection, and then to be completely resorbed into the body after serving its function [56–58, 78, 79]. Figure 14.7a represents exploded, graphic images of a transient piezoresistive pressure sensor with a magnified view of the critical sensing region in the inset [78]. The key design concept of the whole system involves the configuration of the diaphragm (most widely used microelectromechanical systems) to enhance mechanical/physical responses to forces, vibration, heat, fluid flow, and other effects of possible surroundings, whose constituents include diverse biodegradable components and materials. The supporting layer of nanoporous silicon (60–80 μm thick; ~70% porosity) contains a vertical cavity in a square geometry (depth, 30–40 μm), which is covered by a thin sheet of poly(lactic-co-glycolic acid) (PLGA, thickness ~30 μm) via sealing procedure at increased temperature. In a separate procedure, the meander element and electrodes of highly doped silicon nanomembrane (Si NM, ~300 nm), and deposition/pattering of evaporated silicon dioxide layer (SiO_2, ~100 nm) forms active sensing components with connection pads. Transfer printing of these layers to an edge of the air cavity leads to mechanical deformations of the

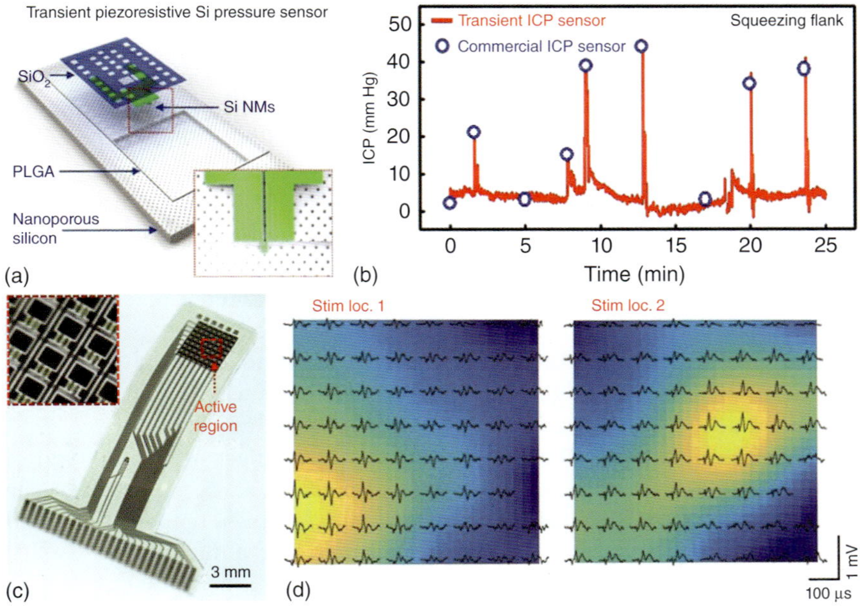

Figure 14.7 Transient, bioresorbable systems. (a) Exploded view illustration of a flexible, bioresorbable electronic system, based on ultrathin silicon nanomembranes (Si NMs), nanoporous silicon, silicon oxide, and poly (lactic-co-glycolic acid) (PLGA). The system utilizes a thin diaphragm structure with a piezoresistive component to maximize chemical, mechanical responses. Inset shows a magnified view of active component, Si NM, in optimized position of the trench. (b) Comparison of measured intracranial pressures as a function of time via a commercial sensor with a transient monitor. The recorded pressure from both sensors indicates that the performance of implanted wireless, transient brain sensors is comparable to that of a commercial sensor (blue, commercial ICP sensor; red, transient ICP sensor). (c) Optical images of an array of actively addressable, multiplexed bioresorbable neural electrodes for recording high spatiotemporal electrocorticography (ECoG) signals. The actively controlled region of 8 × 8 cells includes 128 n-channel Si NMs-based transistors for operating the whole system as well as measuring neural signals, which connects to 64 channels through ACFs to communicate external peripheral circuits. The inset shows a magnified view of Si active device region. (d) Spatial color maps indicating measured locations of relative, evoked potential via the neural recording array after stimulating the barrel cortex. Each map exhibits good agreement in between stimulated coordinates of barrel cortex and locations of evoked potentials by a bioresorbable ECoG array.

serpentine Si resistor induced by PLGA membrane deflections. The position of a piezoresistive sensing element is critical to achieve maximized sensitivity from which the underlying mechanics can be predicted by numerical calculation and finite element analysis (FEA). The evaluated results reveal that highest strain in response to diverse pressure alterations arose at the middle of both sides of the edge (left or right) in the trench, based on principal strain distribution as well as displacement in the vertical direction. Implantation of this piezoresistive sensor into the intracranial region of a rat model allows to record both pressure and temperature variations in real time, connected with the wireless connector placed on the top surface of the skull. Wireless connections of the implanted device can be obtained from embedding biodegradable molybdenum wires (~10 μm thick) to the PLGA sheet (except the top surface of the wires) at the near glass transition temperature (65 °C), followed by Mo evaporation (~2 μm thick) to allow formation of electrical contacts between silicon nanomembranes and the Mo wires. Additional encapsulation layers of PLGA film were applied to the top and bottom side of the Mo wires to enhance electrical insulation. These insulated Mo wires enable to electrically couple the implanted sensor system in the intracranial space with an externally located, miniaturized wireless potentiostat for data transmission. Figure 14.7b illustrates the comparative results of measured intracranial pressures (ICP) using a home-made transient sensor with a commercial product during periodic abdominal compression. Pressure spikes at periodic intervals from ICP correspond to the number of stimulations of abdominal region, and the peak values of wireless, transient ICP monitor are accurately matched to the values determined using a wired-type, clinical probe implanted at the same location. Mild changes in position and/or posture generate gradual increase/decrease of pressure and temperature, such as Trendelenburg (30° head-down position) and reverse Trendelenburg (30° head-up position), and temperature alterations using a heating or cooling blanket. An injectable type of similar subsystem in the intracranial place with slight modifications provides needle-like electrical probes to record various physiological parameters in the deep brain tissue that cannot be addressed by electrodes or sensors mounted on the brain tissue. The output pressures and temperatures measured by bioresorbable penetration sensors are in well agreement with those attained by commercial sensors.

Another type of a highly advanced, elaborated biodegradable electronic system offers active multiplexing neural interfaces based on an array of actively addressable n-channel metal-oxide-semiconductor field-effect transistors (MOSFETs), as shown in Figure 14.7c with a magnified image of active region in the inset [79]. The complete biodegradable neural probes comprise 128 n-type transistors with highly doped silicon nanomembranes for semiconducting materials, molybdenum (Mo) as conducting electrodes (source, drain, and gate contacts) and interconnects, SiO_2 (~100 nm) for gate dielectrics, and PLGA for supporting sheets (substrates). Additional layers of $SiO_2/Si_3N_4/SiO_2$ provide ILDs, second metal of molybdenum (Mo) serves as interconnects, and another combination of $SiO_2/Si_3N_4/SiO_2$ forms protective layers. The design layout with an efficient minimum number of readout wires envisions a scalable approach toward silicon-based industrial circuits with the switching and peripheral transistors for large-area and multiple-channel coverage. The electrical properties of a typical transistor exhibit high mobility of ~400 $cm^2 V^{-1}$, on/off ratio of $>10^{-7}$, and stable input/output potential responses as a sine wave during *in vitro* experiments in a aqueous buffer solution (pH 7.4). Dissolution behaviors in various environments, and *in vitro* and *in vivo* toxicity information of individual electronic components have been well studied in previous articles [80, 81]. Implantation of fabricated 8×8 array of transient neural electrodes to the brain provides diverse research opportunities. The colorized maps obtained from the surface of the barrel cortex in Figure 14.7d illustrate the spatial distribution of amplitudes of the evoked potentials that arose from stimulation of predetermined, relative locations at whiskers. Time-resolved somatosensory evoked potentials (SSEP) can also be achieved by stimulating the estimated locations in rectangular coordinates of whiskers, therefore, those measured evoked potentials at the cortical surface are well matched with the corresponding locations of the stimulated whiskers as a barrel cortex. In addition, implantation of the neural probes at the left side (hemisphere) of the brain could observe various epileptic activities such as clockwise spiral, lower-right to upper-left diagonal, upper-left to lower-right diagonal and right-to-left sweep, with spatiotemporal propagation amplitudes and patterns.

14.9 Conclusion and Outlook

Advances in technology innovation provide new options, directions, and foundations for coupling electronic devices with biological systems to realize effective management of human disease and health. Experimental studies on all aspects of synthesis and processing of materials including the chemistry of composites offer unique insight into the mechanical/electrical properties. Theoretical models supporting fundamental principles of structural, geometrical and engineering strategies incorporated with optimized fabrication procedures enable to achieve capabilities of intimately integrating with soft, curvilinear shapes/surfaces of the human body, which is unlikely to be attained with wafer-based, existing hard electronics. Extensive range of electronic components, from individual modules to forefront system-level devices, demonstrates electrical performance and reliability, and mechanical durability in unusual formats.

Future research directions need to focus on the discovery of new materials and/or synthesis for enhanced materials properties, and robust, cost-effective manufacturing procedures. Biocompatible and biodegradable materials/devices for long-term use and minimum interventions will be required. Challenging research areas might include development of ways to control artificial limbs (prostheses) and to communicate with the brain and nerves via electronics, as well as soft robots installed with equipment for sensory feedback.

References

1 Rogers, J.A., Bao, Z., Baldwin, K., Dodabalapur, A., Crone, B., Raju, V.R., Kuck, V., Katz, H., Amundson, K., Ewing, J., and Drzaic, P. (2001) Paper-like electronic displays: Large-area rubberstamped plastic sheets of electronics and microencapsulated electrophoretic inks. *Proc. Natl. Acad. Sci. U.S.A.*, **98**, 4835.

2 Forrest, S.F. (2004) The path to ubiquitous and low-cost organic electronic appliances on plastic. *Nature*, **428**, 911.

3 Someya, T., Sekitani, T., Iba, S., Kato, Y., Kawaguchi, H., and Sakurai, T. (2004) A large-area, flexible pressure sensor matrix with organic field-effect transistors for artificial skin applications. *Proc. Natl. Acad. Sci. U.S.A.*, **101**, 9966.

4 Someya, T., Kato, Y., Sekitani, T., Iba, S., Noguchi, Y., Murase, Y., Kawaguchi, H., and Sakurai, T. (2005) Conformable, flexible, large-area networks of pressure and thermal sensors with organic transistor active matrixes. *Proc. Natl. Acad. Sci. U.S.A.*, **102**, 12321.

5 Sun, Y., Choi, W.M., Jiang, H., Huang, Y., and Rogers, J.A. (2006) Controlled buckling of semiconductor nanoribbons for stretchable electronics. *Nat. Nanotechnol.*, **1**, 201.

6 Khang, D.Y., Jiang, H.Q., Huang, Y., and Rogers, J.A. (2006) A stretchable form of single-crystal silicon for high-performance electronics on rubber substrates. *Science*, **311**, 208.

7 Sun, Y. and Rogers, J.A. (2007) Structural forms of single crystal semiconductor nanoribbons for high performance stretchable electronics. *J. Mater. Chem.*, **17**, 832–840.

8 Sekitani, T., Takamiya, M., Noguchi, Y., Nakano, S., Kato, Y., Sakurai, T., and Someya, T. (2007) A large-area wireless power-transmission sheet using printed organic transistors and plastic MEMS switches. *Nat. Mater.*, **6**, 413.

9 Cao, Q., Kim, H.-S., Pimparkar, N., Kulkarni, J.P., Wang, C., Shim, M., Roy, K., Alam, M.A., and Rogers, J.A. (2008) Medium-scale carbon nanotube thin-film integrated circuits on flexible plastic substrates. *Nature*, **454**, 495.

10 Sekitani, T., Noguchi, Y., Hata, K., Fukushima, T., Aida, T., and Someya, T. (2008) A rubberlike stretchable active matrix using elastic conductors. *Science*, **321**, 1468.

11 Kim, D.-H., Ahn, J.-H., Choi, W.M., Kim, H.-S., Kim, T.-H., Song, J., Huang, Y.Y., Liu, Z., Lu, C., and Rogers, J.A. (2008) Stretchable and foldable silicon integrated circuits. *Science*, **20**, 507.

12 Kim, D.-H., Song, J., Choi, W.M., Kim, H.-S., Kim, R.-H., Liu, Z., Huang, Y.Y., Hwang, K.-C., Zhang, Y.-W., and Rogers, J.A. (2008) Materials and noncoplanar mesh designs for integrated circuits with linear elastic responses to extreme mechanical deformations. *Proc. Natl. Acad. Sci. U.S.A.*, **105**, 18675.

13 Ahn, B.Y., Duoss, E.B., Motala, M.J., Guo, X., Park, S.-I., Xiong, Y., Yoon, J., Nuzzo, R.G., Rogers, J.A., and Lewis, J.A. (2009) Omnidirectional printing of flexible, stretchable, and spanning silver microelectrodes. *Science*, **323**, 1590.

14 Ko, H.C., Shin, G., Wang, S., Stoykovich, M.P., Lee, J.W., Kim, D.-H., Ha, J.S., Huang, Y., Hwang, K.-C., and Rogers, J.A. (2009) Curvilinear electronics formed using silicon membrane circuits and elastomeric transfer elements. *Small*, **5**, 2703.

15 Park, S.-I., Xiong, Y., Kim, R.-H., Elvikis, P., Meitl, M., Kim, D.-H., Wu, J., Yoon, J., Yu, C.-J., Liu, Z., Huang, Y., Hwang, K.-C., Ferreira, P., Li, X., Choquette, K., and Rogers, J.A. (2009) Printed assemblies of inorganic light-emitting diodes for deformable and semitransparent displays. *Science*, **325**, 977.

16 Mannsfeld, S.C.B., Tee, B.C.-K., Stoltenberg, R.M., Chen, C.V.H.-H., Barman, S., Muir, B.V.O., Sokolov, A.N., Reese, C., and Bao, Z. (2010) Highly sensitive flexible pressure sensors with microstructured rubber dielectric layers. *Nat. Mater.*, **9**, 859.

17 Yoon, J., Jo, S., Chun, I.S., Jung, I., Kim, H.-S., Meitl, M., Menard, E., Li, X., Coleman, J.J., Paik, U., and Rogers, J.A. (2010) GaAs photovoltaics and optoelectronics using releasable multilayer epitaxial assemblies. *Nature*, **465**, 329.

18 Chen, Z., Ren, W., Gao, L., Liu, B., Pei, S., and Cheng, H.-M. (2011) Three-dimensional flexible and conductive interconnected graphene networks grown by chemical vapour deposition. *Nat. Mater.*, **10**, 424.

19 Kim, H.-S., Brueckner, E., Song, J., Li, Y., Kim, S., Lu, C., Sulkin, J., Choquette, K., Huang, Y., Nuzzo, R.G., and Rogers, J.A. (2011) Unusual strategies for using indium gallium nitride grown on silicon (111) for solid-state lighting. *Proc. Natl. Acad. Sci. U.S.A.*, **108**, 10072.

20 Wang, C., Chien, J.-C., Takei, K., Takahashi, T., Nah, J., Niknejad, A.M., and Javey, A. (2012) Extremely bendable, high-performance integrated circuits using semiconducting carbon nanotube networks for digital, analog, and radio-frequency applications. *Nano Lett.*, **12**, 1527.

21 Matsuhisa, N., Kaltenbrunner, M., Yokota, T., Jinno, H., Kuribara, K., Sekitani, T., and Someya, T. (2015) Printable elastic conductors with a high conductivity for electronic textile applications. *Nat. Commun.*, **6**, 7461.

22 Jang, K.-I., Chung, H.U., Xu, S., Lee, C.H., Luan, H., Jeong, J., Cheng, H., Kim, G.-T., Han, S.Y., Lee, J.W., Kim, J., Cho, M., Miao, F., Yang, Y., Jung, H.N., Flavin, M., Liu, H., Kong, G.W., Yu, K.J., Rhee, S.I., Chung, J., Kim, B., Kwak, J.W., Yun, M.H., Kim, J.Y., Song, Y.M., Paik, U., Zhang, Y., Huang, Y., and Rogers, J.A. (2015) Soft network composite materials with deterministic and bio-inspired designs. *Nat. Commun.*, **6**, 6566.

23 Dagdeviren, C., Yang, B.D., Su, Y., Tran, P.L., Joe, P., Anderson, E., Xia, J., Doraiswamy, V., Dehdashti, B., Feng, X., Lu, B., Poston, R., Khalpey, Z., Ghaffari, R., Huang, Y., Slepian, M.J., and Rogers, J.A. (2014) Conformal piezoelectric energy harvesting and storage from motions of the heart, lung, and diaphragm. *Proc. Natl. Acad. Sci. U.S.A.*, **111**, 1927.

24 Viventi, J., Kim, D.-H., Moss, J.D., Kim, Y.-S., Blanco, J.A., Annetta, N., Hicks, A., Xiao, J., Huang, Y., Callans, D.J., Rogers, J.A., and Litt, B. (2010) A conformal, bio-interfaced class of silicon electronics for mapping cardiac electrophysiology. *Sci. Transl. Med.*, **2**, 24ra22.

25 Webb, R.C., Ma, Y., Krishnan, S., Li, Y., Yoon, S., Guo, X., Feng, X., Shi, Y., Seidel, M., Cho, N.H., Kurniawan, J., Ahad, J., Sheth, N., Kim, J., Taylor, J.G., Darlington, T., Chang, K., Huang, W., Ayers, J., Gruebele, A., Pielak, R.M., Slepian, M.J., Huang, Y., Gorbach, A.M., and Rogers, J.A. (2015) Epidermal devices for noninvasive, precise, and continuous mapping of macrovascular and microvascular blood flow. *Sci. Adv.*, **1**, e1500701.

26 Dagdeviren, C., Shi, Y., Joe, P., Ghaffari, R., Balooch, G., Usgaonkar, K., Gur, O., Tran, P.L., Crosby, J.R., Meyer, M., Su, Y., Webb, R.C., Tedesco, A.S., Slepian, M.J., Huang, Y., and Rogers, J.A. (2015) Conformal piezoelectric systems for clinical and experimental characterization of soft tissue biomechanics. *Nat. Mater.*, **14**, 728.

27 Xu, L., Gutbrod, S.R., Bonifas, A.P., Su, Y., Sulkin, M.S., Lu, N., Chung, H.-J., Jang, K.-I., Liu, Z., Ying, M., Lu, C., Webb, R.C., Kim, J.-S., Laughner, J.I., Cheng, H., Liu, Y., Ameen, A., Jeong, J.-W., Kim, G.-T., Huang, Y., Efimov, I.R., and Rogers, J.A. (2014) 3D multifunctional integumentary membranes for spatiotemporal cardiac measurements and stimulation across the entire epicardium. *Nat. Commun.*, **5**, 3329.

28 Yokota, T., Inoue, Y., Terakawa, Y., Reeder, J., Kaltenbrunner, M., Ware, T., Yang, K., Mabuchi, K., Murakawa, T., Sekino, M., Voit, W., Sekitani, T., and Someya, T. (2015) Ultraflexible, large-area, physiological temperature sensors for multipoint measurements. *Proc. Natl. Acad. Sci. U.S.A.*, **112**, 14533.

29 Kim, D.-H., Viventi, J., Amsden, J.J., Xiao, J., Vigeland, L., Kim, Y.-S., Blanco, J.A., Panilaitis, B., Frechette, E.S., Contreras, D., Kaplan, D.L., Omenetto, F.G., Huang, Y., Hwang, K.-C., Zakin, M.R., Litt, B., and Rogers, J.A. (2010) Dissolvable films of silk fibroin for ultrathin, conformal bio-integrated electronics. *Nat. Mater.*, **9**, 511.

30 Viventi, J., Kim, D.-H., Vigeland, L., Frechette, E.S., Blanco, J.A., Kim, Y.-S., Avrin, A.E., Tiruvadi, V.R., Hwang, S.-W., Vanleer, A.C., Wulsin, D.F., Davis, K., Gelber, C.E., Palmer, L., Van der Spiegel, J., Wu, J., Xiao, J., Huang, Y., Contreras, D., Rogers, J.A., and Litt, B. (2011) Flexible, foldable, actively multiplexed, high-density electrode array for mapping brain activity in vivo. *Nat. Neurosci.*, **14**, 1599.

31 Nguyen, T.D., Deshmukh, N., Nagarah, J.M., Kramer, T., Purohit, P.K., Berry, M.J., and McAlpine, M.C. (2012) Piezoelectric nanoribbons for monitoring cellular deformations. *Nat. Nanotechnol.*, **7**, 587.

32 Kim, T.-I., McCall, J.G., Jung, Y.H., Huang, X., Siuda, E.R., Li, Y., Song, J., Song, Y.M., An Pao, H., Kim, R.-H., Lu, C., Lee, S.D., Song, I.-S., Shin, G., Al-Hasani, R., Kim, S., Tan, M.P., Huang, Y., Omenetto, F.G., Rogers, J.A., and Bruchas, M.R. (2013) Injectable, cellular-scale optoelectronics with applications for wireless optogenetics. *Science*, **240**, 211.

33 Tee, B.C.-K., Chortos, A., Berndt, A., Nguyen, A.K., Tom, A., McGuire, A., Lin, Z.C., Tien, K., Bae, W.-G., Wang, H., Mei, P., Chou, H.-H., Cui, B., Deisseroth, K., Ng, T.N., and Bao, Z. (2015) A skin-inspired organic digital mechanoreceptor. *Science*, **350**, 313.

34 Jeong, J.-W., McCall, J.G., Shin, G., Zhang, Y., Al-Hasani, R., Kim, M., Li, S., Sim, J.Y., Jang, K.-I., Shi, Y., Hong, D.Y., Liu, Y., Schmitz, G.P., Xia, L., He, Z., Gamble, P., Ray, W.Z., Huang, Y., Bruchas, M.R., and Rogers, J.A. (2015) Wireless optofluidic systems for programmable in vivo pharmacology and optogenetics. *Cell*, **162**, 1.

35 Minev, I.R., Musienko, P., Hirsch, A., Barraud, Q., Wenger, N., Moraud, E.M., Gandar, J., Capogrosso, M., Milekovic, T., Asboth, L., Torres, R.F., Vachicouras, N., Liu, Q., Pavlova, N., Duis, S., Larmagnac, A., Vörös, J., Micera, S., Suo, Z., Courtine, G., and Lacour, S.P. (2015) Electronic dura mater for long-term multimodal neural interfaces. *Science*, **347**, 159.

36 Park, S.I., Brenner, D.S., Shin, G., Morgan, C.D., Copits, B.A., Chung, H.U., Pullen, M.Y., Noh, K.N., Davidson, S., Oh, S.J., Yoon, J., Jang, K.-I., Samineni, V.K., Norman, M., Grajales-Reyes, J.G., Vogt, S.K., Sundaram, S.S., Wilson, K.M., Ha, J.S., Xu, R., Pan, T., Kim, T.-I., Huang, Y., Montana, M.C., Golden, J.P., Bruchas, M.R., Gereau, R.W., and Rogers, J.A. (2015) Soft, stretchable,

fully implantable miniaturized optoelectronic systems for wireless optogenetics. *Nat. Biotechnol.*, **33**, 1280.

37 Takei, K., Takahashi, T., Ho, J.C., Ko, H., Gillies, A.G., Leu, P.W., Fearing, R.S., and Javey, A. (2010) Nanowire active-matrix circuitry for low-voltage macroscale artificial skin. *Nat. Mater.*, **9**, 821.

38 Kim, D.-H., Lu, N., Ma, R., Kim, Y.-S., Kim, R.-H., Wang, S., Wu, J., Won, S.M., Tao, H., Islam, A., Yu, K.J., Kim, T.-I., Chowdhury, R., Ying, M., Xu, L., Li, M., Chung, H.-J., Keum, H., McCormick, M., Liu, P., Zhang, Y.-W., Omenetto, F.G., Huang, Y., Coleman, T., and Rogers, J.A. (2011) Epidermal electronics. *Science*, **333**, 838.

39 Lipomi, D.J., Vosgueritchian, M., Tee, B.C.-K., Hellstrom, S.L., Lee, J.A., Fox, C.H., and Bao, Z. (2011) Skin-like pressure and strain sensors based on transparent elastic films of carbon nanotubes. *Nat. Nanotechnol.*, **6**, 788.

40 Wang, C., Hwang, D., Yu, Z., Takei, K., Park, J., Chen, T., Ma, B., and Javey, A. (2013) User-interactive electronic skin for instantaneous pressure visualization. *Nat. Mater.*, **12**, 899.

41 Yeo, W.-H., Kim, Y.-S., Lee, J., Ameen, A., Shi, L., Li, M., Wang, S., Ma, R., Jin, S.H., Kang, Z., Huang, Y., and Rogers, J.A. (2013) Multifunctional epidermal electronics printed directly onto the skin. *Adv. Mater.*, **25**, 2773.

42 Webb, R.C., Bonifas, A.P., Behnaz, A., Zhang, Y., Yu, K.J., Cheng, H., Shi, M., Bian, Z., Liu, Z., Kim, Y.S., Yeo, W.-H., Park, J.S., Song, J., Li, Y., Huang, Y., Gorbach, A.M., and Rogers, J.A. (2013) Ultrathin conformal devices for precise and continuous thermal characterization of human skin. *Nat. Mater.*, **12**, 938.

43 Kaltenbrunner, M., Sekitani, T., Reeder, J., Yokota, T., Kuribara, K., Tokuhara, T., Drack, M., Schwodiauer, R., Graz, I., Bauer-Gogonea, S., Bauer, S., and Someya, T. (2013) An ultra-lightweight design for imperceptible plastic electronics. *Nature*, **499**, 458.

44 Gao, W., Emaminejad, S., Nyein, H.Y.Y., Challa, S., Chen, K., Peck, A., Fahad, H.M., Ota, H., Shiraki, H., Kiriya, D., Lien, D.-H., Brooks, G.A., Davis, R.W., and Javey, A. (2016) Fully integrated wearable sensor arrays for multiplexed in situ perspiration analysis. *Nature*, **529**, 509.

45 Yokota, T., Zalar, P., Kaltenbrunner, M., Jinno, H., Matsuhisa, N., Kitanosako, H., Tachibana, Y., Yukita, W., Koizumi, M., and Someya, T. (2016) Ultraflexible organic photonic skin. *Sci. Adv.*, **2**, e1501856.

46 Larson, C., Peele, B., Li, S., Robinson, S., Totaro, M., Beccai, L., Mazzolai, B., and Shepherd, R. (2016) Highly stretchable electroluminescent skin for optical signaling and tactile sensing. *Science*, **351**, 1071.

47 Yoon, J., Baca, A.J., Park, S.-I., Elvikis, P., Geddes, J.B. III, Li, L., Kim, R.H., Xiao, J., Wang, S., Kim, T.-H., Motala, M.J., Ahn, B.Y., Duoss, E.B., Lewis, J.A., Nuzzo, R.G., Ferreira, P.M., Huang, Y., Rockett, A., and Rogers, J.A. (2008) Ultrathin silicon solar microcells for semitransparent, mechanically flexible and microconcentrator module designs. *Nat. Mater.*, **7**, 907.

48 Fan, Z., Razavi, H., Do, J.-W., Moriwaki, A., Ergen, O., Chueh, Y.-L., Leu, P.W., Ho, J.C., Takahashi, T., Reichertz, L.A., Neale, S., Yu, K., Wu, M., Ager, J.W., and Javey, A. (2009) Three-dimensional nanopillar-array photovoltaics on low-cost and flexible substrates. *Nat. Mater.*, **8**, 648.

49 Qi, Y. and McAlpine, M.C. (2010) Nanotechnology-enabled flexible and biocompatible energy harvesting. *Energy Environ. Sci.*, **3**, 1275.

50 Qi, Y., Kim, J., Nguyen, T.D., Lisko, B., Purohit, P.K., and McAlpine, M.C. (2011) Enhanced piezoelectricity and stretchability in energy harvesting devices fabricated from buckled PZT ribbons. *Nano Lett.*, **11**, 1331.

51 Kettlgruber, G., Kaltenbrunner, M., Siket, C.M., Moser, R., Graz, I.M., Schwodiauer, R., and Bauer, S. (2013) Intrinsically stretchable and rechargeable batteries for self-powered stretchable electronics. *J. Mater. Chem. A*, **1**, 5505.

52 Lee, H.S., Chung, J., Hwang, G.-T., Jeong, C.K., Jung, Y., Kwak, J.-H., Kang, H., Byun, M., Kim, W.D., Hur, S., Oh, S.-H., and Lee, K.J. (2014) Flexible inorganic piezoelectric acoustic nanosensors for biomimetic artificial hair cells. *Adv. Funct. Mater.*, **24**, 6914.

53 Xu, S., Zhang, Y., Cho, J., Lee, J., Huang, X., Jia, L., Fan, J.A., Su, Y., Su, J., Zhang, H., Cheng, H., Lu, B., Yu, C., Chuang, C., Kim, T.-I., Song, T., Shigeta, K., Kang, S., Dagdeviren, C., Petrov, I., Braun, P.V., Huang, Y., Paik, U., and Rogers, J.A. (2013) Stretchable batteries with self-similar serpentine interconnects and integrated wireless recharging systems. *Nat. Commun.*, **4**, 1543.

54 Ko, H.C., Stoykovich, M.P., Song, J., Malyarchuk, V., Choi, W.M., Yu, C.-J., Geddes, J.B. III, Xiao, J., Wang, S., Huang, Y., and Rogers, J.A. (2008) A hemispherical electronic eye camera based on compressible silicon optoelectronics. *Nature*, **454**, 748.

55 Song, Y.M., Xie, Y., Malyarchuk, V., Xiao, J., Jung, I., Choi, K.-J., Liu, Z., Park, H., Lu, C., Kim, R.-H., Li, R., Crozier, K.B., Huang, Y., and Rogers, J.A. (2013) Digital cameras with designs inspired by the arthropod eye. *Nature*, **497**, 95.

56 Bettinger, C.J. and Bao, Z. (2010) Organic thin-film transistors fabricated on resorbable biomaterial substrates. *Adv. Mater.*, **22**, 651.

57 Irimia-Vladu, M., Troshin, P.A., Reisinger, M., Shmygleva, L., Kanbur, Y., Schwabegger, G., Bodea, M., Schwödiauer, R., Mumyatov, A., Fergus, J.W., Razumov, V.F., Sitter, H., Sariciftci, N.S., and Bauer, S. (2010) Biocompatible and biodegradable materials for organic field-effect transistors. *Adv. Funct. Mater.*, **20**, 4069.

58 Hwang, S.-W., Tao, H., Kim, D.-H., Cheng, H., Song, J.-K., Rill, E., Brenckle, M.A., Panilaitis, B., Won, S.M., Kim, Y.-S., Song, Y.M., Yu, K.J., Ameen, A., Li, R., Su, Y., Yang, M., Kaplan, D.L., Zakin, M.R., Slepian, M.J., Huang, Y., Omenetto, F.G., and Rogers, J.A. (2012) A physically transient form of silicon electronics. *Science*, **337**, 1640.

59 Symon, K.R. (1971) *Mechanics*, 3rd edn, Addison-Wesley.

60 Kiefer, A.M., Paskiewicz, D.M., Clausen, A.M., Buchwald, W.R., Soref, R.A., and Lagally, M.G. (2011) Si/Ge junctions formed by nanomembrane bonding. *ACS Nano*, **5**, 1179.

61 Rogers, J.A., Lagally, M.G., and Nuzzo, R.G. (2011) Synthesis, assembly and applications of semiconductor nanomembranes. *Nature*, **477**, 45.

62 Chung, H.-J., Kim, T.-I., Kim, H.-S., Wells, S.A., Jo, S., Ahmed, N., Jung, Y.H., Won, S.M., Bower, C.A., and Rogers, J.A. (2011) Fabrication of releasable

single-crystal silicon–metal oxide field-effect devices and their deterministic assembly on foreign substrates. *Adv. Funct. Mater.*, **21**, 3029.

63 Kim, T.-I., Jung, Y.H., Chung, H.-J., Yu, K.J., Ahmed, N., Corcoran, C.J., Park, J.S., Jin, S.H., and Rogers, J.A. (2013) Deterministic assembly of releasable single crystal silicon-metal oxide field-effect devices formed from bulk wafers. *Appl. Phys. Lett.*, **102**, 182104.

64 Hwang, S.-W., Kim, D.-H., Tao, H., Kim, T.-I., Kim, S., Yu, K.J., Panilaitis, B., Jeong, J.-W., Song, J.-K., Omenetto, F.G., and Rogers, J.A. (2013) Materials and fabrication processes for transient and bioresorbable high-performance electronics. *Adv. Funct. Mater.*, **23**, 4087.

65 Fan, Z., Ho, J.C., Jacobson, Z.A., Yerushalmi, R., Alley, R.L., Razavi, H., and Javey, A. (2008) Wafer-scale assembly of highly ordered semiconductor nanowire arrays by contact printing. *Nano Lett.*, **8**, 20.

66 Kim, S., Wu, J., Carlson, A., Jin, S.H., Kovalsky, A., Glass, P., Liu, Z., Ahmed, N., Elgan, S.L., Chen, W., Ferreira, P.M., Sitti, M., Huang, Y., and Rogers, J.A. (2010) Microstructured elastomeric surfaces with reversible adhesion and examples of their use in deterministic assembly by transfer printing. *Proc. Natl. Acad. Sci. U.S.A.*, **107**, 17095.

67 Kim, S., Su, Y., Mihi, A., Lee, S., Liu, Z., Bhandakkar, T.K., Wu, J., Geddes, J.B. III, Johnson, H.T., Zhang, Y., Park, J.-K., Braun, P.V., Huang, Y., and Rogers, J.A. (2012) Imbricate scales as a design construct for microsystem technologies. *Small*, **8**, 901.

68 Fan, J.A., Yeo, W.-H., Su, Y., Hattori, Y., Lee, W., Jung, S.-Y., Zhang, Y., Liu, Z., Cheng, H., Falgout, L., Bajema, M., Coleman, T., Gregoire, D., Larsen, R.J., Huang, Y., and Rogers, J.A. (2014) Fractal design concepts for stretchable electronics. *Nat. Commun.*, **5**, 3266.

69 Iijima, S. and Ichihashi, T. (1993) Single-shell carbon nanotube of 1-nm diameter. *Nature*, **363**, 603.

70 Hata, K., Futaba, D.N., Mizuno, K., Namai, T., Yumura, M., and Iijima, S. (2004) Water-assisted highly efficient synthesis of impurity-free single-walled carbon nanotubes. *Science*, **306**, 1362.

71 Kim, R.-H., Kim, D.-H., Xiao, J., Kim, B.H., Park, S.-I., Panilaitis, B., Ghaffari, R., Yao, J., Li, M., Liu, Z., Malyarchuk, V., Kim, D.G., Le, A.-P., Nuzzo, R.G., Kaplan, D.L., Omenetto, F.G., Huang, Y., Kang, Z., and Rogers, J.A. (2010) Waterproof AlInGaP optoelectronics on stretchable substrates with applications in biomedicine and robotics. *Nat. Mater.*, **9**, 929.

72 Baciewicz, F.A., Penney, D.G., Marinelli, W.A., and Marinelli, R. (1991) Torsional ventricular motion and rotary blood flow. *Card. Chronicle*, **5**, 1.

73 Rushmer, R.F. (1995) Length-circumference relations of the left ventricle. *Circ. Res.*, **3**, 639.

74 McHale, P.A. and Greenfield, J.C. (1973) Evaluation of several geometric models for estimation of left ventricular circumferential wall stress. *Circ. Res.*, **33**, 303.

75 Streeter, D.D. and Hanna, W.T. (1973) Engineering mechanics for successive states in canine left ventricular myocardium. I. Cavity and wall geometry. *Circ. Res.*, **33**, 639.

76 Morgan, R.M., Patterson, M.J., and Nimmo, M.A. (2004) Acute effects of dehydration on sweat composition in men during prolonged exercise in the heat. *Acta Physiol. Scand.*, **182**, 37.

77 Bai, Y., Chen, B., Xiang, F., Zhou, J., Wang, H., and Suo, Z. (2014) Transparent hydrogel with enhanced water retention capacity by introducing highly hydratable salt. *Appl. Phys. Lett.*, **105**, 151903.

78 Kang, S.-K., Murphy, R.K.J., Hwang, S.-W., Lee, S.M., Harburg, D.V., Krueger, N.A., Shin, J., Gamble, P., Cheng, H., Yu, S., Liu, Z., McCall, J.G., Stephen, M., Ying, H., Kim, J., Park, G., Webb, R.C., Lee, C.H., Chung, S., Wie, D.S., Gujar, A.D., Vemulapalli, B., Kim, A.H., Lee, K.-M., Cheng, J., Huang, Y., Lee, S.H., Braun, P.V., Ray, W.Z., and Rogers, J.A. (2016) Bioresorbable silicon electronic sensors for the brain. *Nature*, **530**, 71.

79 Yu, K.J., Kuzum, D., Hwang, S.-W., Kim, B.H., Juul, H., Kim, N.H., Won, S.M., Chiang, K., Trumpis, M., Richardson, A.G., Cheng, H., Fang, H., Thompson, M., Bink, H., Talos, D., Seo, K.J., Lee, H.N., Kang, S.-K., Kim, J.-H., Lee, J.Y., Huang, Y., Jensen, F.E., Dichter, M.A., Lucas, T.H., Viventi, J., Litt, B., and Rogers, J.A. (2016) Bioresorbable silicon electronics for transient spatiotemporal mapping of electrical activity from the cerebral cortex. *Nat. Mater.*, **15**, 782.

80 Hwang, S.-W., Park, G., Cheng, H., Song, J.-K., Kang, S.-K., Yin, L., Kim, J.-H., Omenetto, F.G., Huang, Y., Lee, K.-M., and Rogers, J.A. (2014) 25th anniversary article: materials for high-performance biodegradable semiconductor devices. *Adv. Mater.*, **26**, 1992.

81 Hwang, S.-W., Park, G., Edwards, C., Corbin, E.A., Kang, S.-K., Cheng, H., Song, J.-K., Kim, J.-H., Yu, S., Ng, J., Lee, J.E., Kim, J., Yee, C., Bhaduri, B., Su, Y., Omennetto, F.G., Huang, Y., Bashir, R., Goddard, L., Popescu, G., Lee, K.-M., and Rogers, J.A. (2014) Dissolution chemistry and biocompatibility of single-crystalline silicon nanomembranes and associated materials for transient electronics. *ACS Nano*, **8**, 5843.

15

Implantable Flexible Sensors for Neural Recordings

Shota Yamagiwa, Hirohito Sawahata, and Takeshi Kawano

Toyohashi University of Technology, Department of Electrical and Electronic Information Engineering, 1-1, Hibarigaoka, Tempaku-cho, Toyohashi 441-8580, Japan

15.1 Introduction

"The brain is an extremely complex system." The current understanding of how the brain works is very poor, making it difficult to discover effective cures for brain diseases. One way to increase the knowledge about the brain is to explore the activity of a large number of neurons within the brain tissue.

Neurons, which are excitable cells in electrochemical signals, are the signaling unit of the nervous system. A typical neuron has four regions: cell body, dendrites, axons, and presynaptic terminals. The cell body (or *soma*) has a diameter $\geq 50\,\mu m$, while the axon in the central nervous system has a diameter of 0.2–20 μm (Figure 15.1) [1]. Optical, magnetic, and electrical measurement methods have been proposed to observe neuronal activities [2]. Since the spatial and temporal resolutions of invasive electrical measurements [electrocorticography (ECoG), local field potentials (LFPs), and single-neuron action potential recordings (single units or spikes)] are better than the noninvasive methods [e.g., electroencephalography (EEG) and functional magnetic resonance imaging (fMRI)] (Figure 15.2) and the system can be minimized (microelectronics, wireless system), electrical measurement can be applied for *in vivo* recordings such as free moving measurements and brain–machine interfaces (BMI).

Neurons in the nervous system communicate with each other via electrical signals, called action potentials. The recording amplitude of the action potential is $<100\,mV$ in intracellular (inner cell) recording and $<1\,mV$ in extracellular (outer cell) recording methodologies with a frequency of approximately 1 kHz. Using microscale extracellular electrodes, the synchronized electrical activity of either neuron ensembles (field potentials, FP) or single neurons (single units or spikes) can be detected.

Advances in microelectrode technology using microelectro-mechanical systems (MEMS) offer new possibilities to realize high spatial resolution mappings of the electrical activity within a tissue *in vitro* and *in vivo*, allowing the neuron network to be explored [3, 4]. The section reviews recent advances in MEMS-processed microelectrode devices with a focus on flexibility, which is a

Flexible and Stretchable Medical Devices, First Edition. Edited by Kuniharu Takei.

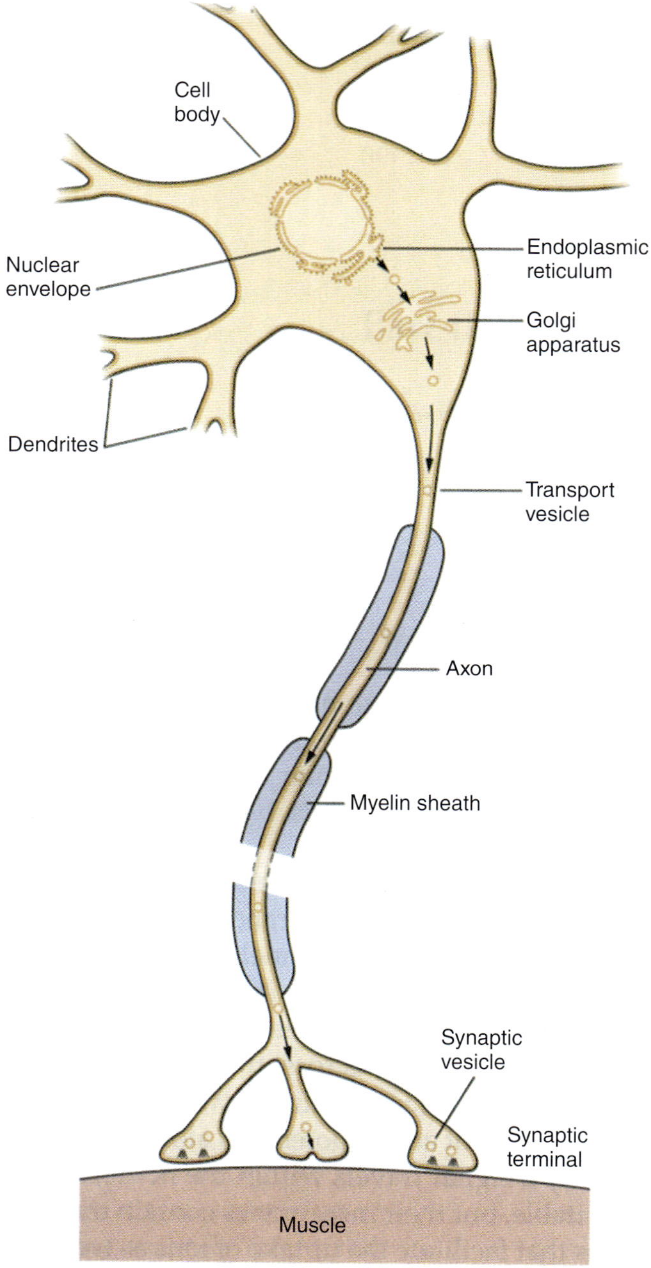

Figure 15.1 The structure of a neuron. A typical neuron has four regions: cell body, dendrites, axons, and presynaptic terminals. (Kandel *et al.* 2012 [1]. Reproduced with permission of John Wiley & Sons.)

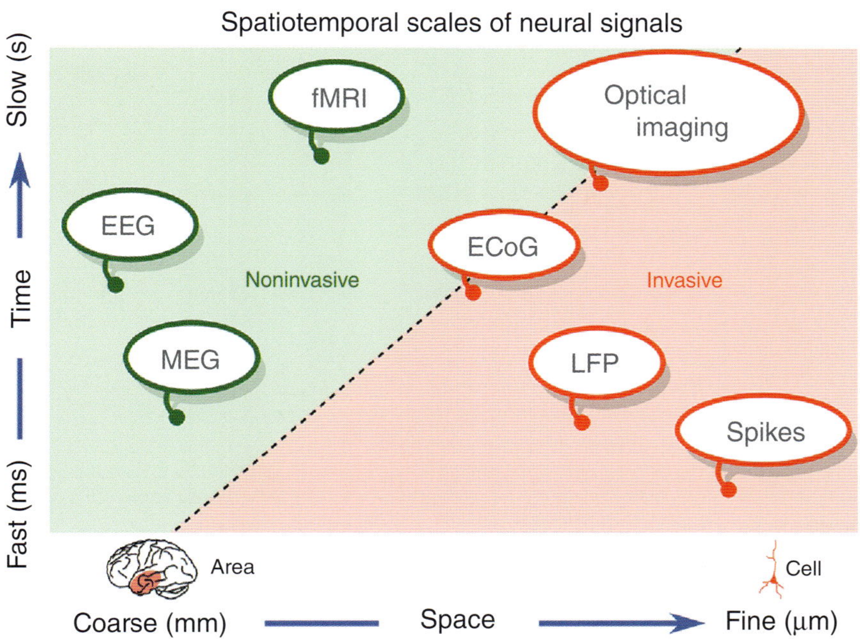

Figure 15.2 Spatiotemporal resolutions of noninvasive methods [e.g., EEG, fMRI, and magnetoencephalography (MEG)] and invasive electrical measurements [e.g., optical imaging, ECoG, LFPs, and single-neuron action potential recordings (single units or spikes)].

powerful feature to realize highly biocompatible and low-invasive tools for use in biological tissues with three-dimensional (3D), deformable, and soft properties.

15.1.1 Neuronal Signal Recordings

The signal quality in a neuronal recording such as the spatiotemporal resolution and the signal-to-noise ratio (SNR) is an important characteristic of a recording device for subsequent signal usages, including epileptic seizure detection and BMI technology [5]. Because the signal source originates from a neuron within brain tissue, the signal quality significantly depends on the recording methodology (distance from the signal source) and the electrode device (geometry, electorate–electrode interfacial impedance, etc.).

Extracellular electrical recording of brain activity is categorized into four primary modalities: EEG, ECoG, LFPs, and single-neuron action potential recordings (single units or spikes) (Figure 15.3). Although nanotechnology has significantly contributed to intracellular recordings, the section here focuses on extracellular devices, which offer stable and long-term (chronic) recording applications. Reviews of intracellular devices employing nanotechnology can be found in the literature [6].

15.1.1.1 EEG

As a safer methodology, noninvasive EEG recordings are used to detect brain activity. Millimeter-scale electrodes placed on the scalp can detect the EEG signal

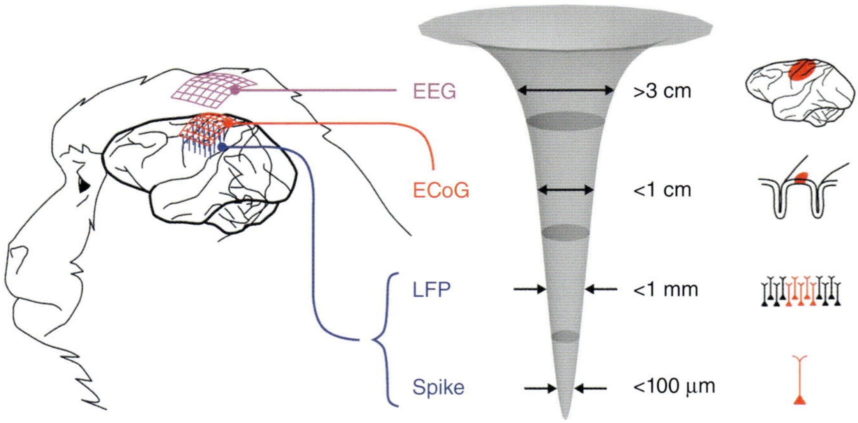

Figure 15.3 Extracellular electrical recordings of brain activities categorized into four primary modalities: EEG, ECoG, LFPs, and single-neuron action potential recordings (single units or spikes).

generated from a large neuronal population of synchronously active neurons. In a human, the scalp is 2–3 cm away from the cortex, providing an EEG signal with a spatial of ~3 cm. A normal human EEG signal shows activity between 1 and 30 Hz. The signal amplitude is in the range of 20–100 μV [1]. These frequencies have been divided into several groups: alpha (8–13 Hz), beta (13–30 Hz), delta (0.5–4 Hz), and theta (4–7 Hz) [1]. EEG recordings are most often used to diagnose epilepsy, which causes abnormalities in the EEG readings.

15.1.1.2 ECoG

Invasive ECoG electrode technology can provide a higher spatial and temporal resolution of the brain activity than EEG. The ECoG electrode is placed directly on the cortical surface and detects the signal of synchronized neuronal potentials (LFPs). Compared to EEG, the ECoG signal is composed of higher frequencies, ranging from alpha to high-gamma (8–100 Hz) with a spatial resolution on the millimeter order [7]. The signal amplitude of ECoG ranges from hundreds of μV to 1 mV. ECoG recordings are categorized into two methodologies: outside the dura mater (epidural) and under the dura mater (subdural), depending on the application. ECoG signal recordings with a high spatial resolution have been used in medical applications to detect the location of a seizure, especially in patients with epilepsy.

15.1.1.3 LFPs and Spikes

LFP (intracortical LFP or depth LFP) and single-neuron action potentials (single units or spikes) are recorded by penetrating a microscale metal electrode, glass electrode, or MEMS-based needle electrode into brain tissue. Recording the signals at a direct current up to ~40 kHz contains both the action potentials and other membrane potentials such as the synaptic potential [8]. LFPs are typically band-pass filtered (e.g., 300 Hz–5 kHz [7]). Lower-frequency LFPs reflect the action potentials in many neurons, but do not reflect spikes in a single neuron, which is an individual action potential with a higher frequency (500 Hz–1 kHz [1]). Electrodes typically have recording sites with 10–50 μm diameters, and the needle (or shank) lengths are 1–5 mm. Because the electrode located near neurons detects neuronal activities, LFP and single-neuron action potential recordings provide spatial resolutions of <1 mm and <0.2 mm [7], respectively, while the signal amplitudes are <1 mV.

15.1.2 Electrode Materials

Electrode materials must have a low impedance for the neuronal recording or safe reversible charge injection for stimulation applications. Biocompatibility is also required for long-term (chronic) recordings and stimulations. Candidate materials for the recording electrode include stainless steel, tungsten, platinum, platinum–iridium (alloy), platinum black, iridium oxide, titanium nitride, and poly(ethylenedioxythiophene) (PEDOT). Recording electrodes are typically characterized by their electrolyte–electrode interfacial electrical impedance measured in saline at 1 kHz, which varies from approximately 50 kΩ to 1 MΩ [9].

For the stimulation, the electrode is required to mediate the transition from electron flow in the electrode to ion flow in a tissue. These types of reactions can be categorized into capacitive or faradaic. Capacitive reactions involve charging and discharging of the electrode–electrolyte double layer, while faradaic reactions oxidize and reduce the surface-confined species. Candidate materials of the stimulating electrode include tantalum/Ta_2O_5 (capacitive), titanium nitride (capacitive), iridium oxide (faradaic), and PEDOT (faradaic). Stimulation electrodes are typically characterized by cyclic voltammetry, impedance spectroscopy, and potential transient measurements [9].

15.1.3 Electrode Impedance in Neural Recordings

The electrical impedance of the recording-site is an important electrode characteristic for neural recordings, especially for high impedance microelectrode devices (e.g., >1 MΩ at 1 kHz) connected to a recording buffer amplifier via a cable line. Because the electrode and embedded parasitic impedances in the recording system construct the voltage divide configuration, both the detected neural and phase delayed signals are attenuated [10, 11].

The parasitic impedances are explained by considering the parasitic capacitances of a microelectrode device and the cable line between the device and the external buffer amplifier.

Figure 15.4 shows an equivalent circuit of the recording system in extracellular neural recordings. Z_e is the metal–electrolyte (electrode–saline) interfacial impedance at the recording site (microelectrode), which consists of the spread resistance (R_{sp}), charge transfer resistance (R_{ct}), and constant phase element (CPE) shown in Figure 15.4. CPE is defined as

$$\mathrm{CPE} = \frac{1}{(j\omega Q)^n} \tag{15.1}$$

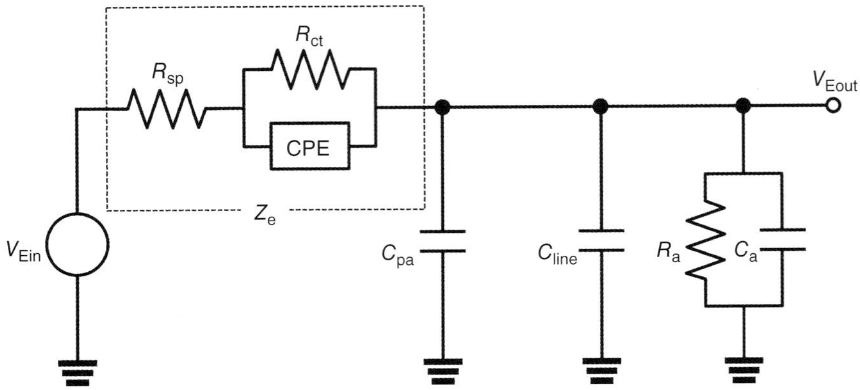

Figure 15.4 Equivalent circuit model of the recording system in extracellular neural recordings.

where Q is the measured magnitude of CPE and n is a constant parameter that depends on the inhomogeneous surface of the electrode. C_{pa} is the parasitic capacitance of the microelectrode device between the metal interconnection and the electrolyte. C_{line} is due to the recording cable from the electrode device (e.g., device-bonding pad) to the external buffer amplifier. The detected signals during a neural recording can be calculated using the voltage divide configuration of the recording system as

$$H(j\omega) = \frac{V_{Eout}(j\omega)}{V_{Ein}(j\omega)} = \frac{Z_p}{Z_e + Z_p} \tag{15.2}$$

$$Z_p = \frac{R_a}{j\omega R_a(C_{pa} + C_{line} + C_a) + 1} \tag{15.3}$$

where $V_{Ein}(j\omega)$ is the input signal, which is the voltage due to the extracellular neural activity. $V_{Eout}(j\omega)$ is the output signal obtained as the input voltage of the buffer amplifier through the electrode device and the cable line. Z_p is the shunt impedance. The configuring parasitic capacitances (C_{pa} and C_{line}) and input impedances of the buffer amplifier (R_a, C_a) are defined in Eq. (15.3). The transfer function in a neural recording $H(j\omega)$ is expressed as

$$H(j\omega) = \frac{V_{Eout}(j\omega)}{V_{Ein}(j\omega)} = |H(j\omega)| \arg H(j\omega) = \frac{|Z_p|}{|Z_e + Z_p|}\{\cos(\theta) + j\sin(\theta)\} \tag{15.4}$$

$$|H(j\omega)| = \frac{|V_{Eout}(j\omega)|}{|V_{Ein}(j\omega)|} = \frac{|Z_p|}{|Z_e + Z_p|} \tag{15.5}$$

$$\begin{aligned}\theta &= \arg H(j\omega)\\ &= \frac{\mathrm{Im}(Z_e)\mathrm{Re}(Z_p) - \mathrm{Re}(Z_e)\mathrm{Im}(Z_p)}{\mathrm{Re}(Z_e)(\mathrm{Re}(Z_e) + \mathrm{Re}(Z_p)) + \mathrm{Im}(Z_e)(\mathrm{Im}(Z_e) + \mathrm{Im}(Z_p))}\end{aligned} \tag{15.6}$$

The absolute value of the transfer function $H(j\omega)$ depicted in Eq. (15.5) indicates that the output/input signal amplitude ratio depends on the microelectrode's impedance (Z_e) and the system's embedded parasitic impedance (Z_p). In addition, Eq. (15.6) indicates the delays in the output/input signals. Both the amplitude attenuation and delay of signal should be minimized to record neuronal signals without the signal degradation. System noise due to the recording system should also be minimized for a high SNR.

15.2 Flexible Needle Electrodes

MEMS fabrication technology can minimize the neural recording needle electrodes [3, 4] for high spatial resolution and low-invasive recordings of neuronal signals. Microscale-needle electrodes penetrated into a tissue record both LFP and spikes; a spike shows a greater spatiotemporal resolution (~100 μm for spatial and ~1 ms for temporal resolution) compared to other types of signals (EEG, ECoG, and LFP). However, since a stiff needle shaft induces large tissue damage (see Section 15.5.1), which limits the long-term recording ability, the needle portion of the electrode should be flexible.

In 2001, Rousche *et al.* proposed the flexible polyimide-based penetration electrode (Figure 15.5) [12]. Gold/chromium were used and patterned as the electrodes and interconnections. The thickness of the substrate was less than 20 μm. The device had two electrodes on one shank.

This configuration may realize re-growth of the astrocyte through the device for implanted device stabilization. Firstly, a planar device is fabricated and released from the silicon substrate. Then, a 3D structure is formed by folding to form the penetration electrodes. Since the device substrate lacks sufficient stiffness for penetration, a pial incision was created by a scalpel or a 100-μm-diameter tungsten needle for device penetration.

As a unique fabrication process of a 3D penetration electrode, Takeuchi *et al.* proposed a flexible electrode device, which can be folded with a magnetic field (Figure 15.6) [13]. Their probe has a total thickness of the polyimide substrate and a probe length of 25 μm and 1.2 mm, respectively. Their device has a nickel layer underneath the insulator of the electrode. By applying a magnetic field, the probes stand up toward the magnetic field with magnetizing nickel, where the strength of the magnetic field can control the bending angle (e.g., 380 mT for 90°). In animal experiment, their device was inserted into the cortex of a rat after peeling back the dura matter. Then the neural signals were recorded through the electrodes (20 μm × 20 μm, 200 μm spacing). The electrode can easily be inserted by pushing the polyimide substrate because the nickel layer has sufficient strength for insertion. However, nickel is a toxic material. The authors claim that, in future work, the nickel layer can be covered with a good biocompatible material (e.g., parylene).

Cheung *et al.* also proposed a flexible needle electrode (Figure 15.7) [14]. They used 15-μm-thick polyimide as the main material of the substrate and integrated 16 channel electrodes. The device was implanted into brain tissue, and neural

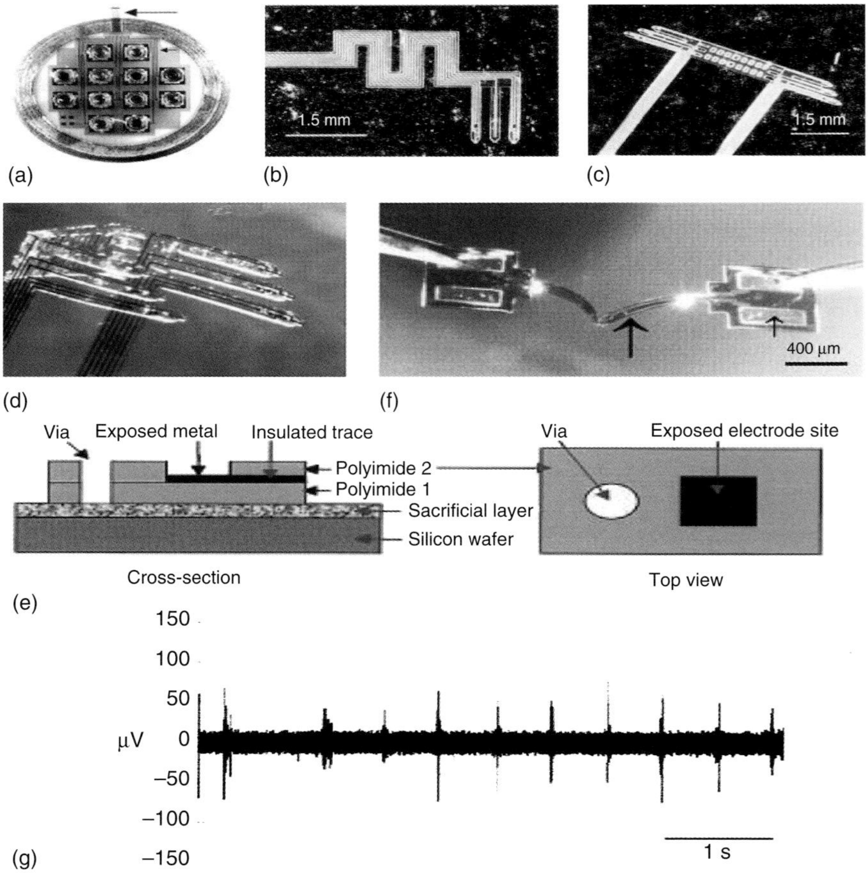

Figure 15.5 A polyimide-based flexible intracortical needle-electrode array. (a) The interconnect system in place on the backside of a 12-pin Microtech connector. The integrated polyimide cable (large arrow) leads from the device, while the single traces (small arrow) break out to individual connector posts. (b) A six-site, three-shaft device with an "S"-curve for strain relief engineered directly into the cable (Scale bar, 1.5 mm). (c,d) A 2D structure (c) (scale bar, 1.5 mm) and a similar structure "bent" into a 3D configuration (d). (e) Schematic views of the layered construction used in the manufacture of a polyimide electrode array. (f) View of a prototype single-shaft electrode array without an integrated cable "flexed" against a mirrored surface. (g) A continuous six-second sample showing multiple unit activity recorded from rat whisker barrel cortex from one site of a polyimide electrode array (site size 40 μm × 40 μm) [12].

signals were recorded through the electrode array. This device reduces the tissue reaction (glial fibrillary acidic protein, GFAP), confirming the low-invasive device structures. In this case, the substrate shows sufficient stiffness for the device penetration without guides.

In 2015, Liu *et al.* proposed another type of penetration electrode array with a mesh structure for flexibility (Figure 15.8) [15]. It can be contained in a syringe and injected into brain tissue. They used SU-8, chromium/gold, and platinum for the mesh substrate, metal interconnection, and exposed electrodes, respectively, while the total thickness was ~1 μm. The best width of the mesh structure

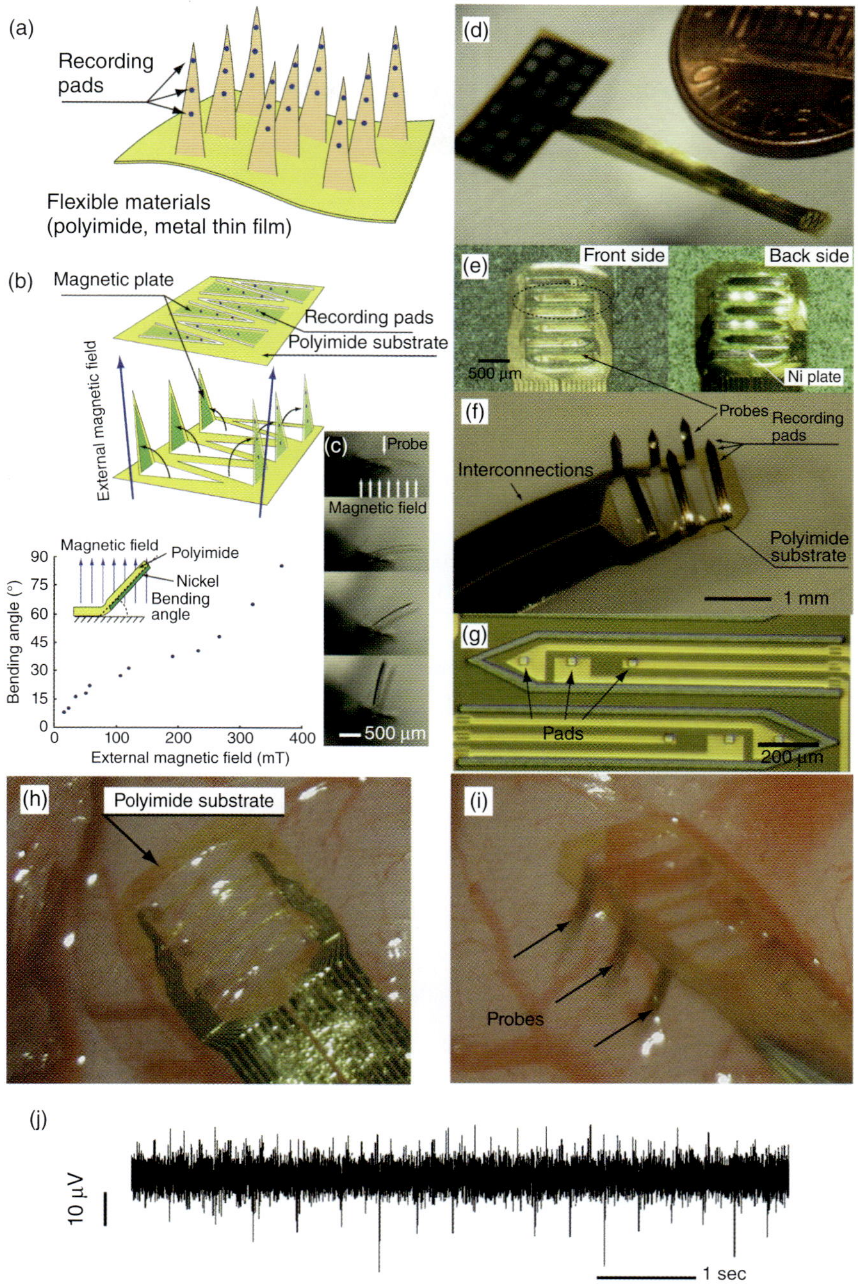

Figure 15.6 A 3D flexible mulichannel polyimide needle electrode array fabricated by magnetic batch assembly process. (a) Schematic illustration of a flexible multichannel 3D needle array. (b) 2D planar needles of polyimide formed to 3D needles by the magnetic batch assembly process. (c) Photos of the bending experiment. Photos of a fabricated needle array: (d) the needle array with 2 cm interconnection cable, (e) front and back side of the array before folding, (f) 3D flexible needle array after folding, and (g) recording pads, (h) photos of an insertion experiment: after the electrode insertion to rat's brain, and (i) the inserted regions after the detachment of the needles by tweezers. (j) Neural signals (spontaneous action potentials) recorded via the flexible needle array. The needle array was inserted to the rat's visual cortex [13]. Takeuchi *et al.* 2004 [13]. With permission from IOP PUBLISHING, LTD.

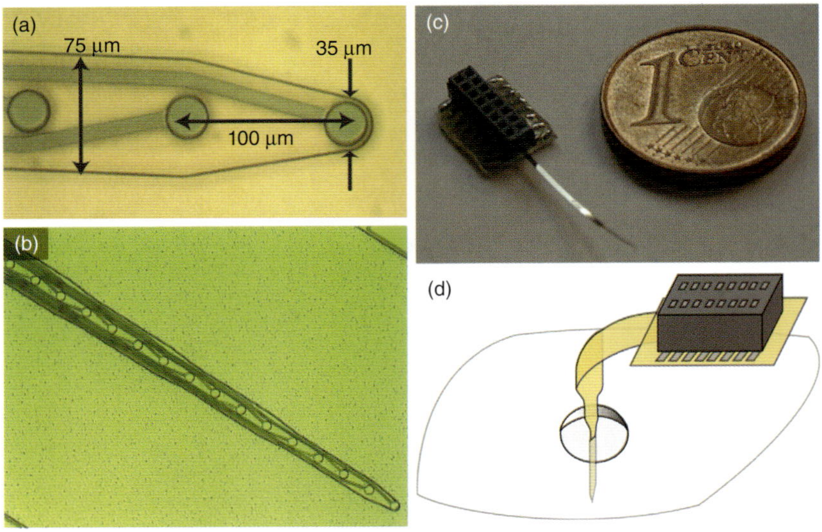

Figure 15.7 A flexible needle electrode by Cheung *et al*. (a,b) Images of the microfabricated needle structures. The needle thickness is 15 μm. Each electrode is a circle of 25 μm diameter. The polyimide is transparent and the overlapping stacked metal lines are visible. (c) A micro surface-mount connector is soldered to the polyimide needle. (d) During recording, the microelectrodes are connected to a head-mounted preamplifier, which is mounted on the distal end of the recording cable and main amplifier. (Cheung *et al*. 2007 [14]. Reproduced with permission of Elsevier.)

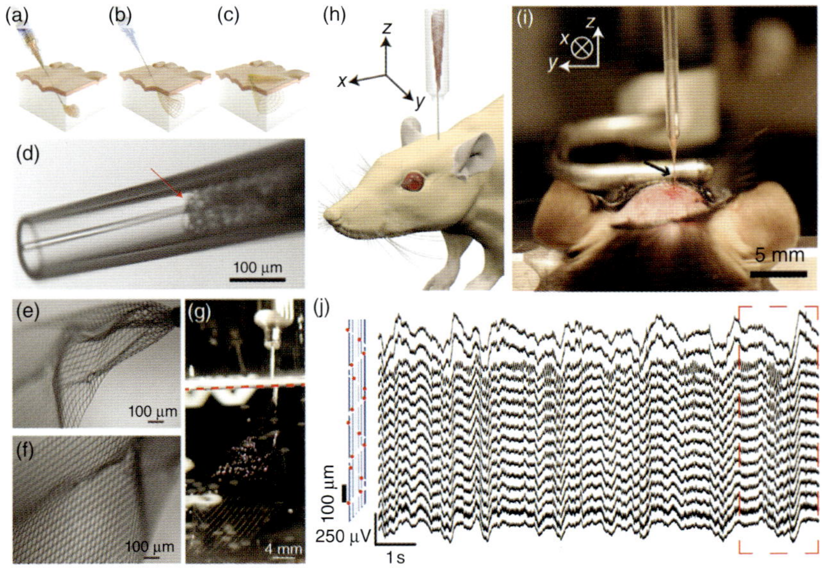

Figure 15.8 Syringe-injectable flexible mesh electronics. (a–c) Schematics of injectable electronics. (d) Bright-field microscopy image of the electronics immediately before injection into solution. (e–g) Injection of mesh electronics into aqueous solution (e,f), (g) Optical image of a 15 mm total width mesh electronics partially injected through a 20 gauge (ID = 600 μm) needle into solution, (h,i) Schematic and optical image of *in vivo* stereotaxic injection of mesh electronics into a mouse brain. (j) Acute *in vivo* 16-channel recording using mesh electronics injected into a mouse brain. (Liu *et al*. 2015 [15]. Reproduced with permission of Nature Publishing Group.)

was characterized by glass pipettes with different inner diameters. They demonstrated a syringe injection of the mesh electronics into a PDMS and/or Matrigel and used a syringe to inject mesh electronics into live rodent brains. The neuronal signals were recorded from 16 electrodes, and the GFAP and NeuN, which is a marker of neurons, were observed to be similar to the background. Since the flexibility of the substrate is closer to the flexibility of the tissue, the mechanical trauma is minimized due to the relative motion between the probe and surrounding tissue. In addition, they demonstrated that the nanowire FETs can be integrated on the same substrate.

15.3 Flexible ECoG Electrodes

ECoG recording affords a low-invasive way to record the neuronal activities from cortical surfaces and is used in medical applications such as diagnostics of diseases (e.g., epilepsy) and BMI. The conventional device consists of a silicone-based ECoG-electrode array. However, device implantation is problematic because the electrode has a thick substrate (e.g., ~800 μm) and must be large enough for mechanical stability. Issues include brain compression, difficulty in applying to an animal brain, low flexibility, and low spatial resolution of the ECoG signals. Recent advances in neuroscience employ microscale ECoG (micro-ECoG) electrode arrays fabricated by MEMS technology.

In 2009, Rubehn *et al.* proposed a MEMS-based flexible ECoG-electrode array [16] with 252 electrodes (1 mm diameter with 2, 2.5, and 3 mm pitch) on 14 "fingers," which were patterned to realize flexibility to fit onto a three-dimensionally spherical brain surface (Figure 15.9). A 300-nm-thick platinum layer was sandwiched between polyimide layers for a total thickness of about 10 μm. This electrode was packaged with solder paste and implanted on a monkey's brain. Then the ECoG signals were detected from each electrode for 4.5 months.

Toda *et al.* proposed a parylene-C-based micro-ECoG electrode array (Figure 15.10) [17]. Parylene-C was selected as the substrate due to its biocompatibility. After gold patterning, subsequent parylene-C deposition and its patterning, platinum black was formed with electrical plating on the electrode sites (50 μm × 50 μm, 1 mm spacing). This electrode device with a mesh structure has three advantages. (i) The substrate flexibility can be increased for a three-dimensionally curved spherical brain. (ii) The device is prevented from disturbing an exchange of biological materials. (iii) Other penetrating electrodes can be inserted through the mesh structure to record the neuronal signals from a deep site and the surface of the brain simultaneously. By using this electrode device, the ECoG signals were recorded from rat brain acutely. Additionally, neuronal signals, including the action potentials and intracortical LFPs, were also recorded to determine the signal sources.

In 2015, Khodagholy *et al.* [18] proposed an ECoG electrode named "NeuroGrid," which has an ultrahigh spatial resolution, for recording action

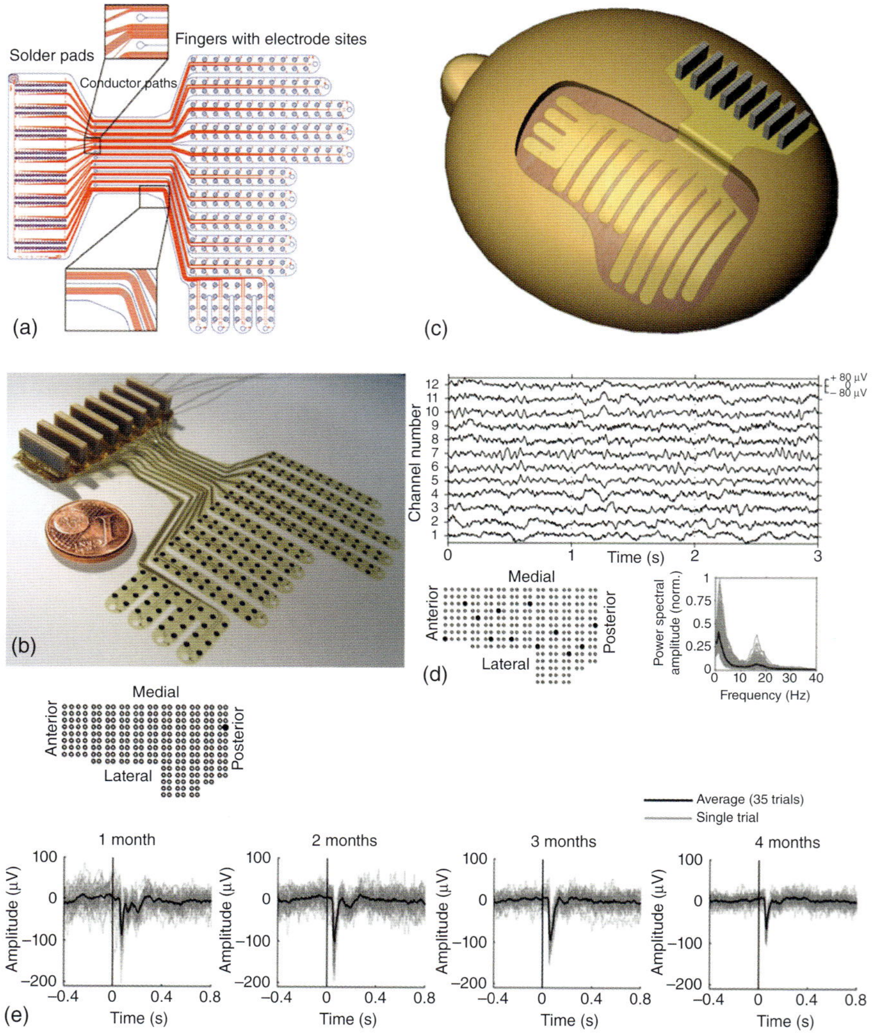

Figure 15.9 MEMS-based flexible ECoG electrode array. (a) Layout of the ECoG-array with 252 electrodes on 14 fingers (right), the ribbon cable (middle) and solder pads (left). (b) Picture of a fully assembled electrode array. The picture also shows a 16-mm-diameter coin for comparison. (c) Schematic diagram of the flexible foil and its position. (d) Example of local field potential (LFP) activity observed in 12 of the 252 channels of the ECoG electrode array. LFPs were recorded in an awake monkey during the performance of a visual task [lower left: layout of the ECoG electrode array (bold dots represent the electrodes chosen for displaying in the upper panel), lower right: the power spectrum of 252 channels is plotted in gray and the average value in black]. (e) Comparison between average and single trials of stimulus-locked LFPs after implantation surgery. The gray lines represent 35 single trials. The black line shows the average over the 35 trials. (Rubehn *et al.* 2009 [16]. With permission from the Nature Publishing Group.)

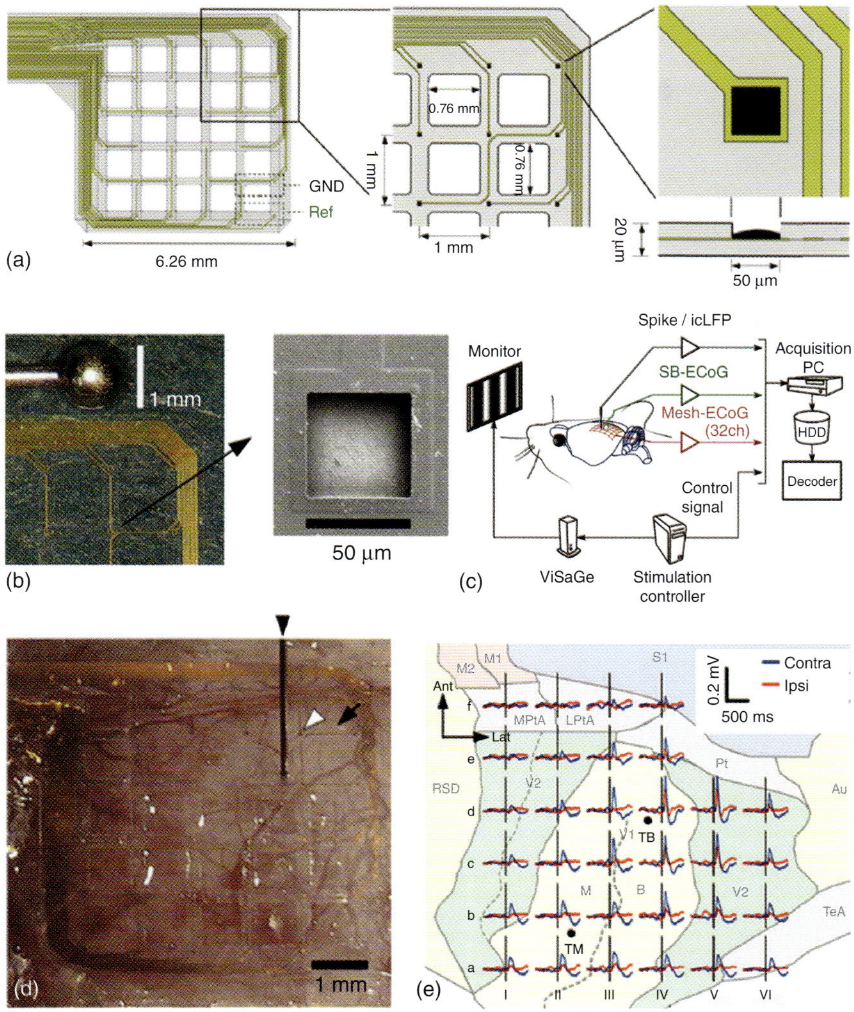

Figure 15.10 A parylene-C based micro-ECoG electrode array with a mesh design. (a) The device structure showing a 6 × 6 array of gold electrodes (50 μm × 50 μm, 1 mm spacing). (b) Picture of the fabricated device with a 1-mm-diameter silver-ball ECoG electrode for comparison. A scanning electron microscopy shows an individual electrode. (c) Experimental set-up for *in vivo* recording of multichannel ECoGs from the rat's visual cortex (Mesh-ECoG). (d) Epidural placement of a micro-ECoG electrode array and a tungsten microelectrode (white arrowhead: a single ECoG electrode, black arrowhead: a tungsten microelectrode, arrow: gold beam for wiring). (e). Visually evoked ECoG signals recorded from the micro-ECoG electrode array. (Toda *et al*. 2011 [17]. Reproduced with permission of Elsevier.)

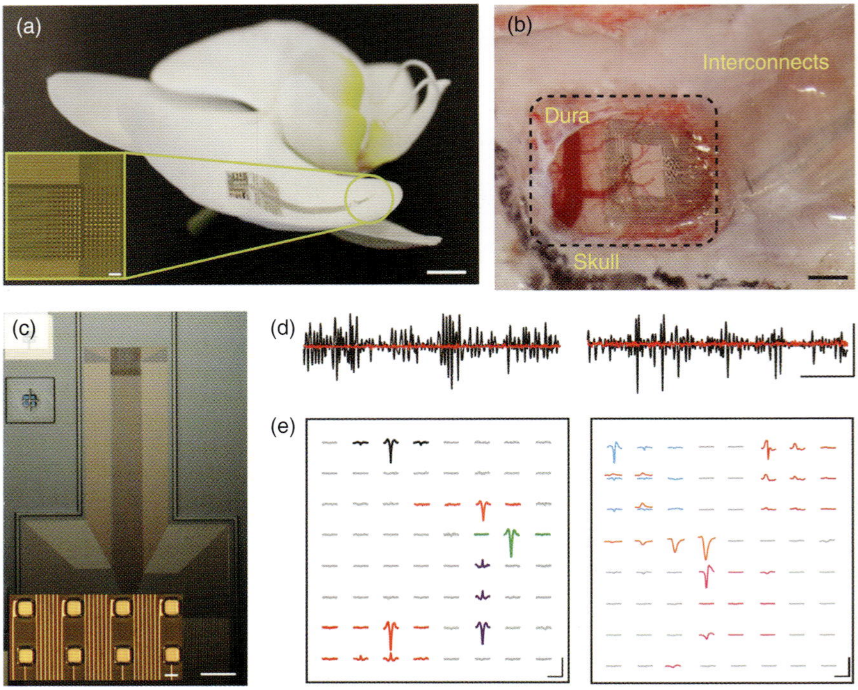

Figure 15.11 An ultrahigh spatial resolution ECoG electrode array named "NeuroGrid" for recording action potentials from the surface of the brain. (a) The NeuroGrid conforms to the surface of an orchid petal (scale bar, 5 mm). Inset shows an optical micrograph of a 256-electrode NeuroGrid (scale bar, 100 μm). Electrodes are $10 \times 10\,\mu m^2$ with 30-μm interelectrode spacing. (b) The NeuroGrid conforms to the surface of the rat somatosensory cortex (scale bar, 1 mm). (c) Optical micrograph of a 256-channel NeuroGrid (scale, 1 mm). Inset shows an optical micrograph of PEDOT:PSS-based recording sites (scale, 10 μm). (d) High-pass-filtered (f_c = 500 Hz) time traces recorded in a freely moving rat from the surface of cortex (left) and hippocampus (right) in black. (e) Examples of the spatial extent of extracellular action potentials in cortex (left) and hippocampus (right) over the geometry of the NeuroGrid by spike-triggered averaging during the detected spike times (scale bars, 1.5 ms × 50 μV). (Khodagholy *et al.* 2015 [18]. Reproduced with permission of Nature Publishing Group.)

potentials from the surface of the brain (Figure 15.11). This NeuroGrid, which contains 10 μm × 10 μm 256-electrode sites with 30-μm interelectrode spacings, is much smaller than other ECoG electrode devices. On the electrode site, poly(3,4-ethylenedioxythiophene) doped with poly(styrenesulfonate) (PEDOT:PSS), which shows a low electrical impedance, was used as the interface material. By using such a low impedance material with a high spatial resolution, they recorded high frequency signals (>500 Hz). Additionally, they recorded the intracortical spikes/LFPs with penetration electrodes and a NeuroGrid, which had a hole for the penetration electrodes, to determine the sources of the spike signals.

15.4 Functionalities of Flexible Substrates

15.4.1 Active Matrixes

A flexible array of passive microelectrodes, which are individually connected to the device interconnections, has been used for multichannel recording of neuronal signals. One requirement of future neural recording devices is that the configuration must have more recording sites with a high spatial resolution. However, the number of the recording sites is limited by the number of the device interconnections, which occupy the area in a small device geometry (e.g., millimeter square).

Viventi *et al.* [19] have overcome this issue by fabricating a flexible active-matrix-based multisite ECoG electrode array device (Figure 15.12). They demonstrated a 360-channel high density mapping of the ECoG signals from cat brain using an electrode size and spacing of 300 μm × 300 μm and 500 μm, respectively. The active matrix circuit design contained two metal-oxide-semiconductor field-effect transistors (MOSFETs) per unit cell. The flexible MOSFET was fabricated using single-crystalline silicon membranes (260 nm thick) [20]. The other materials were polyimide (~1.2 μm) for a metal insulator, epoxy (~4 μm) for device encapsulation, and platinum (~50 nm) for the ECoG electrode. The MOSFET, which was connected to the ECoG electrode, buffered the neuronal signals, while the other multiplexing MOSFET selected the electrode in the array.

15.4.2 Dissolvable Films

As a functionality of the flexible substrate, Kim *et al.* have proposed a dissolvable device substrate by using silk fibroin, a water-soluble material (Figure 15.13) [21]. Silk fibroin, which can be obtained from the cocoons of the larvae of *Bombyx mori*, is biocompatible and water soluble with programmable rates. The dissolution speed of the silk in contact with water is on the order of 50% in volume per 10 min [21]. The dissolution time can be increased to days or weeks using water or methanol-treated silks [22].

Compared to other film devices such as >2.5-μm-thick polyimide, the substrate-dissolved ECoG electrodes realize well conformal wrapping on a spherical brain surface and improve ECoG signal quality (e.g., signal amplitude) [21]. Other candidates for dissolvable materials include polyethylene glycol (PEG) [23], which also has high biocompatibility. In addition to dissolvable substrates, dissolvable silk has been used as a coating material to increase the stiffness of the penetrating electrodes composed of fragile flexible needle [24]. The silk dissolves after penetration of the flexible needle into a brain tissue.

The concept of a dissolvable substrate has been expanded to entirely dissolving electronics, which consists of ECoG electrodes, device interconnections, and MOSFETs (Figure 15.14) [25]. Materials for the interconnection, recording site, and interlayer dialectics are molybdenum, doped silicon, and multilayered silicon dioxide (<300 nm)/silicon nitride (<400 nm)/silicon dioxide (<300 nm),

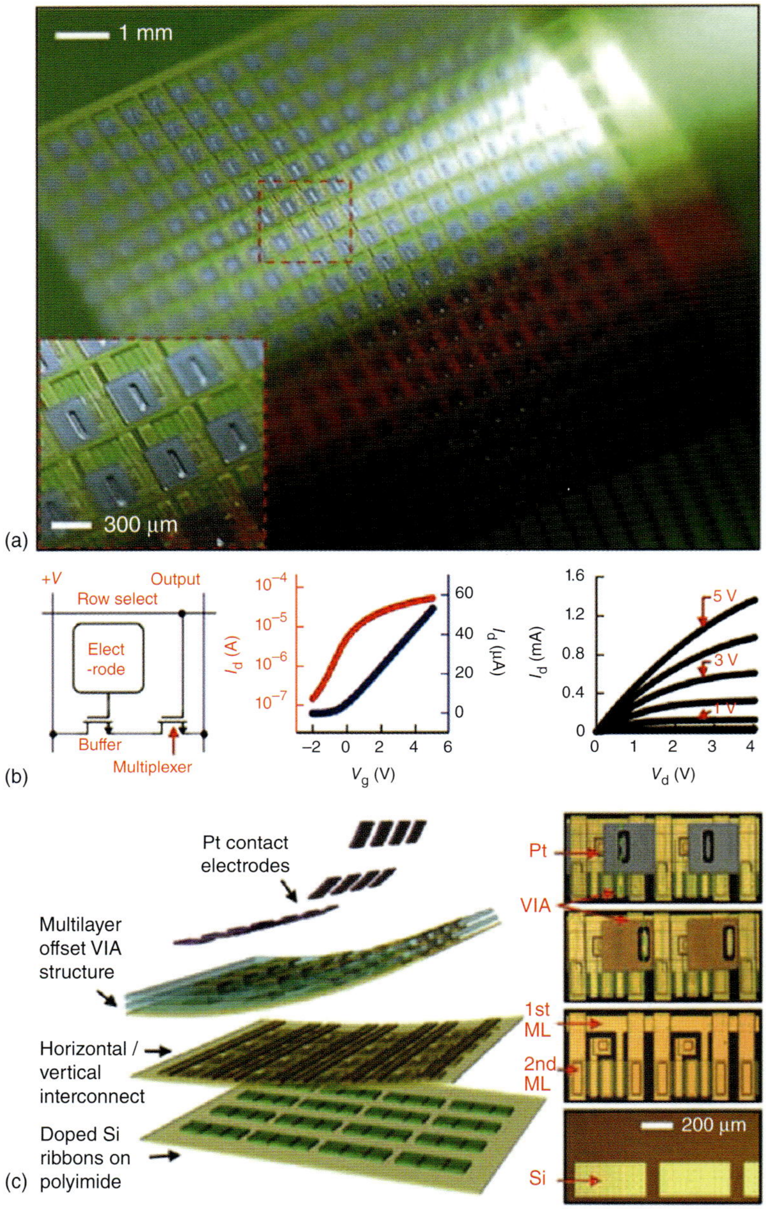

Figure 15.12 A flexible active matrix-based multisite ECoG electrode array device. (a) Photograph of a 360-channel high-density active electrode array. (b) Schematic circuit diagram of single unit cell containing two matched transistors (left), transfer characteristics of drain-to-source current (I_d) from a representative flexible transistor as gate-to-source voltage (V_g) was swept (center). Right, I_d was plotted as a function of drain-to-source voltage (V_d) while V_g was varied. (c) Schematic exploded view (left) and corresponding microscope image of each layer (right). (d) Images of folded electrode array around low modulus polydimethylsiloxane (PDMS) insert. (e) An active electrode array was placed on the visual cortex. (f) Left, folded electrode array before insertion into the interhemispheric fissure. Right, flat electrode array inserted into the interhemispheric fissure. (g) A typical spindle recorded from a representative channel. Negative is plotted up by convention. Arrows point to individual spikes of the spindle (I–IV). (Viventi *et al.* 2011 [19]. Reproduced with permission of Nature Publishing Group.)

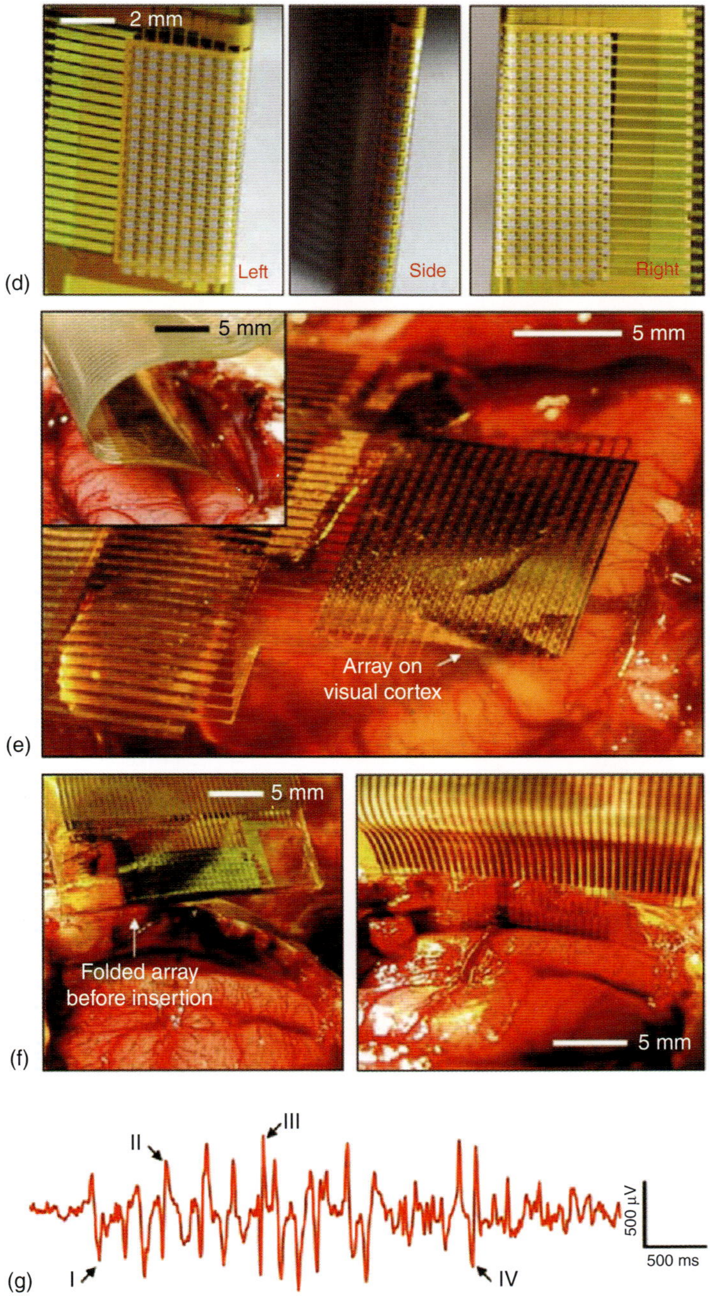

Figure 15.12 (*Continued*)

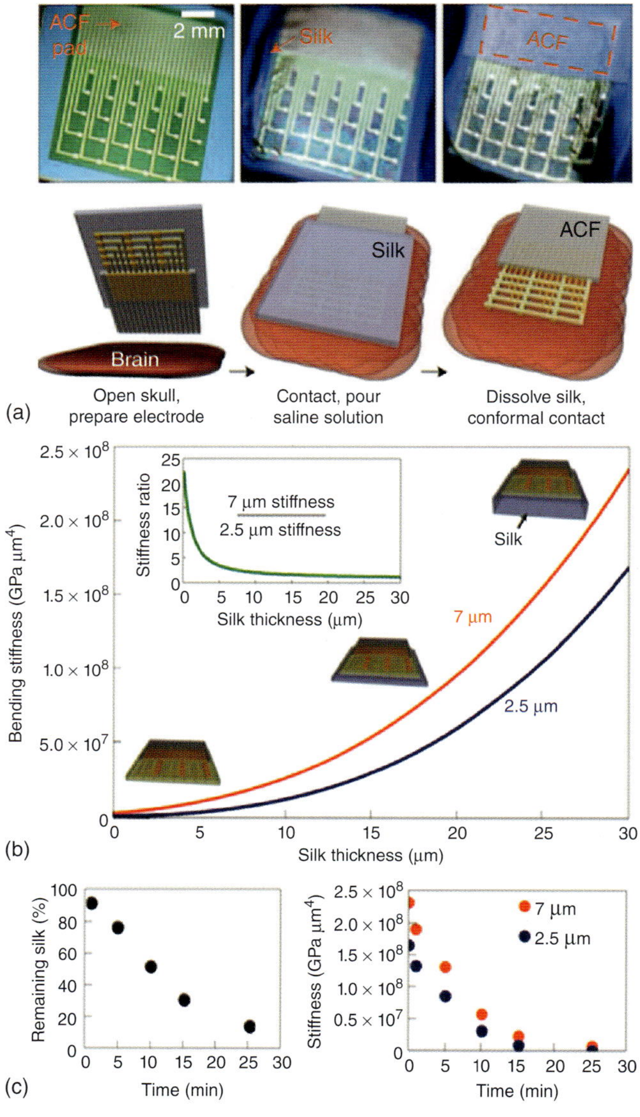

Figure 15.13 A dissolvable device substrate by using silk fibroin. (a) Schematic illustration of a device in an ultrathin mesh geometry with a dissolvable silk support. (b) Bending stiffness of 7 and 2.5 μm electrode arrays on silk films. (c) Time-dependent change in the volume of a silk film during dissolution (left) and bending stiffness calculated for silk (70% ethanol for 5 s) (right). (d) Pictures of electrode arrays of varying thickness on brain models. (e) Images of electrode arrays (76 μm sheet in left top, 2.5 μm sheet in right top, and 2.5 μm mesh in bottom panel) wrapped onto a glass hemisphere. (f–h) Image of an electrode array on a feline brain (left) and the average evoked response from each electrode (right) for a 76 μm (f), 2.5 μm (g) and 2.5 μm mesh (h) electrode array. (i) Representative voltage data from a single electrode in a 2.5 μm mesh electrode array showing a sleep spindle. (Kim *et al*. 2010 [21]. Reproduced with permission of Nature Publishing Group.)

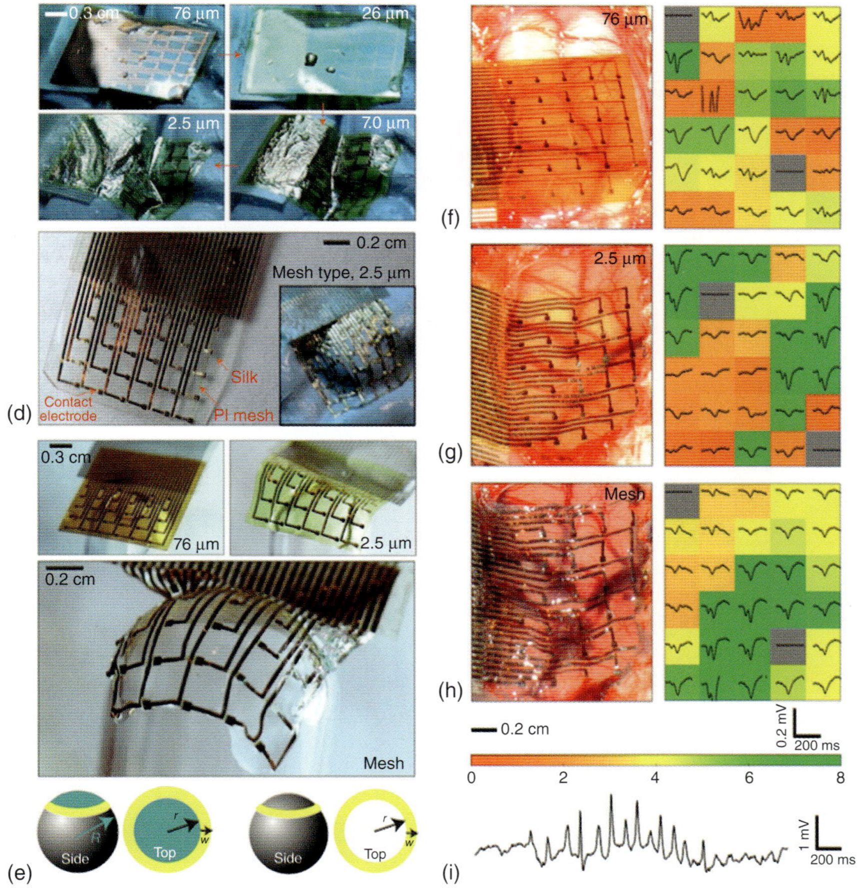

Figure 15.13 *(Continued)*

respectively, while materials for the MOSFETs are Mo for the source/drain and gate electrodes, and silicon dioxide (<100 nm) for the gate dielectrics. Dissolution times of the electronics in biofluids at 37 °C are approximately 4–6 weeks for silicon, molybdenum, and the device substrate of poly(lactic-coglycolic) acid (PLGA), and 6 months for silicon dioxide and silicon nitride. The advantages of dissolvable implantable electronics include minimizing the invasiveness and eliminating risks and costs associated with surgical extraction of an implanted device.

15.4.3 Stretchable Films

Another important characteristic of flexible devices is stretchability, which further expands the opportunities of neural recording applications. Biological samples, including the body, organs, and tissues, have 3D shapes and show large and rapid changes in the volume and the surface of the sample. To realize a stable neural recording using microelectrodes (e.g., micro-ECoG electrodes), the film device must be conformally wrapped on a biological sample by a stretchable film.

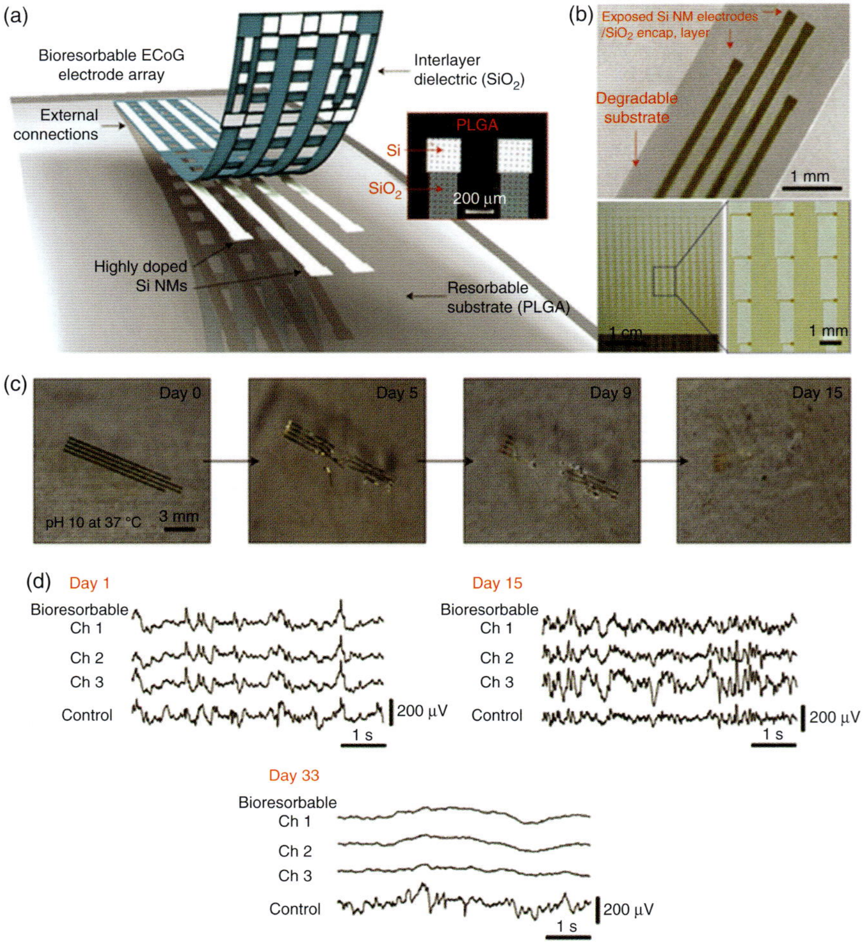

Figure 15.14 Bioresorbable silicon electronics. (a) Schematic illustration of the construction of a passive, bioresorbable neural electrode array for ECoG and subdermal EEG measurements. (b) Photographs of bioresorbable neural electrode arrays with four channels (top) and 256 (16 × 16 configuration) channels (bottom). (c) Images collected at several stages of accelerated dissolution induced by immersion in an aqueous buffer solution. (d) Representative ECoG signals recorded by the bioresorbable array and the control electrode (1, 15, and 33 days). (e) Schematic exploded-view illustration of an actively multiplexed sensing system for high-resolution ECoG, in a fully bioresorbable construction. (f) Optical micrograph images of a pair of unit cells at various stages of fabrication (left) and a picture of a complete system (right). (g) Left, linear (red) and log scale (blue) transfer curves for a representative *n*-channel MOSFET (channel length and width are 15 and 80 μm, respectively). Right: Current-voltage characteristics. (h) Output response of a unit cell with respect to an input sine wave (200 mV peak to peak) on insertion in aqueous phosphate buffer solution (PBS, pH 7.4, room temperature). (i) Images collected at several stages of accelerated dissolution of a system immersed into an aqueous buffer solution. (Yu *et al*. 2016 [25]. Reproduced with permission of Nature Publishing Group.)

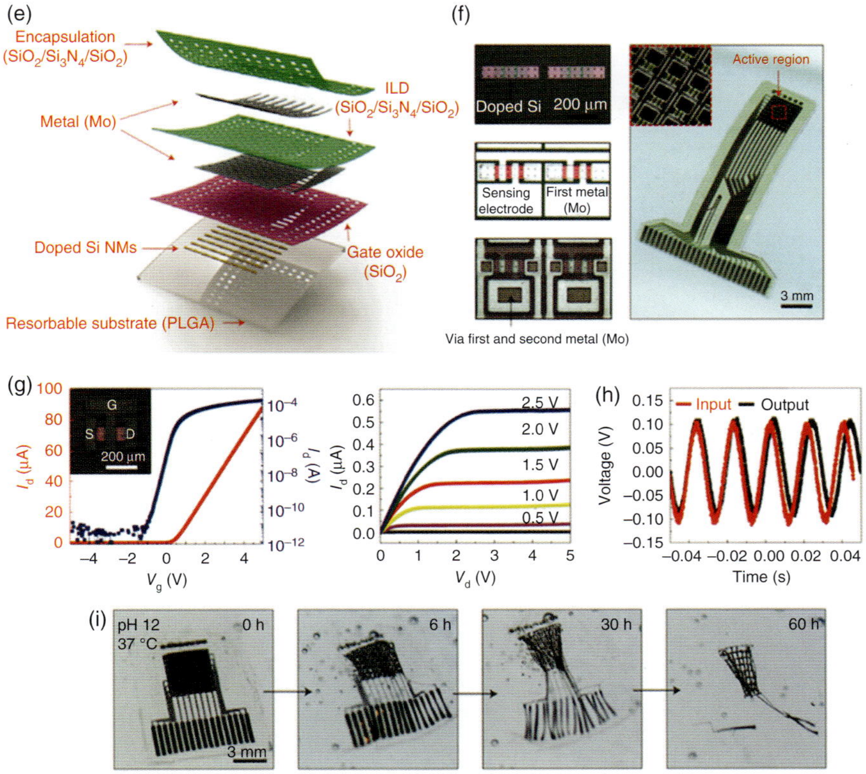

Figure 15.14 (*Continued*)

For example, the surface of *in vivo* brain shows pulsation-induced movements and increase/decrease in the volume due to growth and disease of the tissue (e.g., Alzheimer's).

One potential strategy to realize stretchable devices is to utilize an elastic material as the device substrate, such as polydimethylsiloxane (PDMS), silicone, and rubber, while the device interconnections deform. For example, Kim *et al.* have proposed a balloon catheter device using a PDMS substrate [26]. In addition, a stretchable conductive interconnection has been realized using an elastic composite material such as single-walled carbon nanotubes (SWNTs) [27, 28] with 100% stretchability and conductive ink such as silver flakes [29] with a stretchability of ~215%.

A "Kirigami"-based film design further increases the stretchability of the device substrate. In Japanese culture, "Kirigami" (kiri meaning "cutting") is an artistic transformation of a flat sheet/film into a numerous two-dimensional (2D) and/or 3D sculptures through cutting, folding, and gluing techniques. Kirigami designs have been used in material science and engineering to show ultrastretchable 2D materials, including graphene [30] and nanocomposites [31].

Morikawa *et al.* demonstrated a Kirigami-based stretchable film using a highly biocompatible material of parylene (Figure 15.15) [32]. The film shows

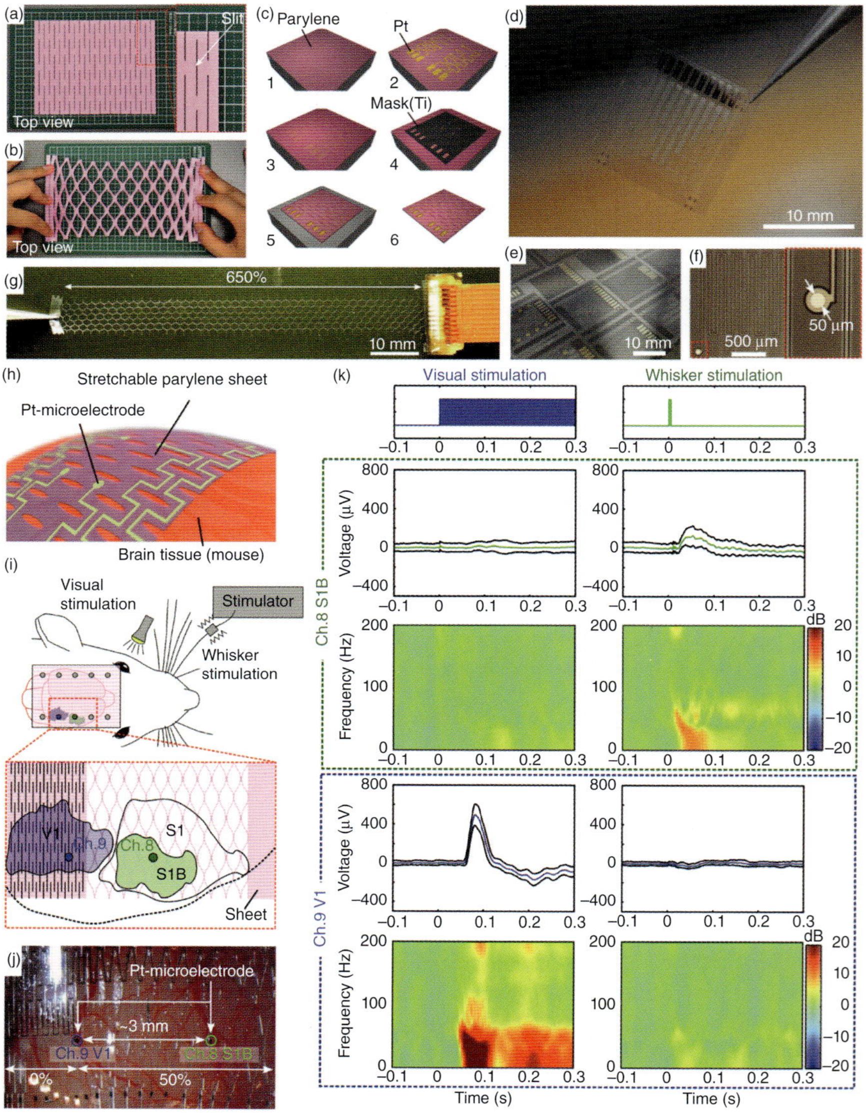

Figure 15.15 "Kirigami"-based stretchable bioprobe film using a highly biocompatible material of parylene. (a) Normal state and (b) stretched state of a Kirigami paper. (c) Device fabrication steps. (d) Photograph of the fabricated device. (e) Photograph showing batch-processed device on a silicon substrate. (f) Photograph showing the 50 μm diameter planar Pt-electrode site in a device connected with a zigzag Pt-interconnection. (g) Photograph showing a fabricated device [3 × 91 slits design] stretched to 650% by tweezers. (h) Schematic of the Kirigami device placed over mouse brain tissue. (i) Schematic shows device placement. (j) Picture shows two electrodes on the visual and barrel cortices while the device stretched. (k) Recorded signals from the visual and barrel cortices of a mouse's brain. Two electrodes detect neuronal activities evoked by visual stimulation and whisker stimulation, respectively [32].

a stretchability of ~1100%, depending on the Kirigami (slit) design. Based on this Kirigami parylene film, an array of ECoG microelectrodes was embedded into the film and the *in vivo* recording of ECoG signals from mouse brain was demonstrated while the film device stretched.

15.4.4 Other Functionalities

Another common issue of flexible devices that are thin (<10 μm) and a large area, including ECoG electrodes, is addressing difficulties during device placement. Yamagiwa *et al.* proposed a way to overcome this by facilitating an actuating film based on a curled film by sandwiching between parylene-N and -C, which have different linear expansion coefficients (Figure 15.16) [33]. However, the curled film is flattened when the film comes in contact with a brain surface due to the surface tension between the film and the brain surface.

Kim *et al.* proposed a multifunctional flexible device for optogenetic applications with four functional layers: (i) a microelectrode for neural signal recordings, (ii) silicon μ-IPD for optical measurements, (3) μ-inorganic light emitting diode (LED) chips for light stimulations, and (iv) a serpentine platinum resistor for temperature sensors [34]. They used polyester as the substrate. Each layer was fabricated individually and aligned/stuck using an aligner. The total thickness of the device was 8.5 μm, and this fabricated device was then adhered on a releasable base with silk fibroin for the thin device injection.

They demonstrated a wireless power supply for a microscale LED (μ-LED) and measured the temperature while turning on the LEDs. Upon modulating the μ-LED driving method, changes in the temperature associated with μ-LED are less than 0.10 °C and the measured power of μ-LED is more than $1\,mW\,mm^{-2}$. Finally, the neural recording capability with a platinum microelectrode and wireless power supply was demonstrated. In addition, optical stimulation with the integrated μ-LED was demonstrated. The tissue reaction (gliosis) can be reduced using a μ-LED integrated on an ultrathin PET substrate. These results show that this device is suitable for optogenetic applications.

15.5 Flexible Devices for Chronic Applications

15.5.1 Tissue Damage

Reducing the damage of tissue and neuron allows long-term neuronal activity recordings and safer device implantation. In the case of needle-electrode penetration, tissue damage due to penetration and movement of the needle arrays should be reduced. The damaged area, which is occupied by glial cells, is proportional to the needle size (cross-sectional area) [35, 36]. Encapsulation of the needle-electrode site with glial cells makes long-term recordings of neuronal activities difficult [36].

Tissue damage in rat brain due to implantations of different types of microscale needles was reported by Szarowski *et al.* by investigating astrocytes and microglia for ~12 weeks [36]. They demonstrated that the volume of the reactive tissue involved in the early stage (i.e., <1 week) is proportional to the cross-sectional

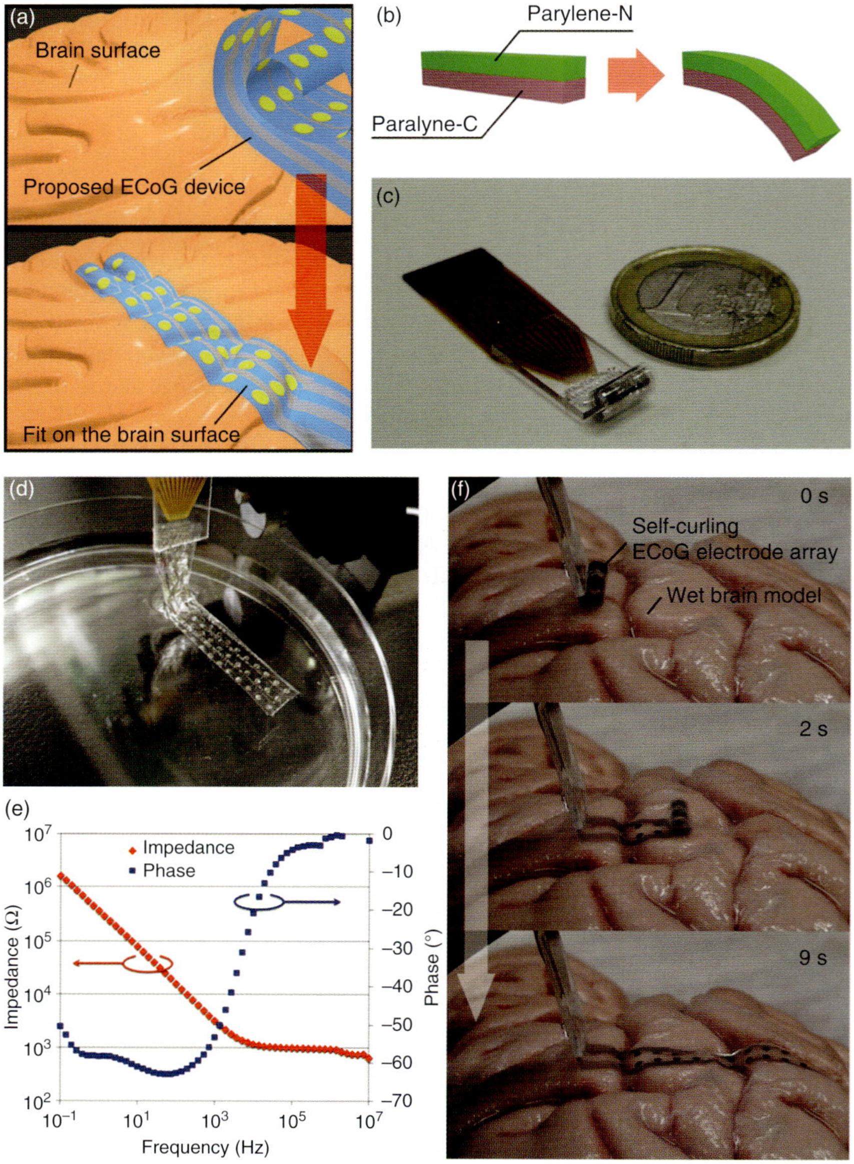

Figure 15.16 An actuating bioprobe (ECoG) film device. (a) Schematic illustration of an actuating ECoG film device. Thermally self-curled ECoG device (blue) is flattened on a wet brain surface by the surface tension between the parylene and the brain. (b) Schematic illustration of the device substrate consisting of parylene-N and -C with different linear expansion coefficients. (c) Fabricated curled parylene-N/-C ECoG electrode array with a curvature radius of ~2 mm. (d) Fabricated ECoG electrode array device sticking to solution surface. (e) Magnitude and phase of impedance taken from a 1-mm-diameter platinum-ECoG electrode [33]. (f) Pictures showing an actuating ECoG film device on a brain model (Yamagiwa, S., *et al.*, unpublished data).

area of the implanted needles (Figure 15.17). By investigating the reactions of astrocytes, microglia, endothelial cells, and neurons two weeks after implantation, Kozai *et al.* reported that penetration of a 8.5-μm-diameter carbon-fiber electrode [7-μm-diameter carbon fiber with a 800-nm-thick poly(*p*-xylylene) insulator layer] causes tissue damage in rat brain [37]. Fujishiro *et al.* evaluated the distribution of microglia using small diameter needles [11].

Consequently, the needle diameter should be minimized to reduce tissue damage. Furthermore, because the movement of a stiff needle-electrode array in soft brain tissue enlarges the damaged area (or "kill zone"), the mechanical mismatch between a stiff needle array and soft brain tissue may be resolved using flexible materials as the needle shafts.

15.5.2 Packaging Technologies

15.5.2.1 Rivet-Like Electric and Mechanic Interconnections

For the connections between the fabricated thin-film device and other substrates (e.g., rigid/flexible printed circuit, amplifier/stimulator chip), Meyer *et al.* proposed rivet-like electric and mechanic interconnections (Figure 15.18a) [38]. The bonding pad of a flexible thin device had a hole, which makes an intermediary structure. As the packaging phase, a gold ball was placed on this hole of the thin-device bonding pad. This ball bonds with both the thin device and the other substrate electrically and mechanically.

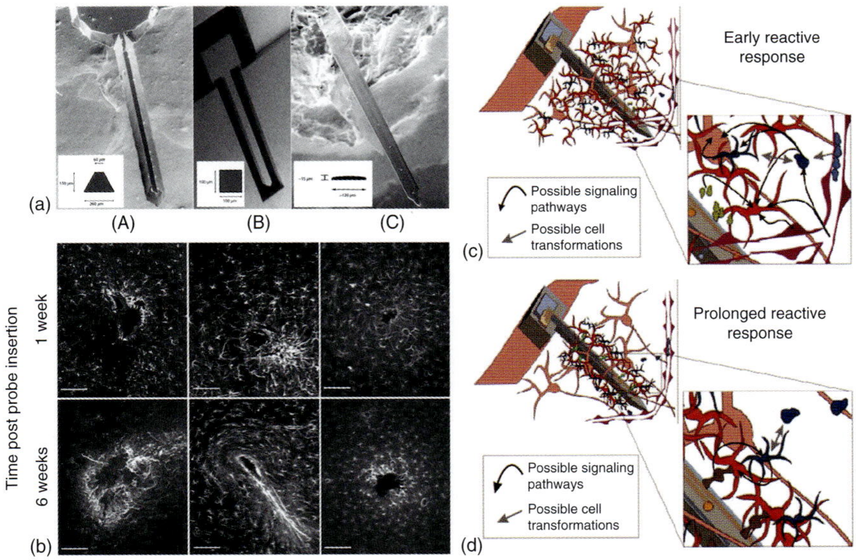

Figure 15.17 Tissue damage in rat brain due to implantations of different types of microscale needles. (a) Comparison of devices used in this study. (b) GFAP immunohistochemistry of tissue slices from brains inserted with the three devices in (a) (Scale bars, 100 μm). Cartoons depicting cellular responses during (c) early and (d) sustained reactive responses observed following device insertion. Neurons (pink), astrocytes (red), monocyte derived cells including microglia (blue), and vasculature (purple) are depicted. (Szarowski 2003 [36]. Reproduced with permission of Elsevier.)

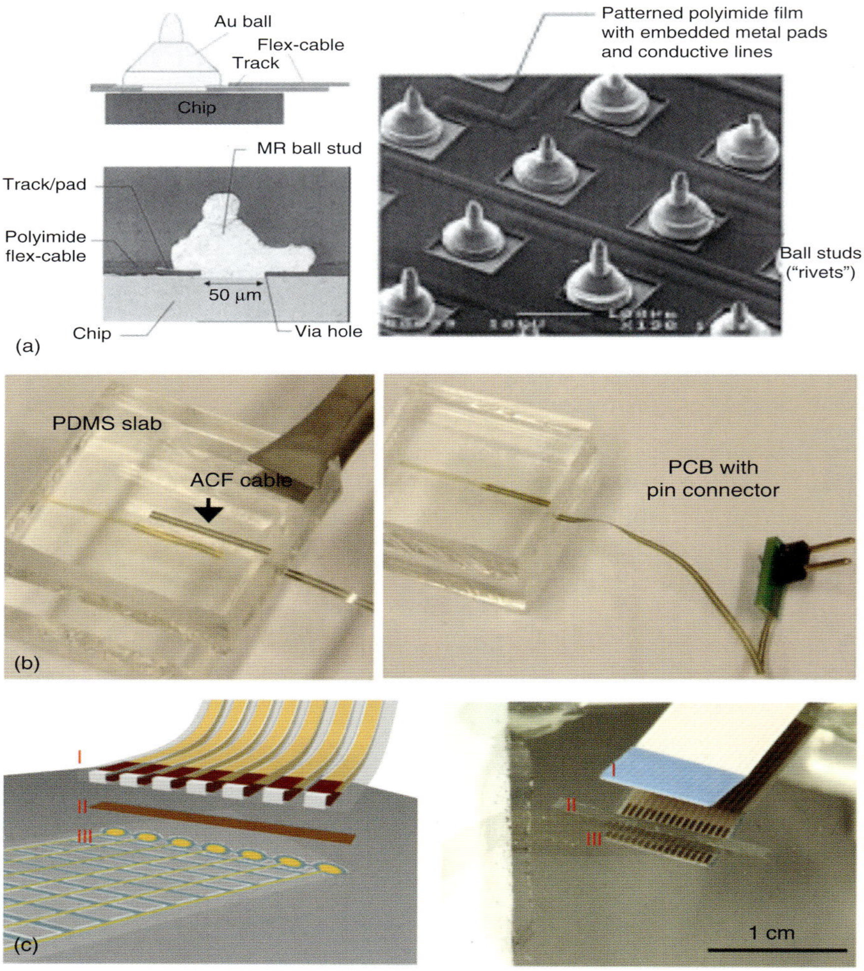

Figure 15.18 Packaging technologies for flexible implantable devices. (a) Rivet-like electric and mechanic interconnections. Top, schematic illustration of the rivet-like electronic and mechanic interconnection between the thin (15 μm) polyimide flexible ribbon substrate and the chip underneath. Middle, metallurgic micrograph showing a vertical cut through the interconnected microstructures. Bottom, SEM image of the patterned polyimide/metal film with rivet-like ball studs placed in arrays. (Meyer *et al.* 2001 [38]. Reproduced with permission of IEEE.). (b) Anisotropic conductive film (ACF) cable. Left, a device is electrically connected to the ACF cable. The PDMS slabs on the top and bottom are compressed using high temperature (~150 °C) to bond the ACF cable. Right, the other side of the ACF cable is connected to a PCB with pin connector [39]. (c) Schematic (left) and corresponding photograph (right) of the overall process of bonding a flexible cable to the I/O pads. In both the schematic and photograph, the flexible cable, ACF, and I/O region of the mesh electronics are indicated by I, II, and III, respectively. (Liu *et al.* 2015 [15]. Reproduced with permission of Nature Publishing Group.)

15.5.2.2 Anisotropic Conductive Paste/Films

Anisotropic conductive paste/films (ACP/ACF) are known to connect the electrical connection pads in an anisotropic manner. Such films have been used to connect high-density electrical connection pads. Both ACP and ACF are often used for flip chip bonding. In particular, the use of ACF for electrical connections between thin-film devices and other cable/printed circuits has recently progressed (Figure 15.18b,c) [15, 39].

15.5.3 Wireless Technologies

Neural recording systems that use wire lines between an implanted microelectrode device and an external device can cause infections through the opening in the skull and the dura. Although the skull can typically be sealed with cement after surgery, holding the wire and dura in place would be difficult. Consequently, there is a risk of infection and leakage of the cerebrospinal fluid during long-term measurements. Therefore, using fully implantable neural interfaces are necessary.

Advances in techniques employed in wireless sensor systems have enabled the creation of novel biomedical applications. Muller *et al.* reported a wireless micro-ECoG system for chronic recordings and wireless transmissions of neural signals from the surface of the cerebral cortex [40]. The device comprises a highly flexible high-density polymer-based 64-channel electrode array and a flexible antenna bonded to 2.4 mm × 2.4 mm silicon-CMOS integrated circuit (IC) that performs 64-channel acquisition, wireless power, and data transmission. The IC consumes 225 μW and can be powered by an external reader transmitting 12 mW at 300 MHz.

15.6 Summary

As discussed earlier in this chapter, the brain is an extremely complex system, and our understanding of how the brain works is very poor. Toward this understanding, this chapter has reviewed the recent advances in MEMS processed microelectrode devices, which may play an important role in exploring the activity and network of a large number of neurons within brain tissue.

Device flexibility and stretchability are powerful features to realize highly biocompatible and low-invasive tools for use in brain and other biological tissues with 3D, deformable, and soft properties. Chronic applications of the microdevices, in which small device packages, biocompatible materials, and wireless systems are necessary to realize the microdevices as implantable tools have also been discussed.

Although these devices are still under development, these flexible device technologies will become powerful tools not only in neuroscience research but also in medical applications including diagnostics of diseases (e.g., epilepsy) and BMI technology.

References

1 Kandel, E.R., Schwartz, J.H., Jessell, T.M. *et al.* (2012) *Principles of Neural Science*, 5th edn, McGraw-Hill, New York.
2 Thakor, N. (2012) Building Brain Machine Interfaces – Neuroprosthetic Control with Electrocorticographic Signals. *IEEE Life Sciences Newsletter.*
3 Rousche, P.J. and Normann, R.A. (1998) Chronic recording capability of the utah intracortical electrode array in cat sensory cortex. *J. Neurosci. Methods*, **82** (1), 1–15.
4 Bai, Q., Wise, K.D., and Anderson, D.J. (2000) A high-yield microassembly structure for three-dimensional microelectrode arrays. *IEEE Trans. Biomed. Eng.*, **47** (3), 281–289.
5 Hochberg, L.R., Bacher, D., Jarosiewicz, B. *et al.* (2012) Reach and grasp by people with tetraplegia using a neurally controlled robotic arm. *Nature*, **485** (7398), 372–375.
6 Spira, M.E. and Hai, A. (2013) Multi-electrode array technologies for neuroscience and cardiology. *Nat. Nanotechnol.*, **8** (2), 83–94.
7 Schwartz, A.B., Cui, X.T., Weber, D., and Moran, D.W. (2006) Brain-controlled interfaces: movement restoration with neural prosthetics. *Neuron*, **52** (1), 205–220.
8 Buzsáki, G., Anastassiou, C.A., and Koch, C. (2012) The origin of extracellular fields and currents–EEG, ECoG, LFP and spikes. *Nat. Rev. Neurosci.*, **13** (6), 407–420.
9 Cogan, S.F. (2008) Neural stimulation and recording electrodes. *Annu. Rev. Biomed. Eng.*, **10**, 275–309.
10 Harimoto, T., Takei, K., Kawano, T. *et al.* (2011) Enlarged gold-tipped silicon microprobe arrays and signal compensation for multi-site electroretinogram recordings in the isolated carp retina. *Biosens. Bioelectron.*, **26** (5), 2368–2375.
11 Fujishiro, A., Kaneko, H., Kawashima, T. *et al.* (2014) *In vivo* neuronal action potential recordings via three-dimensional microscale needle-electrode arrays. *Sci. Rep.*, **4**. 4868.
12 Rousche, P.J., Pellinen, D.S., Pivin, D.P. *et al.* (2001) Flexible polyimide-based intracortical electrode arrays with bioactive capability. *IEEE Trans. Biomed. Eng.*, **48** (3), 361–370.
13 Takeuchi, S., Suzuki, T., Mabuchi, K., and Fujita, H. (2004) 3D flexible multichannel neural probe array. *J. Micromech. Microeng.*, **14** (1), 104–107.
14 Cheung, K.C., Renaud, P., Tanila, H., and Djupsund, K. (2007) Flexible polyimide microelectrode array for *in vivo* recordings and current source density analysis. *Biosens. Bioelectron.*, **22** (8), 1783–1790.
15 Liu, J., Fu, T.-M., Cheng, Z. *et al.* (2015) Syringe-injectable electronics. *Nat. Nanotechnol.*, **10** (7), 629–636.
16 Rubehn, B., Bosman, C., Oostenveld, R. *et al.* (2009) A MEMS-based flexible multichannel ECoG-electrode array. *J. Neural Eng.*, **6** (3), 036003.
17 Toda, H., Suzuki, T., Sawahata, H. *et al.* (2011) Simultaneous recording of ECoG and intracortical neuronal activity using a flexible multichannel electrode-mesh in visual cortex. *Neuroimage*, **54** (1), 203–212.

18 Khodagholy, D., Gelinas, J.N., Thesen, T. *et al.* (2015) NeuroGrid: recording action potentials from the surface of the brain. *Nat. Neurosci.*, **18** (2), 310–315.

19 Viventi, J., Kim, D.-H., Vigeland, L. *et al.* (2011) Flexible, foldable, actively multiplexed, high-density electrode array for mapping brain activity *in vivo*. *Nat. Neurosci.*, **14** (12), 1599–1605.

20 Viventi, J., Kim, D.-H., Moss, J.D. *et al.* (2010) A conformal, bio-interfaced class of silicon electronics for mapping cardiac electrophysiology. *Sci. Transl. Med.*, **2** (24), 24ra22.

21 Kim, D.-H., Viventi, J., Amsden, J.J. *et al.* (2010) Dissolvable films of silk fibroin for ultrathin conformal bio-integrated electronics. *Nat. Mater.*, **9** (6), 511–517.

22 Jin, H.J., Park, J., Karageorgiou, V. *et al.* (2005) Water-stable silk films with reduced β-sheet content. *Adv. Funct. Mater.*, **15** (8), 1241–1247.

23 Takeuchi, S., Ziegler, D., Yoshida, Y. *et al.* (2005) Parylene flexible neural probes integrated with microfluidic channels. *Lab Chip*, **5** (5), 519–523.

24 Tien, L.W., Wu, F., Tang-Schomer, M.D. *et al.* (2013) Silk as a multifunctional biomaterial substrate for reduced glial scarring around brain-penetrating electrodes. *Adv. Funct. Mater.*, **23** (25), 3185–3193.

25 Yu, K.J., Kuzum, D., Hwang, S.-W. *et al.* (2016) Bioresorbable silicon electronics for transient spatiotemporal mapping of electrical activity from the cerebral cortex. *Nat. Mater.*, **15** (7), 782–791.

26 Kim, D.-H., Lu, N., Ghaffari, R. *et al.* (2011) Materials for multifunctional balloon catheters with capabilities in cardiac electrophysiological mapping and ablation therapy. *Nat. Mater.*, **10** (4), 316–323.

27 Sekitani, T., Noguchi, Y., Hata, K. *et al.* (2008) A rubberlike stretchable active matrix using elastic conductors. *Science*, **321** (5895), 1468–1472.

28 Sekitani, T., Nakajima, H., Maeda, H. *et al.* (2009) Stretchable active-matrix organic light-emitting diode display using printable elastic conductors. *Nat. Mater.*, **8** (6), 494–499.

29 Matsuhisa, N., Kaltenbrunner, M., Yokota, T. *et al.* (2015) Printable elastic conductors with a high conductivity for electronic textile applications. *Nat. Commun.*, **6** (May), 7461.

30 Blees, M.K., Barnard, A.W., Rose, P.A. *et al.* (2015) Graphene kirigami. *Nature*, **524** (7564), 204–207.

31 Shyu, T.C., Damasceno, P.F., Dodd, P.M. *et al.* (2015) A kirigami approach to engineering elasticity in nanocomposites through patterned defects. *Nat. Mater.*, **14** (8), 785–789.

32 Morikawa, Y., Yamagiwa, S., Sawahata, H. *et al.* (2017) Ultrastretchable Kirigami Bioprobes. *Adv. Healthc. Mater. in press*. http://onlinelibrary.wiley.com/doi/10.1002/adhm.201701100/full.

33 Yamagiwa, S., Ishida, M., and Kawano, T. (2013) Self-curling and -sticking flexible substrate for ECoG electrode array. Proceedings of the IEEE International Conference Micro Electro Mechanical Systems, pp. 480–483.

34 Kim, T., McCall, J.G., Jung, Y.H. *et al.* (2013) Injectable, cellular-scale optoelectronics with applications for wireless optogenetics. *Science*, **340** (6129), 211–216.

35 Edell, D.J., Toi, V.V., McNeil, V.M., and Clark, L.D. (1992) Factors influencing the biocompatibility of insertable siliconmicroshafts in cerebral cortex. *IEEE Trans. Biomed. Eng.*, **39** (6), 635–643.

36 Szarowski, D.H., Andersen, M.D., Retterer, S. *et al.* (2003) Brain responses to micro-machined silicon devices. *Brain Res.*, **983** (1–2), 23–35.

37 Kozai, T.D.Y., Langhals, N.B., Patel, P.R. *et al.* (2012) Ultrasmall implantable composite microelectrodes with bioactive surfaces for chronic neural interfaces. *Nat. Mater.*, **11** (12), 1065–1073.

38 Meyer, J.U., Stieglitz, T., Scholz, O. *et al.* (2001) High density interconnects and flexible hybrid assemblies for active biomedical implants. *IEEE Trans. Adv. Packag.*, **24** (3), 366–374.

39 McCall, J.G., Kim, T., Shin, G. *et al.* (2013) Fabrication and application of flexible, multimodal light-emitting devices for wireless optogenetics. *Nat. Protoc.*, **8** (12), 2413–2428.

40 Muller, R., Le, H.P., Li, W. *et al.* (2014) A minimally invasive 64-channel wireless μECoG implant. *IEEE J. Solid-State Circuits*, **50** (1), 344–359.

16

Perspective in Flexible and Stretchable Electronics

Kuniharu Takei

Osaka Prefecture University, Department of Physics and Electronics, 1-1 Gakuen Nakaku, Sakai, Osaka, Japan

This book introduces the fundamental characteristics of flexible and stretchable device components such as transistors, memories, capacitors, and sensors using organic and inorganic materials and presents some healthcare, medical, and neural applications. Although the developments have progressed significantly to move forward toward realizing the practical use of flexible and stretchable electronics, there are still many challenges to be overcome such as in signal processing and wireless circuits and batteries to be mechanically flexible, without increasing their cost. In addition to the active components, the reliability and stability of the devices also need to be considered depending on the applications. This is because macroscale flexible electronics have high potential for applications pertaining to the internet of things (IoT) society. For some IoT applications, such as in vehicles and life-lines (water, gas, etc.), to detect stress and crack information for example, long-term reliability and stability are very important parameters since the sensors cannot be replaced for many years. To test such important parameters, collaboration and/or help from industries are essential because it is hard to conduct these tests in universities. It should be noted that even if the device can be disposed for some applications, the reliability of the sensing results is still important for market sustainability. Another important contribution to the future of healthcare and medical applications is to build the consortium and/or alliance and to gather and share many measured health conditions as well as compile activity information into a database to analyze big data. Right now, for inflexible wearable devices, data sets are kept by the company that sells the products. This independent data correction limits the diagnosis pertaining to health conditions, which is a big barrier to demonstrating the usefulness and possibility of the wearable devices. If we can diagnose the health conditions based on big data, wearable devices may be strong candidates for future electronics. In addition to these, there are other things to be addressed and challenges to be overcome for realizing practical application. We welcome all of you to join this new field of flexible and stretchable medical/healthcare electronics to change the world of human lives.

Flexible and Stretchable Medical Devices, First Edition. Edited by Kuniharu Takei.

Index

Flexible and Stretchable Medical Devices, First Edition. Edited by Kuniharu Takei.